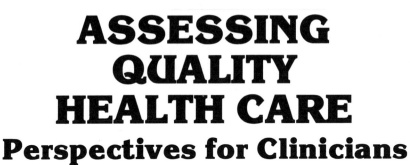

ASSESSING QUALITY HEALTH CARE
Perspectives for Clinicians

ASSESSING QUALITY HEALTH CARE
Perspectives for Clinicians

Edited by

Richard P. Wenzel, M.D., M.Sc.

Professor and Director
Division of General Medicine
Clinical Epidemiology and
Health Services Research
Department of Internal Medicine
University of Iowa College of Medicine
and
Hospital Epidemiologist
University of Iowa Hospitals and Clinics
Iowa City, Iowa

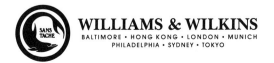

WILLIAMS & WILKINS
BALTIMORE · HONG KONG · LONDON · MUNICH
PHILADELPHIA · SYDNEY · TOKYO

Editor: Laurel Craven
Managing Editor: Carol Eckhart
Copy Editor: Klementyna L. Bryte
Designer: Saturn Graphics
Illustration Planner: Lorraine Wrzosek
Production Coordinator: Barbara J. Felton

Copyright © 1992 except for Chapter 2.
Williams & Wilkins
428 East Preston Street
Baltimore, Maryland 21202, USA

Chapter 2 was written by Federal Government employees. As such, this chapter is in the public domain and cannot be copyrighted. It may be reproduced without permission.

Accurate indications, adverse reactions, and dosage schedules for drugs are provided in this book, but it is possible that they may change. The reader is urged to review the package information data of the manufacturers of the medications mentioned.

Printed in the United States of America

Library of Congress Cataloging-in-Publication Data

Assessing quality health care : perspectives for clinicians / edited by
  Richard P. Wenzel.
      p.   cm.
  Includes bibliographical references and index.
  ISBN 0-683-08924-2
  1. Hospitals—Quality control.   I. Wenzel, Richard P. (Richard
Putnam), 1940–   .
  [DNLM: 1. Epidemiology. 2. Hospitals—standards.
3. Outcome and Process Assessment (Health Care). 4. Quality
Assurance, Health Care.   WX 153 A846]
RA971.A85   1992
362.1'1'068—dc20
DNLM/DLC
for Library of Congress   91-15339
                                                              CIP

                              91   92   93   94   95
                 1   2   3   4   5   6   7   8   9   10

To Jo Gail Hunt Wenzel
whose grace inspires a search for truth
and whose love provides new horizons

Preface

Much has been written recently about the modern revolution in medicine and medical care. Important questions about the value of American health care relative to its costs have been framed in social, ethical, economic, and political perspectives. Considerably less has been written from the perspective of the practitioner. Surely, it must seem ironic to devoted clinicians that, in a country working so diligently to provide the most technically advanced care, there could be so much focus on medicine's shortcomings. Moreover, the same clinicians who are the product of medical schools committed to biotechnology find it incredible that there is currently a veritable tidal wave of regulatory, insurance, credentialing, and consumer demands for evidence of high quality health care.

In discussions with friends and colleagues, it seemed obvious that the time was propitious for the publication of a book that could unify the tasks necessary to meet the demands of the current revolutions. *Assessing Quality Health Care: Perspectives for Clinicians* was written by practicing experts providing state-of-the-art information with a clinical perspective. It is directed to health care providers and the hospital administrators who work with them. It is devoted to continually improved care of our patients. Importantly, it is the clinical perspective that distinguishes this book from other publications, and it is the amalgamation of the disciplines of clinical practice, epidemiology, and health services that provides its basis.

As editor, I have been greatly rewarded by working with an internationally recognized team of contributors. Each has given up a great deal of precious time from both academic and avocational pursuits to prepare for this book. I value their scholarship and their friendship.

I wish to acknowledge the academic atmosphere in the Department of Internal Medicine at the University of Iowa College of Medicine. The support for scholarship provided by our chairman, François M. Abboud, M.D., and my co-division heads is outstanding. In addition, the University of Iowa Hospitals and Clinics, led by John Colloton, has made a major commitment to applying science in the pursuit of quality health care.

Special thanks extend to current and former fellows who have taught me so much. I hold them all in high esteem. I also acknowledge the skill and energy of Cathy Chavez in preparing manuscripts and working with authors, and two wonderful experts at Williams & Wilkins, Carol Eckhart and Tim Satterfield.

Richard P. Wenzel, M.D., M.Sc.
Iowa City, Iowa

Contributors

Willie A. Andersen, M.D.
Associate Professor
Division of Gynecologic Oncology
The University of Virginia Health Sciences
  Center
Charlottesville, Virginia

David A. Ansell, M.D.
Division of General Medicine
Department of Medicine
Cook County Hospital
Chicago, Illinois

Robert C. Brown, M.D.
Professor Emeritus
Department of Radiology
Former Chairman
Quality Assurance Committee
University of Iowa College of Medicine
Iowa City, Iowa

John P. Burke, M.D.
Chief
Infectious Diseases
LDS Hospital
Salt Lake City, Utah

Robert J. Corry, M.D.
Head
Department of Surgery
Director of Transplant Services
University of Iowa College of Medicine
Iowa City, Iowa

James J. Crall, D.D.S., M.S., S.M.
University of Connecticut Health Center
Farmington, Connecticut

Sidney T. Dana, M.D.
Chairman
Department of Otolaryngology
Community-General Hospital
Clinical Professor
Department of Otolaryngology
State University of New York
Upstate Medical Center
Syracuse, New York

Michael D. Decker, M.D., M.P.H.
Assistant Professor
Department of Preventive Medicine
Division of Infectious Diseases
Department of Medicine
Vanderbilt University
Hospital Epidemiologist
St. Thomas Hospital
Nashville, Tennessee

Bradley N. Doebbeling, M.D., M.S.
Assistant Professor
Division of General Medicine, Clinical
  Epidemiology, and Health Services
  Research
University of Iowa College of Medicine
Iowa City, Iowa

Dennis M. Domsic, M.B.A.
Assistant to Chairman
Department of Surgery
University of Iowa College of Medicine
Iowa City, Iowa

Avedis Donabedian, M.D.
Nathan Sinai Distinguished Professor
  Emeritus of Public Health
School of Public Health
University of Michigan
Ann Arbor, Michigan

Bernard Fallon, M.D.
Professor
Department of Urology
University of Iowa Medical School
University of Iowa College of Medicine
Iowa City, Iowa

Michael A. Fauman, Ph.D., M.D.
Director of Quality Assurance
Director of Ambulatory Care Services
Institute of Psychiatry and Human Behavior
University of Maryland School of Medicine
Baltimore, Maryland

David Goldberg, M.D.
Division of General Medicine
Department of Medicine
Cook County Hospital
Chicago, Illinois

Peter A. Gross, M.D.
Chief
Infectious Diseases Section
Professor of Medicine
Department of Internal Medicine
New Jersey Medical School
Hackensack Medical Center
Hackensack, New Jersey

Robert M. Heyssel, M.D.
President and Chief Executive Officer
Johns Hopkins Health System
Johns Hopkins Hospital
Baltimore, Maryland

Joan H. Howanitz, M.D.
UCLA Medical Center
Los Angeles, California

Peter J. Howanitz, M.D.
Director of Clinical Laboratories
UCLA Medical Center
Los Angeles, California

John W. Hoyt, M.D.
Chairman
Department of Critical Care Medicine
St. Francis Medical Center
Clinical Professor of Anesthesiology and
   Critical Care Medicine
University of Pittsburgh
Pittsburgh, Pennsylvania

Marguerite M. Jackson, R.N., M.S., C.I.C.
Director
Medical Center Epidemiology Unit
UCSD Medical Center
San Diego, California

William F. Jessee, M.D.
Former Vice President for Accreditation
   Surveys
Joint Commission on Accreditation of
   Healthcare Organizations
Vice President
Quality Management
Humana, Inc.
Chicago, Illinois

Ronald V. Keech, M.D.
Associate Professor
Department of Ophthalmology
University of Iowa College of Medicine
Iowa City, Iowa

Deborah J. Leisifer, R.N., C.C.R.N.
Nurse Manager
Medical Surgical Intensive Care Unit
St. Francis Medical Center
Pittsburgh, Pennsylvania

Edward E. Mason, M.D., Ph.D.
Professor Emeritus
Department of Surgery
University of Iowa College of Medicine
Iowa City, Iowa

R. Michael Massanari, M.D., M.S.
Director
Hospital Epidemiology
Associate Director
Professional Practice Review Group
Henry Ford Health System
Detroit, Michigan
Adjunct Professor
School of Public Health
University of Michigan
Ann Arbor, Michigan

Hamilton Moses III, M.D.
Vice President for Medical Affairs
Associate Professor of Neurology
The Johns Hopkins Medical Institution
Baltimore, Maryland

Mary D. Nettleman, M.D.
Henry J. Kaiser Family Foundation
Faculty Scholar in General Internal
  Medicine
University of Iowa College of Medicine
Iowa City, Iowa

Dennis S. O'Leary, M.D.
President
Joint Commission on Accreditation of
  Healthcare Organizations
Chicago, Illinois

Stanley L. Pestotnik, R.Ph.
Clinical Pharmacist
Division of Infectious Diseases
LDS Hospital
Salt Lake City, Utah

Michael A. Pfaller, M.D.
Professor and Vice Chairman
Medical Director, Clinical Laboratory
Department of Pathology
Oregon Health Sciences University
Portland, Oregon

Harry S. Rafkin, M.D.
Head
Clinical Investigation and Quality
  Assurance
Department of Critical Care Medicine
St. Francis Medical Center
Clinical Assistant Professor
Anesthesiology and Critical Care Medicine
University of Pittsburgh
Pittsburgh, Pennsylvania

Donald L. Renfrew, M.D.
Department of Radiology
Rusch-Presbyterian-St. Luke's Medical
  Center
Chicago, Illinois

Beverly J. Ringenberg, M.D.
Department of Emergency Medicine
Oregon Health Sciences University
Portland, Oregon

James S. Roberts, M.D.
Senior Vice President for Research and
  Standards
Joint Commission on Accreditation of
  Healthcare Organizations
Chicago, Illinois

Leslie L. Roos, Ph.D.
Professor
Department of Community Health
  Sciences
Faculty of Medicine
University of Manitoba
Director
Research Data Bank
Manitoba Centre for Health Policy and
  Evaluation
Winnipeg, Manitoba
Canada

Noralou P. Roos, Ph.D.
Professor
Department of Community Health
  Sciences
Faculty of Medicine
University of Manitoba
Director
Manitoba Centre for Health Policy and
  Evaluation
Winnipeg, Manitoba
Canada

Martha J. Ryan, R.N., M.H.A.
Quality Assurance Coordinator
Community-General Hospital
President
Central North Association of Quality
  Assurance Professionals
Syracuse, New York

Franklin L. Scamman, M.D.
Associate Professor
Department of Anesthesia
University of Iowa College of Medicine
Iowa City, Iowa

Robert L. Schiff, M.D., M.S.
Assistant Professor of Medicine
Course Director, Medicine II
Division of General Internal Medicine
Loyola University Medical Center
Maywood, Illinois

Paul M. Schyve, M.D.
Vice President for Research and Standards
Joint Commission on Accreditation of
   Healthcare Organizations
Chicago, Illinois

Mitzi W. Sprouse, R.N., C.P.Q.A.
Director
Quality Assurance and Utilization
   Review
St. Thomas Hospital
Nashville, Tennessee

Timothy R. Townsend, M.D.
Associate Professor of Pediatrics
Senior Director for Medical Affairs
The Johns Hopkins Hospital
Baltimore, Maryland

Frank H. Weigelt, F.A.C.H.E.
Assistant to the Chairman
Department of Radiology
University of Iowa College of Medicine
Iowa City, Iowa

Thomas A. Weingeist, M.D., Ph.D.
Professor and Chairman
Department of Ophthalmology
University of Iowa College of Medicine
Iowa City, Iowa

Robert F. Weir, Ph.D.
Professor and Director
Program in Biomedical Ethics
University of Iowa College of Medicine
Iowa City, Iowa

Richard P. Wenzel, M.D., M.Sc.
Professor and Director
Division of General Medicine
Clinical Epidemiology and Health Services
   Research
University of Iowa College of Medicine
Hospital Epidemiologist
University of Iowa Hospitals and Clinics
Iowa City, Iowa

Kerr L. White, M.D.
Former Deputy Director for Health
   Sciences
The Rockefeller Foundation
Charlottesville, Virginia

Raymond P. White, Jr., D.D.S., Ph.D.
School of Dental Medicine
The University of Connecticut Health
   Center
Farmington, Connecticut

Contents

Section IV. Approaches and Examples for Specific Departments

Introduction

Kerr L. White, M.D.

Concerns about the benefits of medical ministrations have a long history. Others preceded us in developing the mosaic of ideas that has lead to this compendium of essays describing theories and methods for assessing the quality of medical care. Although a number are mentioned in the succeeding chapters, a brief chronology of some important intellectual milestones may help the reader to see the current "Perspectives for Clinicians" in historical perspective.

The first contribution may have been that of Sir William Petty (1623–1687), a brilliant young physician who at age 28 was appointed Professor of Anatomy at Oxford. Widely regarded as the father of epidemiology, economics, social surveys, and what we now call health services research, Petty was the author of a notable treatise entitled *Political Arithmetic*. In it he asked, for the first time, whether value was being received for expenditures on health, welfare, and social services. Petty contended that the outcomes of the services, and especially medical care, should be assessed with the same precision accorded the financial expenditures. If Petty introduced us to hospital epidemiology, he was also the first to enunciate the need to assess the outcomes of medical care. Among his impertinent questions, for that period, were the following:

Of 1000 patients to the best physicians, aged of any decade, do not as many die as out of the inhabitants of places where there dwell no physicians?
Of 100 sick of acute diseases who use physicians, do not as many die and in misery, as where no art is used, or only chance?

London Hospitals are better . . . than those of Paris, for in the best at Paris there die two out of 15, whereas at London there die out of the worst two out of 16, and yet but a fiftieth part of the whole die out of the hospitals at London, and two fifths or 20 times that proportion die out of the Paris Hospitals which are of the same kind. (1)

Two centuries later, Florence Nightingale (1820–1910) demonstrated the practical utility and political necessity of meaningful social statistics, especially hospital statistics. Among her many contributions was the introduction of the first Model Hospital Statistical Abstract Form and a plan to produce Uniform Hospital Statistics (2). New ideas take a long time to achieve general acceptance—some say 50 years. Hers was the revolutionary idea that much could be learned from the collective experiences of hospitals, especially about that most personal of professional services, the care of individual patients by individual physicians—one at a time. Aided and abetted by the doyen of health statisticians and another father of modern epidemiology, William Farr (1807–1883), uniform systems for classifying diseases and presenting vital statistics were developed. These became models not only in Britain but also in Europe and America, but the adoption of Farr's principles for assessing hospital care, as Florence Nightingale urged, was slow to emerge.

Fifty years after Nightingale introduced her Uniform Hospital Discharge Form, a

British surgeon, one E. W. Groves urged that the results of all operations be registered.

If . . . a surgeon makes a specialty of some disease or operation and tabulates all his own results, or another by chance has some notable successes and records them, or the author of a textbook collects published records of various writers and summarizes them, is it not obvious that such a collection of figures will represent the best and not the average results? (3)

Groves' ideas included the need for long-term follow-up of patients to determine the outcome of the surgery in terms of mortality, morbidity, disability, and functional capacity.

About the same time, an American surgeon, E. A. Codman, attempted to introduce a similar system. He wrote:

It would be supposed that in the annual reports of hospitals some account of their products would be found. To a certain extent this is true, but often much of the material in annual reports is but a mere account of money subscribed and the proportionate amounts which are spent on the different departments.

I recently collected the annual reports of many of the large hospitals in America and endeavored to compare them with a view, if possible, to obtaining some definite form of report which would be available for all institutions and which would enable those interested to compare the work done by the different ones. (4)

For his troubles, Codman was ousted from the Massachusetts General Hospital, a major teaching hospital of the Harvard Medical School, but he is still remembered for his pioneering efforts to assess the quality of medical care—one more celebrated contributor to the development of hospital epidemiology.

In 1938, another pioneer, J. Alison Glover, M.D., a health officer in Britain, began to document the existence of wide variations in rates for common procedures among otherwise similar small geographic areas. In what has come to be known as the "Glover Phenomenon" he showed conclusively the marked differences for chil-

dren's tonsillectomy rates in different (small area) jurisdictions. For example:

. . . [A] child in Birmingham was more than four times more likely to be tonsillectomised than one in Manchester; and, while Bristol in 1948 trebled her prewar rate, Leeds reduced hers to one fifth. (5).

Then there were the unsung contributions of Professor Paul Lembcke, M.D., who many regard as the originator of both the term and the idea of the "medical audit." Starting about 1950, he undertook a series of studies showing that the feedback to clinicians of their collective experience derived from the analysis of hospital records modified their practices. Lembcke observed:

The purpose of medical auditing is to make certain that the full benefits of medical knowledge are being applied effectively to the needs of patients. A medical audit employing objective criteria is an important addition to such methods of insuring good medical care as the hospital standardization program carried on for many years by the American College of Surgeons and now continued by the Joint Commission on Accreditation. . . . (6)

About the same time, Mindel C. Sheps, M.D., published a classic paper that reviewed most of the empirical American literature up to that time on "quality assessment" and "quality assurance." Emphasizing the importance of developing a theoretical base for the emerging field as well as the need to refine methods, she wrote:

The development of practical and valid methods of measurement will involve the expenditure of considerable money and time. However, in view of efforts and money now being spent on programs to raise quality, it would seem essential to direct some of those resources toward the development of appropriate methods with which to judge their effects. Collaboration of clinicians, administrators, and statisticians is necessary for such a development. (7)

An essential ingredient in any national scheme to improve the quality of care in hospitals, and eventually in ambulatory settings and long-term care facilities, was the need to implement Florence Nightingale's idea of a Uniform Hospital Discharge Abstract with an agreed upon minimum Uniform Hospital Discharge Data Set (UHDDS). To that end, an international conference to address the problem was convened in 1968. Recommendations from that Conference moved the United States National Center for Health Statistics to establish a committee that eventually produced the UHDDS (8). Everything moves slowly. If anyone doubts that access to information is "power," they should examine the history of backing and filling by bureaucrats and their myriad committees and agencies, to say nothing of straightforward opposition from representatives of hospitals, physicians, and insurance carriers to the nationwide adoption of a UHDDS consisting of 14 items as part of every hospital discharge abstract. It took 17 years for the United States Department of Health and Human Services to adopt the final version for national use. More recent developments in the assessment, and especially Professor Avedis Donabedian's seminal construct distinguishing between "structure," "process," and "outcome" (see Chapter 4), in assessing the quality of care are well recounted in the following chapters.

Most physicians are familiar with the "placebo effect" mentioned in several of the essays that follow. On balance, it accounts for some 30–40% of the benefits associated with most medical maneuvers. What is less well known is the extent to which the placebo effect varies among similar studies conducted at different sites. Professor Howard M. Spiro, M.D., of Yale, confirms Professor Howard K. Beecher's figure of 35% (9) as a reasonable estimate of the placebo effect's overall beneficial influence, but notes that in clinical trials of duodenal ulcer the benefit may amount to 60% with an overall rate of at least 50%. More interesting still are the variations in the placebo effect among countries and institutions:

The healing rate on placebo for duodenal ulcer craters in controlled clinical trials runs from 20

percent in London to 70 percent in Switzerland. In the United States it ranges from 50 to 60 percent. A very interesting study was conducted in the United Kingdom a few years ago. An anti-ulcer drug was compared to a placebo in a trial carried out in Dundee and in London. The study was identical at both hospitals, but the healing rates for placebo were quite different: in Dundee 73 percent of ulcers healed on a placebo, in contrast to only 44 percent in London. The reasons for the differences in the healing rates in the two centers were unclear to the observers, who wondered whether there was a difference in the patients, in the doctors taking care of the patients, or in someone's expectations of cure. A study in the United States foreshadowed this observation. In one hospital . . . antacids relieved pain 79 percent of the time, but in another hospital the same antacids were effective only 17 percent of the time. In one hospital placebos gave relief to 45 percent of the patients, but in another only 25 percent were helped. In both the British and American studies the experimental design, definition of terms, and criteria were the same, but the responses were different, suggesting there are fundamental differences in responses to placebo as well as therapy. (10)

These findings suggest the presence of influences on the outcomes of care other than specific therapeutic maneuvers and the placebo effect. They may well be associated with the Hawthorne effect referred to in Chapter 8 (Doebbeling). A series of classic experiments first documented objectively the existence of a significant factor that affected behavior and feeling states. This factor, best described as "caring," constituted a beneficial and therapeutic force in its own right. Investigators from Harvard University and the Western Electric Company's Hawthorne plant near Chicago during the decade 1927 to 1937 documented their unexpected finding. During the 1930s the Western Electric and Bell Laboratories had also given us the theoretical base and many of the methods for quality control through the work of Walter A. Shewhart and W. Edwards Deming (see Chapter 10). The second series of Western Electric's landmark studies was designed initially to determine the extent to which variations in the conditions and physical environment of the workplace affected the productivity of employees. The investigations were extensive and complex. They involved six women who formed a discrete social group in a dedicated working environment; the women assembled telephone relays—the dependent variable—that measured productivity. In brief, the investigators found, to their great surprise, that no matter what changes were introduced by the company in the experimental situation, productivity improved. When the wattage of light bulbs was increased, production went up; when it was decreased, production went up! This ubiquitous phenomenon has been referred to ever since as the Hawthorne effect—a Heisenberg effect in human interactions. In other words, the observer's influence is always present in the clinical, research, and educational environments. Whatever else they did, the company "cared," and caring became the operative influence in the work environment. The Hawthorne effect permeates health services at both the micro and macro levels; to ignore it is to omit an essential part of reality.

The vital role it plays in the commercial and industrial worlds was placed in context by the guiding intellect behind the Western Electric studies, Elton Mayo (1880—1949), Professor of Industrial Research in the Harvard Graduate School of Business Administration. He described the research in a classic volume, *The Human Problems of an Industrial Civilization* (11). On balance, the Hawthorne effect was associated with increases in productivity at the Western Electric plant ranging from 8.3% to 17.5% in one series, and from 5.9% to 24.1% in a second series. The mean increases were 12.6% and 15.6%, respectively. In recent years the studies have been criticized methodologically, but it still seems reasonable to attribute to the Hawthorne effect some 10–15% of the observed benefits from general and specific interventions at the individual and population levels (12).

Lawrence J. Henderson (1878–1942), renowned Harvard biochemist, physiologist, and sometime social scientist, is best known to scholars who view medicine as part of larger social systems that influence health and disease. His famous 1941 article in *Science* was entitled "The Study of Man" (13). Henderson, however, is less well-known for his close association with Elton Mayo and the team conducting the Hawthorne experiments. Knowledge of both the natural and social sciences and Henderson's "systems approach" to understanding complex human phenomena made him an ideal collaborator. These interests had been prompted initially in Henderson by his early work as head of the Fatigue Laboratory established in the Harvard Graduate School of Business Administration to study physical and mental stress in workers (14). This interest, in turn, had been stimulated by World War I research at the British Industrial Health Research Board (later a branch of the Medical Research Council). Their ideas, in turn, may have originated with one, Charles Turner Thackrah (1795–1833), a surgeon in Leeds and founder of that city's medical school, who in 1835 published a volume on *The Effects of Arts, Trades and Professions on Health and Longevity*. He documented the deleterious impact of contemporary working conditions on health with resulting incapacity, permanent disabilities, and premature death. Among the noxious influences he associated with a wide range of accidents, diseases, and disabilities were dust and other atmospheric pollutants, unnatural body postures, excessive muscular effort, "close work" affecting vision, high temperature, "anxiety and mental worry," and "low, varied, and uncertain wages" (15).

My purpose in recounting this history and noting the role played by these ideas in the evolution of hospital epidemiology is to emphasize that, in addition to the ministrations of physicians and other health professionals and personnel, there are institutional and organizational factors that have a bearing on the outcomes of care. These too constitute an important dimension of quality, beyond patient "satisfaction."

Consider Sir William Osler's observation in the *British Medical Journal* of 1910:

Faith in *St. Johns Hopkins*, as we used to call him, an atmosphere of optimism, and cheerful nurses, worked just the same sort of cures as *Æscupalius* at Epidaurus. (16)

"Caring is part of the cure!" read the message on buttons worn by the staff of the Johns Hopkins Hospital 60 years later. An institutionwide campaign to make both professional and support personnel recognize their own therapeutic powers was perhaps unknowingly based on scientific knowledge. Those who regard this as a public relations ploy would do well to consider the studies conducted by Professor Reginald Revans of Manchester University. In the 1960s he showed that, when size and other factors were controlled, hospitals where supervisors employed authoritarian attitudes and behavior, compared to those where permissive and supportive management styles prevailed, had much higher rates of staff turnover (especially for nurses) and longer lengths of stay for six common medical conditions and six common surgical conditions (17).

All of this implies the need for additional "indicators" of institutional quality. These could include rates for personnel turnover, absenteeism, tardiness, medication errors, patient calls for assistance, waiting times for tests, procedures, pharmacy responses, admissions, etc. Noise levels measured in decibels should be recorded regularly. Such indicators should be enhanced by the monitoring of sentinel events as Decker and Sprouse point out in Chapter 10. In other words, the total institutional ambience in which patient care is conducted requires monitoring as closely as does the work of individual physicians and other health professionals. Everything and everyone matters in the extremely complex human enterprise that comprises the contemporary hospital.

"Quality" has many dimensions. The "structure," i.e., the hospital or health services system and all of its departments or subunits have an impact on the services provided and the outcome of each individual patient's care. "Processes" are not confined to the specific interventions of physicians and other health professionals; they include the attitudes, behavior, enthusiasm, support, dress, and concern of everyone in the organization. Industry,

especially those concerned with the "quality" of their services and products, are well aware of these dimensions. "Outcomes," however defined and measured, can be enhanced only when everyone's morale and esprit de corps are high and their presence is manifested throughout the organization.

Much is said about the application of epidemiological concepts and methods in the chapters that follow. Indeed they are essential for tracking the quality of care in institutions. They are also important at the population level as Glover first showed and Professors Noralou and Leslie Roos (see Chapter 13), Jack Wennberg, and others have demonstrated so elegantly. To the extent that hospitals and health care institutions accept responsibility for the care of populations defined by geography, the institutional and population approaches are identical. However, when several institutions serve a geopolitical jurisdiction, such as a municipality, county, or state, both sets of measures are required to appreciate fully the overall quality of care for the entire population. All of these dimensions are now coming under increasing scrutiny but the responsible agencies, data sets, terms, definitions, and measures still require effective coordination in the interests of enhancing comparability and reducing costs. To that end, the inordinate preoccupation that now prevails with collecting billing data to the exclusion of clinical data would have distressed William Petty. What is the point of emphasizing charges and costs without an equal emphasis on benefits and outcomes of the services rendered? Much greater attention needs to be given to collecting useful and usable data at the same time that billing and claims data are generated. Much more important from the patient's viewpoint than a diagnosis is a statement about the level of severity, disability, and impairment—so-called functional capacity—experienced by the patient before and after an encounter with the health care system. There is much room for the development of innovative software for use by hospitals and physicians in what is bound to become an important aspect of future hospital and health information systems.

To this end, medical and health sciences centers may well want to consider incorporating many aspects of a quality assessment program into a Health Intelligence and Analysis Unit responsible for coordinating and monitoring the health status of the surrounding population, as well as keeping the faculty, community practitioners, and the public abreast of new medical interventions, ongoing developments, and needed research, etc. (18).

But population-based studies, whether of general populations or of an institutions' patients, demonstrate only *where* the problems lie, not *what* the problems are. They do not indicate the precise nature of the problems with equipment, facilities, records, communication, etc. and the respective roles and activities of different personnel. Macro approaches are not substitutes for a micro approach. Once problems are identified, those responsible for assessing the quality of care will need to examine individual patient records and the contributions of a variety of factors including those of individual health personnel, be they physicians, clerks, or janitors. Patient care is provided one patient at a time as the authors of the following chapters repeatedly emphasize. Misadventures of whatever nature need to be investigated in depth. As in the case of an airline infraction, mishap, or crash, the probable sequence of events or "causes" should be established and individual or systemic improvements or changes introduced.

This brings us to one of the central issues characterizing this volume. Assessing the quality of care is essentially an educational and behavioral enterprise. The object is to "shift the entire curve to the right." Even a few weak players can improve their contributions. Far better to help all the institution's personnel (professional and support) to improve, than to identify a few laggards. Quality assessment or assurance (an improbable term rapidly being replaced by the former term) must not become or be perceived as a rascal-hunting

exercise. It is designed to promote institutional and individual improvements as the studies at Hawthorne demonstrated more than half a century ago. Caring is really part of the cure and the implementation of a truly effective system for assessing the quality of care is an essential ingredient in the provision of compassionate, science-based, effective, and efficient health services.

References

1. Greenwood M. Medical statistics from Graunt to Farr. Cambridge: Cambridge University Press, 1948.
2. Woodham-Smith C. Florence Nightingale (1820–1910). London: Constable, 1950.
3. Groves EW. A plea for a uniform registration of operation results. British Med J 1908;2:1008–1009.
4. Codman EA. The product of a hospital. Surg Gynecol Obstet 1914;April:491–496.
5. Glover JA. Tonsillectomy in the school medical service. IV. Increased incidence in 1948. Monthly Bull Ministry Health 1950;9:62–68.
6. Lembcke PA. Medical auditing by scientific methods. JAMA 1956;162:646–655.
7. Sheps MC. Approaches to the quality of hospital care. Public Health Rep 1955;70:877–886.
8. Murnaghan J, White KL, eds. Hospital discharge data: Report of a conference on hospital discharge abstract systems. Med Care 1970;8(4)(Suppl).
9. Beecher HK. The powerful placebo. JAMA 1955;159:1602–1606.
10. Spiro HM. Doctors, patients and placebos. New Haven and London: Yale University Press, 1986.
11. Mayo E. The human problems of an industrial civilization. New York: Macmillan, 1933.
12. Roethlisberger FJ, Dickson WJ. Management and the worker. Cambridge, MA: Harvard University Press, 1939.
13. Henderson LJ. The study of man. Science 1941;94:1–10.
14. Barber B, ed. L. J. Henderson on the social system. Chicago and London: University of Chicago Press, 1970:102,209.
15. Newman G. The rise of preventive medicine. London: Oxford University Press, 1932:172–173.
16. Cushing H. The life of Sir William Osler. London and New York: Oxford University Press, 1940:909.
17. Revans RW. The measurement of supervisory attitudes. Manchester: Manchester Statistical Society, 1961:32.
18. White KL, Connelly JE. The medical school's mission and the population's health. New York and Heidelberg: Springer-Verlag, 1991.

Section I

Revolution in Health Care Delivery

1

Historical Perspectives

Richard P. Wenzel, M.D., M.Sc.

The concerns for quality medical care have become a major public issue in the United States. Just a decade ago, this would have been an unusual situation, but now health and health care delivery have become a focus of important social magnitude. One cannot read a leading newspaper without encountering at least weekly a featured article on medical care. For example, *The New York Times, The Washington Post,* and *The Wall Street Journal* have focused on the spiraling costs of medical care, the lack of access for millions of medically uninsured Americans, recurrent questions about the level of appropriateness of commonly performed procedures, and the current dissatisfaction of physicians with intensified governmental regulations of medical care delivery (1–6). The point is not only that there are the usual scholarly reviews of the medical system in peer-reviewed literature but that also these concerns have become so widespread that they are the grist for newspaper editorials, television specials, and public debate.

The irony of the current situation is that the country acknowledged by many to have the most technologically sophisticated health care system in the world is coming under greatest scrutiny and criticism by its citizens. In addition, there are frustrations voiced by business and industry, Congressional members, and federal agencies. The criticism and frustrations focus on the value of the care and particularly the value relative to the cost of that care. In large part, the negative views of United States health care are in response to its escalating costs and the perceived failure of the health care profession to develop effective measures to control those costs.

In an attempt to deal with the growing economic burden of medical care, the United States government has imposed a number of sanctions on medical care delivery and medical care deliverers. In turn, the nation's health care delivery team has expressed some anguish regarding both the sanctions and the perceptions of the general public. Physicians, in particular, think that the government has become too intrusive and too bureaucratic and, as a result, the paperwork required by professional review procedures has interfered with optimal patient care and professional time—time to think, read, attend conferences and learn, and time to spend with the patient. Moreover, the continued scrutiny, debate, and documentation of care, physicians argue, have led to less respect in the community for both the medical and nursing professions.

The current frustrations have reached so great a pitch that there have been numerous calls to change the health care system. A particularly recurrent theme is the development of a national health care system, perhaps similar to the one in Canada (7), and the introduction of a centralized form of rationing of health care (8, 9). Those who are so vocal for a centralized system of rationing argue that we currently have an economic—and thus unfair—system of health care rationing. Many others who favor the concept of centralized rationing think that it is a necessary and just step in providing some system of health care delivery for all of our citizens. Industry is especially concerned because the cost of health care benefits is eroding corporate profits significantly. Despite the clamor, the Secretary of Health and Human Services has responded by noting that no change should be made until the pitfalls of the current versus the proposed system are fully explored and understood (10). Moreover, Arnold Relman, an outspoken authority on health care delivery, has argued that such federal rationing will not solve our current economic problems (11).

The purpose of this chapter is to describe how a number of forces have evolved to interact and impact on health care and health care providers. The commonly expressed concern is whether quality health care is being provided. The major point to be stressed is that quality assessment and quality enhancement are key issues through which the nation's health care

systems will be evaluated and ultimately defined. This chapter will present a paradigm for visualizing quality health care and offer a working definition of health itself. Thereafter, the issue of measuring quality care, the current problems with measurement, and options for organizing for quality assessment will be discussed. One of the goals of this chapter is to expand on the classic works of Donabedian (12, 13), bringing the issues up to date for the practicing clinician.

The issues noted above are frequently discussed under the umbrella term of "quality of care." However, all acknowledge that the basis of the major concern is the economic burden posed by the existing health care system. Some might frame this issue more directly: the new emphasis on quality is a proxy for squeezing costs. Since the most expensive health care delivery is in inpatient care and large outpatient facilities, much of the focus of current debate is on health care delivery in hospitals and clinics. In fact, the resulting changes in medical care have become so different in the last decade compared to earlier ones

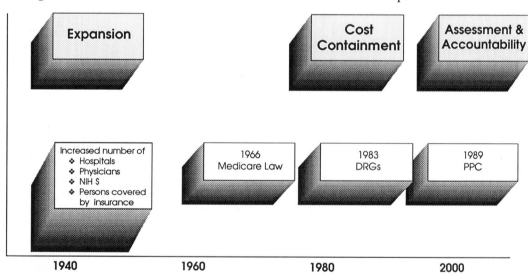

Figure 1.1.   Revolutions in health care. The period of expansion began in the 1940s and continued for over two decades. Increased numbers of persons were covered by health insurance during this period. The period of cost containment was highlighted by the passage in 1983 of a new Medicare payment, fixing fees on a limited number of diagnoses—the diagnosis related-groups (DRGs). The period of assessment and accountability began in the 1980s and continues. In late 1989, the Medicare fees of physicians were fixed by the passage of the Omnibus Budget Reconciliation Act, recommended by the Congressionally appointed Professional Practice Commission (PPC). (Adapted from Relman AS. The trouble with rationing. N Engl J Med 1990;323:911–913.)

that the editor of the *New England Journal of Medicine* has referred to it as a third modern revolution in medical care (14).

In Relman's view, the three periods signifying modern revolutions occurred as follows: expansion (1940–1960s), cost containment (early 1980s), and assessment and accountability (late 1980s) (Fig. 1.1). The expansion period was characterized by rapid growth in the numbers of hospitals, physicians, technical advances, National Institutes of Health dollars for basic research, and United States citizens who were covered by a health insurance plan. Evidence for the nagnitude of the expansion is that between 1960 and 1990 the proportion of the gross national product (GNP) for which health care accounted increased from 4.4 to almost 12%. Furthermore, it has been estimated that national spending for health will exceed $1.5 trillion by the year 2000 (15), accounting for perhaps 20% of the GNP (16). In the meantime, such inflationary changes inevitably led to cost containment, highlighted by the development of the reimbursement system for hospitalization's costs based on a limited number of diagnosis-related groups (DRGs). In large part this change in cost reimbursement was stimulated by the fact that Medicare, the largest federally funded health care program, consumed a major portion of the health care budget. Thus, the government became keenly interested in cost containment and switched from a retrospective cost-based method to prospective pricing as the fundamental hospital payment system.

In addition to the institution of DRGs, other methods to control costs were introduced including managed care, especially with second opinions, and insurance cost-sharing between beneficiaries and the insurance companies via coinsurance and deductibles (17). Industry also has been concerned that the cost of health care is eroding corporate benefits significantly. Most recently, we have encountered increasing regulatory, insurance and consumer demands for assessment of quality and accountability for more and more of the common medical practices. Whether or not one thinks that there is a separate and independent third revolution or whether the latter is a part of the second is unimportant. What is important is tht there is no doubt about the national preoccupation for monitoring health care and health care providers. The sentiment is that, with respect to runaway costs for health care, nothing so far has worked!

THE DRGs AND BEYOND

One question is whether or not the DRGs had any effect on medical costs. Davis and colleagues (18) have outlined their perspective of the impact of prospective payment:

1. Lengths of stay have shortened greatly;
2. Hospital admissions for the elderly did not rise as predicted but have decreased slightly;
3. There was not massive cost shifting to the private sector;
4. There was moderation of the previously noted rates of increase in real hospital spending;
5. Real hospital costs per day have, nevertheless, continued to increase markedly;
6. Fees for physician services continued to increase faster than the Consumer Price Index.

Nevertheless, even in 1985 the total United States health care spending was $425 billion, which was 1.5 times greater than the defense budget. The main point is that the DRGs provided the mechanism that jolted the medical community from its traditional acceptance of a cost-based reimbursement system whose changes were automatically passed on to third party payers, including the government. Obviously, the DRGs had an important impact on institutional spending. Some suggest, however, that this was subsequently offset by the increased volume of services provided. The latter doubled between 1978 and 1988 from 12 to 24 per beneficiary (19).

In the meantime, the government agency that oversees the spending of Medicare, the Health Care Financing Administration (HCFA), transformed the already existing Professional Standard Review Organization (PSRO) to the Peer Review Organizations (PROs). These agencies administer a peer review process organized to deny payment of admissions that are not considered to be medically necessary. Many hospitals have responded by scrutinizing admissions themselves more closely, creating more outpatient units, and encouraging shorter hospital stays, resulting in a decline in inpatient census. Their existing utilization review committees now audit critically their own physicians' decisions regarding admission and discharge of patients, often within specialty services, in the best sense of the term "peer review." Thus, the increased bureaucracy in the hospital is economically driven and is a response to the regulatory process evaluating "appropriate" medical care. So far, however, we have no evidence that these steps have either controlled costs or improved quality.

One might question the extent of the bureaucracy and address the concern that some for-profit institutions, especially, would intrude in traditional medical affairs in the self interest of the institution. A recent care study is encouraging (20). Campbell and Kane studied the physician-management relationships at Hospital Corporation of America. The latter institution in fact recognized that, although community hospitals are locally driven businesses, physician-management relations are at the heart of any hospital strategy to increase its market share or its earnings. Moreover, the authors concluded, "those relationships cannot be forged by corporate boilerplate" (20).

An offshoot of quality assurance (QA) programs is the more easily measurable and negative component, risk management. Quality assurance proposes to create appropriate frameworks to monitor the quality of care that patients receive, with a promise of altering suboptimal practices. Risk management has as its goal the reduction of potential risk for patients and ultimately of costs associated with negative outcomes, specifically, payable malpractice suits. As summarized succinctly by Massanari: "An ounce of prevention is worth a ton of money" (21).

What we have witnessed so far is only the tip of a huge iceberg of regulations. Congress, having already developed a method to limit costs related to hospitalization (the DRGs), has in turn also created the Physician Payment Review Commission to advise the legislature regarding proposals to reform Medicare physician payment. Specifically, the mission is to revise the ways in which fees are set and to devise methods to control the growth of expenditures for physicians' services (22). Moreover, while developing a strategy to curb costs for services, the Commission is also developing an approach to improve quality of care by increasing the appropriateness of services provided for Medicare beneficiaries. The point is that, whereas the DRGs were created to limit costs related to hospitalization, new laws are being created to limit payment for physicians' fees. It will be important to measure the effect of this new step.

RISING COSTS

The causes of the rising costs are many, including the changing demographics of our population, the high costs of new technology, the existing medical culture in the United States, which thrives on using the new technology, and the lack of incentives to curb costs. In the United States, a greater proportion of our population is old, and the older group consumes greater resources when they become ill, including the newest and most expensive technologies and life-saving medications. An important factor in the current governmental thinking, therefore, relates to the demographics of the elderly (10): between 1970 and 1984 the proportion of those ≥65 years old and those ≥85 years old increased from approximately 10 to 12% and from 7 to 9%, respectively. With respect to the utilization of medical resources by the elderly, it is noteworthy that discharge rates for short-stay hospitals for persons aged 65–74 have increased 55% since Medicare began in 1965; in 1981, persons aged 45–54 averaged 4.7 medical office visits annually compared to 6.3 visits per year for those aged 65–74; Americans over the age of 60 comprise 16% of the population but consume 38% of all prescribed medications, filling 560 million prescriptions annually. It may well be, however, that the influence of the aging population on current health care costs is minor. Evans (23) has suggested that age-adjusted per capita costs fell between 1983 and 1984 by 2%, but that spending on hospital care rose by 6.1% due to price increases. Moreover, the difference in health care costs in the United States and Canada could not be explained by population demographics.

In a recent report, Iglehart (19) has reviewed the new law on Medicare's payments to physicians. In the review, he noted that "although the payment-reform policies will initially apply only to Medicare, they will certainly influence the relationship between physicians and private health insurers as well." Additionally, in the past, Congress allowed physicians to charge Medicare patients a fee greater than the approved limit, but the new bill clearly limits the amount. The current law states that, if Medicare expenditures for physicians' services exceed the rate of growth projected according to the volume standard, future increases in fees will be reduced to compensate for the excess. The Secretary of Health and Human Services and the congressionally appointed Professional Practice Review Commission (PPRC) will send target volume recommendations to Congress each year. The bill authorizes physicians' fee schedules according to resource costs (25), thus reducing the disparity of payment between those physicians performing procedures and those in the "cognitive" disciplines. The resource costs take into account equipment, supplies, time expended, and the previous costs of education of the health care provider. A critical observation underscored by Iglehart is that the Resource Based Relative Value Scale (RBRVS) does not take into account a physician's competence or the quality of service delivered.

In his critical review of health care costs in the United States, Evans (23) underscores other issues. In particular, compared to the Canadian system, the United States costs for program administration and overhead are six times as great. Specifically, these costs increased from $14.5

billion in 1983 to $19.1 billion in 1984 and to $26.2 billion in 1985. According to Evans, approximately one-fourth of the difference between health care costs (as a percent of GNP) between the United States and Canada is the cost of running the payment system itself. If this pattern persists, says Evans, "it may be that the U.S. experience after 1983 represents merely a transfer of outlays and incomes from hospital patient care staff to managers and investors, with no net savings to payors" (23).

Evans also points out that much of the remaining discrepancy between health care costs in the United States and Canada reflects the increasing physician fees and intensity of services in the United States. Of interest is that the increased number of physicians, the more competitive environment, and the continuing high average workloads per physician have had no influence on physician fees.

There is also no question that the increased costs of medical care have been fueled by the health care deliverers' desire to use expensive technology and by the consumers' perceptions of need. Medicine's appetite for the development and use of the latest technology has been matched by the public's sense of entitlement for optimal care. In part, it is argued that both physicians and patients have come to expect 100% certainty in diagnoses and therapy (26), perhaps because of our basic culture but also—from the physicians' point of view—because of a concern for lawsuits. Ours is a litigious society, and "defensive medicine" and escalating costs of malpractice insurance have been the result.

Other forces have also been operative, including the evolution of accreditation agencies and the introduction of the competitive health care model. Thus, *more is being done* in the name of modern medicine. Many have questioned the United States' approach that more is better. For example, Callahan summarized the frustrations of many by noting that "the United States spends 2.8 times as much per capita on health care as Great Britain, with essentially identical outcomes . . ." (27). Other data from the American Medical Association and Population Reference

Bureau cited recently by *The New York Times* indicate that the infant mortality rate and life expectancy are no better in the United States than in countries that spend considerably less on health: Australia, Austria, Italy, the Netherlands, Norway, and Sweden (6). The current emphasis on appropriateness of expensive procedures is a reflection of the concern and doubt that increased volume of procedures is correlated with better outcome.

QUALITY HEALTH CARE

So much effort is expended in meeting the guidelines and requirements of regulatory agencies and accrediting bodies that it is easy to forget that the real issue is quality care. This has been broadly defined as desirable and achievable health care (28). Clearly then it is a function of both perceptions and knowledge. Certainly a patient has a perception of the worst case-best case situation and perhaps some preconceived notions about the style and content of communications between him or her and the patient care deliverer. The patient may also have a perception about the evaluation time needed for diagnosis, therapy, and favorable outcome, which is very much culturally determined. Nevertheless, patients will vary greatly with respect to their knowledge of a reasonable workup for a given condition, the therapeutic options available, and the spectrum of outcomes. Moreover, with reflection it should be obvious that one cannot define quality solely from the vantage point of a patient: a perfectly content patient may not be receiving quality care. It is a necessary but not sufficient element.

What is also needed for quality is the highest achievable—the optimal—health care outcome defined from the vantage point of existing medical technology. Since the latter can be assessed only by an informed segment of the medical profession, the involvement of the profession is essential. Thus, the information needed to assess the technical aspects of optimal health must derive from careful observations subject to scientific rigor and analyzed skillfully in the aggregate. Quality

therefore is based not only on patients' perceptions (a function of their attitudes based on culture and experience) but also on an accurate synthesis of modern medical care observations.

If the latter statements are true, then important questions include how one makes observations and how one learns and synthesizes available data. It is a basic assumption that it is necessary to recognize all important data, and that it is important to recognize that in medicine one learns in three ways (29). (*a*) In a *clinical setting*, an astute physician makes a new observation while caring for individual patients. The results of such work are often published as case reports or a series of cases. (*b*) In a *laboratory setting*, basic biophysical events give clues to the mechanisms of the interaction of host (or host cellular components) and external stimuli. Such work is published in basic science journals and currently is illustrated by the popularity of molecular biology. (*c*) In a *population setting*, cases and controls are compared, risk factors defined, and new approaches tested in groups of people. Such work is best exemplified by epidemiological reports, clinical trials, and studies involving patients' choices when offered therapeutic options, each with different risks and benefits (30).

If one agrees that the observations of all three types contribute to medical progress, it is incumbent upon those interested in quality to be able to assemble information from all three disciplines in an accurate manner. Such skill requires a great deal of training (26) and might best be accomplished by those exposed to all three medical disciplines. Essentially the synthesis of medical information is as critical to achieving quality as it is to the study and measurement of the delivery of quality, i.e., quality assessment.

It should perhaps be stated that quality health care might be viewed in light of what a reasonable medical person(s) could do. This is to acknowledge human effort on the one hand and human frailties on the other. Perhaps this is important to state early since so much of quality health care has had a negative connotation, in large part because of the apparent desire of health care recipients for a "perfect" outcome and a risk-free process (31). This is clearly unrealistic, and the communication between caregivers and the public needs to be realistic. Moreover, those delivering health care do so with a great deal of uncertainty, for the "truth" is often unknown. Existing quality health care is, therefore, based on the best available studies, but the resulting data are often quite limited. Thus, the art of quality care includes the application of limited science and common sense to a specific patient whose individual value system must be incorporated into the management plan.

So far, quality health care has been discussed as an encounter directly between a patient and a physician. Although this may be the most common situation, it is obvious that more complex encounters occur between a patient and the health care system. There is an entire medical care bureaucracy that influences and defines health care; and issues of access, expedient and careful diagnosis, and the use of ancillary services are important. All of this is to emphasize what Donabedian (32) has referred to as the structure and process of medical care. Thus, the determinants of quality health care are a function of not only the skill and compassion of the physician and the value system of the patient but also the state of the art of medicine, a country's resources allocated to health care, the structure of the health care delivery system, and the attitudes and governance of the health care team.

HEALTH

It is beyond the scope of this chapter to discuss health in depth; however, a few comments and personal views are in order. It is this author's perception that health could best be viewed as a state of harmony between a person and his or her environment. Whenever that harmony is missing—to a greater or lesser extent—health is not optimal. In order to restore health, one must alter the individual or change the environment. According to Kovacs, "The healthy form of the relationship between the body and its environment is character-

ized by a dynamic, steady state which can be maintained by the living being in spite of certain changes in the environment. This requires the quality of adaptation" (33). The implications of this view are several: (a) health cannot be defined for all people from a single perspective; (b) health cannot be defined in a mechanistic, i.e., deterministic model alone such as the model of molecular biology; (c) there is no need to separate the mind and the body of the patient as though they were independent functions; they are preserved as a whole; and (d) improved health states can occur as a function of altering either aspect of the relationship of the person and the environment, not merely the biophysical state of the person. The phrasing of Kovacs is again helpful: ". . . health is that physical or mental state, function or reaction, which is capable of adapting to the natural and social-environmental surroundings of the individual with the appropriate advantage/disadvantage ratio for the body and spirit" (33). From a clinical perspective, the health care provider may be tempted to "bend" the patient to his or her environment. However, within the current paradigm, quality health care might be better served by altering the environment to provide a more harmonious match with the patient.

To extend the paradigm of health to populations, one would conclude that, in its broadest sense, public health has as its major function to seek an optimal harmony between groups of men and women in society and their environment. This goal can be approached in three ways: (a) by methods to improve host resistance of populations to environmental "hazards"; (b) by effective plans to improve the safety of the environment; and (c) by improving health care systems designed to increase the likelihood, efficiency, and effectiveness of the first two goals (Table 1.1). The purpose of mentioning this view of health is that it offers an expanded view of health care and new opportunities to measure the value of health care delivery in individuals and in populations. It is important to underscore the idea that the term "environment" is used broadly to include not only the biological and physical environment of a person or a population but also

Table 1.1.
**Methods to Improve Public Health Control
of Diseases**

Improved resistance to environmental hazards
  Hygiene and hygienic behavior
  Nutrition
  Immunity
  Antimicrobials and other medications
  Psychological factors
  Exercise
  Genetic alteration
Improved environmental safety
  Sanitation
  Air
  Water
  Food
  Infectious agents, vectors, and animal
    reservoirs
  Industrial hazards
Public health systems
  Access
  Efficiency
  Resources
  Priorities
  Containment
  Contact tracing for prophylaxis and therapy
  Education
  Social forces
  Laws
  Measurement of problems and of
    efficiency and effectiveness of control

the social, economic, political, and cultural environment. Much of this is consistent with an earlier definition of the World Health Organization (WHO): "Health is a state of complete physical, mental and social well-being and not merely the absence of disease and infirmity" (quoted in Clare (34)).

Woods and Edwards (35) highlight the central issue in health from a patient's perspective: how is ill-health experienced? They underscore the burden of not only the new illness but also the psychological reaction. In the current paradigm, both are determinants of the lack of harmony between a patient and the environment. According to these authors,

The basic human desires, hopes, fears, the image one has of oneself, the vitality of the ego, all are suddenly at stake when illness threatens. These feelings of a lack of control, the loss of self, that are so often manifested in illness are

compounded in serious illness. By having to turn to others, to give up certain rights, to become passive and accept the decisions that others make about our lives, we adopt the role of the patient. (35)

If we can define health as a harmony of a person (or a population) with the environment, then quality health care defines our ability to create that harmony in a desirable and achievable fashion. Moreover, the concept of the individual's inseparability of mind and body, of the broad view of the environment and the meaning of ill health, or of being a patient frees us to examine the determinants of health and health care. Given a full understanding of the state of the art of medicine, the goals of individuals and groups of people, and the components of the environment, including the institutions created to deliver health care, one can begin to measure quality care.

MEASURING QUALITY CARE

From an epidemiological perspective, quality assessment might be viewed as the study of the distribution and determinants of desirable and achievable health care in a hospital or clinic setting (36). One could begin with some type of routine and orderly collection of rates of occurrence of quality care, i.e., with surveillance. Once the end points are identified, operationally useful definitions could be employed and surveillance begun. Certainly, before the data are taken at face value, the surveillance system would have to be evaluated by a concurrent "gold standard." Thereafter, one could determine the estimates and precision of the measured rates of occurrence, and eventually the independent risk determinants for quality (or lack thereof) could be identified and some of those subjected to intervention studies.

Epidemiological and clinical skills are disciplines necessary for quality assessment. No system for measuring quality care can exclude either. Nevertheless, if structure, process, the attitudes of physicians and patients, and the political and economic climate of a country are important, then other disciplines are also necessary to measure quality health care. These include social psychology, health economics, health policy, and others. The point is, however, that it is not only important to employ these disciplines in new and creative ways to improve the health of a society, but it is essential to *measure* the effects of our efforts.

Quality assessment begins with access (37–40) to the health care system and continues through the discharge process (Fig. 1.2). It is important to emphasize that quality care does not end at the point of discharge, but rather at some time afterwards. From the patient's point of view there is an assumed warranty for reasonable health after discharge. From both the patient's and the technological points of view one might assess the adequacy of access to the health care system and, of course, access in a "timely" fashion. Additionally, one might ask questions about the distribution of access to care: is it similar for all groups regardless of age, race, income, or illness? Similarly, one could evaluate a number of other attributes related to the process: the rates of satisfac-

tory communication, an appreciation of the cleanliness of the hospital or clinic, the sense of privacy, the level of apprehension created or avoided, the utility of support services, and others. The measure of performance could be expressed in terms of expected benefit or side effects.

From the technical point of view, one could examine access in terms of the distribution of transferred patients in stable conditions to a second hospital from a referring institution (37). Moreover, after admission one could examine whether or not a complete history and physical examination were performed, if a follow-up note was sent to the referring physician, or if a complete blood count was performed on all new inpatients. The latter might be referred to as "process-oriented" monitors. Alternately, one could monitor occurrences that directly lead to some morbidity or mortality. These would be referred to as "outcome" measurements and might include rates of infection, bleeding, drug errors, and others (Table 1.2). Within the paradigm of health presented above, one might also wish to design measures of patients' sense of control over their health

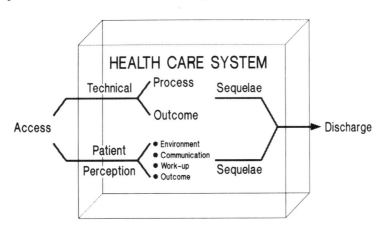

Figure 1.2. Quality assessment begins with measuring the patients' access to the health care system and proceeds to involve the experience within the system until discharge. Both technical aspects of optimal health care as well as patients' perceptions can be assessed. Within the technical aspects there are both process-oriented and outcome-oriented end points and sequelae to each. Patients may be concerned about the perceived quality of communication, workup, environment, and outcome. All may influence the patient-health care system interaction with possibly important sequelae. The type of discharge (involving the competent patient's right to die) and its timing are also quality issues. (Reprinted by permission of the publisher from Wenzel RP. Quality assessment: An emerging component of hospital epidemiology. Diagn Microbiol Infect Dis 1990;13:197–204. Copyright 1990 by Elsevier Science Publishing Co., Inc.)

Table 1.2.
Examples of End Points for Measuring Quality of Care[a]

Access
  Access to an emergency service
  Access to a subspecialty clinic
  Admission to hospital for acute abdomen/
    AIDS/etc. regardless of income
  Access to particular services and technology
Process
  Complete history and physical
  Complete blood count on all inpatients
  Discharge summary within 24 hours
  Daily note by all physicians
Outcome
  Infection
  Bleeding
  Drug error
  Fall
  Pulmonary embolus
  Myocardial infarction
  Hypo-/Hypernatremia
  Patient satisfaction and symptom relief
  Functional status
Consequence of outcome
  Excess stay in hospital
  Stroke
  Allergic reaction
  Fractured hip
  Mechanical ventilation
  Cardiac arrest
  Coma
  Out of pocket expenses

[a]Reprinted by permission of the publisher from Wenzel RP. Quality assessment: An emerging component of hospital epidemiology. Diagn Microbiol Infect Dis 1990;13:197–204. Copyright 1990 by Elsevier Science Publishing Co., Inc.

care process, their sense of anxiety or depressed mood as a consequence of hospitalization, and their sense of estrangement within the medical care system. Such approaches might measure what has been referred to as harmony between a person and his or her environment. If the patient were having trouble coping, it could be a sign of failure of the health care system to provide a comfortable environment. In addition, one might want to extend the view of outcome occurrences to look at attributable consequences of these outcome measurements such as excess stay in the hospital, stroke, loss of function, and others. Lastly, the quality of discharge

could be evaluated in terms of the patient's right for death with dignity or for a discharge to a private home rather than to a nursing institution.

The major point to be stressed is that one can examine structure, process, or outcome anywhere from access to discharge and follow-up. However, whatever focus is chosen, some quality indicator can be measured. It should be understood that the quality of the measurement tool must be assessed as well, i.e., one must test the test. It is no longer acceptable to say that a hospital or clinic is a high quality institution; we must instead say *how much* quality is present.

CURRENT ISSUES

Several problems exist nationally with respect to current quality assurance programs and have been identified earlier. A few are highlighted below. First, most utilization review is now based on statistical norms rather than on appropriate medical care. The concerns that surround the publication of crude mortality rates by institution, with insufficient adjustment for severity of underlying diseases, are examples. These concerns are beginning to be addressed (41–43).

Second, few tasks arouse physician anger and frustration as greatly as the "hassle" of preadmission screening based on superficial guidelines, especially when administered by nonprofessionals. In part, this is a reflection of the fact that there is virtually a complete lack of evidence that current guidelines influence favorably the quality of patient care (44). Some clinicians and administrators have been quite sensitive to this issue and, in fact, have divorced utilization review from quality assessment. Each is a different activity with a different purpose, and the two activities should probably not be linked.

Third, there is an obvious increase in physician pressure with respect to his or her allocation of time—time to read and synthesize the literature, to go to conferences, or learn about new technology. Moreover, if there is a continual erosion of time to spend with patients, quality care will suffer. This has become a sensitive issue. Thus, the physician feels "nickle-and-dimed" by his or her perceptions of the scientifically unsound quality assurance process. Unfortunately, it is ironic that some have used this perception to argue for still greater health care "guidelines" for patient management.

Fourth, with respect to outcome measures, from either the patients' perspective or that of the professionals, there are shortcomings. No programs setting guidelines have systematically presented information on outcomes to *patients* and directly elicited their responses. Few programs explicitly evaluate outcomes (rather than process), and still fewer have validated the program with a "gold standard."

From a more noble perspective, one could argue that a major goal for all in medicine is to provide a better health care system. Because we have so little measure of the value of our current system, it is imperative to pursue studies of its appropriateness. This will require a great commitment of resources but would represent a significant investment for the future.

ORGANIZING FOR QUALITY ASSESSMENT

One might view organization from a national (or macro-) level to the institution (or microlevel). From a national perspective, Levey and Hill (45) have estimated that for 1989 the federal investment for general research and development was $62 billion; only $8 billion was directed to the health field. Only $75 million went to health services research. Whereas some may consider this an astonishingly low figure, it may in fact reflect the way American businesses act in general. For example, many industries spend a great deal of resources on bench science to develop new products. They probably spend little on research to find more cost-effective ways to organize their retail stores delivering the product to the customer. Should we think it is odd that our government operates in the same manner? Levey and Hill point out, however, that current concerns over the high health care

costs have led to the development of the Agency for Health Care Policy and Research, an organization equivalent to such Public Health Service agencies as the National Institutes of Health or Centers for Disease Control. Thus, there is some reason for modest optimism that funding will increase for those who wish to test alternative hypotheses to deliver quality health care. This optimism should be placed in perspective. Surely there must be strong governmental support for all types of research: clinical, biomedical, or population-based. On the other hand, there is no clear proof for the idea—however popularly supported by all interest groups—that increasing money either for the individual or the project correlates with increasing progress. This was articulately stated decades ago by the famous English statistician, Major Greenwood:

It is . . . ridiculous to believe that the offer of a price of a million will cause a better play than "Hamlet" to be written or finer researches than those of Pasteur to be accomplished; it is . . . but elementary common sense to believe that a nation which condemns poets or research chemists to hopeless poverty is unlikely to breed Shakespeares and Pasteurs (46).

At the individual hospital level, the three major paradigms currently espoused for organizing quality assessment activities are the industrial model (47–49), the hospital epidemiology model (26, 36, 50), and the outcomes management model (51). The various proposals undoubtedly reflect the fact that people from diverse disciplines have recognized the issue of quality health care and the problems of quality health care delivery and assessment. The only sensible approach is to encourage experimentation with all new ideas and the measurement of their relative value. One of the key elements of the industrial model is the emphasis on creating a new medical "culture," one that continually works toward quality at all levels of the system. Most authors espouse a positive attitude and positive feedback to employees, decrying the "bad apple" approach (49). It is assumed that system (structure) changes could correct many of the problems associated with an individual's performance.

The epidemiological and outcomes models are part of a continuum that: examines health care delivery; asks why the distributions are what they are; and emphasizes measurement, development of new hypotheses, new tests, and follow-up measurements. Perhaps all of this was succinctly summarized by Otis Bowen in the 1987 Shattuck Lecture. In Bowen's estimation, the pursuit of quality care "constitutes a developing field that often makes use of a new approach called the epidemiology of medical care" (52). Donabedian would agree with the idea. Writing on the contributions of epidemiology to quality assessment and monitoring, Donabedian (53) states that "the result of a marriage between epidemiology and health care administration would be the emergence of a new health professional: one who might be called a clinical-performance epidemiologist."

SUMMARY

In this chapter it is reasoned that the current emphasis on quality health care has been driven by overriding concerns about runaway costs of our health care system. What is really being asked is if the quality is worth the costs. The government's response to the question has been to develop legislation that is designed to reduce the costs. So far, such legislation has been ineffective: the costs continue to escalate. Nevertheless, the effects of the legislation have been to create escalating bureaucracy and highlight the conflicts between patients and physicians, physicians and hospital administrators, and physicians and both accreditation agencies and third party payers. It is fair to say that there has been a drastic shift of power away from the clinicians and toward administrators. This is surely not a simple dissatisfaction with physicians but a much more complex interaction of social forces creating a more uniform process of medical care, the accreditation and credentialing of professionals, and competition among providers. Moreover, the very fabric of the

medical care culture has been exposed, and all of its inequities and imperfections have been identified. Perhaps this latter fact alone explains why the term "quality care" has been used to symbolize recent events.

What is clear is that no civilized society can exist unless *all* of its citizens have appropriate access to health care. So far this situation does not apply to the United States. Access must be followed by reasonable efforts to prevent illness and promote health and by compassionate and competent care when needed. The amount of any country's spending power that is allocated to health versus other areas needs to be a popular decision, and if there are limitations to our national budget, these limitations should not affect basic health care.

The activities of the modern health care provider will be evaluated by measures of knowledge, reasonable options applied, humanitarian skills, and outcome. Whatever the shortcomings of measurement, there will be no turning back: All health care and health care delivery will be measured. We have the potential to have the best health care system in the world; to attain that goal, we will need to find a way to use advanced technology appropriately. Those clinicians of the modern era who believe in quality care, who can adapt to the current environment of accountability, who might therefore be themselves called healthy, will find identity, rewards, and adventure ahead.

References

1. The New York Times: The health cost explosion, evaded [Editorial]. March 29, 1990; p. A12.
2. The Washington Post. Caring for the Poor: Who pays. June 5, 1990; p. A24.
3. The New York Times: The honesty gap on medigap: Closed [Editorial]. November 21, 1990; p. A14.
4. The New York Times: Access for medically uninsured [Editorial]. Dr. Axelrod's potent health plan. September 11, 1989, p. A26.
5. The Wall Street Journal. Blue Cross to help pay for clinical test of controversial breast cancer therapy. October 30, 1990; p. 84.
6. The New York Times: Changes in medicine bring pain to healing profession. February 18, 1990, p. A1.

7. Iglehart JK. Canada's health system faces its problems. N Engl J Med 1990;322:562–568.
8. Aaron H, Schwartz WB. Rationing health care: The choice before us. Science 1990;247:418–422.
9. Schwartz WB, Aaron AJ. Rationing hospital care: Lessons from Britain. N Engl J Med 1984;310:52–56.
10. Sullivan LW. 1989 Statement of the Society of Health and Human Services before the Medicare and Long Term Care Subcommittee on Finance. United States Senate, June 16, 1989; and in Aging America Trends and Protection, 1987–89 edition. US Department of Health and Human Services, Published LR3377(188).D12198.
11. Relman AS. The trouble with rationing. N Engl J Med 1990;323:911–913.
12. Donabedian A. Explorations in quality assessment and monitoring, Vol. I: The definition of quality and approaches to its assessment. Ann Arbor, MI: Health Administration Press, 1980.
13. Donabedian A. Explorations in quality assessment and monitoring, Vol. II: The criteria and standards of quality. Ann Arbor, MI: Health Administration Press, 1982.
14. Relman AS. Assessment and accountability: The third revolution in medical care. N Engl J Med 1988;319:1220–1222.
15. Fuchs VR. The health care sector's share of the gross national product. Science 1990;247:534–538.
16. National Leadership Commission on Health Care: For the health of a nation: A shared responsibility. Ann Arbor, MI: Health Administration Press, 1989.
17. Relman AS. Reforming the health care system. N Engl J Med 1990;323:991–992.
18. Davis K, Anderson GH, Rowland D, Steinberg EP. Health care cost containment. Baltimore: The Johns Hopkins University Press, 1990:34–55, 162–180.
19. Iglehart JK. The New Law on Medicare's payments to physicians. N Engl J Med 1990;322:1247–1252.
20. Campbell A, Kane NM. Physician-management relationships at HCA: A case study. J Health Polit Policy Law 1990;15:591–605.
21. Massanari RM. Risk management: An epidemiologic approach. Infect Control 1987;8:3–6.
22. Roper WL. Perspectives on physician-payment reform. The Resource-Based Relative-Value Scale in context. N Engl J Med 1988;319:865–867.
23. Evans RG. Finding the levers, finding the coverage: lessons from cost containment in North America. J Health Polit Policy Law 1986;11:587–615.
24. Deleted in proof.
25. Hsiao WC, Braun P, Yntema D, Becker ER. Estimating physicians' work for a Resource-Based Relative Value Scale. N Engl J Med 1988;319:835–841.
26. Wenzel RP. The development of academic programs for quality assessment. Arch Intern Med 1991;151:653–654.
27. Callahan D. What kind of life. The limits of medical progress. New York: Simon & Schuster; 1990:74.
28. Donabedian A. Quality assessment and assurance: Utility of purpose, diversity of means. Inquiry 1988;25:173–192.
29. White KL. Physician and professional perspective. In White KL, ed. The task of medicine. Menlo Park, OR: The Henry J. Kaiser Family Foundation, 1988:4–46.
30. Wennberg JE. Outcomes research, cost containment, and the fear of heath care rationing. N Engl J Med 1990;323:1202–1204.
31. Eddy DM. Variations in physician practice: The role of uncertainty. Health Aff (Millwood) 1984; 3:74–89.
32. Donabedian A. Evaluating the quality of medical care. Milbank Memorial Fund Q: Health Soc 44(July, 1966, Part 2):166–203.
33. Kovacs J. Concepts of health and disease. J Med Philos 1989;14:261–267.
34. Clare A. Psychiatry in dissent. London: Tavistock, 1976.
35. Woods S, Edwards S. Philosophy and health. J Adv Nurs 1989;14:661–664.
36. Wenzel RP. Quality assessment: An emerging component of hospital epidemiology. Diagn Microbiol Infect Dis 1990;13:197–204.
37. Schiff RL, Ansell DA, Schlosser JE, Idris AH, Morrison A, Whitman S. Transfer to a public hospital. A prospective study of 467 patients. N Engl J Med 1986;314:552–557.
38. Access to Health Care. American College of Physicians Position Paper. Ann Intern Med 1990; 112:641–661.
39. Greenberger NJ, Davies NE, Maynard EP, Wallerstein RO, Hildreth EA, Jever LH. Universal access to health care in America: A moral and medical imperative. Ann Intern Med 1990;112:637–639.
40. Welch HG. Health care tickets for the uninsured: First class, coach, or standby? N Engl J Med 1989; 321:1261–1264.
41. Horn SD. Validity, reliability, and implications of an index of inpatient severity of illness. Med Care 1981;19:354–362.
42. Greenfield S, Aronow HV, Elashoff RM, Watanabe D. Flaws in mortality data: The hazards of ignoring comorbid disease. JAMA 1988;260:2253–2255.
43. Green J, Wintfeld N, Sharkey P, Passman LJ. The importance of severity of illness in assessing hospital mortality. JAMA 1990;263:241–246.
44. Imperiale T, Siegal A, Crede WB, Ramens EA. Preadmission screening of Medicare patients: The clinical impact of reimbursement disapproval. JAMA 1988;259:3418–3421.
45. Levey S, Hill J. A new era for health services research. Hosp Health Services Admin 1990; 4:493–504.
46. Greenwood M. Medical research science. LVIII 1923;133–135.
47. Laffel G, Blumenthal D. The case for using industrial quality management science in health care organizations. JAMA 1989;262:2869–2873.
48. Batalden PB, Buchanan ED. Industrial models of quality improvement in providing quality care: The challenge to clinicians. Goldfield N, Nash

DB, eds. Philadelphia: American College of Physicians, 1989:133–159.

49. Berwick DM. Continuous improvements as an ideal in health care. N Engl J Med 1989;320: 53–56.

50. Wenzel RP, Pfaller MA. Infection control: The premier quality assessment program in United States hospitals. Am J Med 1991, in press.

51. Ellwood PM. Outcomes management: A technology of patient experience. N Engl J Med 1988; 318:1549–1556.

52. Bowen OR. Shattuck Lecture. What is quality care? N Engl J Med 1987;316:1578–1579.

53. Donabedian A. Contributions of epidemiology to quality assessment and monitoring. Infect Control Hosp Epidemiol 1990;11:117–121.

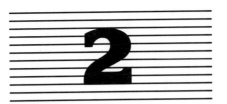

The New Accreditation System

An Overview from the Joint Commission on Accreditation of Healthcare Organizations

James S. Roberts, M.D., Dennis S. O'Leary, M.D., Paul M. Schyve, M.D., and William F. Jessee, M.D.

BACKGROUND

The Decision to Improve

In December 1986, following a searching strategic and programmatic evaluation, the Board of Commissioners determined that it was necessary to improve and refocus all components (standards, surveys, and monitoring mechanisms) of the Joint Commission's accreditation system. From its inception in 1987, this multiyear developmental effort—the Agenda for Change— has been designed to create evolutionary, but substantive, improvement of the accreditation system. Thus, considerable effort has been devoted both to development of a more contemporary conceptual framework for accreditation and to rigorous design and testing of the new approach.

A New Focus: Continual Improvement in Patient Outcomes

The vision that has guided this effort is that Joint Commission accreditation should more directly address and tangibly influence the *results* of the care. The intent is to make the improvement of patient outcomes an important and visible objective of the new accreditation system.

As this vision of an outcomes-oriented accreditation system was being more fully conceptualized, another important and complementary concept surfaced—that the philosophies and methods of continual improvement represented the next appropriate progression in the approaches health care organizations should use to address quality internally. Emanating in the form of the Joint Commission's "Principles of Organization and Management Effectiveness," this new framework is based on two interrelated premises.

The first is that there is an identifiable set of *key functions* in a health care organization that must be performed well if its patients are to receive maximum benefit from the organization's services. Ranging from direct care activities such as patient assessment and use of diagnostic and therapeutic procedures, to support processes such as dispensing of medications and provision of laboratory and imaging services, to managerial and governance responsibilities such as the implementation of quality-monitoring mechanisms and the use of quality-related data in resource allocation decisions, these key functions are understood to have an important impact on patient outcomes.

The related premise is that these key functions are carried out through the performance of a set of *critical governance, managerial, clinical and/or support processes*—processes whose effectiveness can and must be measured and continually improved if patient outcomes are to be maximized.

OVERARCHING OBJECTIVE OF THE NEW ACCREDITATION SYSTEM

Linking the desire to influence positively patient outcomes with the value of widespread adoption of continual improvement form the basis for the following overarching objective for the accreditation system being created through the Agenda for Change:

The new accreditation system must stimulate continual improvement in the outcomes achieved by the patients cared for in accredited health care organizations.

Certain components of this objective merit emphasis. "Continual improvement" means the well-described set of philosophies and methods that have been used for decades in other sectors of our economy and have recently been introduced into health care. "Outcomes" are those physical, psychological, social, functional, and other patient results that are potentially influenced by the governance, management, clinical and support processes of health care organizations. These outcomes will be monitored by the Joint Commission through the indicator monitoring system now under development, by other external agencies and, in a more detailed fashion, by each accredited organization through its own internal quality assessment and improvement system.

Achievement of this objective requires careful and coordinated redesign of each component of the accreditation system. The next section reviews the weaknesses of current approaches and the goals and the design characteristics for each of the three tracks of the Agenda for Change developmental efforts. It should be borne in mind that what is being described is an *accreditation* system, the purposes of which are (a) to determine whether a health care organization evidences a demonstrable level of commitment to providing appropriate care in an effective and efficient fashion in a safe environment, and (b) to stimulate all organizations, irrespective of their current level of performance, to continually improve those processes that affect patient outcomes.

Accomplishment of these purposes requires the application of accepted measures (standards and indicators), accurate and consistent measurement (on-site surveys and indicator monitoring activities), and effective feedback and education (on-site education during surveys, accreditation survey reports, and periodic feedback of comparative indicator data).

The Agenda for Change should lead to a substantially improved accreditation system. However, as with health care itself, the accreditation of health care organizations is an inherently complex endeavor, and evaluation methods are continuing to evolve. Recognizing this, the Joint Commission has made a long-term commitment to use its own internal quality improvement program to enhance continually the effectiveness and value of accreditation.

THE NEW ACCREDITATION SYSTEM: WHAT IS BEING DEVELOPED AND WHY

Refocusing Accreditation Standards

A. Current Weakness of Joint Commission Standards

Historically, Joint Commission hospital standards have been organized into department-specific chapters and have, for each department, described the structures and processes felt to affect the quality of care most. This approach creates fragmentation and considerable duplication in the standards. Further, by prompting professional groups to think only of "their chapter," the standards manual format creates a barrier to the cross-professional coordination that is so central to the quality of care. These design flaws have been magnified as the implications of implementing continual improvement systems become better understood. Effective continual improvement systems require effective cross-departmental and interprofessional coordination and cooperation in measuring and improving key processes.

B.   Developmental Goals and Plans

A substantial reconfiguration and enhancement of the *Accreditation Manual for Hospitals* is now underway. This initiative is to proceed in two major phases. First, the 1992 *Accreditation Manual for Hospitals* (*AMH*) will be revised to:

a.   Reduce some of the duplication that now exists across chapters;
b.   Eliminate major portions of standards that are not surveyed or that are surveyed but are judged to have little influence on patient outcomes;
c.   Remove or modify standards that represent barriers to a hospital's adoption of continual improvement methods.

Efforts will then be undertaken toward revision of the 1994 *AMH* which will:

a.   Be organized into chapters whose headings identify key functions and which describe the processes judged most important to patient outcomes;
b.   Describe the characteristics of a process measurement and improvement system that is focused

on continual enhancement in performance, as demonstrated by improved patient outcomes;
c.   Eliminate both the remaining duplication and standards that are judged not to have an important impact on patient outcomes.

During both of these phases, priority attention is to be given to retention of deemed status; the parallel development of "scoring guidelines" that describe alternative methods to achieve standards compliance; and the education of surveyors and the field to assure a smooth transition with respect to this aspect of the accreditation process.

Survey Process Redesign

A.   Weaknesses in the Current Survey Process

The current survey process is in need of redesign. Its flaws include inconsistency in evaluation methods and results; variation in the extent and value of on-site education; insufficient attention to the unique characteristics of each organization; and inadequate ability to assess the degree to which an innovative approach to standards compliance matches the intent, if not the letter, of the standards.

The root cause of these problems is often perceived to be the surveyors. Yet, it is clear that at least equally important contributing factors are the demands placed on the surveyor by the nature of the survey process itself. The Joint Commission asks its surveyors to assess increasingly general standards consistently using scoring guidelines that may not clearly articulate the intent of the standards and may not provide a sufficient array of possible approaches to meet the standards intent. Further, surveyors are asked to be both good evaluators and helpful educators when, for many surveyors, their backgrounds equip them, not as skilled organizational assessors or expert consultants, but as good doctors, nurses, or managers. Current approaches to initial and ongoing surveyor training are not uniformly effective in developing the desired surveyor talents.

B. Developmental Goals and Plans

Resolution of these issues requires that a triennial (regular) survey provide:

1. Consistent and objective evaluation of the organization's performance of the key functions described in the standards;
2. Education that is relevant to the organization and effective in helping it to measure and continually improve its key functions.

In addition, surveys that follow up on indicator data should provide consistent and objective evaluation of the effectiveness with which the health care organization examines and improves the key functions that relate to its patient outcomes, as well as practical education concerning methods for evaluating and improving the processes relevant to the organization's outcome performance.

These objectives, coupled with the acknowledged flaws in the current survey process, form the basis for potential alternative designs for the future survey process. Appropriate models are to be prepared and initially tested in several settings between 1991 and 1993. Current thinking is that the new survey process should incorporate the following broad parameters:

1. Increased Presurvey Analysis of Hospital-Specific Information

Staff would gather and analyze a wide variety of organization-specific descriptive information and data prior to the survey. Such information and data might include: (*a*) descriptive materials about the organization's mission, structure, service mix, and quality improvement systems; (*b*) historical levels of compliance with

Joint Commission standards; and (*c*) as they become available, organization-specific and comparative indicator data. Certain traditional information, such as medical staff bylaws, might also be included. Consideration may also be given to asking each organization to conduct a self-evaluation of its current level of compliance with key standards. The analyzed presurvey information would be used to tailor the actual on-site evaluation of the organization.

2. More Targeted On-Site Evaluation and Educational Assistance

The on-site survey would be conducted by individuals, likely including some of the current surveyor and central office staff, who have demonstrated skills in organizational assessment. The purpose of the survey would be to gather the information needed to judge compliance with standards and to provide relevant assistance and advice to the organization where compliance is found to be weak. In most if not all cases, the findings from this survey would lead to an accreditation decision. It is possible that, in some organizations, there will be areas where more specific expertise is needed to judge compliance. When this occurs, individuals with in-depth knowledge in the area, perhaps regionally based, could conduct a second on-site visit, with the accreditation decision being based on the results of both evaluations. An alternative to a second visit would be to have experts available by phone to aid the on-site surveyor in working through a problematic or contentious issue.

3. Decision Making, Reporting and Interim Monitoring

The results of the evaluation process would lead to both an accreditation decision and a tailored monitoring mechanism that could range from continued routine submission of indicator data to intense short-term follow-up not unlike that now used for conditionally accredited organizations.

An important objective in this phase is to assure that the report is clear and useful to the organization. At a minimum, this will require enhancements in the current report; more specific information about the nature of the weaknesses found during the survey; and relevant suggestions for improvement. It may also be feasible to have the report delivered by an individual having the expertise to review and clarify the findings of the survey and to provide specific advice on actions needed to improve standards compliance.

At this stage, this is but a conceptual outline. There are potential alternative approaches for each step of the process.

Whatever its final design, the new survey process must be sensitive to maintenance of deemed status; have demonstrable interrater reliability in all of its evaluation and decision-making phases; be as objective as the state-of-the-art allows; provide educational assistance that is relevant and useful to each organization; and be judged by the field to have sufficient value (the balance of cost and quality) to assure continued, widespread support for voluntary participation in the accreditation process.

General though the conceptual framework is, some may be tempted to equate the model described above with that used to accredit educational institutions and residency training programs. Whereas such approaches have much to offer, it is clear that the accreditation of health care organizations has features that contrast sharply with accreditation in other arenas. For example, the burden of an extensive self-assessment mechanism would be difficult for most small health care organizations to undertake. It is also clear that Joint Commission accreditation is conducted under a much more intense spotlight than accreditation of academic institutions or residency training programs. The standards are subject to broad and critical analysis both inside and outside the health care field; the objectivity and rigor of the survey and decision-making processes are the subject of constant scrutiny by consumer groups, legislators, and governmental investigators and agencies at both the state and federal levels; and the confidentiality of organization-specific survey data is steadily being eroded. The unique challenges faced by the Joint Commission must constantly be considered in the design of the new survey process.

Development of an Indicator Monitoring System

A. Weaknesses in the Current Monitoring System

Over the last several years, the Joint Commission has developed and refined its approach to monitoring organizations between full surveys. The current system involves two activities. The first is a structured follow-up of an organization's correction of the major standard's compliance issues that were identified during its full survey. Taking the form of focused on-site visits and written progress reports, this approach has generally been effective in prompting correction of specific weaknesses.

The second mechanism involves the evaluation of specific concerns or complaints about an accredited organization. These surface in the form of letters, media investigations, complaints to governmental agencies, etc. While most of the issues identified are not of great consequence, some are. In these cases, the Joint Commission has found problems that are relevant to its standards—issues that either were not identified during the full survey or that developed subsequent to it.

While useful, these approaches do not provide predictable early warning of new problems that surface during the

3-year period between full surveys. The contemplated indicator monitoring system should largely remedy this deficiency by creating a powerful outcome-oriented data base. Use of this national resource will help accredited organizations to examine the effectiveness of key governance, clinical, managerial, and support processes, most of which will be identified in the Joint Commission standards, and to improve those that are weak. Just as important, for those organizations already performing well, comparative data will provide a useful stimulus to continual improvement.

In addition to requiring properly tested and valid indicators and a feasible data exchange mechanism, this new monitoring system must be supported by standards that relate to the reliable collection and timely submission of indicator data and mechanisms that organizations should use to examine and improve processes that the indicator data signal may be weak.

B.   Developmental Goals and Plans

Representing the newest and most innovative component of the Agenda for Change, the Joint Commission is examining the feasibility and value of creating an outcomes-based monitoring system—a process of data collection and comparative feedback that would help accredited organizations to improve continually the levels of their patients' outcomes. The specific goals of this project are to:

1. Identify and test indicators that are judged to reflect the performance of those governance, management, clinical, and support processes that significantly influence patient outcomes.
2. Examine the feasibility, both for health care organizations and for the Joint Commission, of collecting, submitting, analyzing, comparing, and feeding back data concerning these indicators.

3. Integrate this monitoring system into the other components of the Joint Commission's accreditation system. Data from the system should be helpful in targeting the content of the on-site evaluations. Standards must not only address indicator data collection methods and the reporting of indicator data, but also the mechanisms organizations should use to conduct in-depth assessments of processes related to "outlier" indicator data.
4. Create the capability to support internal and collaborative research that will enhance knowledge of the relationship between key processes and patient outcomes. The results of such research will be used to modify accreditation standards, enhance the survey process, and improve indicators.

To create this new monitoring system, the Joint Commission is using expert panels and a two-phased on-site testing process that have been designed to produce:

1. Indicators that have been shown to raise important quality-of-care questions within health care organizations, i.e., valid indicators.
2. Indicators for which data can be collected in a reliable fashion.
3. Cost-effective mechanisms for data collection, submission, analysis, and feedback.
4. Feedback reports that are useful to accredited organizations.
5. A mechanism through which indicators can be periodically updated.
6. Standards, or some other form of Joint Commission requirement, and a related survey process that permit evaluation of an organization's indicator data handling capability and assessment of the rigor and effectiveness of an organization's follow-up of indicator data.

CONCLUSION

The accreditation system described in this paper is intended to enhance the effectiveness of the Joint Commission in stimulating continual improvements in patient outcomes. Using such a system, the Joint Commission can continue to play a central role in meeting the compelling societal demand for effective and efficient health care services.

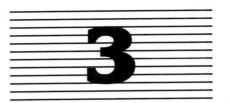

Clinical Quality

The Effective Relationship of Hospital Management and the Medical Staff

Hamilton Moses III, M.D., and Robert M. Heyssel, M.D.

BACKGROUND

Nearly everyone related to the practice of medicine is interested in quality; either hoping and expecting it exists, maintaining that it does not, reassuring the public that it does, or arguing that such discussions are fruitless and unnecessary. Despite so many conflicting opinions, a reasonable consensus has begun to develop about the desirability of using sound epidemiological principles to describe formally and quantitatively the quality of medical care, allowing the evaluation of hospitals, individual practitioners, and other varieties of medical organizations (1). Unfortunately, despite its far greater importance, much less attention has been devoted to decribing the optimum way to improve the quality of medical care and practice. Likewise, an effective theoretical or organizational framework that allows the emerging quantitative information to be truly useful in improving quality has yet to be developed. Because of this, nearly everyone—doctors, nurses, hospital directors, trustees, regulators, and insurers—is in a quandry about the large and growing field of quality measurement of medical practice.

Medical practice lacks a uniform definition of quality (2, 3). Ideally, the definition would be general and broad yet specific enough to be truly useful, simply applied, and uniformly accepted without controversy. Such a definition is not at hand. The Supreme Court struggled with just such difficulty when attempting to define pornography, giving rise to the late Justice Potter Stewart's definition (to paraphrase): "I can't define pornography, but I know it when I see it." Similarly, those who argue over good art versus bad art maintain that the difference between the two is readily apparent, at least to the trained and discerning eye. Whereas certain arcane statistical techniques can be applied to such subjective observations, they are not easily adapted to the evaluation of medical practice, using chart review, case abstraction, or other bureaucratic ways of collecting data. Such a "know it when I see it" definition of quality does, however, have the advantage of being widely believed and easily understood by almost everyone, particularly within academic medical centers where "higher quality" is a shibboleth that is nearly universally believed.

Even if quality is not defined, the constituents that comprise it can be articulated. As Eddy has written:

The quality of medical care is determined by two main factors: the quality of the decisions that determine what actions are taken and the quality with which those actions are executed— what to do and how to do it. If the wrong actions are chosen, no matter how skillfully they are executed, the quality of care will suffer. Similarly, if the correct actions are chosen but the execution is flawed, the quality of care will suffer. (4)

This distinction between making the decision to act and the execution of the action is critical of our thinking about the quality of medical practice, and it is increasingly being articulated by numerous researchers in the field. Furthermore, it also suggests an organizational structure that can support the improvement of quality within large hospitals and other complex medical organizations.

For the past decade, we at The Johns Hopkins Hospital have dealt with all of these conflicts, issues, and opportunities, building upon a conviction that optimum care will be best provided by individuals in an organization that has a commitment and strives to provide and teach exemplary care, while always trying to improve. Fortunately, most doctors, nurses, and hospitals share this commitment. Furthermore, we generally believe—and correctly so— that the traditional mechanisms (however informal) of peer pressure, hallway conversation, and across-the-operating-table criticism remain remarkably effective in both discovering where improvement is desirable and accomplishing it. However, there is also a growing belief that we cannot solely rely on such informal mechanisms as medical practice becomes more complex and continues to change rapidly. With the advent of shortened lengths of stay, home care, same day and outpatient surgery, and the myriad other changes that are certain to be on the horizon, a more formal and reliable system must be developed (5).

In this chapter we will explore the changes that are evolving at Johns Hopkins. Though these are emerging in an academic medical center, the issues, judgments, preferences, and conflicts are inherent to any group of practitioners as well as to all hospitals and other medical organizations, both large and small.

HISTORICAL PERSPECTIVE

Concerns about the quality of medical practice have been a part of the American scene for well over a century. Osler, Weir Mitchell, Herrick, and many other academic physicians wrote and preached about the importance of improving the quality of one's personal medical practice in the late 19th century and in the pre-Flexnerian era. Flexner and those who incorporated his views into what became the modern American medical school and academic hospital did so largely because of concerns about quality, both of the quality of physicians and their education, as well as their practice. In the modern era, however, questions of quality, cost, access, and perception have become muddled as a large, bureaucratic, formal, and largely ineffective "quality assurance" structure has evolved.

In the decades before the cost of medicine became an issue, attempts at improving quality were aimed at quality per se, without consideration of cost. The situation began rapidly to change with the advent of Medicare in the 1960s. Over the ensuing 30 years, issues of quality and cost have become hopelessly confused, in part by design, so that now even the bureaucracies are interchangeable. In most hospitals, quality assurance, utilization review (now called utilization management), and risk management are usually combined to some degree under one organizational umbrella. Within government, the Health Care Finance Administration has had responsibility both for reimbursement and for overseeing quality of care, although recent legislative changes that recognize the inherent conflicts have begun to remedy this to some degree. The blur between cost and quality has led to confusion, suspicion, and great imprecision about just what is meant by "quality." As Donabedian has written:

If costs were no object, health care practitioners would be obligated simply to provide maximally effective care—that is, the kind of care that could be expected to bring about the greatest improvement in health that science and technology are able to offer. True, they would also be obligated to treat their patients with tact and understanding and to provide care under circumstances that are congenial and convenient . . . "quality" and "effectiveness" would become almost synonyms. (6)

In addition to this confusion over the quality and cost, regulatory forces have also entered the fray, particularly in the late 1980s. Led by a variety of state agencies, most notably in New York State and Massachusetts, as well as by the Joint Commission on Accreditation of Health Care Organizations, the Health Care Financing Administration, and a variety of state Medicaid programs, quality has become a watchword. Regulators have entered this arena both because of a genuine concern over quality (given added impetus by a number of unfortunate incidents exploited by the press) and in part by a need to decrease financial costs. Also, because of their ready access to claims data bases, large insurers and the federal government can readily make simple calculations of mortality, readmission rates, and adverse outcomes allowing direct comparison of hospitals and, potentially, of practitioners (7). The Medicare administration's yearly list of hospital mortality rates is the best example to date of the use of such general clinical information. The understandable fear that initially met the Medicare mortality data and Medicare's progressive understanding of the inherent limitations of such information have been instructive, for Medicare's comparison is one of the first examples that shows the importance of obtaining reliable information and also of recognizing the pitfalls of how it is applied. Furthermore, since mortality in the first 6 months after discharge is paired to hospitalization, the Medicare mortality figures represent the most ambitious attempt to date at describing the *outcome* of medical care rather than the *process*. This distinction between outcome and process represents a major change of the late 1980s (8).

The Joint Commission on Accreditation of Health Care Organizations began, in 1987, to embark on an "Agenda for Change." Since the beginning of the Joint Commission's days, it focused primarily on the organization of the hospital, the staff committee structure, and the operation of the quality assurance process. As the Joint Commission has broadened its focus, and as both patients' and payers' influences have become stronger, the Joint Commission has begun to shift attention to measures of outcome. A series of demonstration projects has ensued in a number of areas including obstetrics, anesthesia, cardiovascular disease, trauma, and cancer, though none has yet been broadly applied within the Joint Commission accreditation surveys. The project has been hindered by the slow evolution of quantitative measures, and the Commission's realization that their development is much more difficult than had been anticipated. Both Medicare and the Joint Commission's experience and the lessons learned illustrate the potential pitfalls in this arena, particularly the importance of having correct, truly valuable clinical information, applied in ways that are easily understood and developed by wide consensus.

In response to Medicare's efforts and those of the Joint Commisssion, a number of other groups have begun projects involving the quality of care. These include efforts by the Maryland Hospital Association, the Inter Mountain Hospital Group, and a variety of academic consortia who share a willingness to combine information and to pool resources to develop more meaningful quantitative descriptors of quality. The success or failure of these efforts will remain undetermined for some time. Even if successful, the means by which such quantitative, normative information is applied at the individual's bedside remains to be discerned.

At this juncture and as the field evolves, it will be extremely important to separate the different—and often conflicting—aims of regulators, cost containers, and managers from the wishes and needs of patients, so that the physicians, nurses, and other practitioners can best serve their patients' needs.

HOSPITAL MANAGEMENT'S PERSPECTIVE

Within the hospital, physicians, nurses, and a variety of technicians and technologists have primary responsibility for the minute-to-minute conduct of clinical care, as well as for its day-to-day quality. However, the hospital's trustees and the hospital's management also have responsibility for the overall quality of care provided within the hospital. Similarly, within HMOs, other managed care organizations, and some large group practices, practitioners both provide care and monitor quality while the boards, owners, and managers share responsibility (in a corporate sense) for its quality. The perspectives of the practitioner, the manager, and the trustees, while distinct, are for the most part parallel and congruent. Nevertheless, both the clinician and the manager often suspect that they are in conflict, for the potential of conflict is very real; particularly when finances enter the arena of quality, the likelihood for conflict becomes more probable. Maintaining the congruence of interest between clinician and management and minimizing the opportunity for conflict are the most important functions of the quality assurance mechanism within the hospital.

Managing a hospital is a very complex task. As Drucker (9) repeatedly has written, hospitals are among the most complex organizations, where a large number of technical and nontechnical employees share a need to be tightly coordinated to provide optimal care of patients. Just as physicians and nurses have become highly specialized, so, too, have a panoply of technicians and technologists, many of whom belong to professional societies or organizations that have an interest in both furthering their own specialty and setting standards for those who wish to practice it. As these medical, nursing, and other professional groups have become further "professionalized," the potential for conflict among them has also grown. Furthermore, as the domains of the various medical, nursing, and technical groups have grown, areas of their respective responsi-

bilites have become better defined and more narrowly limited. In most hospitals this has had the unintended consequence of greatly complicating the relationships between groups, which, in turn, requires the hospital's management to be certain that communications, coordination, and planning for care all occur in a more rigid and formal way so that the care of patients can be optimally provided. Another unintended and unfortunate consequence of growth of specialization and the narrowing of focus is that many groups believe that their franchise extends only so far in a given domain, leaving unsaid and unstated just who is to have responsibility for the remainder. All groups—physicians, nurses, and technicians—share responsibility for this unfortunate development, not withstanding the fact that the quality of care within a narrow area may well have improved among the specialties. The hospital's management must recognize these forces.

Regulatory Pressures

Regulatory pressures also fall primarily on hospital management. In nearly every state over the past decade, hospitals have become a highly regulated group. Even in those states where regulation has been less onerous, the federal government introduced throughout the 1980s a myriad of regulations and new laws that affect hospitals and medicine more generally. While the initial focus was primarily on finance and cost, more recent regulations have focused on employee safety, the work environment, the physical plant, capacity, as well as patient safety and quality. Hospitals have not traditionally been thought of as heavily regulated bodies as have, say, banks or the airlines, though now they have become so. At the same time, the growth of regulation of individual practitioners has added to the burden of hospital management, for hospitals have usually been chosen to be the vehicle for regulations to be applied. For instance, in California, Illinois, Maryland, Massachusetts, and New York, the regulations aimed at individual physicians and nurses have been enforced via hospitals, and hospital managers are expected to play a major role in both educating their staffs and monitoring their compliance. This effort has been aided by the Joint Commission under the rubric of "self-policing." These regulatory forces place the hospital's management in a position of potential conflict with members of the professional staff. In some states, because of pressure by hospitals, efforts have begun to shift responsibility for monitoring and oversight to state health departments, licensing bureaus, or other agencies of the state government where monitoring and enforcement are more properly located, rather than have hospitals be the primary vehicle. Whether these efforts will be successful is very much an open question.

Fiscal Responsibility

Fiscal responsibility does properly fall primarily to hospital's management. In the domain of finance, distinguishing between quality and cost is a crucial issue and one that also may give rise to conflict. As the era of prospective hospital payment has evolved since 1983, hospital managers keenly feel the need to provide both ongoing yearly operational revenue, as well as to provide funds for investment in new capital equipment and the development of new clinical programs. As we enter the 1990s, nearly all hospitals, both not-for-profit and proprietary, are feeling and will continue to feel pressure on both operating revenues and those for investment.

To date, Medicare, the states, and large insurance companies have all asserted and assumed that cost and quality are not synonymous, that high cost does not mean high quality, and that costs can be cut and monies saved without hindering, and may even improve, the quality of medical practice or outcome. This has been a comforting assumption that has been convenient to assert. It is also a notion that needs testing. The view that we can cut the fat without sacrificing the lean will be sorely tested over the coming decade.

In this arena, the hospital and its management has again been caught in potential conflict with its medical staff. Since the advent of prospective payment by Medi-

care in 1983, the hospital has had a strong incentive to decrease utilization, decrease length of stay, and decrease the number of procedures performed on hospital inpatients. On the other hand, the traditional financial incentives for physicians have remained unchanged—providing financial inducements to increase utilization and the number of procedures performed, with little incentive to decrease length of stay. It is surprising that this conflict between the incentives for hospitals and physicians has not grown more strident over the past few years. It is also likely that the changes contemplated by Medicare for physician reimbursement may diminish the conflict to some degree. Also, with respect to quality, financial forces (particularly the growth of HMOs and managed care) are likely to develop that again place hospitals and physicians in more directly parallel positions.

Hospital Boards and Trustees

Hospital boards and trustees also have an interest in quality (10). Because of recent legal events arising from a number of malpractice cases, the role and responsibilities of trustees in assuring quality within the hospital are often keenly felt. This important change represents a relatively new development and one that is further complicated by the numerous changes in regulations that have previously been described. Traditionally, money and building were left to the board, operations to management, and clinical practice to doctors and nurses. Since the 1980s, however, trustees have shared general responsibility for the quality of care conducted within the hospital, but at least for the nonphysician trustees they have not had the medical knowledge to make accurate judgments or take appropriate action. Even if knowledge were available, it would be both inappropriate and undesirable for the board to be very active. Nevertheless, because trustees, management, and clinicians all share differing responsibilities for quality, it has become extremely important to delineate carefully the respective domains of each group. In some hospitals these distinctions have been formal and rigid, whereas in others they remain fluid and indistinct.

Nevertheless, the trustee is often uncomfortable being told that he or she has responsibility for quality, without knowing whether care is optimal and without knowing whether mechanisms are in place to be certain that quality improves. Because of this dilemma, many trustees, hospital associations, and the Joint Commission itself have pushed for the development of quantitative means of expressing quality and outcome, which ultimately could be used in a manner analogous to routine financial information to judge quality of practice. As the argument goes, just as we have succinct standard balance sheets showing assets and liabilities or statements of income and expense, why can there not be reports of medical outcome showing mortality, readmission rates or other quantitative markers of quality? This analogy to financial information has grown very attractive to numerous regulatory groups, not just trustees, and will likely evolve over the coming few years. Unfortunately, as viewed from the clinician's perspective, such information has mostly focused on the negative—adverse outcome such as mortality—making such information punitive and inherently unpopular. Therefore, the need to develop positive indicators of desired quality becomes clearer and more imperative. Efforts to define these indicators are underway in a number of centers and hospitals.

The trustees' interest in quality is currently served by overseeing a variety of hospital and medical staff committees that report to the board, either directly or indirectly, about aspects of care within the hospital. In some hospitals, particularly in those states where regulation has been more burdensome, trustees, management, physicians, nurses, and other professionals meet together, often weekly, in order to review cases and take appropriate action. In some cases, such quality oversight committees are actually chaired by trustees or by senior management rather than by doctors or nurses. Whether such an organization, which is not the norm, is more successful than traditional peer review remains very much an open question.

Several areas of responsibility for quality fall specifically on hospital management:

Interdepartmental Issues

Many clinical problems can be solved only by concerted efforts on a number of fronts within separate departments or divisions. The hospital's management must assure that cases, issues, and conflicts among departments are worked through in a way to keep the patients' needs paramount. Situations arise in the everyday conduct of clinical care within a hospital that require well-coordinated efforts in numerous departments. Perhaps the best example is in the conduct of the emergency service in trauma. Here, the emergency room staff, surgeons, radiologists, internists or pediatricians, respiratory therapists, blood gas technicians, and other professionals must be tightly coordinated in order to provide minute-to-minute care to gravely ill individuals. Coordinating that care requires constant interdepartmental review, adjustment of protocols and procedures, and above all else, careful communication of individuals responsible for various facets of care. Insuring such communication falls directly to the hospital's management and the coordinator of the emergency trauma team. In many hospitals the evolution of the trauma team became the prototype for the development of communication and conduct of care within other groups such as between cardiology and cardiac surgery, neurology and neurosurgery, vascular surgery and interventional radiology, and so on. These opportunities will undoubtedly become more numerous as technology evolves and as practitioners become more dependent on one another for specific aspects of care. The hospital management's role is particularly important where, because of close collegial relationships and interdependence of these practitioners, areas of conflict are apt not to be resolved because of an understandable wish to avoid conflict and confrontation. It is hospital management's job to overcome such impediments in a constructive way.

Impaired Practitioner

Another area that resides within the domain of hospital's management is that of the impaired practitioner. Although there is self-policing by physicians and nurses, impairment is frequently first brought to the attention of a manager or the hopital's administrator—often anonymously—as the result of aberrant behavior or faulty judgment within a clinical arena or sometimes because of behavior elsewhere within the community outside of the medical setting. The latter incidence is often first known to trustees, who may either observe or hear from others of the physician's or nurse's conduct within the community. These awkward situations may have a clear bearing on quality of care and fall within hospital managers' purview. Because these situations are delicate and threatening, the skill with which the manager deals with these issues is paramount. Such situations highlight the apparent conflict between manager and practitioner and, depending on how deftly handled, may hinder or help the overall efforts to improve quality within an organization.

CLINICIAN'S PERSPECTIVE

Many practicing physicians and nurses view formal efforts to improve quality as colossal distractions. Some even believe that these efforts are dangerous; they assert that, by substituting a formal bureaucratic organization for a series of time-honored informal mechanisms that improve quality, quality will decline (11). This invocation of the law of unintended consequences is widely believed and has much merit. Within the traditional physician's practice, particularly when based in a hospital, and when the perspective is for a single hospitalization or other episode of illness, traditional informal mechanisms usually suffice. But in the emerging era, these informal mechanisms will almost certainly be inadequate.

The single greatest barrier to the development of more sophisticated means to improve quality is the view that changes are unnecessary. Medicine, nursing, and many other disciplines have time-honored traditions of furthering quality. Moreover, most practitioners have a strong dedication to improve quality; they remain vigilant, willing, and eager to improve, and therefore they resent any heavy-handed or bureaucratic admonition to do so by a hospital manager, a state regulator, or a federal agency. They assert, "I try every day to do better, so you need not tell me how to do so." This view is not easy to address, and the resentment is not easy to overcome.

The thoughtful clinician will raise a number of other objections to changes in the quality arena that have a similar origin and that are also highly pertinent. These include the following:

Lack of Useful Information and Inclusion of Data of Poor Quality

Over the past decades, hospitals have tabulated much numerical information about such things as patterns of blood utilization, numbers of drug reactions, length of stay, readmission or mortality rates, etc., which are often called *clinical indicators*. Such data have nearly universally been poorly received and largely disregarded. With few exceptions, such clinical indicators are not felt to be truly useful or applicable to improving the actual quality of medical practice. In many instances, such indicators were developed by administrators, quality assurance staff, or others with a minimum of direction or leadership by physicians. In others, particularly in those states where regulation has been most burdensome, indicators have actually been specified by the legislature or various regulatory groups. Clinicians quarrel with the quality of information because, after even cursory review, much of the clinical information is found to be faulty. Either the chart was incorrectly reviewed, the conclusions drawn were erroneous, or other inaccuracies of information were uncovered. In general, the quality of such information has been poor and without rigorously validated case abstraction, coding, and analysis. (Coding of clinical information for billing purposes has been more successful because it has received more attention, however.) The antidote to this shortcoming is the use of sound epidemiologic methods, using highly trained staff, with rigorous testing of reliability and validation in order to provide data of maximum quality that can truly be useful in improving quality of care.

Arbitrary Action by Hospitals or Regulators

Information is power. Clinicians fear that information available in a computerized database or elsewhere will be misused. This fear is not at all groundless, and numerous examples of misuse of information can be cited in nearly every large and small hospital. Unfortunately, it is now a fact of life that much clinical information is available in a great number of places, such as in insurance companies' records or in various discharge abstracts provided (by law) to the federal government under Medicare or to many state regulators as part of rate-review process. Such information can be manipulated to draw conclusions, correctly or incorrectly, about quality. The Medicare mortality information, which was previously cited, is a case in point. Clinicians fear that adding to this data within the hospital will simply complicate their lives. Understandably, they resist doing so. Overcoming this objection requires an understanding that the hospitals' and clinicians' aim should be to improve the quality of information, not to resist efforts to obtain it. Both the hospital and physician should strive to be certain that the data are accurate and draw only those conclusions that are justified by the information available. Inaccurate data should be weeded out and the proper precautions taken to be certain that faulty data are not misused. This requires constant vigilance and a close working relationship between hospital and clinicians.

But even correct, reliable, and accurate information about clinical quality can be misused. Whereas this is true of all information, information on quality itself is particularly threatening. Because most clinicians feel that quality is in their domain while finance is in the hospital's, the need for information on quality outside of a practice or department is poorly understood. More specifically, most physicians fear that action of one kind or another will be taken that will hurt their practice or limit their freedom in some way. This argument often takes a slightly different focus:

Misuse of Information on Quality to Make Financial Decisions

The fear is that financial decisions disguised as decisions made on the basis of quality will be based on information that the clinicians themselves have provided. Trust and clear ground rules are the only antidote to this problem.

Arbitrary Regulatory Efforts Furthered by Providing Information on Quality

Clinicians understandably feel and fear a loss of control. Providing information and developing a sophisticated quality assurance process that is designed by and run by clinicians is the best foil to arbitrary regulatory efforts. To date, state and federal regulators have sought information not about individual practitioners or individual conditions but rather about individual hospitals, departments, or groups: have they taken the steps necessary to improve quality and to ascertain whether serious or systematic errors of one kind or another are being made? They wish to see that *the process* of improving quality is underway, not so much the content of those efforts.

Loss of Confidentiality

Physicians also fear the loss of privacy. To have others oversee their work, either directly or indirectly, is a tacit threat. Just as most physicians have a strong inbred imperative to improve, likewise they have a wish to practice without undue scrutiny. A tradition of scrutiny is not inherent in medical practice, at least after internship and residency have been completed. The formal mechanisms to review quality are an understandable threat.

All of these concerns are legitimate. However, they are fostered in an atmosphere where a we/they mentality has developed between various forces—between the physician or nurse, between the practitioner and hospital, between the hospital and regulatory body—all of which often operate singly or in combination.

NEED FOR A NEW PERSPECTIVE

Can clinicians and hospitals continue to rely on the traditional informal mechanisms for maintaining quality? Almost certainly, traditional mechanisms will be inadequate as the health care arena continues to change.

The inadequacies stem from several sources:

As Practice Changes, a Perspective Broader than One Episode of Illness or Hospitalization Is Required. The care of a single patient now nearly always occurs in several settings including the traditional office, a variety of laboratories for imaging, blood work, and special studies, in outpatient surgery, within a hospital bed, via care at home, and with numerous consultants and other personnel involved. The mechanism to monitor quality and improve outcome must recognize that a single physician or other individual can rarely oversee all of these components of care unless more specific information that is clinically useful becomes available.

Because Many Organizations Are Involved in an Individual Patient's Care, a Unifying Means to Observe and Improve the Quality of Care Is Required. The organizational complexity requires new ways of overseeing all aspects of a patient's care. Since a single physician is rarely directly responsible for care everywhere it is provided, new ways of observing and monitoring quality are desirable. If properly mounted, such efforts can be extremely reassuring to both physicians and patients. Also, since many individuals and organizations are involved in aspects of care, it is of utmost importance to be certain that discussions occur among the groups when problems are encountered. Such discussions can rarely be undertaken in the absence of a formal mechanism for doing so, using highly specific, clinically usable information as everyday material for the organization of the discussions.

The Focus on Outcome Rather Than Process Requires a Change in Orientation. Outcome can be assessed only after care has been provided. We can express the outcome of a procedure or the outcome of the care of an illness after the fact, at one week, one month, six months, or later. Doing so requires a mechanism to relate the status of an individual at a later time to events that occurred when the procedure was conducted or the care provided. Such links must be highly specific in order for information to be truly usable in future patients to improve the process and improve the success of a given intervention. Thinking of this kind has long been part of the methods used to construct formal clinical trials, but only recently has it been adapted to day-to-day efforts of quality improvement. As with clinical trials, much development is needed to ensure that the attributes (both positive and negative) that contribute to favorable outcome be properly assessed and built into the mechanisms of information gathering.

The Patient's Judgment Is Important to Gauge (12). Patients' perceptions are often neglected. A focus primarily on the process of care and even including clinical outcomes is not sufficient because these ignore the patient's view of whether he or she is truly better, worse, or unchanged. Because our time for observation is often short, the perspective is limited and the patient's view can be easily neglected. By focusing on outcome with a longer perspective using later observations, it becomes more difficult to ignore a patient's perceptions and forces us to include this important measure of how well we are doing.

Systematic Errors in Care Are Rarely Addressed Unless a Longer Perspective Is Taken. Again, clinical trials have highlighted the importance of using systematic observations to ensure that apparent short-term gains are not eclipsed by longer term detrimental effects. Forcing the discipline of systematic observation after an interval of days, weeks, or months is the best safeguard against this error.

Without Formal Quantitative Ways of Expressing the Quality of Care and Outcome, We Lack a Way to Demonstrate Favorable Outcome. Traditionally informal mechanisms of quality assessment concentrate on the negative. The development of new mechanisms driven by epidemiological principles allows us to focus on the positive. Rates of favorable outcome provide quantitative measurements of success while providing the raw material to improve and diminish the likelihood of unfavorable outcomes in the future. Eventually this may prove to be the most positive incentive for a major overhaul of traditional mechanisms of quality assurance and quality assessment and provide the impetus for quality improvement. But perhaps the inability to quantitate acceptable measures of quality of care may stem in part from the absence of a discipline to define the desirable outcomes of tests or therapy, as seen by both patient and physician. In most encounters, neither the patient nor the physician clearly defines and articulates the desired outcome. The inability to do so stems in most instances from an inherent uncertainty as to the nature and depth of the problem, but it also may stem from the lack of specific goals set by patient and physician.

Managed Care Is on the Rise. Unlike traditional fee-for-service medicine, managed care is closely monitored from the financial standpoint. Utilization rates, expense per physicians, and expense per episode of care are all closely watched. Clinical measurements are much less further developed, though several large managed care organizations and employers have begun to examine closely both quality and outcome. Even before clinicians and hospitals have developed sophisticated clinical information systems, managed care organizations, unions, and employers have done so. Doctors and hospitals are quite far behind. Not only must we catch up, but we must be certain that our data are of superior quality. Since we are closer to the patient, it should not be difficult for us to be more precise and accurate, providing more truly useful information. Furthermore, almost certainly such important specific and worthwhile information will be highly desirable to have as hospitals and doctors negotiate with managed care organizations. Highly accurate and specific data that are clinically useful will be an important part of all negotiations, and those groups that have such information early on will have a decided competitive advantage. In fact, it is not an overstatement to assert that the development of accurate and useful clinical information on quality and outcome will be critical to compete successfully for patients, reimbursement, and managed care contracts.

Use of Sophisticated Information Systems is Increasing. Automated systems have long been a part of the medical financial arena. In the clinical arena, they have been much later arriving. Although automated clinical abstracts, reporting of laboratory results, registration, and indexing of patients exist, at present, the use of automated charts and clinical records is in its infancy. That situation will not be true for long, however. Automated clinical systems are rapidly developing using voice recognition, optical storage, and other technical advances. Soon, the ability to abstract such charts in an automated fashion will be available; this in turn will allow clinical information to be scored, coded, and otherwise manipulated in ways that may or may not be clinically valid. The anticipation of this eventuality is another important reason why mechanisms need to be developed for the sophisticated analysis of clinical information so that quality and outcome can be accurately expressed.

EMERGING PROGRAMS AT THE JOHNS HOPKINS

Our thinking about clinical quality at Hopkins has moved through several stages over the past decade and a half. In the late 1970s, we, like most hospitals, had a traditional quality assurance mechanism that confused the goals and aims of insurance carriers with the true maintenance and improvement of clinical quality. Predictably, that approach resulted in skepticism of the system and ongoing frustration among members of the medical, nursing, and other clinical staff. Beginning in the early 1980s, the limitations of this approach became evident to the hospital's management, and changes were made to emphasize the distinctive needs to improve clinical quality. By the mid-1980s, further changes were made due to the more restrictive regulatory environment. Once again, frustration over the heavy-handedness of the regulatory approach became evident, and by the late 1980s, focusing on ways to improve clinical quality again became of paramount importance. Thus, over the past 15 years we have seen two cycles in which the emphasis alternated between the external environment (insurance companies and regulators) and internal needs (for improving quality). These cycles have been instructive because they emphasize the distinctly different agendas and needs of outside and inside groups.

Recently there has been a gradual clarification of the specific needs of three similar, overlapping, though distinct, arenas: insurance liaison, risk management, and quality assurance. All three of these areas depend upon highly specific clinical information that is up-to-date and that can readily be expressed and interpreted to those who require it. In order to meet those needs, in the mid-1980s Hopkins established a computerized clinical data base that used commercially available software to allow the uniform collection and abstraction of clinical information. Quality assurance nurse-coordinators now collect clinical information in a standard format, which is then made available via the software to the central quality assurance staff, the quality assurance committees in each department, and the hospital's risk management and legal staff. Several layers of security procedures are built into the system to guard against unauthorized access, and additional precautions are taken to disguise the names, patient numbers, and other identifiers when the information is used in the hospital. The software provides a great deal of flexibility to sort different kinds of cases, develop specific customized reports in a variety of formats, and likewise can be used to track many other activities, such as the use of specific medications or blood products or to moni-

tor adverse reactions. More importantly, highly specific targeted reviews are facilitated by this flexible system, so that specific clinical data can be quickly made available. Clinical research has also been aided by the system, for the need for much chart abstracting has been obviated by the specificity of the information contained in the data base and the use of the sort-merge features that the system allows. This ability to help clinical research has made it particularly attractive to the medical and nursing staff, who readily embraced the system after appreciating its role in research.

Insurance Liaison

Insurance companies, third party administrators, and claims review organizations now require highly specific and detailed clinical information before paying a claim. At times this occurs before hospitalization, but it now extends to many occasions both during and after a hospitalization. For instance, a company's nurse-reviewer may call one, two, or five or six times during a hopitalization to ask for specific information about medications, intravenous rates, ventilator settings, and so forth, in order to grant authorization for continuing stay. We rely on the insurance liaison staff within the quality assurance organization to provide this information in a uniform way. This allows an economy of effort, because one nurse can often answer many questions about many patients. We have chosen to provide this service centrally within the hospital for inpatients and outpatients rather than have individual physicians provide the information themselves or through their offices; likewise we have chosen not to have the floor nursing staff involved in this burdensome activity.

Risk Management

Risk management is a major feature in every hospital. While risk management is distinct from quality assurance, its needs are nearly exactly parallel to those that serve quality. We believe that the best way to minimize risk is to practice medicine as well as possible. Therefore, risk management and quality assurance are exactly parallel. Efforts to support one will aid the other. However, since we are not perfect, and since both preventable and nonpreventable misadventures do occur, the hospital must have a mechanism to protect itself and its staff. These are the discrete activities of risk management per se. Risk management also requires highly specific clinical information, both for minimizing risk as well as for supporting legal and administrative proceedings that may follow an untoward event. The clinical information data base provides much of the raw material for the risk management apparatus serving that need very effectively. It allows immediate identification of events to facilitate prompt and timely investigation. Perhaps the most important role of risk management occurs via its link to quality assurance: untoward events serve as markers of areas to be examined, which at Hopkins we choose to do in a highly individual, decentralized fashion within each department.

The Johns Hopkins Hospital is a highly decentralized organization (13). The hospital is divided into eight clinical departments, four ancillary clinical units, and 12 central support groups. Each of the clinical and ancillary departments has control over its personnel, budget, and all aspects of day-to-day operations. Each of the clinical departments is headed by a physician who works closely with a director of nursing and an administrator. This trio is responsible for quality of care within its domain, as well as for its financial operations.

Quality Assurance

Quality assurance is likewise conducted in a decentralized fashion. Each department has a quality assurance committee with representative physicians (both attending and housestaff), nurses, social workers, the administrator, and others who have special responsibilities within each unit. The week-to-week and month-to-month review of cases, practices, and other areas occurs via the quality assurance committee within each department. The central coordination of the quality assurance mechanism falls to several com-

mittees of the medical staff, which in turn are coordinated by the chairman of the hospital's medical board and the vice president for medical affairs. Our philosophy of decentralized quality assurance is consistent with the overall organization of the hospital. In keeping with our philosophy, each department is responsible for the quality of care within it.

The Hopkins decentralized structure has the advantage of tailoring the approach within each department to the particular clinical field. Our experience suggests that the review of cases, exploration of problems, and other such reviews can be done only by a specialist within a field, and we encourage such highly specific reviews. However, the finely tailored decentralized structure also may inhibit the review of cases among departments. Medical staff committees and hospital's management see that cases are reviewed when more than one department is concerned. Such two-, three-, or five- or six-way discussions, apropos specific issues, are among the most important reviews that can take place. We have chosen to conduct such interdepartmental activities on a centralized basis via both the risk management and quality assurance mechanisms.

The Hopkins approach of decentralized quality assurance with centralized control of risk management and interdepartmental review has served us well for the past decade. However, its limitations are now becoming apparent. We have begun to rethink our approach and to modify the quality assurance mechanism using new methods of hospital epidemiology and outcomes assessment in a new program of *clinical measurement*.

One limitation of our traditional system stems from emphasis on the negative. Over the past years, Hopkins has used a series of *clinical indicators*. As previously discussed, these markers of mortality, readmission, etc. all highlight adverse events. As such, they are inherently negative. They pinpoint areas that *may* indicate a focus of concern. The idicator itself, marking an untoward event, cannot answer whether the event was expected, unexpected, preventable, or not preventable. Such analysis usually requires more information and judgment. Therefore, this approach is extremely cumbersome because much raw information must be analyzed and distilled for it to become useful. The ratio of usable information to total information is undesirably low. For this reason, we have attempted to limit the number of clinical indicators obtained, analyze them more thoroughly, and gradually revise the process to distill to absolute minimum the number of indicators that remain useful to the process. Also, because of the cumbersome nature of this technique, it is unlikely that such indicators will be useful when applied more broadly or indiscriminately, without such analysis. This may prove to be a limitation of the Joint Commission's Agenda for Change and other similar approaches, which provide normative data by which hospitals can be compared.

As Hopkins develops new means of clinical measurement, it has become apparent that clinical quality has several components. We have focused on three: quality of service, perception of quality, and quality of care. Each of these areas is distinct. *Quality of service* refers to general attributes such as timeliness of an appointment, attitude of secretaries, clerks, and staff, cleanliness, ease of parking, and other aspects of the nature of the patient's encounter with the physician, hospital, or clinic. Many of these have been called the "hotel" functions of the organization. *Perception of quality* concerns the patient's (and referring physician's) evaluation of the care provided. Perception, per se, is the focus. This can be measured by a variety of means including questionnaires, telephone surveys, and other means of inquiry. The patient's perception and referring physician's perception may or may not be guided by true knowledge of the actual quality of care provided, but clearly is influenced by perception of the interaction. *Quality of care* refers to the objective assessment of the medical, nursing, and other clinical actions that the patient undergoes. Assessment of clinical quality can occur both via analysis of individual patients and by groups of them. Furthermore, analysis of the quality of care can be divided into other components, such as quality of diagnostic decisions, quality of the conduct of a procedure, response to therapy, and outcome. Each component of quality can be analyzed using separate methods. Of these components, assessment of outcome has received a great deal of attention and is growing in importance as the methods of outcome assessment become more refined. Also, assessment of outcomes and expression of rates of favorable and unfavorable outcome are attractive both to clinical staff of the hospital, as well as to outside regulatory groups and to insurers. Therefore, we are emphasizing outcomes assessment and plan gradually to supplement the cumbersome clinical indicators and case-by-case analysis with the more useful and popular analysis of outcomes.

ISSUES ON THE HORIZON: A SUMMARY

What will be the attributes of a program that serves both the needs of the hospital as well as the needs and desires of its clinicians? Furthermore, what will be the needs of large and complex integrated systems that include not just doctors and hospitals, but also home care agencies, nursing homes, and newly emerging managed care organizations? Several general attributes are apparent.

First, clinically accurate information on quality and outcome must be collected, coded, and expressed in an easily understood format so that it will be useful to clinicians and hospital managers. This requires the application of principles of hospital epidemiology, with a high degree of thoughtfulness and rigor both in design and execution. Such information must be specific enough to be useful by highly specialized clinicians in very narrow specialties, yet expressed in a simple and broad enough way to be easily understood by the nonspecialist.

Second, sophisticated clinicians must guide the process. Specialists within the field can best judge when information is truly important. They must guide the development of the procedures for data collection, analysis, and evaluation as well as be prepared to act on information once it becomes available. Appropriate clinicians need to be involved at the very first phases of the development of epidemiologic-based quality programs in any hospital or health organization. An endocrinologist cannot do the work of a vascular surgeon. However, guidance and direction from clinicians in other fields should be part of the process in its development, for other perspectives are very useful and frequently very incisive.

Third, areas of conflict between hospital management and the clinical staff need to be continually recognized, aired, and resolved. On an ongoing basis, the structure that develops in each hospital should support the month-to-month resolution of new areas of conflict that are encountered, for they will be numerous. Dealing with these areas of conflict requires a smoothly working committee structure, a series of informal discussions, and a high degree of trust among all of those involved in the process. It is perhaps most important that from the start the senior management of the hospital and senior members of the medical and nursing staff all agree on the need for close collaboration in an ongoing strong working relationship. That message then needs to be shared wisely among all members of the staff.

Fourth, regulatory requirements must be recognized. Because the regulatory world is rapidly changing, it is largely impossible to anticipate the specific needs and wants of the Joint Commission, state health departments, and the federal government. Nevertheless, as changes in the quality assurance process occur, each hospital should anticipate as far as possible the local and national regulatory climate. Furthermore, since regulators are usually in a quandary about what is desirable and useful, hospitals may well be in a position to influence regulatory policy in its formative stages especially within states and at the local level. Having a carefully formulated and well-functioning sophisticated quality and outcomes system is a potent antidote to regulatory zeal.

Finally, one indicator of the maturity of an organization—as with the maturity of an individual—is the willingness to recognize imperfections and errors, just as it is to be proud of accomplishments and success. This requires that the aims of assessing quality and outcome need to be kept clearly in mind, both as programs develop and as day-to-day affairs are conducted. These efforts should support the hospitals', physicians', and nurses' ability to care for their patients and to help overcome obstacles in doing so.

References

1. Donabedian, A. The quality of care: How can it be assessed? JAMA 1988;260(12):1743–1748.
2. Rutstein DD, Berenberg W, Chalmers TC, Child CG, Fishman AP, Perrin EB. Measuring the quality of medical care: A clinical method. N Engl J Med 1976;294(11):582–588.
3. Steffen GE. Quality medical care: A definition. JAMA 1988;260(1):56–61.
4. Eddy, DM. Clinical decision making: From theory to practice—Anatomy of a decision. JAMA 1990; 363(3):441–443.
5. Eisenberg JM, Kabendl A. Organized practice and the quality of medical care. Inquiry (Blue Cross and Blue Shield Association) 1988;25:78–89.
6. Donabedian A. Quality and cost: Choices and responsibilities. Inquiry (Blue Cross and Blue Shield Association) 1988;25:90–99.
7. Hartz AJ, Krakauer H, Kuhn EM, Young M, Jacobsen SJ, Gay G, Muenz L, Katzoff M, Bailey RC, Rimm AA. Hospital characteristics and mortality rates. N Engl J Med 1989;321(25):1720–1725.
8. Berwick DM. Health services research and quality of care: Assignments for the 1990s. Med Care 1989;27(8):763–771.
9. Drucker PF. Managing the nonprofit organization: Principles and practices. New York: Harper Collins Publishers, 1990.
10. Sheldon A. Managing Doctors. Illinois: Dow Jones-Irwin, 1986:131ff.
11. Jaffe BM. Does quality assurance assure quality? [Editorial]. Surgical Rounds, November 1989:13–14.
12. Cleary PD, McNeil BJ. Patient satisfaction as an indicator of quality care. Inquiry 1988:25–36.
13. Heyssel RM, Gaintner JR, Kues IW, Jones AA, Lipstein SH. Decentralized management in a teaching hospital. New Engl J Med 1984;310–1477.

Section II

Organizing for Change

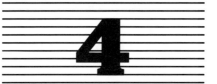

Defining and Measuring the Quality of Health Care

Avedis Donabedian, M.D.

There are some who believe that quality in health care is a property so subtle and mysterious, and one so variable in meaning from situation to situation, that it is not amenable to prior specification. For that reason, they argue, quality is best left to experienced clinicians to determine, case by case. Some others hold the opposite view, believing quality to be capable of such precise specification that it can be bought and sold, as it were, by the pound. The viewpoint to be offered in this chapter is between these two extremes. Quality in health care will be shown to be a complex property indeed, but one amenable to systematic analysis, and permitting a degree of accuracy in assessment which, though far from perfect, is still sufficient for most practical purposes. It is in this more modest sense, that the word "measurement" is to be interpreted.

THE NATURE OF QUALITY

To assess quality it is necessary, first, to define it, so that one can understand what it is. Moreover, if the assessment is meant to precede a concerted effort to safeguard and promote quality, the definition of quality must be accepted as legitimate by those expected to act upon it. That is why a chapter on measurement begins, inevitably, with a conceptual exploration.

The key properties of health care that constitute quality are listed and briefly defined in Table 4.1. They are: effectiveness, efficiency, optimality, acceptability, legitimacy, and equity. Each will be discussed in somewhat greater detail below.

Table 4.1.
Some Attributes of Quality in Health Care

Effectiveness
  The ability to attain the greatest improvements in health now achievable by the best care
Efficiency
  The ability to lower the cost of care without diminishing attainable improvements in health
Optimality
  The balancing of costs against the effects of care on health (or on the benefits of health care, meaning the monetary value of improvements in health) so as to attain the most advantageous balance
Acceptability
  Conformity to the wishes, desires, and expectations of patients and responsible members of their families
Legitimacy
  Conformity to social preferences as expressed in ethical principles, values, norms, mores, laws, and regulations
Equity
  Conformity to a principle that determines what is just or fair in the distribution of health care and of its benefits among the members of a population

Effectiveness

Effectiveness is the degree to which the care proposed or received has achieved, or can be expected to achieve, the greatest improvement in health now possible, given the patient's condition and the current state of the science and technology of health care. The concept of effectiveness is illustrated in Figure 4.1.

The abscissa of Figure 4.1 represents time; the ordinate represents a measure of health or wellness. The solid, undergirding line represents the course of a self-limiting illness that begins sharply, causes a rapid reduction in healthiness, lasts a short time, and rapidly improves, permitting the patient's health to return to its original state. The topmost, interrupted line in the figure represents the course of the illness when managed in the best way now known. The intermediate, dotted line represents the course of the illness with the kind of care whose relative effectiveness is to be assessed as one step in assessing its quality. Under this formulation, relative effectiveness is represented by (Area A) ÷ (Area A + B).

This formulation calls for some comment, first, on the method of presentation used. A self-limiting disease has been chosen only to simplify the figure; the basic relationships depicted would emerge no matter what the course of the illness, with and without care, is projected to be. Also for simplicity, the course of the illness and the effects of care have been represented as certainties. In fact, they are probabilities or expectations. In assessing the quality of care, one is guided by information about what would be expected to occur in a large number of cases of similar kind, rather than by what has happened in a particular patient. In that sense, care can indeed be excellent although the patient has died; it is excellent because in patients of that particular kind it accomplishes the best results, on the average.

Second, it should be noted that, according to Figure 4.1, effectiveness as a property of the quality of care is bounded by what the science and technology of health care can achieve at their best. Therefore, quality is not assessed relative to unattainable ideals, but relative to what is currently attainable. As science and technology im-

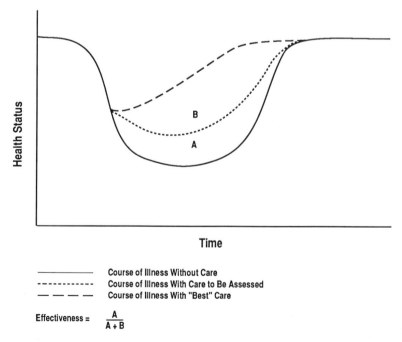

Figure 4.1.   Graphic presentation of effectiveness in a self-limiting disease. (Donabedian A. The quality of care: Can it be assessed? JAMA 1988;260:1743–1748.)

prove, the standards by which relative effectiveness is judged will be raised accordingly.

Third, Figure 4.1 calls for prior conceptualization and measurement of health status. Since the purpose of health care is to safeguard health, it is not surprising that one must ask: What kind of health? The answer could determine whether care is judged good or not. The more technical issues of measurement, including validity, reliability, specificity, and sensitivity also bear heavily on the ability to assess quality. The definition and measurement of health status can be regarded, therefore, as a preliminary step to the definition and measurement of quality. But, although this is the case, only some introductory comments on the measurement of health status can be made here. For more, the reader is referred to the extensive literature on the subject (1, 2).

Health status would be measured most comprehensively by a measure of longevity, with appropriate adjustments for functional capacity and degree of satisfaction, so that years at less than full capacity to function and enjoy would be given proportionately less value (3–5). Considerable progress has been made in developing such measures, but their usefulness in quality assessment is not yet established. Ordinarily, rather simple, more traditional measures of health status are used in quality assessment. Examples are the percent of patients who have survived, or who are free of specified laboratory abnormalities or symptoms, at specified intervals after a clinical intervention. So-called "negative" measures of health, such as mortality and morbidity may also be used; Figure 4.1 would then be reversed in direction, without losing its essential characteristics.

In general, rather discrete measures of health status, selected to represent the goals of care for particular types of patients (e.g., lower blood pressure values, fewer asthmatic attacks, normal urine cultures, etc.), can be expected to be more specific and sensitive measures of the relative effectiveness of care. They do represent, however, only restricted segments of the broader concept of health. The more inclusive measures of longevity-adjusted-for-functional-capacity (sometimes called "quality-adjusted" years of life) have the advantage of comprehensiveness, but are expected to be less sensitive to variations in the quality of care and more likely to reflect the effects of factors additional to health care.

Fourth, the formulation depicted in Figure 4.1 calls for a considerable amount of information, much of it unavailable, or available in less than fully validated form. The effects on health of alternative regimens or strategies of care are not well understood; even less often can the effects be plotted for long periods of time after the onset of care. The natural course of an illness, with no treatment at all, is usually unknown. Often, it is unknowable, since treatment cannot be intentionally withheld. This being the case, one must proceed on two fronts: using to best effect what is currently known, while additional information is being sought.

If there is no information about the curves of Figure 4.1 in their entirety, useful assessments can still be made if one knows the situation at any given time, so that corresponding points on each of the three curves can be compared. If information about the untreated state of the illness is not available, comparisons can be made among alternative methods of care, perhaps holding initial health status as the benchmark. To be most sensitive to differences in effectiveness, such comparisons would be done at the optimal "time window," which is the time when the curves diverge the most from each other (6). But all these comparisons provide only partial, and perhaps biased, information. Relative effectiveness is likely to be underestimated if the untreated course of the illness is progressive, and overestimated if it tends to spontaneous improvement. For better estimates, we need to know more.

The kinds of information envisaged in Figure 4.1 are obtained through appropriate research, including clinical trials and carefully designed epidemiological observations (7). These investigative efforts do not contribute only to quality assessment. Rather, they are necessary to establishing the scientific base on which rational health care should rest. It must be understood that the knowledge needed to assess the relative effectiveness of health care is no different from the knowledge needed to provide that care in the first place.

Efficiency

Efficiency is expressed as a ratio of actual or expected improvements in health to the cost of care responsible for these improvements. Therefore, efficiency could be enhanced by only improving the effects of care, by only lowering costs, or, best of all, by accomplishing both at once. Still another possibility, that improvements in health would be reduced, but costs reduced even more, will be excluded for now, seeing that established values and traditions in health care require a constant striving for the best results.

Some would say that efficiency is not an integral part of the concept of quality; it is simply the cost at which quality in health care is obtained. Others would argue that unnecessary care or unnecessarily costly care, even in the unlikely event of not interfering with the attainment of maxi-

mum improvements of health, suggest ineptitude, carelessness, or social irresponsibility. For that reason they reflect on the competence of the care giver.

Optimality

Optimality is represented as a ratio of the effects of care on health, or of the financial benefits of these effects, to the cost of care. This means that improvements in health are valued, not in absolute terms, but relative to the cost of care. Figure 4.2 is a simplified schematic depiction of the meaning of optimality; it also shows some of the consequences of including optimality as a component of quality.

The *top panel* of Figure 4.2 depicts the consequences of making progressive additions to care. Although, to simplify the figure, all these additions have been assumed to be useful, the curve of effects (or of benefits) shows an eventual flattening, whereas the cost of care continues to rise. The result of relating benefits to cost is shown in the *lower panel* of the figure. Clearly, beyond a certain point in the progression of useful care, the balance of

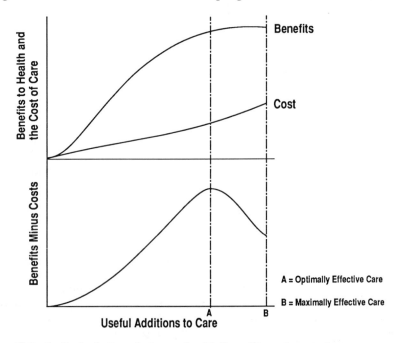

Figure 4.2. Hypothetical relations between health benefits and cost of care, as useful additions are made to care. (Donabedian A. The quality of care: Can it be assessed? JAMA 1988;260:1743–1748.)

benefits to costs becomes adverse. Thus, two specifications of the most desirable level of quality emerge. The regimen or strategy of care designated *A* represents optimally effective care; the strategy designated *B* represents maximally effective care. Subject to considerations to be described below, either can be set as the standard in quality assessment.

Besides raising issues of public policy, the inclusion of optimality as a component in the definition of quality adds to the burdens of measurement. In addition to measuring effects, as already described, one will need to measure costs if either efficiency or optimality are to be determined, and to measure the benefits of care, if these benefits are to be compared to cost in determinations of optimality. The methods required are in the specialized province of health economics (8, 9).

Acceptability

A fourth constituent of quality in health care is the acceptability of that care to patients or their surrogates, usually members of their families. The degree of acceptability, in its turn, hinges on at least the following five properties: (*a*) accessibility, (*b*) the patient-practitioner relation, (*c*) amenities, (*d*) patient preferences as to the effects of care, and (*e*) patient preferences as to the cost of care.

Accessibility

Experts tend to debate whether accessibility is a component of goodness in care, or only a factor that contributes to receiving care, that care, itself, liable to being good, bad, or indifferent in quality. It is likely, however, that potential patients are unimpressed by such fine distinctions. To them, the ability to obtain care easily and conveniently is likely to be an important mark of quality. As will become clear soon, accessibility also contributes to equity in the distribution of care, a key requirement for its social acceptability.

The Patient-Practitioner Relation

When patients gain access to care and get to use it, their impression of its quality depends very much on how their medical attendants behave toward them. It is difficult to catalogue all the properties that might be regarded to constitute goodness in the patient-practitioner relation. Table 4.2 provides a partial listing, offered mainly as an example. To put it briefly, personal concern, empathy, respectfulness, avoidance of condescension, willingness to explain, and plain good manners are all essential to goodness in care. They are essential in several ways.

First, these are properties desirable in their own right, since they characterize socially acceptable interaction among equals. Second, patients take them as evidence, which they understand, of the goodness of technical care, which they may not understand so well. Third, a good patient-practitioner relation can, in fact, contribute to greater effectiveness in care, motivating the practitioners to be more assiduous and the patient more cooperative. Fourth, in some situations, particularly when psychological disorders are treated, the patient-practitioner interaction is, itself, a rather formal technique. When that is the case, the distinction between technical care and the management of interpersonal process may be too small to matter.

Amenities

Amenities are the desirable aspects of the circumstances under which care is given. They include convenience, comfort, cleanliness, privacy, good food, and so on. Patients value these attributes, but they also recognize that effectiveness and a satisfactory patient-practitioner relation are more important. If possible, they would, of course, like to have all three (10).

Patient Preferences as to the Effects of Care

We have already seen how important to assessing quality the effects of care on health are. Now, it is necessary to add that patients may value these effects differently from the valuations of professionals. Various states of health and ill health mean different things to different persons, per-

Table 4.2.
Some Attributes of a Good Patient-Practitioner Relationship[a]

Congruence between therapist and client expectations, orientations and so forth

Adaptation and flexibility: the ability of the therapist to adapt his or her approach not only to the expectations of the client but also to the demands of the clinical situation

Mutuality: gains for both therapist and client

Stability: a stable relationship between client and therapist

Maintenance of maximum possible client autonomy, freedom of action, and movement

Maintenance of family and community communication and ties

Maximum possible degree of egalitarianism in the client-therapist relationship

Maximum possible degree of active client participation through (a) sharing knowledge concerning the health situation, (b) shared decision making, and (c) participation in carrying out therapy

Maintenance of empathy and rapport without undue emotional involvement of the therapist

Maintenance of a supportive relationship without encouragement of undue dependency

Confining the therapists' and the clients' influence and action within the boundaries of their legitimate social functions

Avoidance of exploitation of the client and of the therapist economically, socially, sexually, or any other way

Maintenance of the clients' and therapists' dignity and individuality

Maintenance of privacy

Maintenance of confidentiality

[a]Donabedian A. Models for organizing the delivery of personal health services and criteria for evaluating them. Milbank Memorial Fund Q 1972;50(part 2):117.

haps reflecting their occupational requirements, social situations, or psychological makeup. Therefore, when faced with a choice among alternative treatments, offering significantly different prospects of benefits and risks, a properly informed patient or surrogate ought to be consulted. Quality assessments should reflect the principle that the course of action considered by one patient to be best may differ from that preferred by another patient, and that both could be different from what is best in the practitioner's opinion.

Patient Preferences as to the Cost of Care

In addition to placing different, personal valuations on the effects of care, patients are unequal in their susceptibility and averseness to bearing its costs. They differ in susceptibility because of variations in coverage by health insurance or other third party payments. They differ in averseness to bearing the cost of care because of economic circumstances, as well as the relative attractiveness, to them, of alternative ways of spending their own money.

Comments on Acceptability as a Component of Quality

In summary, including acceptability to patients or their surrogates as a component of quality modifies its meaning in two ways. First, the concept of quality is broadened to embrace the accessibility of care, the amenities of the settings in which care is provided, and, most importantly, the attributes of the patient-practitioner relation. Second, estimates of effectiveness, efficiency, and optimality are altered, sometimes radically, by the interposition of personal valuations of effects, costs, or both.

Another consequence is that personal judgments on quality are likely to vary considerably among individuals. Accordingly, the methods for assessing quality need to provide for eliciting patient preferences for and satisfaction with the aspects of care detailed above. This calls for yet another set of measurement tools, this time contributed mainly by the behavioral sciences (11–15).

More fundamental still, is an understanding of the limitations of including patient satisfaction as a component of quality. Patient satisfaction cannot be a final arbiter of quality. Patients may be satisfied with less than is their due, or expect too much. They may be misled by a pleasing "bedside manner." They may make choices that are not in their own best interests, are against the ethical principles of the practitioner, or are contrary to the public interest. When there are such discords, there may not be a single measure of quality. Rather, the judgment of quality may have to be differentiated to indicate in which of its aspects care is approved and in which it is not.

Legitimacy

Legitimacy is taken to mean conformity to social preferences as expressed in ethical principles, values, norms, mores, laws, and regulations. Legitimacy may be regarded as acceptability to the community or to society at large, making this attribute a counterpart to the acceptability of care to individuals.

In a democratic society, all the features of care important to individuals are expected to be also matters of social concern. But, at the societal level, there must be concern for the welfare of the collectivity as well. In some cases, this means that what could be best for any given individual might not be best for everyone as a group.

If one excludes the more obvious forms of antisocial behavior, one finds that the disparity between social and individual acceptability often arises from differences in valuations of the costs and effects of care. Costs are estimated differently whenever care is at least partly financed by government programs or by health insurance. In that case, individuals may wish to have more care than society is willing to pay for. In Figure 4.2, the social optimum would fall to the left of the individual optimum.

As to the effects of care, social and individual valuations are likely to disagree when others are benefited or harmed by an individual's receiving care or failing to receive it. Examples include genetic counseling, family planning, immunization, care for communicable diseases, and health supervision of those who, if their capacities fail, might endanger others. The reporting of communicable diseases and aggressive behaviors might be added as interventions distasteful to the individuals concerned but signifying quality from the social perspective. The same could be said of policies that imply a lesser valuation on some, for example the aged, in order to differentially favor others, for example children. Such differential valuations may simply reflect estimates of what is more effective and efficient for society as a whole. But, sometimes, an additional principle is invoked, one that is a key contributor to legitimacy, but is also sufficiently distinctive to be singled out as the final entry in the list of attributes that constitute quality.

Equity

Equity is the principle of fairness or justice in the distribution of care and of its benefits among the members of a population. As such, it should contribute to acceptability of care to individuals as well as to society at large. But individuals, unless exceptionally altruistic, are expected to seek what is best for themselves. Society, by contrast, must make equity a deliberate consideration in social policy, quite distinct from the pursuit of the greatest collective improvement in health at lowest cost. Equity is a moral commitment in obedience to which some may receive more care even if that increment of care would have yielded greater improvements in health when used by others.

Comment on Legitimacy and Equity as Components of Quality

The inclusion of societal considerations in assessing quality creates serious problems for both clinical practice and its assessment. The dominant ethical principles and traditions of the health care professions require practitioners to do what is best for individual patients under their care. To say that care ought to be acceptable to patients, merely implies that the practitioner confirm what patients consider best for themselves. Although practitioners and patients might disagree on what is best for patients, the divergence of opinions is not often large, or can be narrowed by a sharing of information. By contrast, social and individual specifications can be large and difficult to reconcile, the usual difference being that individuals want more care than society affords to provide, though in some cases the reverse can happen. This is not the appropriate place to discuss how these differences might be handled in practice (16). Insofar as quality assessment is concerned, it might be necessary to provide alternative judgments, specifying the perspective from which each judgment derives.

THE MEASUREMENT OF QUALITY

Having established the range of attributes that quality in health care might embrace, it is possible to move on to the task of measurement itself. The steps entailed will be described as follows: (a) specification of the attributes to be measured, (b) choice of an approach to measurement, (c) choice of the phenomena to be assessed, (d) formulation of criteria and standards, and (e) obtaining information about care.

Attributes To Be Assessed

One might wonder if an assessment of quality is at all possible, seeing the multiplicity of attributes relevant to the concept of quality, and the possibility that goodness in one might conflict with goodness in another. Fortunately, the principle of "contextuality" offers a way out of the difficulty. By contextuality I mean that in any given situation certain components are more important and relevant; other components can be left out, although in a different situation, those excluded components would be the very ones to include. For example, in most clinical situations, we ask if the care provided is calculated to be the most effective, in the light of contemporary knowledge. Sometimes we ask if care is given efficiently. Attention to the factors that contribute to acceptability to patients is less often in evidence, although it ought to be. As yet, determinations of social optimality and equity have not been required in clinical settings; in the future they might be. But, of course, the social perspective on quality would dominate if the assessment is made for national planning.

One may conclude that the first step in moving from broad conceptual formulations to measurement would be to specify the smaller subset of components that is to be the focus of attention. But this should be done with a clear understanding of what has been left out and a reasonable justification of why.

Approach to Measurement

It was suggested almost 25 years ago that there are three approaches to assessing the quality of care: "structure," "process," and "outcome" (17). The meaning of these terms, the relationship among the approaches, and their use in quality assessment are the subjects that follow.

Definitions of the Three Approaches

Structure is taken to comprise properties of personnel and facilities, including their financing and organization, that either increase or decrease the probability of good care being given. Structure includes human, material, and organizational resources. Process is a designation of what is done for patients and by patients. It includes the content of care and the skill with which care is executed. Outcome signifies what is accomplished for and by individual patients, patients as a group, or populations as a whole. Most importantly, outcomes are improvements in health and well-being attributable to antecedent health care—the variable placed on the ordinate in Figure 4.1. Changes in health-related knowledge and behavior may also be included as outcomes. Table 4.3 provides a more complete classification supported by many examples.

In some ways, patient satisfaction belongs among the outcomes of care, since it is a type of well-being that results from acceptable care. But satisfaction or dissatisfaction can also be taken as the patients' judgments on certain aspects of care, calibrating the degree of their acceptability. To the extent that satisfaction contributes to the success of future care, it can also be considered as a structural feature or input.

In thinking about how the three approaches are to be used, one must remember that they are not, themselves, proper-

Table 4.3.
Classification of Health Care Outcomes[a]

A. Clinical
  1. Reported symptoms that have clinical significance
  2. Diagnostic categorization as an indication of morbidity
  3. Disease staging relevant to functional encroachment and prognosis
  4. Diagnostic performance—the frequency of false positives and false negatives as indicators of diagnostic or case finding performance
B. Physiological-biochemical
  1. Abnormalities
  2. Functions
    a. Loss of function
    b. Functional reserve—includes performance in test situations under various degrees of stress
C. Physical
  1. Loss or impairment of structural form or integrity—includes abnormalities, defects, and disfigurement
  2. Functional performance of physical activities and tasks
    a. Under the circumstances of daily living
    b. Under test conditions that involve various degrees of stress
D. Psychological, mental
  1. Feelings—include discomfort, pain, fear, anxiety (or their opposites, including satisfaction)
  2. Beliefs that are relevant to health and health care
  3. Knowledge that is relevant to healthful living, health care, and coping with illness
  4. Impairments of discrete psychological or mental functions
    a. Under the circumstances of daily living
    b. Under test conditions that involve various degrees of stress
E. Social and psychosocial
  1. Behaviors relevant to coping with current illness or affecting future health, including adherence to health care regimens, and changes in health-related habits
  2. Role performance
    a. Marital
    b. Familial
    c. Occupational
    d. Other interpersonal
  3. Performance under test conditions involving varying degrees of stress
F. Integrative outcomes
  1. Mortality
  2. Longevity
  3. Longevity, with adjustments made to take account of impairments of physical, psychological, or psychosocial function: "full-function equivalents"
  4. Monetary value of the above
G. Evaluative outcomes
  1. Client opinions about, and satisfaction with, various aspects of care, including accessibility, continuity, thoroughness, humaneness, informativeness, effectiveness, cost

[a]Donabedian A. Exploration in quality assessment and monitoring. Vol. II: The criteria and standards of quality. Ann Arbor: Health Administration Press, 1980:367–368.

ties of quality. They are only kinds of information that can lead to inferences about the degree of goodness in one or more attributes of quality. Furthermore, the three approaches represent rather rough subdivisions in a chain of events, each event in the chain being the consequence of a preceding event as well as the cause of a subsequent one. In such a chain, it may not be easy to say, for example, where process ends and outcome begins. A useful rule for identifying an outcome is to ask if it is a change, temporary or permanent, in the patient. Thus, not every consequence of care is, strictly speaking, an outcome. But, a clear understanding of the chain of events to be assessed is more important than precisely what each juncture is to be called.

Interrelationships among Approaches

Three approaches to obtaining information about the degree of quality are possible if, and only if, good structural properties increase the likelihood of the process of care being good; good process increases the likelihood of good outcomes occurring; and good outcomes are more likely to have been preceded by a good process of care. It is important to note that: the relations between adjacent pairs in this sequence are only probabilities, not certainties; these probabilities can be high or low; and our knowledge of the probabilities is often incomplete. All these features cause a lesser or greater degree of uncertainty in judgments of quality, particularly on the technical component of care. This kind of uncertainty cannot be reduced by refinements in methods of assessment; only advances in basic knowledge can reduce it.

Relative Usefulness of the Three Approaches

There is no doubt that structure is important to the quality of care, since the way a health care program or system is set up and run shapes behavior in that program or system. But the relation between structural features and either process or outcome is seldom strong. Consequently, assessments of structure usually produce presumptive judgments on quality. Nevertheless, assessments of structure are valuable and necessary. Although the more abstract properties of organizational structure and behavior are difficult to measure (18), many of the more concrete features are stable and rather easily observed. Consequently, assessments of structure have been the chief tool in the armamentarium of licensing and accrediting agencies. Besides being useful indicators of quality, assessments of structure are often necessary if one is to explain how deficiencies in process and outcome of care arise.

Assessments of process provide more direct information about quality, but the validity of the information, in the case of technical care, depends on how certain one is, based on prior scientific information, of the relative efficacy of alternative methods of care. Given a reasonable degree of certainty, another advantage of process assessment is the relative availability of timely information, usually in the medical record. But the medical record suffers from deficiencies, to be described later in this chapter, and the special studies needed to supplement the medical record can be time consuming and costly.

Information about outcomes that occur during the process of care is rather easy to obtain, but it is difficult to get information about outcomes that occur later, sometimes after many years have gone by. Still, assessments of outcome are often favored

because it is argued, quite justifiably, that what matters most in care is its effect on health and well-being, as shown in Figure 4.1. Moreover, outcomes have the remarkable property of representing the total, interactive effects of all contributions to care, including those of the patient, weighted by their relative importance to health and well-being. But there are drawbacks, as well, to outcome assessment.

Outcomes very often do not show, as process assessments can, precisely in what way care has been good or not. Furthermore, changes in health may occur for reasons unrelated to quantity or quality of health care. These include the initial severity of illness as well as other innate or acquired characteristics of patients. These differences can be addressed by two methods; one is statistical and the other could be called "clinical."

It is possible to make adjustments, through proper study design or statistical manipulation or both, for differences in type of patient and type of illness before outcomes are compared. But, I believe, we do not now have a workable statistical tool for removing the effects of extraneous factors so completely that one can rely entirely on outcome measurement to assess the quality of care. And even if such a tool were available, one would still not know precisely in what ways, for what reasons, quality had failed.

More credible and detailed judgments can be obtained by the "clinical" method, by which is meant the verification, through review of the antecedent process of care, of the reasons that account for the outcomes observed. Still, prior correction for differences in outcome unrelated to quality, either by study design or statistical adjustment, can markedly reduce the burden of unnecessary case review. Therefore, in addition to the more generally applicable methods of research, the specific tools of case mix adjustment are important members of the family of methods pertinent to quality assessment (19–22).

Conclusions about Choice of an Approach

Seeing the mix of advantages and disadvantages that attend each of the approaches to assessment, it would seem best to use elements of all three in any strategy of assessment, especially if the purpose is constant surveillance leading to corrective action. In that way, if outcomes are unsatisfactory, one can discover what, if anything, was deficient in antecedent care; and if care is defective, one can see what structural features may have contributed to that deficiency, so improvements can be made. Concurrent information obtained by the three approaches also allows the judgments on quality inferred from each to be compared. Agreement among them is reassuring, but if they disagree, one is alerted to the likelihood of error.

Disparities between judgments based on process and outcome are taken by some to signify that process cannot be trusted to indicate quality (23). Actually, there are many reasons for such disparities, including the following: (*a*) when the relation between process and outcome is represented by a rather small probability, the number of cases observed may have been too small to reveal the relation; (*b*) when the effect of care is most evident during a rather short period of time, or is delayed, outcomes may not have been observed during the optimal time window, or for long enough; (*c*) the outcome measure contains more information than is contained in the aspects of process assessed, since outcomes represent all contributions to care, including skill in the execution of care; (*d*) the aspects of process measured are irrelevant to the outcomes of care, or the outcomes measured are not, nor could have been, the objectives of care; (*e*) case mix adjustment, either through study design or statistical corrections, has been defective; (*f*) the knowledge from which the presumptions about expected relations between process and outcome were derived is defective at the source, so to speak; and (*g*) the information about process, or outcome, or both was inaccurate to begin with, or may have been tampered with later.

There is more to be said about the relationships among structure, process, and outcome, but more detailed sources should be consulted for that (23–26).

Choice of Phenomena To Be Assessed

Assuming one has been asked to devise a method for assessing, episodically or continuously, the quality of care in an enterprise, the following might be the first questions to ask: What is done here? How is it done? What is the purpose of doing it? How would one know if one has failed or succeeded? More abstractly stated, one would try to elucidate the functions, processes, products, and objectives of the enterprise. These preliminaries are illustrated in Figure 4.3, a flow diagram of the steps of care in a hospital's emergency care unit, and Table 4.4, a list of specific objectives that those who operate that unit might have. The choice of what structures, segments of care, or outcomes to assess is suggested by a prior exploration of this kind. It is also influenced, to some degree, by whether one is interested in judging performance under ordinary circumstances, or in verifying the capacity to perform under more severe challenge to competence.

Excluding structural features, the most common categories of phenomena selected for assessment are listed in Table 4.5. There can be, of course, many others, depending on what aspect of the health care system is being assessed, and there is an abundance of items within each category. How is one to choose?

As shown in Table 4.5, the choice of phenomena to be assessed is influenced by importance, representativeness, and feasibility. Importance can be gauged, mainly, by Williamson's principle of "maximum achievable benefit" (27). This means: how frequent the phenomenon is, how subject it is to error in management, how injurious to health the error is, and how amenable to correction and prevention, respectively, the error and the injury are. If one were interested to test the limits of clinical competence, one would include conditions that severely challenge that competence. In addition, the need to monitor certain things is heightened for administrative or political reasons, for example, the need to satisfy governmental regulations, to avoid litigation, to accommodate to the configu-

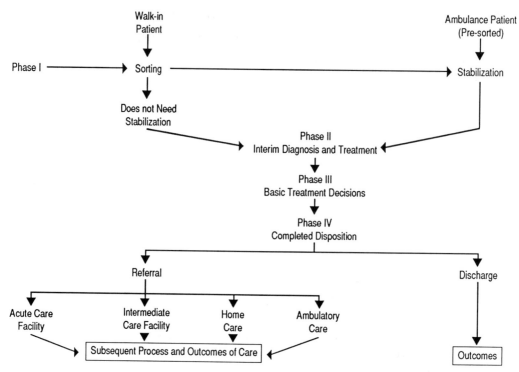

Figure 4.3.   A specification of functions and processes in a hospital's emergency unit. (Rhee KE, Donabedian A, Burney RE. Assessing quality of care in a hospital's emergency unit: A framework and its application. Qual Rev Bull 1987;13:4–16.)

ration of power and influence in an organization, or to ensure fairness.

True representative sampling, as statisticians understand it, is necessary for research intended to ascertain the actual state of affairs in a population. It is not a usual strategy in quality assessment for administrative purposes, unless it is to select cases within a category already chosen on other grounds. Probability samples tend to include too many cases whose assessment reveals few significant errors in care. For administrative purposes, a strategy that could be called "illustrative sampling" may be more feasible, while garnering more critical information. If one has already specified functions, processes, products, and objectives, it is often possible to select one or two diagnoses, conditions, events, or activities that, if examined, would give a feel of how the system is performing with regard to each of these prespecified features. Figure 4.4 is a hypothetical example corresponding to the

specification provided earlier in Figure 4.3 and Table 4.4. The strategy it illustrates, introduced by Kessner et al. (28, 29) as the "tracer" method, is an ambitious undertaking seldom fully implemented. But I believe it to be valuable if prudently used.

Feasibility is always a consideration in choosing what to assess and how. Because quality assessment is often resisted, one is often dependent on opportunities of access and cooperation. Information needs to be available at reasonable cost. The state of knowledge should permit the formulation of criteria and standards sufficiently valid and acceptable to permit measurement.

Less attention seems to have been paid to devising criteria for the systematic selection of structural features. Partly, this may be because many structural requirements are clearly spelled out in the conditions for licensing, accreditation, and approval for advanced training. Perhaps it is because the features of structure that contribute to safety and amenability are thought to be rather obvious, as are the prerequisites for providing specified kinds of care. It is possible, nevertheless, to set up for the choice of structural features, a prioritizing scheme very similar to that already described. In particular, the features selected should be amenable to administrative intervention and be closely related to process and outcome in ways critical to quality.

Formulation of Criteria and Standards

All measurement requires something analogous to a yardstick. Criteria and standards are the yardstick for quality assessment. "Criterion" is taken to mean an attribute of structure, process, or outcome that, if recorded and measured, would lead to an inference about quality. A "standard" is taken to mean a precise, quantitative statement that stands for goodness in any criterion. These definitions, accompanied by some examples, appear in Table 4.6. An additional word,

"norm," is often used to mean a standard derived from actual practice, rather than from notions of what ought to be. All these terms need to be defined in any discourse because the nomenclature has not been standardized as yet.

Criteria and standards are important because they are the means by which the general concepts and attributes chosen to represent quality are translated to actual measures. The construction, evaluation, and application of criteria and standards are complicated matters that cannot be fully described in this chapter. Only a few of the more important aspects of the subject will be briefly presented under the following headings: (a) sources, (b) derivation, (c) degree of prior specification, (d) format, (e) evaluation, and (f) procedure for formulation. For more, the reader is

Table 4.4.
Specification of Some Objectives in a Hospital's Emergency Unit[a]

Expeditiousness, timeliness, and duration of care
Appropriateness of diagnostic and therapeutic interventions as judged by the greatest net benefit at lowest cost
The validity of diagnostic decisions
Skill in the execution of diagnostic and therapeutic interventions
Reliability and validity of diagnostic information and monitoring data
Appropriateness of referral
Maintenance of continuity in care through successful linkage with, and transfer of adequate information to, a more stable source of care
Appropriate recording and management of information
Patient education and motivation with a view to prevention
Discharge of legitimate organizational and social obligations with due regard to responsibilities toward individual patients

[a]Rhee KE, Donabedian A, Burney RE. Assessing quality of care in a hospital's emergency unit: A framework and its application. Qual Rev Bull 1987;13:4–16.

Table 4.5.
Phenomena to be Assessed and Criteria for Choice and Sampling[a]

A. Phenomena that could be used to assess clinical practice
  1. Diagnostic categories
     Examples: pneumonia, myocardial infarction
  2. Conditions
     Examples: abdominal pain, headache
  3. Clinical procedures: therapeutic, diagnostic, medical, surgical
     Examples: liver biopsy, use of antibiotics, coronary bypass
  4. Adverse outcomes, events, "critical incidents"
     Examples: deaths, complications, accidents, complaints
B. Criteria for choice and sampling
  1. Importance
     a. "Maximum achievable benefit"
        Phenomenon frequent
        Error frequent, serious, costly
        Error correctable
     b. Administrative, "political"
  2. Representativeness
     a. Proportionate sampling
     b. "Illustrative sampling"
  3. Feasibility

[a]Donabedian A. A primer of quality assurance and monitoring. In: Law practice quality evaluation: An appraisal of peer review and other measures to enhance professional performance. Philadelphia: American Law Institute and American Bar Association, October 1988:131.

Phases and Components of the Process of Care		Aspects of Illness, Health, and Health Care		
		Physical-Physiological	Psychological	Social, Environmental
Phase I Sorting and Stabilization		Cardiac Arrest Multiple Trauma	Acute behavioral disturbance	Acute behavioral disturbance
Phase II Diagnosis and Interim Management	Interim Treatment	Cardiac Arrest Multiple Trauma	Acute behavioral disturbance	Acute behavioral disturbance
	Diagnosis	Chest Pain Abdominal Pain Musculoskeletal pain "sick child"	Depression Acute psychosis Bronchial asthma	Child abuse Bronchial asthma
Phase III Basic Treatment Decisions	Therapeutic	Bronchial asthma Poisoning Upper respiratory infections Lacerations	Bronchial asthma Poisoning	Bronchial asthma Rape Assault
	Preventive	Poisoning Foreign body Hypertension	Poisoning Foreign body Bronchial asthma	Poisoning Foreign body Bronchial asthma Child abuse, spouse abuse
Phase IV Completion of Disposition	Referral-Linkage	Any of the above Specified illnesses among "vulnerable": (eg, aged, poor, isolated)	Any of the above "Vulnerable" population groups	Any of the above "Vulnerable" population groups Substance abuse
	Societal Functions	Reportable infections: Conditions requiring genetic counseling Acts of violence Motor vehicle accidents	Cases requiring commitment	Child abuse Spouse abuse Rape Assault Suicide
	Information Management	Any of the above	Any of the above	Any of the above

Figure 4.4. A proposed application of the "tracer method" to assessing care in a hospital's emergency unit. (Rhee KE, Donabedian A, Burney RE. Assessing quality of care in a hospital's emergency unit: A framework and its application. Qual Rev Bull 1987;13:4–16.)

referred to the extensive literature on the subject (30, 31).

Sources

If one excludes aspects of construction and safety, the criteria and standards of the goodness of structure come mostly from the sciences of health care administration. They are limited, therefore, by the relatively undeveloped nature of these sciences. They are also limited by the highly contingent nature of the relation between structure and process. Structure is almost never a sufficient cause and may not even be always a necessary one.

The criteria and standards of the technical process of care come from the clinical sciences. They suffer, therefore, from weaknesses in the scientific basis of current practice. It cannot be emphasized too strongly that if the scientific foundation of clinical practice is weak, judgments on the quality of technical care will be correspondingly open to question.

The criteria and standards of acceptability to clients and to society derive mainly from personal preferences and social values. Whatever legitimacy these possess is transmitted to the criteria and standards that represent them; any lack of legitimacy is also transmitted.

Derivation

In a more immediate sense, criteria and standards may be derived in two ways: (a) "normatively," which means from the sci-

Table 4.6.
Definitions and Examples of Criteria and Standards[a]

A. Definitions

   Criterion: Attribute of structure, process, or outcome capable of leading to an inference about quality

   Standard: A specific, quantitative measure that defines goodness

B. Examples

	Structure	Process	Outcome
Criterion	Staffing of intensive care unit	Blood transfusion during surgery	Case fatality
Standard	Not less than one R.N. per two occupied beds	Not less than 5% and not more than 20% of "average" cases	Not to exceed 0.1% for a specified procedure

[a]Donabedian A. The process of quality assurance. The Bernard Snell Lecture at the University of Alberta, Alberta, Canada, April 1990.

entific literature, supplemented by the opinions of recognized experts, and (b) "empirically," from examples of actual practice or behavior. That practice may be what is actually done or accomplished by leading experts in the most prestigious institutions, or by practitioners on the average.

Degree of Prior Specification

I have classified criteria into "implicit" and "explicit," a nomenclature now widely accepted (32). Implicit criteria and standards are present in the minds of experts who are asked to provide a judgment on care as observed or portrayed in the medical record. By contrast, explicit criteria and standards are prepared ahead of time, usually by groups of experts assembled for the purpose.

Explicit criteria take time and effort to prepare, but, once formulated, they can be applied rather easily and inexpensively to a large number of similar cases, and they produce replicable measurements. But explicit criteria and standards apply only to the average case in a prespecified category. Unless special modifications are made, they cannot take into account all the variability among patients, diseases, circumstances, and preferences. Implicit criteria, by contrast, are as flexible as clinical judgment itself. Unlike explicit criteria, designed as they are to apply only to prespecified categories of cases, implicit criteria can be used to assess probability samples of entire caseloads, provided the

necessary range of experts is at hand. But implicit criteria are costly to use because they demand a great deal of time from experts. Also, because individual experts can differ in their opinions, or may lose concentration during the lengthy process of review, the judgments that ensue may be unreliable (33).

Judgments based on implicit criteria are more likely to be reliable: if expert assessors experienced in and committed to the task of quality review are used; if the judgments required are confined to a few distinctions, such as between good, fair, and poor; and if the records of care being reviewed are reasonably complete, well organized, and legible. The credibility of judgments is heightened by agreement among the independent judgments of two or more reviewers.

The correspondence between the characteristics of cases and the relevant criteria and standards can be improved by carefully prespecifying narrow, more homogeneous subgroups before the explicit criteria and standards are formulated and by refinements in design to be described below.

Seeing that assessments using either implicit or explicit criteria-standards have both advantages and disadvantages, perhaps the most reasonable strategy in quality assessment for administrative purposes is, first, to use explicit criteria to screen cases. Then, all questioned cases would be subjected to careful review, using implicit criteria. To test the ability of explicit criteria to detect error, a sample of questioned cases would also be reviewed in the same way. The usual measures of screening efficiency (sensitivity, specificity, likelihood ratio) could then be derived.

Format

Explicit criteria of the process of care are most often simple listings of requirements that should be met by every case, sometimes supplemented by a list of interventions appropriate for some cases, so that they would not elicit criticism if done. An example is shown in Table 4.7.

A criteria list would usually include criteria to justify the diagnosis and appropriateness of admission to the hospital, the essential historical information to be ob-

tained, the key steps and findings in the physical examination, the diagnostic tests to be performed, and the treatment recommended. Each of the required items in this listing may have equal weight. Alternatively, differential weights may be assigned (as in the example shown) based on how important to successful diagnosis and treatment the expert panel judges each item to be.

Given a weighted or unweighted listing of items required in all cases, it is easy to compute a quantitative measure of quality as a percent of requirements met. This measure, called a "physician performance index" (34), is very useful for statistical purposes, but its correspondence to judg-

Table 4.7.
Criteria List for Cholecystitis and Cholelithiasis[a]

I. Indications for admission	If dehydrated:	
A. Acceptable criteria for admitting patients suspected of having acute cholecystitis	(1) Serum sodium	0.5
1. Pain, nausea, and vomiting	(2) Serum chloride	0.5
2. Recurrent gallbladder attacks	(3) Serum carbon dioxide	0.5
3. Fever	(4) Serum potassium	0.5
4. Jaundice	If jaundiced:	
5. Right upper quadrant mass	(1) Serum bilirubin	1.0
B. Diagnosis of cholelithiasis or cholecystitis, admitted for operation	(2) Alkaline phosphatase	1.0
	(3) Prothrombin time or partial thromboplastin time	1.0
II. Services recommended	4. Roentgenology	
A. Acute cholecystitis	a. Chest x-ray within 1 year	0.5
1. History: specific reference to: *Weight*	b. Intravenous cholangiogram or cholecystogram unless patient is jaundiced or is operated on within 24 hours after admission	2.0
a. Character of pain 3.0		
b. Recurrence 0.5		
c. Radiation 0.5		
d. Symptoms referable to jaundice 0.5	B. Chronic cholecystitis or cholelithiasis	
e. Time of onset 0.5	1. History: specific reference to:	
2. Physical examination: specific reference to:	a. Food intolerance	1.0
a. Right upper quadrant 3.0	b. Previous gallbladder attacks	1.0
b. Mass 0.5	c. Jaundice	1.0
c. Liver size 0.5	2. Physical examination: none specific	
d. Jaundice 0.5	3. Laboratory	
e. Guarding 0.5	a. Complete blood count (hematocrit, white blood cell count, differential)	0.5
3. Laboratory	b. Urinalysis	0.5
a. Complete blood count (hematocrit, white blood cell count, differential) 0.5	c. Electrocardiogram if over age 50 (within 6 months if normal)	1.0
b. Urinalysis 0.5	4. Roentgenology	
c. Electrocardiogram (if over 50 years of age) 0.5	a. Chest x-ray within 1 year	1.0
d. Serum amylase (if patient is alcoholic or if pain is diffuse in nature) 1.0	b. Cholecystography	3.0

ments such as "good," "fair," and "poor" needs to be established.

Criteria-standards of the type described are sometimes pejoratively referred to as "laundry lists." They are not easily adaptable to case variation and are thought to encourage overservicing by including too many items that might be done, while seldom specifying what would be unwise or unnecessary to do. A simple way to address this problem is not to require that all the criteria-standards be met in every case, but to specify a percentage of compliance, or a percentile range, that would be acceptable, given an average mix of patients in a category. This is not a completely satisfactory solution because it is

difficult to establish the average mix and because percentage compliance reflects not only doing the right thing, but can be also the resultant of doing too much in some cases and too little in others. An additional disadvantage is that one needs to wait until there is a sufficient number of cases before a judgment can be made about the entire group; individual cases cannot be pinpointed.

A better approach would be to "branch" the criteria by introducing contingencies identifying the situations in which specified procedures should be done or should be dispensed with. When branching is fully developed, one obtains the "criteria maps" devised by Greenfield et al. (35), as

Table 4.7.
Criteria List for Cholecystitis and Cholelithiasis *(Continued)*

III. Preoperative
  A. Patients with history of recurrent gallbladder attacks may be admitted for study and operation; up to 5 days preoperative stay may be required.
IV. Probable length of stay
  A. With no surgery: should be discharged on subsidence of present illness
  B. Cholecystectomy, uncomplicated: 5–10 days postoperative
  C. If exploration of common duct is also required and T-tube left for drainage: 5–15 days postoperative
  D. Stay is prolonged and unpredictable if any of the following procedures are done:
    1. Duodenotomy
    2. Sphincterotomy
    3. Cholecystotomy
    4. Repair of common duct stricture
V. Complications that may extend length of stay
  A. Wound infection
  B. Wound disruption
  C. Retained common duct stone
  D. Phlebothrombosis or thromboembolism
  E. Pancreatitis
  F. Pneumonia
  G. Diabetes
  H. Heart disease
  I. Bile peritonitis

  J. Postoperative jaundice
  K. Unexplained jaundice
  L. Fever of unknown origin
VI. Indications for discharge
  A. With no surgery:
    1. Afebrile
    2. Pain, tenderness, nausea, and vomiting subsided
  B. With cholecystectomy:
    1. Afebrile (99.4°F or below) unless explanatory remarks noted in record to justify discharge with temperature 100°F
    2. Wound healing satisfactorily
    3. Return of gastrointestinal function
    4. Complications under control
VII. Prehospitalization: specific reference to:
  A. History: same as hospital
  B. Physical examination: same as hospital
  C. Laboratory: same as hospital
  D. Roentgenology: same as hospital
VIII. Posthospitalization: specific reference to:
  A. Revisit approximately 1 week or less and at 6 weeks postoperative, at which time:
    1. Examine wound
    2. Record temperature
IX. End results of treatment
  A. No jaundice
  B. No recurrence of right upper quadrant pain or indigestion
  C. No incision hernia

*Payne BC, Lyons TF, Dwarshius L, Kolton M, Morris W. The quality of medical care: Evaluation and improvement. Chicago: Hospital Research and Educational Trust, 1976:93–95.

illustrated by Figure 4.5. Such a map takes account of case variability because, as the map unfolds its several branches, beginning with the problem posed for it, it differentiates successively smaller subsets of cases, snugly fitting the criteria of care to each subset. Redundancies in care are readily identified as the most effective pathway is plotted out. Thus, though the map in its entirety can be very extensive, only a small part of it suffices to characterize the management of a particular case. In their earlier work, Greenfield et al. summarized performance as a proportion of mapped items complied with. Later, they developed a system of scoring based on the probability that a given clinical condition exists, given a specified degree of progres-

sion along one or more branches of a diagnostic algorithm (36).

Process criteria-standards include information on outcomes, indirectly, if they specify complications that lengthen stay and the condition of the patient at discharge. But there can also be, as in Table 4.7, a direct specification of the outcomes to be expected if care is appropriate and is skillfully executed. To be more complete, the criteria-standards should also specify the time window during which the outcomes are to be measured. Some outcome criteria-standards select a time subsequent to the initiation of care when virtually every person should have been relieved of the condition that was responsible for seeking care. Single cases that have fallen

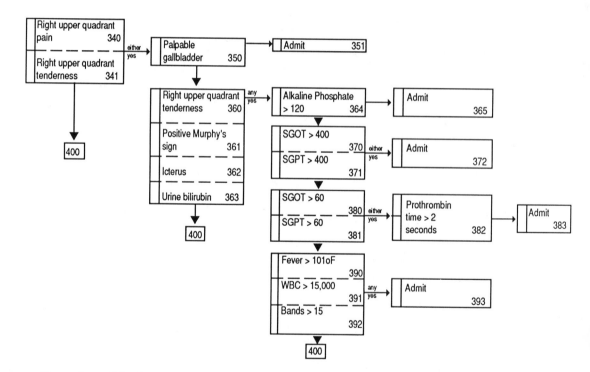

Figure 4.5.   Criteria map for abdominal pain that may be caused by cholecystitis. This is only part of a larger criteria map for abdominal pain that specifies indications for admission to the hospital. This excerpt begins with a notation about right upper quadrant pain or tenderness and seeks to identify the presence of cholecystitis, hepatitis, or any other serious condition in the area of the gallbladder. In the larger map, cholecystitis can be identified through other findings as well. Criteria are numbered to facilitate routing through the map. Positive responses to a criterion lead to the next item to the right. Negative responses and missing information responses are directed down to the next vertical item. (Donabedian A. Explorations in quality assessment and monitoring. Vol. II: The criteria and standards of quality. Ann Arbor: Health Administration Press, 1980:367–368.)

short of the standard can, then, be called in for review (37). This is in contrast to another variety of criteria-standards for which the time window is selected to be both convenient and as revealing as possible of outcome differences among levels of quality in care. Outcome standards are in the form of percentages of cases that attain specified outcomes. Therefore, assessments of quality can be made only when the experience of a group of cases falls short of the standard by a significant margin, significance being established statistically and judgmentally (6, 38).

Evaluation

Many of the issues pertinent to the evaluation of criteria and standards have already surfaced in the preceding discussion of the features of implicit and explicit criteria. But some recapitulation and expansion might be useful. The order in which the evaluative attributes will be discussed is shown in Table 4.8.

Perhaps the first step in evaluating criteria and standards is to note their scope, meaning the extent to which they embody the several attributes of quality described in the first part of this chapter. Quality assessment in clinical settings focuses on the effectiveness of technical care, and the criteria-standards of assessment reflect this preoccupation. Efficiency is taken into account by attention to justification of

Table 4.8.
Some Evaluative Characteristics of Criteria and Standards[a]

Scope
Validity
    Scientific
    Consensual
Currency
Reliability
Adaptability to case variation
Importance and differential weighting
Screening efficiency
Stringency

[a]Donabedian A. A primer of quality assurance and monitoring. In: Law practice quality evaluation: An appraisal of peer review and other measures to enhance professional performance. Philadelphia: American Law Institute and American Bar Association, October 1988:132.

admission and length of stay, particularly in hospitals. Some criteria lists are designed especially with site-of-care appropriateness in view (39, 40). Beyond attention to the site of care, most criteria lists are not good at identifying and down-rating unnecessary or unnecessarily costly care. The aspects of care that contribute to acceptability or legitimacy are almost never reflected in explicit criteria.

After ascertaining the scope of criteria-standards, the most important single attribute to establish is their validity, meaning their ability to represent completely and truthfully whatever attribute of quality they purport to measure. As already pointed out, the validity of criteria-standards for technical care derives from scientifically established prior knowledge about the relations among features of structure, process, and outcome. Where scientific evidence is lacking, it is customary to be guided by the opinion of experts. Consensus among experts is taken partly as interim evidence of validity; partly it is needed to make the criteria-standards acceptable to those who are to be judged by them. But, at the same time, it is important to remain alert to scientific progress, so that the criteria-standards are frequently revised to include innovations of verified usefulness, whereas the less useful or discredited is deleted.

Reliability of measurement, which is the ability of several measurements of the same thing to arrive at the same conclusion, is, of course, a necessary prerequisite to validity. Still, measurements may be reliable, but not valid, if the unintended attribute is being measured. As already pointed out, judgments of quality using implicit criteria tend to be unreliable, although reliability can be improved by observing the precautions described earlier. It also helps if the judges are provided with careful guidelines that structure the task of assessment in advance (41–43).

Judgments based on explicit criteria are very reliable, but, sometimes, the validity of the judgments has been questioned. One contribution to invalidity is inability to adapt to variations in the characteristics of individual cases within a category, a problem already discussed. Another is the tendency to overload the lists of criteria-standards with items of lesser importance to case management and to improved outcomes. Eliminating clearly questionable items and differentially weighting those that remain would seem to be reasonable remedies. Unfortunately, there is, as yet, no clear cut evidence that differential weighting has much effect on the judgments of quality that result (44).

The validity of explicit criteria also influences their usefulness as screens to prepare the way for review by implicit criteria, as already described. Screening efficiency requires that the explicit criteria point to the greatest number of cases in which quality proves to have been poor, while falsely incriminating as poor the fewest cases in which quality proves to have been good. But it should be remembered that, for practical purposes, the optimum balance is not necessarily the one which achieves the cleanest separation of good quality from poor. This is because the penalty associated with calling care bad when, in fact, it is good, is likely to be different from that of calling care good when, in fact, it is bad (45).

The stringency of the criteria is an evaluative characteristic of some practical importance. If the criteria-standards require such a high level of performance that every case is found to have failed, they are likely to be rejected. If the criteria-standards are set at too low a level, so everyone passes, they lose their capacity to stimulate reform. The ability to discriminate among different levels of quality is a property to be valued in criteria-standards.

Procedure for Formulating Explicit Criteria and Standards

Table 4.9 shows the key steps in a procedure for formulating lists of explicit criteria and standards, mainly for the technical process of care, but including outcomes as well.

The first step is to assemble one or more groups of experts, each to be entrusted with developing criteria-standards in the area of care corresponding to its expertise. Besides ensuring expertise, it is useful to make the panels as representative as possi-

Table 4.9.
Procedure for Formulating Criteria and Standards for Technical Care[a]

Selection of panels
  Expertise
  Representativeness, influence, etc.
Selection of method for consensus
  Traditional committee
  "Nominal group process," "Delphi"
Selection of phenomena to be assessed
Selection of criteria/standards
  Assembling inclusive set
  Rating of items
    "Importance," "relevance," "recordability," reliability of information, feasibility, etc.
  Selection of agreed-upon subset
  Weighting, if desired
  Specification of "time window" for outcome criteria
  Specification of achievable standards
Specification of sources of information, procedures and rules for abstracting, etc.
Testing through pilot implementation: feasibility, reliability and accuracy of judgments, etc.

[a] Donabedian A. A primer of quality assurance and monitoring. In: Law practice quality evaluation: An appraisal of peer review and other measures to enhance professional performance. Philadelphia: American Law Institute and American Bar Association, October 1988:132.

ble of relevant professional subgroups and their organizations. It is important to remember that the formulation of criteria and standards has significant political implications as well; those who control them are in a position, through them, to control clinical practice itself.

Next in line is choosing a method for arriving at agreement among the members of each panel. The traditional committee procedures may do, but more structured methods such as the Delphi technique, the nominal group process, or some combination or modification of these are often recommended. In the Delphi method, panels can be large, since the members do not meet. Each member is polled by mail or telephone. The opinions expressed are anonymously assembled, tabulated, and summarized, and the results sent back to each member, with a request to reaffirm or modify the original opinion in the light of the opinions of the members of the panel as a group. After one or more such rounds, individual opinions tend to stabilize, so the polling is terminated (46).

The nominal group process requires that members of each panel attend a meeting, which limits their number somewhat. At the meeting, each member is asked to offer a written opinion without consulting other members. These opinions are assembled, displayed, and discussed. Then each member is asked for a final written opinion, again without consultation (47).

The more structured methods of eliciting group opinion allow a sharing of views; but, by virtue of anonymous polling, they eliminate or reduce the possibility that more forceful members will unduly influence or inhibit the others. The opinion adopted may be that of a specified majority, or it may be expressed as a measure of central tendency, such as mean or median. More complex decision rules may be adopted, for example that a specified, large proportion will strongly approve a specified course of action, but without there being a strongly disapproving minority of significant size.

After these preliminaries are settled, the expert panels can begin their work. Using the methods described, they select the phenomena to be assessed, guided by the principles of importance, representativeness, and feasibility already described. Then it is time to formulate the criteria and standards. To accomplish this, it is useful to begin with a rather large set assembled partly from the literature, partly from preexisting lists, and partly from the recommendations of individual panel members. Next, the items in this intentionally unwieldy set are weighted according to importance to good care and relevance to good outcomes. Sometimes, they are also rated according to "recordability," which is the likelihood that the information needed to ascertain compliance with a criterion-standard will be found in the medical record. On the basis of these initial weights, the subset of highly approved items is assembled. If desired, these are weighted according to relative importance. For outcomes, the time window is specified (6, 48, 49).

Having formulated the criteria and standards, some additional work is needed to help in their implementation. This would include saying where the information about compliance with the criteria is to be found, preparing instructions for abstracting that information, and, perhaps, specifying how case mix is to be standardized (6). Then, there is a period of testing to find out how difficult, costly, reliable, acceptable, and efficient the proposed method of assessment is. When pilot testing is satisfactorily completed, the criteria and standards can be offered for general use.

Sources of Information

It is not possible to measure quality unless one has information about features of structure, process, and outcome that pertain to the attributes of quality to be measured. The accuracy and completeness of that information determine the accuracy and completeness of the corresponding judgments of quality. That is why, in a chapter on measurement, at least a little needs to be said about the sources of information partially listed in Table 4.10.

The medical record is the single most important source of information for assessing the technical process of care and the outcomes of the process that occur before care is terminated. Unfortunately, medical records are not always well kept, are often incomplete, and sometimes inaccurate. Therefore, judgments on quality based on

Table 4.10.
Some Sources of Information

Medical records
Opinion surveys
    Of patients (and family)
    Of providers of care
Population surveys
    Accessibility
    Acceptability
    Measures of health, disability, etc.
Statistical reports
    Vital statistics, etc.
    Data available to programs that finance and
       provide care
Direct observation
    Of structure
    Of process
    Of outcomes

such records are often disparaged, even rejected, for being judgments on recording rather than on the quality of care itself. One might put up some defense by saying that good recording is, in itself, an important contribution to good care. One might add that there is a demonstrable, though small, correlation between good recording and judgments of quality more or less independent of recording (42, 50). But the only real remedy is radical improvement in the records themselves.

In addition to documenting more completely the patient's condition, the care provided, and the results achieved, the record should reveal the objectives of care and how these objectives were influenced by patient preferences and societal directives. In particular, the records ought to say more about the interpersonal process, perhaps to the point of having patients record their own impressions of the care they have received. In practice, none of these improvements is likely to occur soon. Therefore, in many cases it is imperative to talk to the clinicians responsible for care, and to the patient as well, so as to interpret and supplement the record.

More systematic surveys of the opinions of patients and practitioners can also be helpful. Patients can provide credible information about some aspects of technical care, especially if it is recent. But their unique contribution is to tell us about the acceptability of care, in general, and of the interpersonal process in particular. Under certain circumstances, much can be learned from eliciting the opinions of health care personnel and supportive staff, and also of administrators and other knowledgeable persons in the community.

Surveys of the general population can provide information about the accessibility of care and its acceptability once access has occurred. One can also learn about the magnitude and distribution of ill health and disability in the population, these being rough indicators of the outcomes of care. Statistical data compiled by health departments and by agencies that finance care, provide it, or do both can also provide information, most of it presumptive, about problems in quality that might require further study.

Direct observation is, of course, a time-honored method of assessing the physical structure of health settings, including their safety, hygiene, amenities, and capacity to provide good care. The process of care can also be observed, either directly or by videotaping. Observation of care may alter usual behavior, providing a better picture than everyday realities might warrant. Still, it is useful, especially for assessing the finer points of personal interactions, and as an educational tool (41, 48, 51, 52). The outcomes of care are also often amenable to detailed assessment by direct, independent examination of patients.

This sketchy account of sources of information is perhaps enough to suggest that good information is the lifeblood of quality measurement. For more on this subject and on everything else this chapter could only touch upon, readers must look elsewhere. It is hoped that they are now better prepared to undertake that lengthier exploration.

References

1. Lohr KN. Outcome measurement: Concepts and questions. Inquiry 1988;25:37–50.
2. Lohr KN, ed. Advances in health status measurement: Proceedings of a conference. Med Care 1989;27:S1–S294, March supplement.
3. Fanshel S, Bush JW. A health-status index and its application to health-services outcomes. Operations Res 1970;18:1021–1066.
4. Kaplan RM, Bush JW. Health-related quality of life measurements for evaluation research and policy analysis. Health Psychol 1982;1:61–80.
5. Mosteller F, Falotico-Taylor J, eds. Quality of life and technology assessment. Washington, DC: National Academy Press, 1989.
6. Brook RH, Davies-Avery A, Greenfield S, Harris LJ, Lelah T, Solomon NE, Ware JE, Jr. Assessing the quality of medical care using outcome measures: An overview of the method. Med Care 1977;15:1–165, September supplement.
7. Cochrane AL. Effectiveness and efficiency: Random reflections on health services. London: Nuffield Provincial Trust, 1972.
8. Hodgson TA, Meiners MR. Cost-of-illness methodology: A guide to current practices and procedures. Milbank Memorial Fund Health Soc 1982; 60:429–462.
9. Torrance GW. Measurement of health status utilities for economic appraisal: A review. Health Econ 1986;5:1–30.
10. Donabedian A. The clients' view of quality. In: Donabedian A, ed. Explorations in quality assessment and monitoring, Vol. 1: The definition of quality and approaches to its assessment. Ann

Arbor: Health Administration Press, 1980: 36–48.

11. McNeil BJ, Pauker SG, Sox HC, Jr., Tversky A. On the elicitation of preferences for alternative therapies. N Engl J Med 1982;306:1259–1262.

12. Ware JE, Jr, Davies-Avery A, Stewart AL. The measurement and meaning of patient satisfaction. Health Med Serv Rev 1978;1:1–15.

13. Locker D, Dunt D. Theoretical and methodological issues in sociological studies of consumer satisfaction with medical care. Soc Sci Med 1978;12:283–292.

14. Ware JE, Jr, Snyder MK, Wright WR, Davies AR. Defining and measuring patient satisfaction with medical care. Eval Program Planning 1983;6:247–263.

15. Cleary PD, McNeil BJ. Patient satisfaction as an indicator of quality care. Inquiry 1988;25:25–36.

16. Donabedian A. Quality and cost: Choices and responsibilities. Inquiry 1988;25:90–99.

17. Donabedian A. Evaluating the quality of medical care. Milbank Memorial Fund 1966;44:166–203, July, part 2.

18. Scott WR, Forrest WH, Jr, Brown BW. Hospital structure and postoperative mortality and morbidity. In: Shortell SM, Brown M, eds. Organization research in hospitals. Chicago: Blue Cross Association, 1976:72–89.

19. Hornbrook MC. Hospital case mix: Its definition, measurement, and use, Parts 1 and 2. Med Care Rev 1982;39:1–43, 73–123.

20. Cretin S, Worthman LG. Alternative systems for case mix classification in health care financing. Santa Monica: The Rand Corporation, 1986.

21. Blumberg MS. Risk adjusting health care outcomes. Med Care Rev 1986;43:351–393.

22. Thomas JW, Longo DR. Application of severity measurement systems for hospital quality management. Hosp Health Serv Admin 1990;35:221–243.

23. McAuliffe WE. Measuring the quality of medical care: Process versus outcome. Milbank Memorial Fund Health Soc 1979;57:118–152.

24. Donabedian A. Basic approaches to assessment: Structure, process, and outcome. In: Donabedian A, ed. Explorations in quality assessment and monitoring, Vol. 1: The definition of quality and approaches to its assessment. Ann Arbor: Health Administration Press, 1980:77–128.

25. Palmer RH, Reilly MC. Individual and institutional variables which may serve as indicators of quality of medical care. Med Care 1979;17:693–717.

26. Donabedian A. The epidemiology of quality. Inquiry 1985;22:282–292.

27. Williamson JW. Formulating priorities for quality assurance activity: Description of a method and its application. JAMA 1978;239:631–637.

28. Kessner DM, Kalk CE, Singer J. Assessing health quality—The case for tracers. N Engl J Med 1973;288:189–194.

29. Kessner DM, Snow CK, Singer J. Contrasts in health status, Vol. 2: Assessment of medical care for children. Washington, D.C.: Institute of Medicine, National Academy of Sciences, 1974.

30. Donabedian A. Explorations in quality assessment and monitoring, Vol. 2: The criteria and standards of quality. Ann Arbor: Health Administration Press, 1982.

31. Donabedian A. Criteria and standards for quality assessment and monitoring. Quality Rev Bull 1986;99:99–108.

32. Donabedian A. A guide to medical care administration, Vol. 2: medical care appraisal. New York: American Public Health Association, 1969:70 ff.

33. Donabedian A. Advantages and limitations of explicit criteria for assessing the quality of health care. Milbank Memorial Fund Health Soc 1981;59:99–106.

34. Payne BC, Lyons TF, Dwarshius L, Kolton M, Morris W. The quality of medical care: Evaluation and improvement. Chicago: Hospital Research and Educational Trust, 1976:15 ff.

35. Greenfield S, Lewis CE, Kaplan SH, Davidson MB. Peer review by criteria mapping: Criteria for diabetes mellitus: The use of decision-making in chart audit. Ann Intern Med 1975;83:761–770.

36. Greenfield S, Cretin S, Worthman LG, Dorey FJ, Solomon NE, Goldberg GA. Comparison of a criteria map to a criteria list in quality-of-care assessment for patients with chest pain: The relation of each to outcome. Med Care 1981; 19:255–272.

37. Mushlin AI, Appel FA. Testing an outcome-based quality assurance strategy in primary care. Med Care 1980;18:1–100, May supplement.

38. Williamson JW. Assessing and improving health care outcomes: The health accounting approach to quality assurance. Cambridge, MA: Ballinger Publishing Company, 1978.

39. Gertman PM, Restuccia J. The appropriateness evaluation protocol: A technique for assessing unnecessary days of hospital care. Med Care 1981;19:69–85.

40. Kreger BE, Restuccia JD. Assessing the need to hospitalize children: Pediatric appropriateness evaluation protocol. Pediatrics 1989;84:242–247.

41. Peterson OL, Andrews LP, Spain RS, Greenberg, BG. An analytical study of North Carolina general practice, 1953–54. J Med Educ 1956;31:1–165, part 2 of December.

42. Rosenfeld LS. Quality of medical care in hospitals. Am J Public Health 1957;47:856–865.

43. Dubois RW, Brook RH. Preventable deaths: Who, how often, and why? Ann Intern Med 1988;109: 582–589.

44. Lyons TF, Payne BC. The use of item weights in assessing physician performance with predetermined criteria indices. Med Care 1975;13:432–439.

45. McClain JO. Decision modeling in case selection for medical utilization review. Management Sci 1972;18:B706–B717.

46. Dalkey NC, Rourke DL, Lewis R, Snyder D. The quality of life: Delphi decision-making. Lexington, MA: Lexington Books, D.C. Heath and Company, 1972.

47. Delbecq AL, Van de Ven AH. A group process model for problem identification and program planning. J Appl Behav Sci 1971;7:466–492.

48. Riedel RL, Riedel DC. Practice and performance: An assessment of ambulatory care. Ann Arbor: Health Administration Press, 1979.

49. Hulka BS, Romm FJ, Parkerson GR, Jr, Russell IT,

Clapp NE, Johnson FS. Peer review in ambulatory care: Use of explicit criteria and implicit judgments. Med Care 1979;17:1–73, March supplement.

50. Lyons TF, Payne BC. The relationship of physicians' medical recording performance to their medical care performance. Med Care 1974;12:714–720.

51. Hinz CF. Direct observation as a means of teaching and evaluating clinical skills. J Med Educ 1966;41:150–161.

52. Royal College of General Practitioners. What sort of doctor: Assessing quality of care in general practice. London: Royal College of General Practitioners, 1985;3:20–21.

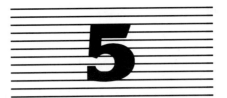

Setting Standards

Marguerite M. Jackson, R.N., M.S., C.I.C.

The attempt to regulate health care practices with standards had its origins with Florence Nightingale when she began to establish standards regarding food, noise, and patient care conditions for wounded troops at Scutari in 1859 (1). From this beginning, the setting of standards and the measuring of actual practice have become an integral part of the health care delivery system.

This chapter will discuss the use of standards in three contexts: (*a*) licensure of health care providers and agencies, (*b*) government regulation of the health care environment, and (*c*) the relationship to accreditation of facilities by the Joint Commission on Accreditation of Healthcare Organizations (JCAHO). The standards for setting standards, developed by an expert panel commissioned by the National Academy of Sciences Institute of Medicine in 1989, will also be presented. Finally, as an example of the interplay among these contexts, together with the influence of consumer pressures to make changes in standards, the care of the elderly in long-term care facilities will be discussed.

STANDARDS FOR PROFESSIONAL LICENSURE

In Starr's (2) analysis of the social transformation of American medicine, licensure was tightly connected with the movement toward professionalism in medicine, the creation of the first medical schools and societies, and agitation for protective medical legislation. In fact, the first licensure law calling for prospective examination of physicians was enacted in New York City in 1760. The first medical school in the United States was opened in Philadelphia in 1765 at what is now The University of Pennsylvania; however, regulation of the newly emerging schools began only in the early 1900s (2, p. 118) and was greatly strengthened when results of the Flexner Report were published in 1910 (3). The initiative for new medical schools in the 19th century came from groups of physicians who approached local colleges with proposals. These faculty members were unsalaried and were paid by their students only if they passed. Although some medical school faculty wanted to raise the American profession to the prestige and status level of physicians in Europe, there was no evidence that, even with licensure, sanctions were ever enforced against unlicensed practitioners for many years (4). The reasons why licensing persisted for several decades, in spite of its lack of effectiveness, were similar to reasons why medical schools multiplied: they both served the immediate interests of the parties to the transaction (2, p. 45).

Concurrently, efforts were being made to establish medical societies and in 1781, the Massachusetts Medical Society was incorporated, but the closed corporate culture proved impossible to maintain, and in 1803 it ceased to be a closed corporation.

Although the initial intent of the Society was to limit the number of fellows, it became less exclusive in order to maintain viability and admitted anyone who passed an examination and practiced for 3 years in good repute (5).

The American Medical Association

The American Medical Association (AMA) also had its early beginnings in the mid-19th century with a primary goal of raising and standardizing the requirements for medical degrees. It also enacted a code of professional ethics intended to exclude sectarian and untrained practitioners; however, the AMA had little impact for at least 50 years. The AMA's efforts at voluntary reform of medical education also failed, as the schools would not comply (2, p. 91). As Vanderpoel (6) stated in 1883, "[the AMA was] a purely voluntary organization without any chartered privileges and with no authority to enforce its own edicts."

Contributing to the difficulty of maintaining exclusivity for licensed physicians was the dialectic between professionalism and the nation's democratic culture. Although many physicians attempted to raise standards, dignity, and privileges through medical schools, societies, and licensing, the democratic ideals of America encouraged an openness that was difficult to control. The result was that the position of physicians became less secure (2, p. 54). State legislatures that had enacted licensing laws into the 1820s began rescinding them in quick succession, and by midcentury, there were few states that still had licensure statutes. What fundamentally destroyed licensure in the early 19th century was an interpretation of it as an expression of favoritism rather than of competence. This was at variance from the democratic ideals of the time and was interpreted by many as an attempt by physicians to recreate English institutions in America. In Friedson's (7, p. 20) discussion of the evolution of the profession of medicine, he commented that egalitarianism in the 19th century led to the belief that freedom to heal others should not be hampered by licensing laws, and that the rapid expansion of the United States precluded the enforcement of rules about who could heal others. In fact, by the end of the century there were many persons on the frontier who called themselves "doctor" who had no formal training.

Between 1850 and 1880, conflicts intensified between practitioners of homeopathy (founded by the German physician Samuel Hahnemann), who saw disease fundamentally as a matter of spirit, and orthodox medicine, which insisted that homeopaths be expelled from the profession. These conflicts consumed considerable energy and time and had an effect on the profession that cannot be measured in numbers; as long as physicians were divided, any move by orthodox medicine to bring back licensing or to reform medical education seemed self-serving. Public resistance to orthodox claims eventually brought concessions and compromises, and beginning in the 1870s and 1880s, there was common support for restoration of medical licensing.

Over the next few decades, a much better basis for legitimacy of the medical profession turned out to be scientific progress in understanding the complexities of illness. This rapidly expanding scientific data base provided a growing complexity and specialization to medical information such that the pubic, through its legislators and individual decisions, gradually acknowledged that "every man could not be his own physician . . ." (2, p. 59). This led to legitimization of the profession of medicine, increasing professional independence and autonomy, and eventual reenactment of licensure laws that were based on uniform standards of medical education (8). With uniform training, licensed physicians could be expected to have a basic technical education that was distinct from that of other kinds of healers. With a sound technical basis for training and political consolidation of the nation, physicians could win public confidence. Thereafter, enforcing licensing laws became possible (7, p. 21).

The Licensing Movement

The licensing movement in the late 19th century was not restricted to physicians or those in professions, but was also extended to many different types of tradespeople. Historically, the purpose of licensure was to insure safety of the public, and this benefit could logically be applied to licensure for any occupations that provided services to the public (e.g., barbers, plumbers, pharmacists, embalmers). More importantly, the occupations in which their leaders pursued interests through licensing were distinguished less by their political power than by their distinctive structural position within the economy. Most of these individuals were self-employed, their trades or professions were easy to enter, and competition for business could be intense. Most important, however, none of the occupations seeking licensure faced organized buyers or employers who stood to lose by the monopoly that licensing would create because most services were provided to individuals, not organizations. These factors helped minimize political opposition to licensing legislation; the people most immediately affected by licensure were generally unorganized and unskilled competitors. Since most licensure statutes provided for "grandfathering" of persons in business at the time, there was little opposition to the legislation (2, p. 103). By 1901, all states and jurisdictions had a licensing statute (medical practice act) of some sort for physicians (9).

In the same year, the AMA revised its constitution, created the House of Delegates, and developed an organizational structure that neatly forced all physicians who wanted to belong to their county medical society or to the national AMA to become dues-paying members of their state association. This led to rapid transformation of state medical societies and provided resources for reorganization on a uniform plan. In a remarkably short period, physicians began to achieve the unity and coherence so long desired. By 1920, membership in the AMA had reached 60% of practicing physicians, and the power of "organized medicine" was well established (2, pp. 109–110).

By 1987, 35 health professions and occupations were licensed by one or more states. Individual licensure is a complex matter and represents a contract between the professional group and the state legislature granting control over individuals' entrance into, maintenance of good standing in, and exit from the profession. Most professions are responsible for defining the content of their work, and they gain virtual monopoly over the provision of that work to the public. In return, the profession theoretically guarantees to the state legislatures that the work will be of good quality. Enforcement of licensure agreements is through the criminal justice system (10). There is little evidence that the criteria used in licensing actually predict the quality of care to be delivered or protect the public (11); however, there is ample evidence that licensure serves to protect the professional group and its members from competition and public scrutiny.

Physician Dominance in Health Care Arena

Physicians are in an unusual professional position because they not only control their own work but are the dominant profession in the health care arena directing the work of others. In fact, Freidson states that, in order to escape subordination to medical authority, other licensed health care personnel must find some area of work over which they can maintain a monopoly because, to attain the autonomy of a profession, the occupation must control a fairly discrete area of work that can be separated from the main body of medicine and practiced without dependence on medicine. Few of the licensed health care professions deal with such potentially autonomous areas, although many claim to do so. Even an aggressive occupation like nursing with its own schools, graduate programs, and control of many licensing boards finds that much of the work performed by its members remains subject to the requirements of another occupation, professional medicine (7, pp. 67–70). A paradox of this hierarchical arrangement is that those with the most authority (physicians) have the least regulation through licensure because the authority to practice medicine, once licensure has been obtained, is generally for life. Although many states have instituted certain continuing medical education (CME) requirements for license renewal, attendance is generally sufficient to meet the statutory mandate (12), whereas there are strict limitations placed on most other health professionals subject to licensure (13, p. 270).

In response to growing concerns that licensure of physicians has not met the objectives for which it was intended, and in order to make it an effective tool in the pursuit of quality care, the Health Care Quality Improvement Act of 1986 (Public Law 99-660) included provisions to establish a National Practitioner Data Bank (NPDB). Data to be deposited in the NPDB include information about malpractice payments on behalf of any licensed health practitioner as a result of a court judgment or out-of-court settlement, disciplinary actions against licensed physicians or dentists by state medical and dental boards, adverse actions taken by health care entities against physician's or dentist's clinical privileges (when actions will last more than 30 days), and adverse actions taken against members by professional societies when they have been reached by peer review assessing practitioner competency and/or professional conduct. Members of other health care fields may also be reported, but it is not mandated except for malpractice data (14). The NPDB is intended to facilitate sharing of information among states and to close loopholes that permit interstate movement of marginal practitioners.

The authority to mandate such data collection at the federal level stems from increasing federal involvement in all aspects of health care initiated in the 1960s with the Medicare and Medicaid programs. When the government assumed major responsibility for paying the bills of the elderly and the poor, the cost of health care rose much faster than other segments of the economy. Controlling costs became a dominant force in the public and political arena.

A variety of administrative and review mechanisms for monitoring physician practice has developed over the past two decades and many believe that the changes were long overdue. Freidson noted "It was the profession's own failure to regulate itself in the public interest that created the legal, economic, and political pressures of the past twenty years . . ." (7, p. 390). Even though the regulations will limit technical autonomy of practitioners, the practice standards that are created and administered remain within the control of the profession at large. However, they are intended to reduce discretionary choices of practitioners and limit patients to services only within the limits that are officially approved. Freidson states

It is true that the closer the methods of controlling cost and quality come to resemble those employed in the industrial production of goods, the lower the monetary cost per standardized unit . . . such "efficiency" is gained at the cost of transforming most patients and their problems into industrial objects and withholding service from others . . . . In order to provide a truly human service, practitioners must have a significant degree of autonomy within reasonable limits dictated by patients' rights, official standards, and autonomy . . . [while] stopping well short of reducing practitioners to passive cogs in a rationalized system . . . . (From Freidson E. Profession of medicine: A study of the sociology of applied knowledge. Chicago: University of Chicago Press, 1988:391. © 1970, 1988 by Eliot Freidson.)

ADDITIONAL EXTERNAL CONTROLS OF THE HEALTH CARE SYSTEM

Licensing of major health care facilities did not become common until the 1940s (15); however, all states now license hospitals, nursing homes, and pharmacies (10). In addition, states may also license homes for the mentally retarded and services such as ambulances and home health care. State agencies generally license facilities, and health departments of most states are responsible for licensure of health care facilities. Institutional licenses may be granted for varying periods of time, the minimum usually being 1 year.

Although licensing as a role of government is viewed as a critical component to protecting the public, voluntary self-regulation through accreditation and professional certification is another dominant theme in the development of standards. Examples include the JCAHO that accredits health care organizations (16) and boards for certification of individuals with medical and other specialties (11, p. 372).

Licensure, accreditation, and professional certification make up a combination of external controls that are more extensive in the United States than anywhere else in the world. Vladeck (17) describes two primary reasons why they are also more extensive, intrusive, and complex: first, precisely because the American system is so decentralized, pluralistic, and fragmented; and second, because, to a large degree, the nature of external controls is not well understood by the providers due to the nature of the American legal system. In the context of external control over the quality of health services, subjective clinical judgment rarely generates the kind of documentable, objective, testable evidence that is needed for legal sanctions. Although for many years the legal system often deferred to entities such as the JCAHO by delegating extraordinary autonomy to them, the public willingness to accept unquestioningly the unsupervised decision making of professionals is increasingly being challenged. Many question whether this eroding confidence might have been prevented had professionals done a better job at self-regulation in the past, but more relevant is the notion that experience, subjectivity, and judgment do not fit with standards and biases of formalized, legalized external controls. Because of the difficulties presented by these dilemmas, external controls have traditionally focused on aspects of service quality that may not constitute high-quality service but are relatively objective in nature and lend themselves to some form of objective measurement.

Process of External Control

The process of external control of health services has three steps. First, the adoption of formal standards that define a set of common expectations about the basic characteristics of the system in which they all participate. As suggested by current activities by the JCAHO, the Health Care Financing Administration (HCFA) requirements for receipt of Medicare funds, and federal conditions of participation for nursing homes, the standards-setting process and the policy-making process have become one. "Formal standards adopted by authoritative external control agencies not only embody policy, they *are* policy . . ." (17).

The second step, surveillance of providers to assess the degree of compliance with those standards, is based on the belief that people perform better when other people are watching. Indeed, this is the rationale pioneered by Cruse (18) over two decades ago when he reported on the probable beneficial effect of providing surgeons with incidence data and secular trends on their own patients' wound infection rates. This strategy has also been widely promoted by Haley (19) and others as a way of reducing surgical infection rates. Vladek (17) comments that the benefits of surveillance, in terms of eliciting improved compliance, probably diminish with increased surveillance activity and coincident increased cost. In addition, excessively intrusive surveillance may engender hostility on the part of providers. Perhaps most damaging is the potential for surveillance to become an end in itself and a substitute for more effective or more relevant activities that external control agencies are not capable of, or willing to, perform (17).

The third step is imposition of whatever sanctions or incentives the external control agency may use in response to reported deviations from standards. The existence of sanctions, and the possibility that they may be invoked, is a powerful incentive for many health care facilities. Indeed, agencies that can impose sanctions have considerable power. For example, the Joint Commission (in exercising its option to withhold accreditation from facilities failing to comply with JCAHO standards) or HFCA (in determining that a facility has failed to comply with its rules for conditions of participation) can have direct impact on the facility's financial base and ability to continue to deliver health care services (17, 20).

Federal Program Sanctions

The use of sanctions is an integral part of federal programs designed to address incentives for the prevailing financing mechanisms for health care. These programs have included the Experimental Medical Care Review Organizations (EMCROs) (in existence between 1970 and 1975), which was a prototype for Professional Standards Review Organizations (PSROs), now replaced by Utilization and Quality Control Peer Review Organizations (PROs). Although the PROs theoretically have a considerably stronger hand in sanctioning physicians and hospitals than the PSROs, a recent Institute of Medicine study found that their regulatory power has not been demonstrably enhanced (13, p. 145).

In summary, as knowledge and understanding of the complexities of good health care increase, so does understanding of the multiple factors that apparently impinge on the quality of health care. Historically, professionalism has been relied on as the primary mechanism to assure quality (21, 22). Regulatory efforts have attempted to use and support professionalism, but at times they have been perceived as hostile or actively detrimental to it. The ideals of professionalism are in direct conflict with ideals of competition and market forces and with the atmosphere created by malpractice litigation. Some professionals believe that these forces result in an erosion of the provider-patient relationship. Nonetheless, professional self-examination has fostered the development of standards, criteria, and efforts at continuing professional growth. Participation in voluntary accreditation programs such as those of the JCAHO reflects a broader institutional and corporate provider perspective of professionalism (13, p. 33).

CRITERIA FOR SETTING STANDARDS FOR QUALITY OF CARE

In 1986, the Congress of the United States called upon the Secretary of the United States Department of Health and Human Services to solicit a proposal from the National Academy of Sciences (NAS) to conduct a study to design a strategy for quality review and assurance in Medicare. This charge was part of the Omnibus Budget Reconciliation Act (OBRA 1986: Section 9313, Public Law 99-509). The purpose of the study was to address eight legislative charges, including among them one to "develop prototype criteria and standards for defining and measuring quality of care." With general oversight from the Institute of Medicine (IOM) Committee to Design a Strategy for Quality Review and Assurance in Medicare (Steven A. Schroeder, Chair), a special expert panel (11 members with staff support from the IOM) was convened in 1989 to develop recommendations concerning standards by which quality-of-care criteria and appropriateness of practice guidelines might be evaluated. Some results of their work are presented in Tables 5.1 and 5.3 and will be discussed here (13, pp. 303–342).

Good criteria for distinguishing appropriate from inappropriate care and for assessing quality of care can be used to strengthen the clinical basis for review activities intended to detect and avoid unnecessary care and avoid costs. In addition, they can be used to identify or prevent underuse of care that might be an undesirable effect of financial incentives, review programs, or other cost control methods.

A prerequisite for developing useful and acceptable criteria for standards was to gain agreement on desirable attributes of quality-of-care criteria. The panel first identified three broad types of criteria sets: (a) appropriateness guidelines, (b) patient care evaluation and management criteria, and (c) case-finding screens.

Appropriateness Guidelines. Appropriateness guidelines are used to describe accepted indications for medical interventions and technology such as surgical procedures and diagnostic studies. Guidelines may specify under what circumstances a particular service is indicated (appropriate) and may identify areas of uncertainty where there is lack of agreement among clinicians. Appropriateness is an integral part of quality health care, and in the context of developing criteria sets, the service in question should have demonstrated clinical benefit with a likelihood that benefits clearly outweigh harm.

Third party payers and Medicare also develop standards for appropriate indications for various technologies and procedures. Their primary purpose is to use these standards for utilization review or coverage decisions intended to control costs. PRO preadmission review criteria are a type of appropriateness guidelines. Independent organizations such as the RAND Corporation have also used various research methodologies to develop guidelines for appropriate use of various technologies.

Patient Care Evaluation and Patient Management Criteria Sets. These criteria sets have evolved to help guide and assess management of particular medical problems rather than specific services or technology. Traditionally, criteria developed for evaluating patient care have dealt with the complexity and variability presented by patients with differing clinical presentations, sociodemographic characteristics, and treatment preferences by identifying the minimum process elements for managing a particular condition. Substantial clinical judgment is allowed beyond the minimum, partly because clinical research and resources are lacking to provide greater specificity. Computerized software, detailed algorithms, decision trees, criteria maps, and other approaches have been suggested as ways of increasing objectivity in patient management; however, many of these approaches are complex and lack practicality in normal clinical or crisis situations.

Case-Finding Screens. Potential quality-of-care problems that warrant further evaluation can be identified using case-finding screens, which are objective, easily used, and possibly related to complications resulting from either provider or system problems. Case-finding screens are also called "occurrence screens" or "generic screens" and have been used by the PROs for several years. These facilitywide process or outcome criteria are intended to be broadly applicable across many departments and specialties and have been adopted by the American Hospital Associ-

ation's "Integrated Quality Assurance" (IQA) program (23).

Specialty-specific clinical indicators now being developed by the JCAHO are another variety of case-finding screens (24–28). The JCAHO clinical indicators are used to assess a measurable aspect of patient care as a guide to assess performance of individual practitioners or the health care organization (see Chapter 2 for further discussion). The indicators may be either adverse outcomes linked to a process under the control of the provider or the system, or processes that have been clearly associated with adverse outcomes (25).

Other types of case-finding screens include rates of events above or below a defined level (threshold) to prompt further evaluation of a potential problem. Aggregated rates of other adverse occurrences can also be used as flags for possible institutional quality-of-care problems.

O'Leary (29), speaking for the JCAHO, pointed out in 1988 that "The science that lies within quality assessment is an epidemiologic science. . . . But the epidemiology [of quality assessment] is in its infancy. . . ." However, epidemiologists have been analyzing aggregated data for decades, and Donabedian (30) recently summarized contributions of epidemiology to quality assessment and monitoring. Wenzel also discussed the evolving role of hospital epidemiology, first in a more limited infectious diseases context (31), and later as applied to quality management (32, 33). A more telling comment was made by Jonas and Rosenberg (34, p. 453) who pointed out ". . . the chasm that exists between the academic researchers in the quality field and those professionals who are charged with implementing the quality-control measures on the books. Not only do they generally not talk to each other, but they sometimes don't even speak the same language." Although their comments were specific to the gap between the two groups in understanding Donabedian's structure-process-outcome evaluation schema (35–37), they apply equally well to deficiencies in knowledge of epidemiologic methods by many who are charged with the responsibility of implementing programs for quality of care but lack the proper tools to do so. In 1985, Jackson and Lynch (38) attempted to bridge the gap somewhat in an article about epidemiologic methods for the *Quality Review Bulletin*, a publication of the JCAHO widely read by facility personnel charged with the responsibility of implementing quality management programs.

Relationships Among Criteria Sets. The IOM expert panel noted that appropriateness guidelines, patient care evaluation and management criteria, and case-finding screens are not mutually exclusive categories, nor are they in conflict with one another (13, p. 308). For example, case-finding screens can be used as an initial mechanism to identify cases for a more detailed review to evaluate appropriateness guidelines or patient evaluation and management criteria. Historically, case-review screening methods have been used to identify sentinel events or process of care problems, and have focused primarily on misuse of medical technology rather than over or underuse. Similarly, outcome data have traditionally been used to screen for poor technical quality of services rather than over or underuse.

General Attributes of Criteria Sets

After considerable discussion, the expert panel generated a list of general attributes of criteria sets and divided them into two categories: (*a*) substantive (or structural) attributes that are inherent characteristics of a criteria set, and (*b*) implementation (or process) attributes that focus on the processes of developing and applying a criteria set.

The process of quality review can be seen as having three steps: (*a*) application of an initial case-finding screen, (*b*) in-depth secondary or peer review, and (*c*) appeal. The various attributes of criteria sets are applicable to different steps of the process.

Table 5.1 provides the short labels for attributes, each of which is described in more detail below (13, pp. 311–319).

Substantive and Structural Attributes

Sensitivity, Specificity, and Predictive Value. These terms are usually used in the context of case-finding screens to determine how often the screen detects cases of deficient care that require further review (how *sensitive* is the case-finding method?) while passing over cases of adequate care without prompting further review (how *specific* is the case-finding method?).

Sensitivity. Sensitivity refers to the likelihood that a case that is deficient will be identified as deficient, where deficient care is measured by an outside "gold standard" that reviews all care provided. Criteria that are sensitive have a high likelihood of finding "true positive" (truly deficient) cases. A screen or criterion that is poorly sensitive *misses* many cases where care was deficient.

Specificity. Specificity refers to the degree to which the criteria can identify *only* cases where quality of care problems exist. Criteria that are specific *rule out* cases where adequate care is provided so that only cases with true deficiencies are identified. Screens or criteria that are poorly specific identify many cases for further review where care was actually satisfactory. Using criteria that have low specificity results in unnecessary review of numerous cases that wastes time and resources.

Predictive Value. Predictive value is defined as the proportion of cases identified by the criteria as presenting quality problems that subsequently prove to be *true* quality problems. Predictive value takes into account the prevalence of the quality problem being investigated as well as the sensitivity of the criteria, and because of these relationships, the expert panel elected not to include it in the final list (Table 5.1).

The traditional definitions and formulas for sensitivity, specificity, and predictive value are presented in Table 5.2.

Reliability. A criteria set that is reliable generates consistent results for all users repeatedly. Case-finding criteria that are reliable should identify the same kinds of cases, regardless of who uses the criteria.

Validity. The attribute validity relates to outcomes and scientific evidence of

Table 5.1.
Final List of General Attributes of Criteria Sets for Standards as Developed by an Expert Panel Commissioned by the Institute of Medicine, 1989[a]

Attribute	Definition or Explanation
Substantive and structural attributes	
Sensitivity	High "true positive rate" in detecting deficient or inappropriate care
Specificity	High "true negative rate" in passing over cases of adequate care
Reliability	Known to produce same decisions or evaluations when applied by the user groups for which the criteria set is intended
Validity	Based on outcome studies or other scientific evidence of effectiveness
Documentation	A. Documents methods of development and cites literature (including estimates of outcomes)
	B. Documents how reliability was established
Patient responsiveness	Allows for eliciting or taking account of patient preferences
Flexibility	Respects the role of clinical judgment, with "clinical judgment" explicable
Clinical adaptability	Allows for or takes into consideration clinically relevant differences among different classes of patients; population to which criteria apply is specified
Inclusiveness	Covers all major foreseeable clinical situations and full range of clinical problems
Concordance	Reflects consensus of professionals with extensive experience in field, with input from academic and nonacademic practitioners, generalists, and specialists
Acceptability	Acceptable to majority of professionals
Clarity	Written in unambiguous language; terms, populations, data elements, and collection approach clearly defined
Appropriateness	Specifies appropriate, inappropriate, and equivocal indications (procedure and technology appropriateness guidelines)
Implementation and process attributes	
Pretesting	Guidelines are tested before implementation
Dynamism	Mechanism and commitment exists for reviewing and updating criteria sets to incorporate new information and cover new situations
Evaluation	Mechanism exists to review and evaluate outcome or impact of guidelines
Comprehendability	A. Format understood by nonphysician reviewers
	B. Format understood by practitioners
	C. Format easily understood by patients/consumers
Manageability	A. Not unduly burdensome for nonphysician reviewers to apply
	B. Not unduly burdensome for physician reviewers to apply
	C. Not unduly burdensome for professional to follow
Nonintrusiveness	Minimizes inappropriate direct interaction with treating physicians
Appealability	Allows for appeals process by professionals and patients
Feasibility	Ease of obtaining information
Computerization	Has been or could easily be computerized
Executability	A. Includes instructions for implementation
	B. Includes instructions for scoring and quantification

[a]From Lohr KN, ed. Medicare: A strategy for quality assurance. Vol. 1. Washington, D.C.: National Academy Press, 1990:312–313. © 1990 by the National Academy of Sciences, National Academy Press, Washington, D.C.

Table 5.2.
Computational Definitions of Sensitivity, Specificity, and Predictive Value[a]

Screen or Criterion	Standard	
	Poor Care	Good Care
Poor care	a True positive	b False positive
Good care	c False negative	d True negative

NOTE:
Sensitivity = True positive/(True positive + False negative), or $a/(a + c)$
Specificity = True negative/(False positive + True negative), or $d/(b + d)$

Predictive value (positive) = true positive/(true positive + false positive), or $a/(a + b)$
Predictive value (negative) = true negative/(false negative + true negative), or $d/(c + d)$

[a]From Lohr KN, ed. Medicare: A strategy for quality assurance. Vol 1. Washington, D.C.: National Academy Press, 1990:313. © 1990 by the National Academy of Sciences, National Academy Press, Washington, D.C.

effectiveness (and possibly efficacy). A valid criteria set should be based on scientific evidence or studies of patient outcomes, if such data are available.

Documentation. Documentation for criteria sets should include information about how the criteria were developed, the literature upon which they are based, what is known or not known about the expected outcomes, and how reliability for them was established. The evidence should be very explicit so that the user can evaluate the criteria set objectively.

Patient Responsiveness. This attribute concerns whether there is some mechanism for taking into account patient preferences and values. This is especially critical when the only treatment option (e.g., life-prolonging chemotherapy) has serious side effects (e.g., potential blindness) and the patient's values should be considered in making the treatment decision.

Flexibility. This attribute reflects the extent to which a criteria set identifies and specifies exceptions to criteria. Although this may not be as important in initial case-finding, it is critical at the secondary, peer-review level so that allowances can be made for clinical judgment. The less specific guidelines are to assist in secondary review, the more important is the role of clinical judgment.

Clinical Adaptability. Whereas flexibility deals with more idiosyncratic cases, clinical adaptability takes into account the predictable, clinically relevant differences among groups of patients. The criteria set should specify the groups to which they are intended to apply (e.g., with patients divided into groups based on age, sex, diagnosis, surgical risk, problem severity, or other factors).

Inclusiveness. This attribute implies that criteria sets collectively should cover the full range of surgical and medical problems encountered in the health care setting being reviewed. In addition, a specific criteria set should apply to a large proportion of the patients for which it is intended.

Concordance. This attribute embodies the important concept that guideline development should be based on consensus of persons with extensive and appropriate clinical experience, including generalists, specialists, and nonacademic and academic practitioners. Concordance should be reflected in documentation for the criteria set.

Acceptability. Acceptance by the target user group is a critical attribute. That is, does the criteria set seem to have at least face validity to the professionals who will use them?

Clarity. Criteria sets should be easily understood, and interpreted and applied consistently. Clarity calls for specific definitions of terms, data elements, and target population, as well as the use of unambiguous language.

Appropriateness. This attribute refers to whether the criteria describe explicitly (*a*) what actions are clearly appropriate (indicated), (*b*) where there is divergence of or absence of evidence (equivocal), and (*c*) what actions are clearly inappropriate (not indicated). In addition, alternative approaches that may be appropriate for diagnosis and treatment of the problem should be listed.

The expert panel also noted that appealability and concordance can be classified as either structure or process attributes and elected to include them in the first list (13, p. 316).

Implementation and Process Attributes

Pretesting. Consistent with the implementation of criteria of any sort, pretesting is the first step. Pretesting also provides an opportunity to modify language and format and to improve reliability. In addition, pretesting can also provide information about the extent to which a perceived problem actually exists.

Dynamism. Criteria sets should reflect the most current information and thus require a mechanism for ongoing review and revision. Dynamism means building feedback into the implementation system and using it to make appropriate changes in the criteria sets.

Evaluation. A mechanism for evaluating the impact of criteria should be part of the plan for implementation.

Comprehendability. Although the logic underlying criteria may be complex, their format and elements should be easily understood. In addition, since initial case review is usually done by nonphysicians, the criteria need to be clear to these trained reviewers.

Manageability. This attribute means that criteria should be manageable by nonphysician reviewers, physician reviewers, and practitioners. Particularly with

procedure and management guidelines, the practitioner should be able to internalize the practice standards so that he or she does not need to refer to written criteria frequently.

Nonintrusiveness. The process used to obtain information should be as nonintrusive as possible. The goal of this attribute is to design criteria clearly enough so that interaction with treating physicians (e.g., in utilization and preprocedure review programs) is kept to the essential minimum.

Appealability. This attribute is intended to provide a mechanism where patient uniqueness can be taken into account. That is, even highly valid, sensitive, and specific criteria will not be appropriate for every case in every possible situation because each patient is unique. Appealability is the extent to which exceptions to even the best criteria can be allowed.

Feasibility. How easy is it to obtain information for review? There is often a delicate balance between avoiding burdensome data collection and vitiating pressure needed to improve the quality and availability of information in patient records and from other sources. When the cost of acquiring the information exceeds the value of the information obtained, the data element may be excluded from the criteria; however, a decision to exclude data elements should be made carefully.

Computerization and Executability. Criteria sets should be constructed so that they can be translated into a computerized format for use by both reviewers or practitioners, as appropriate. Executability means that instructions for implementation include information about how to use the data collection form and, if scores are used, information on scoring and quantification.

Expert Panel Assessment of Most Critical Attributes

One of the assignments for the expert panel was to score each attribute on an importance scale (5 = most important, 1 = least important) for the three types of criteria sets: appropriateness, evaluation/ management, and case-finding. Attributes rated 4.5 or higher were defined as "key attributes." *Clarity* was identified as a key attribute for all three types of criteria sets.

Appropriateness Guidelines. Validity was identified as the most important attribute for technology and procedure-specific appropriateness guidelines. Sensitivity was also emphasized as a critical attribute, along with appealability as a key attribute for implementation.

Evaluation and Management. Clarity, flexibility, and clinical adaptability were rated as critical attributes for evaluation and management criteria, along with reliability, validity, and concordance as being very important. More generally stated, criteria sets must recognize valid alternatives to patient evaluation and treatment. Dynamism and executability were the two key attributes for implementation of evaluation and management guidelines.

Case-Finding Screens. Clarity and sensitivity were the two key structural attributes in this category. Because generic screens are intended to identify cases for secondary review using more rigorous criteria, the panel selected three key attributes for implementation: appealability, comprehendability, and evaluation. "The disappointing history of the use of generic screens in the Medicare program may account for the importance accorded these attributes by the expert panel" (13, p. 323).

Priorities for Quality of Care Criteria

The expert panel agreed that, in general, priority for criteria development should be given to high-risk, high-cost, high-volume, or problem-prone services. They used examples that included carotid endarterectomy (high risk), liver transplant (high cost), Pap smears (high volume), or nursing home care (problem prone). They recommended emphasis on guidelines for technology/management problems that could result in serious outcomes (e.g., death or disability) although no clear consensus on standards exists. In fact, guidelines may be most useful where practices are more divergent, partly because they will highlight where practice and data

conflict. The expert panel was also sensitive to the need for cost consciousness in developing and promulgating criteria and warned against "a headlong rush to formulate guidelines for the sake of having guidelines . . ." (13, p. 325).

Finally, at the end of the panel discussion, the group developed Table 5.3 to combine several substantive attributes into four major categories related to their scientific grounding, latitude, design, and efficiency; and the implementation attributes into four other categories related to their implementation, ease of use, appealability, and dynamism.

They concluded their work by stating that most, if not all, criteria sets existing at the time (1989) would fail if evaluated against the attributes listed in Table 5.1, and not all attributes can be maximized simultaneously in any single criteria set. They challenged users of the information presented above to do further work in the area, including evaluating the impact of better criteria sets on patient care and the best way to use criteria sets to assist practitioners, patients, and family members make better health care decisions (13, p. 329). It is indeed gratifying that many of the attributes listed by the expert panel are included among the characteristics of clinical indicators that are currently under development by the JCAHO (24).

CARE OF THE ELDERLY IN LONG-TERM CARE FACILITIES: AN EXAMPLE OF THE INTERPLAY OF POLITICS, REGULATIONS, STANDARDS, AND THE PUBLIC

The passage of the Social Security Act of 1935 included establishing a federal-state public assistance program for the elderly called Old Age Assistance (OAA). The drafters of the legislation opposed the use of the public poorhouse to care for the poor elderly, and thus the Act prohibited the payment of funds from the OAA to residents of public institutions. Accordingly, this stimulated the growth of voluntary

Table 5.3.
Possible "Larger Clusters" of Attributes for Quality-of-Care Criteria as Proposed by an Expert Panel Commissioned by the Institute of Medicine, 1989[a]

Substantive attributes
  Scientific grounding
    Reliability
    Validity
    Documentation
  Latitude (clinical and patient boundaries and judgment)
    Flexibility[b]
    Appealability[b]
    Patient responsiveness
    Clinical adaptability
    Inclusiveness
  Design
    Clarity
    Concordance
    Acceptability
    Appropriateness
  Efficiency
    Sensitivity
    Specificity
Implementation attributes
  Implementation
    Feasibility
    Computerization
    Executability
  Ease of use
    Comprehendability
    Manageability
    Nonintrusiveness
  Appealability
    Flexibility[b]
    Appealability[b]
  Dynamism
    Pretesting
    Dynamism
    Evaluation

[a]From Lohr KN, ed. Medicare: A strategy for quality assurance. Vol. 1. Washington, D.C: National Academy Press, 1990:326. © 1990 by the National Academy of Sciences, National Academy Press, Washington, D.C.
[b]Both flexibility and appealability might be built into the criteria or their application and, depending on the type of criteria set, at various stages of review.

and proprietary nursing homes that could receive payment from the OAA fund. The federal prohibition against payments to public institutions was withdrawn in the early 1950s for public facilities that were licensed by states. After World War II, there was a shortage of hospital beds, and policymakers envisioned nursing homes as proper places for persons who might otherwise have long hospital stays for convalescence. Federal funds to build nursing homes were authorized under the Hill-Burton legislation in 1954. Although Hill-Burton funds were limited to nonproprietary organizations, proprietary facilities lobbied for federal support and were successful before the end of the decade in gaining legislation for loans under the Small Business Administration and for federal loan insurance from the Federal Housing Administration (39, Appendix A; 40, pp. 17–19).

With increasing federal financial involvement in nursing home construction and services, concern about quality issues in nursing homes became a federal concern. Problems with the quality of care in nursing homes were first evaluated by the Council on State Governments in 1955 (41) and by the Commission on Chronic Illness in 1956 (42). In addition, the states were also starting to report problems (43), specifically that the majority of nursing homes used relatively untrained personnel and were functioning with low standards.

Even though an amendment to the Social Security Act in 1950 was intended to be a "standard-setting amendment," it did not specify minimum state licensure standards or procedures, and there was no mechanism to assure enforcement by the states. In fact, in a survey by the United States Public Health Service in 1958, it was found that few states had adequate personnel to conduct surveys and that their qualifications varied widely (44). In response to these findings, a special Senate Subcommittee on Problems of the Aged and Aging was established in 1959. Even though the findings indicated that most facilities were substandard, had poorly trained or untrained staff, and provided few services, the Subcommittee concluded ". . . because of the shortages of nursing home beds, many states have not fully enforced the existing regulations. . . . Many states report that strict enforcement of the regulations would close the majority of the homes . . ." (45).

Faced with this serious dilemma about the quality of care and safety of nursing homes, the Public Health Service began to study state licensing programs in 1957 and work with the states and industry to develop federal guidelines for nursing home licensure. The Nursing Home Standards Guide was first issued in 1963, and although it was mostly concerned with standards, it also included recommendations for regulatory organization and procedures (46). The Special Committee on Aging, created in 1961, also began to hold public hearings on nursing home problems in 1963 (39, p. 240).

Two years later, Medicare and Medicaid programs were enacted by the federal government. This greatly expanded federal funding for nursing home services and gave the United States Department of Health, Education and Welfare authority to set standards for nursing homes choosing to participate. The Medicare Act provided funding for posthospital convalescence in "extended care facilities" (ECFs); Medicaid paid for skilled nursing services.

The Medicare ECF program had immediate problems when the majority of nursing homes could not meet the health and safety standards or provide the levels of service required. Faced with the reality of thousands of elderly persons in facilities that could not meet the Medicare standards, the Medicaid program elected to leave it to the states to decide on nursing home participation. Over the next several years, there were lengthy battles over the scope and substance of nursing home legislation; however, pressure to increase the standards for nursing homes participating in Medicare and Medicaid began to build in the early 1970s. As the Special Committee on Aging (chaired by Senator Frank Moss) continued its hearings (39, pp. 241–245), it became clear by 1974 that the reasons for the variations in nursing homes could be related to the following factors (47):

1. Enforcement meant closure of the facilities, already in short supply, with no place to put the dispossessed patients.
2. States had little leverage other than the threat of license revocation to bring a home into compliance.
3. The license revocation itself was of very little use because of protracted administrative or legal procedures required.
4. Even if the revocation procedure was implemented, judges were reluctant to close a facility when the operator claimed that the deficiencies were being corrected.
5. Nursing home inspections were geared to surveying the physical plant rather than assessing the quality of care.

As a result of these and other findings, the government established the Office of Nursing Home Affairs in 1974. One of the responsibilities of the regional directors was the authority to approve provider agreements with Medicare and Medicare/Medicaid skilled nursing facilities (SNFs) and to monitor state agency certification and agreements with Medicaid-only providers. Methods for monitoring included surprise visits to SNFs during a study of the quality of care in nursing homes, conducted in 1974. The study found great variation in compliance with federal standards of care and safety (48). In addition, they found that surveys looked only at whether facilities had the *capacity* to deliver required services (evaluation of structure) not whether services of adequate quality were being delivered (evaluation of process of care). These findings resulted in additional regulatory activities and recommendations at the federal and state levels that culminated in another major reform effort to revise the nursing home survey program, "Operation Common Sense" in 1976–1978. Results of this program included realization that enforcement problems were still evident in the survey process and that elevating certain requirements to HCFA "conditions of participation" would make them more enforceable. After 2 years of work, HCFA proposed new rules in 1980. The intention of this reform effort was to focus on patient care and the result of that care on individual residents; however, the nursing home industry disputed HCFA's estimates of costs, and the Carter administration that had promoted the regulations was in its final hours. The Reagan administration immediately rescinded the new regulations in 1981 and began a regulatory relief effort. Subsequent political and public maneuvers resulted in leaving the 1974 rules in effect (39, pp. 247–248).

In the summer of 1983, the HCFA and Congress agreed to postpone all changes in regulations until a committee appointed by the Institute of Medicine studied the issues and reported recommendations for changes. The study resulted in a landmark publication, released in March of 1986 (39). The report, representing consensus of various interests involved in nursing home care, called for: major restructuring of the HCFA Conditions of Participation; deleting regulatory distinctions among different types of long-term care facilities; creating requirements for resident assessment, quality of care, quality of life, and administration; developing new standards for discrimination against Medicaid recipients and for nurses' aide training; strengthening social services; increasing nursing staffing; making major improvements in the survey and certification processes; and enforcing by state and federal government.

There was a great deal of public support for the IOM report, led by major support from consumer groups. The National Citizens' Coalition for Nursing Home Reform (NCCNHR), founded in 1975, played a central role. The Coalition, made up of over 300 local, state, and national consumer organizations, launched the "Campaign for Quality Care" in June of 1986 coincident with publication of the IOM report. Over the next year, representatives of 30 national organizations worked together to study the IOM report and to develop detailed positions outlining how nursing home laws and regulations should be changed and strengthened (49). Participants included representatives from general health care organizations including the American Nurses Association, Association of Health Facility Licensure and Certification Directors, National Association of Social Workers, American Occupational Therapy Association, Catholic Health Association, and the American Psychological Association. Several organizations were represented whose mission specifically is to represent the needs of the aged. These included the National Council on Aging, American Health Care Association, American Association of Retired Persons, American Association of Homes for the Aging, Gray Panthers, National Council of Senior Citizens, National Committee to Preserve Social Security and Medicare, and the Older Women's League. Long-term care ombuds programs were represented, along with the American Federation of State, County and Municipal Employees (AFSCME) and the Service Employees International Union (SEIU). In addition to the participating organizations, the Coalition gained endorsement of over 50 national organizations for the consensus positions. Interestingly, however, neither the American Medical Association nor the American Hospital Association participated in any of the consensus decisions.

Considerable pressure was levied on the Congress by the NCCNHR whose Campaign for Quality Care represented a 20-month effort by consumer, provider, and professional groups to implement the 1986 IOM report. This lobbying effort, along with sponsorship of legislation by key elected officials in Washington, resulted in inclusion of Nursing Home Reform Amendments in the Omnibus Budget Reconciliation Act of 1987 (OBRA, Public Law 100-203) in December of 1987 (50). OBRA 1987 added nearly 20 pages of new requirements to the Social Security Act, with a number of detailed provisions; additional amendments were made in 1988, 1989, and 1990, with full implementation intended in October of 1990. Key provisions of amendments included detailed requirements for quality of care, quality of life, residents' rights, survey activities, enforcement, and staffing (51, 52). An important change implemented with the new regulations was the combination of skilled nursing facilities (SNFs) and intermediate care facilities (ICFs) into a single category now called "nursing facilities" (NFs) that will be held to a single standard of care. In addition, to support this new level of quality of care, facilities are required to have licensed nurses around the clock, including registered nurses (RNs) every day for at least one shift. A major triumph for consumer advocates was in the area of residents' rights, including the right for residents to be free from abuse and from use of chemical or physical restraints except when necessary for the safety or medical treatment of the resident (53).

As has often been the case, there was question among various state departments of health regarding the need for additional federal resources to implement these sweeping reforms. This was best exemplified in a September 17, 1990 commentary in *The New York Times* (54) by the deputy director of the California Department of Health Services who was quoted from an interview the previous week as stating ". . . Medicaid does not have the funds to pay nursing homes in this state for the additional costs of implementing the 1987 law. I will not enforce standards if we have not given nursing homes the funds to meet them. That would be unreasonable." Consumers responded immediately by filing a class action suit, Valdivia vs. California, on October 1, 1990 (55), and the California judge granted them a preliminary injunction to stop California from evading the law on January 11, 1991 (56).

In summary, the history of nursing home reform and the development of standards for nursing homes has been a continuing saga of recommendations, regulations, political maneuvers, and fiscal constraints. The Nursing Home Reform Amendments of OBRA are sweeping. In many areas, standards with measurable criteria are included for the first time. The Institute of Medicine reports (13, 39) are comprehensive and thorough. How much impact these reports and new regulations will actually have on nursing home management and quality of care for residents will be seen only as we progress through the next decade. One thing is certain, however: there will undoubtedly be another Congressional charge to evaluate the quality of nursing home care yet another time.

SUMMARY AND CONCLUSIONS

The standards for hospitals developed for government regulation by HCFA and for professional self-regulation by the Joint Commission are intended to assure the quality of care provided in hospitals. As summarized by McGeary, "Both sets of standards have evolved from efforts to assure a minimum capacity to provide adequate care to more ambitious efforts to make hospitals assess and improve their organizational and clinical performance in a comprehensive and continuous manner" (57, p. 296). The federal government has had a much heavier hand in regulations for nursing homes since the implementation of the Medicare and Medicaid regulations a quarter century ago. These regulations have also evolved from a minimum standard of care to a requirement that "Each resident must receive the necessary nursing, medical and psychosocial services to attain and maintain the highest possible mental and physical functional status . . ." (52, p. 5365).

The methods used for regulation, however, are often based on the "Theory of Bad Apples" rather than on the "Theory of Continuous Improvement" described by Berwick (58) who states ". . . professionals must take part in specifying preferred methods of care, but must avoid minimalist 'standards' of care. . . . A company that seeks merely to meet standards cannot achieve excellence. . . ." The HCFA and JCAHO would do well to heed Berwick's final words: "We are wasting our time with the Theory of Bad Apples and our defensive response to it in health care today. . . . The Theory of Continuous Improvement . . . holds some badly needed answers for American Health care" (57, p. 36).

The influence of the Medicare and Medicaid legislation over the past quarter century has been far more encompassing than ever envisioned. At the outset, there was tremendous political pressure to make health care benefits available quickly and universally to all Social Security recipients. The pressures were magnified by the need to develop procedures quickly. The standards could not be too complex because they would be applied by persons surveying for the states who had widely divergent experience and training. Most of the drafters of the 1965–1966 standards probably did not even have access to Donabedian's organizational structure-process-outcome schema as it was not published until 1966 (35).

Despite over 70 years of fairly intense

effort by the hospital industry (represented by the Joint Commission) and the federal government, adequate and valid standards for quality of care are just beginning to emerge. The standards for standards, developed by the Institute of Medicine's expert panel in 1989 and presented in this chapter, can provide an organizational schema that at least has the potential for adequacy and valid measurement.

The methods for surveillance and monitoring for compliance with standards that do exist are heavily dependent upon the certification and accreditation process that is periodic, and still often focused on evaluation of the paperwork associated with the structure and process of care rather than measurable outcomes. This is partly because evaluation of outcomes of care is difficult, and patient outcomes are affected by many factors other than those controlled by health care providers or systems. With the technology of computers now available, it is possible to study proposed standards systematically and determine their validity; however, to perform the studies correctly requires access to highly trained professionals who have knowledge of research methods and statistics. These people command large salaries and are unlikely to be hired by the average facility. Thus validation of standards will undoubtedly continue to rest largely with research facilities, academic medical centers, and studies contracted for by various state and federal agencies. In the last few years, the Joint Commission has also initiated development of clinical indicators for quality using research design and analysis methods that appear to be valid and reliable. The final set of infection control indicators began the alpha testing phase in early 1991 (59).

A third problem with using regulatory or voluntary standards as measures for quality of care is the ambivalent attitude of surveyors, state agencies, and the Joint Commission toward the use of sanctions. The goals of these groups are different: the Joint Commission is interested in professional self-improvement; state and federal officials are motivated by public and political pressures to provide care at the lowest cost while not limiting access for Medicare

and other recipients. One formal sanction, loss of certification or accreditation, is a drastic step that leaders of these groups are often reluctant to take.

In addition, even though for hospitals the federal government has delegated much of the standard-setting and enforcement power to private accreditation agencies, it has also passed on much responsibility to the states. The interpretation of standards by the states can thus be of 50 different varieties; however, given our current political environment, little is being done to increase consistency. Since HCFA is in control of a large proportion of the resources paid for care, they are in a position to take a larger role in setting standards that are consistent for all states and have done so most successfully for nursing homes (52).

Finally, many of the obstacles to the development of standards for more effective quality of care measurement include lack of knowledge about the relationships among structure, process, and outcome, as well as geographic disharmony, and political, economic, and public pressures. These factors are illustrated best by the fact that, when a good hotel room may cost more than $100/day and a hospital room in a community hospital may exceed $400/day, people still expect to find a nursing home room for little more than $50/day. It is a mistake to think that even supervised domiciliary care can be rendered at that cost. Such stringent economics often results in facilities constructed poorly, located in inaccessible places, and staffed by minimum wage personnel with few or no benefits. These factors must result in compromised care. In fact, the facilities and a number of the staff needed to provide skilled care are often similar to those needed by small community hospitals. It is also a mistake to believe that alert, healthy, young people with single-system diseases or injuries are more expensive to care for than confused, chronically ill, frail elderly people with multiple health problems. These expectations are unrealistic and inappropriate. The new HCFA requirements for long-term care facilities (52) offer an opportunity to determine once again whether or not regulatory requirements can lead to improvements in the quality of care for nursing home patients. On behalf of the millions of elderly citizens today and the remainder of us who will join the ranks of the elderly in the future, we are hopeful that the reforms will be successful this time.

References

1. Nightingale F. Notes on nursing. New York: D Appleton & Co, 1860.
2. Starr P. The social transformation of American medicine. New York: Basic Books, Inc, 1982.
3. Flexner A. Medical education in the United States and Canada: A report to the Carnegie Foundation for the advancement of teaching. New York: The Carnegie Foundation, 1910.
4. Duffy J. A history of public health in New York City, 1625–1866. New York: Russel Sage Foundation, 1968:65–66.
5. Fitz RH. The rise and fall of the licensed physician in Massachusetts, 1781–1860. Trans Assoc Am Physicians 1894;9:1–18.
6. Vanderpoel SO. IN: Post AC, et al. An ethical symposium. New York: Putnam, 1883:37–38.
7. Freidson E. Profession of medicine: A study of the sociology of applied knowledge. Chicago: University of Chicago Press, 1988:391.
8. Flexner A. Medical education. New York: Macmillan, 1925.
9. American Medical Association. Laws regulating the practice of medicine in the various states and territories of the United States. JAMA 1901; 37: 1318.
10. Wilson FA, Neuhauser D. Health services in the United States. 2nd ed. Cambridge, MA: L. Ballinger, 1987.
11. Weitzman BC. The quality of care: Assessment and assurance. In: Kovner AR. Health care delivery in the United States. 4th ed. New York: Springer, 1990:353–380.
12. Davis D, Haynes RB, Chambers L, et al. The impact of CME: A methodologic review of the continuing medical education literature. Eval Health Profes 1984;7:251–284.
13. Lohr KN, ed. Medicare: A strategy for quality assurance. Vol. 1. Washington, D.C.: National Academy Press, 1990.
14. Federal Register 1989;54:1956–1967.
15. Hollis G. State licensing of health facilities. Washington, D.C.: National Center for Health Statistics, United States Department of Health, Education and Welfare, 1968.
16. Roberts JS, Coale JG, Redman RR. A history of the Joint Commission on Accreditation of Hospitals. JAMA 1987;258:936–940.
17. Vladek BC. Quality assurance through external controls. Inquiry 1988;25:100–107.
18. Cruse PJE. Surgical wound sepsis. Can Med Assoc J 1970;111:563–573.
19. Haley RW. Managing hospital infection control for cost effectiveness: A strategy for reducing infectious complications. Chicago: American Hospital Publishing, 1986.
20. Kerfoot KM. Regulatory agencies—An impetus for change. In: Johnson M, McCloskey J, eds. Changing organizational structures. Vol. 2. Iowa Nursing Administration Series. Menlo Park, CA: Addison-Wesley, 1989.
21. Donabedian A. Quality assessment and assurance: Unity of purpose, diversity of means. Inquiry 1988;25:173–192.
22. Donabedian A. Monitoring: The eyes and ears of healthcare. Health Progress 1988;69:38–43.
23. Longo DR, Ciccone KR, Lord JT. Integrated quality assessment: A model for concurrent review. Chicago: American Hospital Association, 1989.
24. Joint Commission on Accreditation of Healthcare Organizations (JCAHO). Characteristics of clinical indicators. QRB 1989;15:330–339.
25. Lehman R. Forum on clinical indicator development: A discussion of the use and development of indicators. QRB 1989;15:223–227.
26. Marder RJ. Relationship of clinical indicators and practice guidelines. QRB 1989;16:60.
27. Agency for Health Care Policy and Research (AHCPR). Clinical guideline development. AHCPR Program Note, August 1990.
28. Crede WB, Hierholzer WJ, Jr. Surveillance for quality assessment: III. The critical assessment of quality indicators. Infect Control Hosp Epidemiol 1990;11:197–201.
29. O'Leary DS. Quality assessment: Moving from theory to practice. JAMA 1988;260:1760.
30. Donabedian A. Contributions of epidemiology to quality assessment and monitoring. Infect Control Hosp Edidemiol 1990;11:117–121.
31. Wenzel RP. The evolving art and science of hospital epidemiology. J Infect Dis 1986;153:462–470.
32. Wenzel RP. Expanding roles of hospital epidemiology: Quality assurance. Infect Control Hosp Epidemiol 1989;10:255–256.
33. Garibaldi RA, Wenzel RP. Challenges and controversies [Editorial]. Infect Control Hosp Epidemiol 1989;10:239.
34. Jonas S, Rosenberg SN. Measurement and control of the quality of health care. In: Jonas S, ed. Health care delivery in the United States. 3rd ed. New York: Springer, 1986.
35. Donabedian A. Evaluating the quality of medical care. Milbank Memorial Fund Q 1966;44:166–206.
36. Donabedian A. The quality of medical care. Science 1978;200:856–864.
37. Donabedian A. Commentary on some studies of the quality of care. Health Care Fin Rev 1987; Annual Review:75–85.
38. Jackson MM, Lynch P. Applying an epidemiologic structure to risk management and quality assurance activities. QRB 1985;11:306–312.
39. Institute of Medicine Committee on Nursing Home Regulation. Improving the quality of care in nursing homes. Washington, D.C.: National Academy Press, 1986.
40. Eustis, NN, Greenberg JN, Patten SK. Long-term care for older persons: A policy perspective. Monterey, CA: Wadsworth, 1984.

41. United States Senate. A bill of objectives for older people and a program for action in the field of aging, by the Council of State Governments. In: Committee on Labor and Public Welfare. Studies of the aged and aging. Vol. 1. Washington, D.C.: U.S. Government Printing Office, 1956:183–189.

42. United States Senate. Recommendations of the Commission on Chronic Illness on the care of the long-term patient. In: Committee on Labor and Public Welfare. Studies of the aged and aging. Vol. 2. Washington, D.C.: U.S. Government Printing Office, 1956:75–94.

43. United States Senate. Recommended state action for the aging and aged: A summary of recommendations on problems of the aging as compiled from reports of state agencies, by the council of State Governments. In: Committee on Labor and Public Welfare: Studies of the aged and aging. Vol. 1. Washington, D.C.: U.S. Government Printing Office, 1956:275–309.

44. United States Department of Health, Education and Welfare. Report on National Conference on Nursing Homes and Homes for the Aged, February 25–28, 1958. United States Public Health Service Publication No. 625. Washington, D.C.: U.S. Government Printing Office, 1958.

45. United States Senate. The aged and aging in the United States: A national problem. Report No. 1121, 86th Congress, 2nd Session, February 23, 1950. Washington, D.C.: U.S. Government Printing Office, 1960.

46. United States Department of Health, Education, and Welfare. Nursing home standards guide: Recommendations relating to standards for establishing, maintaining, and operating nursing homes. Washington, D.C.: Nursing Homes and Related Facilities Program, Division of Chronic Diseases, U.S. Public Health Service, 1963.

47. United States Senate. Nursing home care in the United States: Failure in public policy: An introductory report. Senate Report No. 93-1420, 93rd Congress, 2nd Session, December 19, 1974. Washington, D.C.: Special Committee on Aging, Subcommittee on Long-term Care, United States Senate, 1974.

48. United States Department of Health, Education, and Welfare. Interim Report: Long-term care facility improvement study. Washington, D.C.: Office of Nursing Home Affairs, U.S. Public Health Service, U.S. Department of Health, Education and Welfare, 1975.

49. National Citizens' Coalition for Nursing Home Reform. Campaign for quality care in nursing homes. Washington, D.C.: National Citizens' Coalition for Nursing Home Reform, 1987.

50. Anonymous. Congress passes quality care bill; major reforms become law at last. Qual Care Advocate 1988;Jan/Feb.

51. National Citizens' Coalition for Nursing Home Reform. A brief summary of selected key provisions of the nursing home reform amendments of OBRA 1987. Washington, D.C.: National Citizens' Coalition for Nursing Home Reform, October 1990.

52. Department of Health and Human Services: Health Care Financing Administration. Medicare and Medicaid; Requirements for long term care facilities. 42 CFR Parts 405, 442, 447, 483, 488, 489, and 498. Federal Register 54(21):5316–5373, February 2, 1989.

53. Holder E. Long term care ombudsman desk reference. Washington, D.C.: National Citizens' Coalition for Nursing Home Reform, December 1990.

54. Pear R. As deadline nears, U.S. lags on rules for nursing care. *The New York Times*, Monday, September 17, 1990.

55. United States District Court Eastern District of California. Valdivia vs. California. Class Action No. CIV S-90-1226 EJG (EM), filed October 1, 1990.

56. Frank B. Personal communication. National Citizens' Coalition for Nursing Home Reform, January 14, 1991.

57. McGeary MGH. Medicare conditions of participation and accreditation for hospitals. In: Lohr KN. Medicare: A strategy for quality assurance. Vol. II. Washington, D.C.: National Academy Press, 1990:292–342.

58. Berwick DM. Sounding board: Continuous improvement as an ideal in health care. N Engl J Med 1989;320:53–56.

59. Nadzam DM, Mickus K. Memorandum to Infection Control Task Force Membership: Final set of indicators for alpha testing. Chicago: Joint Commission, November 26, 1990.

6

Decision Analysis and Meta-Analysis

Dealing with Information Overload

Mary D. Nettleman, M.D.

How can quality be maximized in a climate of limited financial resources? What standards should be used to measure appropriateness of care? Answers to these questions are often intuitive—based on personal experience and a partial knowledge of the literature. However, important decisions and those likely to have extensive ramifications require a more rigorous and scientific approach. The application of scientific method to clinical decision making is the cornerstone of both decision analysis and meta-analysis.

DECISION ANALYSIS

The virtual explosion of medical technology has led to a bewildering assortment of new tests, treatments, and procedures. Coupled with this are financial restrictions imposed by government or third party payers. Is a new product worth the extra money (1)? Conversely, is cheaper always better? As the proportion of the gross national product spent on health care moves decisively into double digits, physicians are increasingly asked to minimize costs while simultaneously maximizing benefits, a truly herculean task (2–4). Decision analysis is a logical and structured

approach to solving problems in an atmosphere of uncertainty (5–12). Uncertainty arises because tests are not perfect, treatments are not completely effective, and individual outcomes are not predictable. Rooted in game theory (13–15) and used for decades to identify cost-effective strategies in the field of business, decision analysis has only recently been applied to problems in medicine.

Clinicians make decisions by assimilating new data, questioning old practices, and intuitively weighing the risks and benefits of an intervention against those of alternative interventions (16). Flawed decisions result from incomplete data acquisition or insertion of personal biases into the decision-making process. For example, a clinician who has recently seen a patient with a very unusual disease may be tempted thereafter to test for that disease more frequently than logic would deem necessary. Thus, probability estimates may be distorted by an isolated incident. Decision analysis substitutes numerical values for intuition. Steps include structuring the problem in a logical manner, assigning values to benefits, risks, and costs, quantifying differences among alternative solutions, and investigating the impact of reasonable variations in the assigned values (sensitivity analysis). The goal of decision analysis is to identify the alternative that maximizes a specified outcome. That outcome might be cure, survival, quality-adjusted life expectancy, or cost-effectiveness.

Structuring the Problem

Traditionally, problems are structured through the construction of a decision tree, which is a graphic description of alternative interventions, events, and outcomes. Every important alternative should be included and the decision tree structured so that sequential events appear in adjacent branches. For example, a clinician may wish to decide which of two tests is most cost-effective. Figure 6.1 shows an initial decision tree. The two branches representing the two tests spring from a "decision" node represented by a *square*. Decision nodes occur when an active decision on the part of the clinician is required. Obviously, this tree does not completely describe the problem. A more complete tree is shown in Figure 6.2. Note that the nodes before the two test result branches are represented by *circles*. These are called "chance" nodes because the clinician has no control over whether the test result will be positive or negative.

Figure 6.3 shows a tree where branches have been added for treatment decisions. The tree incorporates the assumption that all patients with positive test results will be treated and that patients with negative test results will not be treated. A combination of decisions like this is referred to as a strategy. Thus, the tree depicts the strategy: test all patients, treat if test results are positive and withhold treatment if test results are negative. Note that the tree also

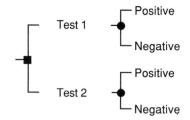

Figure 6.2.   Decision tree: chance nodes.

includes the possibility of no disease being present even though the test was positive (false-positive result) and the possibility of disease being present even though the test was negative (false-negative result). Other branches are added as required to completely describe the problem under study. As might be expected, detailed decision trees may grow bushy and cumbersome (17). To make the tree more compact, unnecessary branches may be eliminated or "pruned." In addition, groups of branches that appear repetitively can be represented by a marker designating a "subtree" containing those branches (8).

Probability and Chance Nodes

Every chance node is associated with uncertainty, which can be expressed as probabilities. For example, what is the probability of a positive test result? In order to perform the analysis, it is necessary to identify the probability of entering each branch following a chance node. To do this, it is best to review the definitions of sensitivity, specificity, and predictive value.

The sensitivity of a test is the probability that the test result will be positive in persons who truly have disease. In shorthand notation, sensitivity is: $P(T^+|D^+)$. Specificity is the probability that the test result will be negative in persons who are truly free of disease: $P(T^-|D^-)$. Values for sensitivity and specificity may be obtained from product literature or from independent studies.

If the test is positive and the patient actually has disease, the result is referred to as a true-positive result. The proportion of patients with true-positive results is simply the sensitivity of the test multiplied

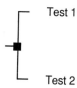

Figure 6.1.   Decision tree: decision nodes.

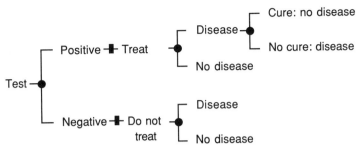

Figure 6.3. Decision tree.

by the prevalence of disease. Conversely, the probability of a true-negative result is the specificity multiplied by the proportion of the population that is not diseased. Few tests are perfect and it is not uncommon for falsely positive or falsely negative results to occur. The probability of a positive test result occurring in a patient who is not diseased is:

Probability of
false-positive result
$$= (1 - \text{specificity}) \cdot (1 - \text{prevalence})$$
$$= [1 - P(T^-|D^-)] \cdot P(D^-)$$

In other words, false-positive results occur in patients who are not diseased when tests are less than 100% specific. Falsely negative tests are a failure of sensitivity:

Probability of
false-negative result
$$= (1 - \text{sensitivity}) \cdot \text{prevalence}$$
$$= [1 - P(T^+|D^+)] \cdot P(D^+)$$

The probability of a positive test is the sum of the probability of a true-positive test result and the probability of a false-positive test result and is abbreviated: $P(T^+)$.

Note that sensitivity and specificity are not very useful to the clinician because they measure the quality of the test in populations known to have disease or to be free of disease. However, there is no way of distinguishing true-positive and false-positive test results. In practice, the clinician is faced with a positive test result and desires to know the probability that the patient truly has disease. The probability of disease given a positive test is the positive predictive value of the test:

$P(D^+|T^+)$. Conversely, the negative predictive value is the probability that a patient with a negative test is actually free of disease: $P(D^-|T^-)$.

To convert sensitivity and specificity into the more useful positive and negative predictive values, it is necessary to have some idea of the prevalence of disease in the population being tested: $P(D^+)$. Disease prevalence may be known from prior cross-sectional studies in the population or may be estimated from studies in other populations. Predictive values are then calculated using the centuries-old Bayes' theorem (18–20):

$$P(D^+|T^+) = \frac{P(T^+|D^+) \cdot P(D^+)}{P(T^+)}$$

Note that the numerator is simply the sensitivity of the test multiplied by the prevalence of infection in the population to be tested. Negative predictive value is:

$$P(D^-|T^-) = \frac{P(T^-|D^-) \cdot P(D^-)}{P(T^-)}$$

To look at this another way, consider the 2 × 2 table:

	Disease	No Disease
Positive test	a	b
Negative test	c	d

Assume that variables a, b, c, and d are probabilities and, being mutually exclusive, sum to 1. Sensitivity is the probability of a positive test in persons with disease: $a/(a+c)$. Note that $(a + c)$ is the probability of disease in the population (prevalence).

Similarly, specificity is the probability of a negative test in persons who are free of disease: $d/(b + d)$. If the sensitivity, specificity, and prevalence of disease are known, the variables a, b, c, and d may be calculated.

For example, consider a test that is 80% sensitive and 95% specific. Assume that the test is to be used in a population that has a 5% prevalence of disease. The 2×2 table for this situation is:

	Disease	No Disease
Positive test	0.04	0.0475
Negative test	0.01	0.9025

Positive predictive value is the probability of disease in persons with a positive test: $a/(a + b)$. In the example, the positive predictive value of the test is 46%. In other words, patients with a positive test have a 46% probability of having disease. In this example, a positive test result is not definitive evidence of disease, but rather an indication that there is an increased probability of disease. Prior to the test, the patient would have been assumed to have a 5% risk of being diseased based on the prevalence in the population. This is sometimes referred to as the "prior probability." After testing, the patient with a positive test has a 46% probability of disease, referred to as a "posterior probability" (9).

Probabilities must be assigned for transitions over each chance node. Often, no agreement exists on the probability of an event. For example, there may be a wide range of probabilities for treatment complications reported in the literature. The decision analyst could rely on an average of reported values, a meta-analysis, an educated opinion, or a Delphi survey. A Delphi survey is a method of obtaining a single opinion from a group of experts (21). Each participating expert is asked to submit his or her best estimate of the exact value of the probability in question and give reasons for the choice. Results of all estimates are fed back anonymously to the group, and the experts are asked to make a second estimate. The process is continued until general agreement is reached. Although this method has been shown to produce a

consensus, there is of course no guarantee that the resulting value is accurate.

Cost

Costs are incurred when tests are performed, treatments are prescribed, side effects occur, uncured disease results in complications, etc. In the example, all patients incur the cost of testing but only those with positive test results incur the cost of treatment. These costs are wholly attributable to the testing strategy and are referred to as direct costs (22, 23).

Indirect costs are measures of the human cost of illness incurred as a result of the implementation of a strategy (23–26). An example would be decreased earnings resulting from time lost from work. Lost wages due to death prior to the age of retirement are sometimes used to estimate the value of lives lost. Here, it is important to realize that strategies that save the lives of the young will be favored over strategies that save the lives of the old (23, 27). In addition, persons in high paying jobs will appear to be worth more than persons in low paying jobs. Therefore, such analyses are best confined to selected groups of similar age and income. A second method of determining the monetary value of morbidity is the "willingness to pay" method, which asks the question: "How much would you be willing to pay to avert this outcome?" The estimation of worth determined by this method is obviously subjective. Because of potential inaccuracies in the measurement of indirect costs, decision analyses are often performed both with and without inclusion of indirect costs.

All costs may not be incurred simultaneously. For example, side effects may be delayed for days or even years. The value of money is sometimes "discounted" if there is a long delay before a debt must be paid or before money will be received. Discounting is a reduction in the value of money over time (23). It is based on the premise that a person who has immediate control of money is better off than a person whose control is delayed until a future date. Therefore, money that will be spent or earned in the remote future is not valued as highly as money that will be spent or earned today.

Although the terms are often used interchangeably, costs and charges are not identical measures of resource consumption. Cost refers to the actual amount of resource consumed, whereas charge refers to the fee set by the marketplace for a service or goods (23, 28). Thus, it may cost a hospital only $5 to perform a test including the cost of labor and materials, but the charge to the patient for the test may be $25. The problem with charges is that they vary considerably according to what the market is willing to pay and may vary from one region of the country to another. However, charges are a measure of resources drained from the consumer or third-party payer, whereas costs are a measure of resources drained from the supplier. In addition, true costs are often difficult to estimate. Thus, the choice between using costs or charges in a decision analysis is dependent upon the availability of the data and the perspective of the analysis, that of supplier or that of consumer.

Measuring Outcome

In order to compare strategies, a scale must be developed to distinguish between good and bad outcomes. In some instances, outcome may be measured as life expectancy or survival. In others, it may be represented by freedom from disease.

In many instances, the investigator will be interested not only in survival, but also in the quality of life. Patients may be willing to trade decreased survival for increased quality of life. Quality-adjusted life years (QALYs) have been used to estimate the value of this trade-off (29–35). In order to calculate QALY, it is necessary to devise a scale that rates quality of life in one state against quality of life in another. Commonly, this is done by asking for an estimate from the patient or a group of patients or a panel of experts (36–38). For example, it may be determined that a year of life with the acquired immunodeficiency syndrome (AIDS) is equivalent to 6 months of life without AIDS. Thus, although survival with AIDS might be 2 years, it would be equivalent to one quality-adjusted life

year. This is referred to as the "time trade-off" method of adjusting for quality. A variation of this method is the "basic reference gamble" approach in which patients are asked if they would trade a fixed survival with disease for a lesser survival without disease. For example, the patient might be asked "Would you rather live 20 years with AIDS or only 1 year without AIDS?" If the patient chooses prolonged survival with disease, he or she is then asked "Would you rather live 15 years with AIDS or only 1 year without AIDS?" The questioning is continued until the point of indifference where the patient considers the trade-off between disease and decreased survival to be equivalent.

Obvious problems arise when calculating QALYs (39). Is the patient making an objective judgment or is the quality scale colored by fear due to limited knowledge about the disease (29)? Certain words like "cancer" and "AIDS" may raise apprehensions to the point where the patient feels he or she would do anything to avoid the disease. Can a panel of experts really determine the impact of disease on a patient (40)? Quality adjustment of life years may also bias an analysis in favor of interventions that maintain life in persons whose quality of life is already high and bias against interventions in persons whose quality of life is perceived to be low prior to the intervention (32). However, in this era when life of questionable quality can be prolonged indefinitely, quality of life has become a topic of importance to most patients and should be considered in decision analyses (41).

In a similar manner, utility scales may be developed to measure the relative value of different outcomes. Thus, the utility of the best outcome might be 1.0 and that of the worst outcome might be 0. Intermediate outcomes must then be placed between these two extremes. Standard reference gamble and time trade-off methods have been used to position intermediate outcomes. Again, difficulties arise when the physician and patient do not agree on the ranking of an outcome (42, 43).

If patients pass through several health states, life expectancy, quality of life, and resources consumed will depend on the duration of time spent in each state. For example, a patient may move from an uninfected state, to an asymptomatic infected state, to a symptomatic state, and finally to death. Only a proportion of the total population will be in each state at a fixed point in time. Models that take transitions between several health states into account are referred to as Markov models (44, 45).

In analogy to cost, some authors have discounted effectiveness, arguing that life years gained now are more valuable than life years gained in the future (46). For example, following a low fat diet may add years to the end of a young person's life, but seat belt use has a higher chance of preventing immediate death and adds years in the near future. This type of analysis will, in a sense, favor interventions that prolong youth and not those that prolong old age (27).

Because estimates of effectiveness, life quality, and even life expectancy are often inexact (47, 48), it is important to perform sensitivity analysis to determine if reasonable variations in these values change the outcome of the analysis.

Cost-effectiveness and Cost Benefit

By dividing the total cost of a strategy by its effectiveness value, a cost-effectiveness ratio is obtained. The result might be expressed in cost per year of life saved, cost per life saved, or cost per quality-adjusted life year saved. It is useful to compare a strategy to a reference strategy to determine the incremental benefit obtained. For example, testing might be compared to not testing.

In some instances, the benefit of a strategy may be converted entirely into a financial value by estimating the willingness of society to pay for a particular outcome. In a cost-benefit analysis, the total cost of a strategy is compared to its financial benefit (29, 41).

Sensitivity Analysis

Decision analysis is based on the estimation of many variables: test parameters,

disease prevalence, probability of complications, etc. Confidence in the result is directly proportional to confidence in the estimates (49). Sensitivity analysis is performed to determine if reasonable changes in the value of these variables impact substantially on the outcome of the analysis. In this way also, the reader may see the effect of inserting his or her own estimates into the analysis. Although controversy may exist over some estimates, sensitivity analysis can highlight areas where wide variations in the values do not affect the outcome. Alternatively, sensitivity analysis may point to values where minor changes may completely overturn the conclusions. Sensitivity analysis is valuable in measuring the robustness of the analysis and in identifying areas where further study is important for guiding health care policy.

Interpretation of the Results

Informal decision analyses are performed by clinicians whenever they choose an intervention or testing strategy. Formal decision analysis is a valuable aid to intuitive judgment (50), but results must be interpreted in the context of the analysis. For example, most analyses are performed from the standpoint of public health. Although it may be cost-effective for the public to restrict resources for expensive interventions, individual patients may feel that the best care should be provided to them regardless of the cost (2, 51, 52). The physician in his or her natural role as patient advocate may not serve as an effective gatekeeper for resource distribution (53).

Of importance, not all costs are borne uniformly by society. A strategy that is shown to be cost-effective may be resisted because it requires input of money from one source while benefiting another source (29, 54, 55).

Decision analysis is not meant to be a substitute for intuitive judgment. Indeed, the clinician may often incorporate a variety of intangible but important aspects of the problem into his or her decision which cannot be easily incorporated into a more formal analysis (56). Decision analysis is also a time-consuming process that is not always well adapted to the many decisions that must be made at the patient's bedside (57–59). Several computer programs have recently been introduced to facilitate analysis (60–63).

Familiarity with decision analysis fosters an acceptance of uncertainty. For example, a positive test does not always indicate disease. The appropriate response is not to order automatically several more tests to relieve the physician's anxiety, but rather to estimate the probability of disease in view of the test result and determine whether the threshold for treatment has been reached.

Uncertainty will always pervade the field of medicine. Resources will always be limited and should not be wasted. Physicians must actively ensure that funds are directed appropriately. Decision analysis is a tool that can help clarify uncertain issues and guide public policy to ensure that the maximum benefit is obtained from limited resources.

META-ANALYSIS

Despite a wealth of data on appropriateness of medical care, current approaches to quality assurance are predominately unstructured and inefficient. In part, this results from information overload brought about by a vast and confusing array of published studies. Meta-analysis is a term coined to describe a structured method of combining data from clinical trials to yield an overall estimation of treatment effect (64). Essentially, data from several trials are pooled and statistical inferences about the intervention under study are drawn from the pooled data base. Chalmers (65) has said that meta-analysis is to the review article as the randomized prospective controlled clinical trial is to the uncontrolled or historically controlled clinical trial. Jenicek (66) has stated: "Meta-analysis is a rigorous and structured approach to health problems across studies, and therefore in direct opposition to an educated guess." Although the method is at times controversial, much of the controversy stems from the mistaken impression that this is a "new" technology that has never been

used before. In fact, every time clinicians change the way they practice medicine, perhaps using a new treatment or eliminating an old test, they are in essence pooling new information with their previous knowledge, judging the relative importance of the new and old data, and drawing conclusions. These are the principles of meta-analysis (65–73). In meta-analysis, however, a review of the entire body of medical knowledge regarding a subject is attempted rather than a recall of just what is known to a specific clinician. In addition, statistical methods for pooling and weighting studies are utilized in place of intuitive judgment, and conclusions are based on the statistical confidence of the result rather than on a subjective impression.

Common synonyms include "overview," "quantitative synthesis," "pooling," and "quantitative review" (65, 66, 74). In the past, however, authors have tended to use or create a number of different eponyms (74, 75). In fact, only 48% of 119 recent meta-analyses could be extracted from a MEDLINE search using "meta-analysis," "pooling," "overview," and "quantitative synthesis" as text words and medical subject headings (74). The inclusion of "META-ANALYSIS" as a medical subject heading by the National Library of Medicine in 1989 and recent pleas for standardization of terminology, it is hoped, will limit confusion.

Importance

Meta-analysis, if done correctly, is demanding and time consuming. Thus, it is logical to choose the subject of the analysis carefully. Meta-analysis is well adapted to questions where many similar randomized clinical trials exist but no consensus of opinion has been possible from any single study. Often, this is a failure of sample size in the individual trials or the result of only a single trial reaching statistical significance. A common scenario would be a series of studies on the benefit of a preventive treatment where outcome events may be rare or where even small treatment effects may be important. For example, a recent meta-analysis of adjunctive therapy to prevent recurrence following surgical removal of breast cancer found 28 trials (16,513 patients) where tamoxifen therapy could be evaluated and 40 trials (13,442 patients) in which chemotherapy could be evaluated (76). Despite this huge amount of data, no consensus existed on the use of adjunctive therapy. Due to the large numbers of women who acquire breast cancer, even a small improvement in survival would result in large numbers of life years saved. Meta-analysis was used to pool data from several trials in order to increase power and therefore increase the likelihood of finding a significant difference if one truly existed.

Individual trials may not have sufficient power to investigate subgroups. In some instances, meta-analysis has been successful in subgroup analysis. For example, the study of breast cancer adjuvant therapy was able to identify a subgroup of women who would benefit most from tamoxifen (those over age 50) and a subgroup who would benefit most from chemotherapy (those under age 50) (76). In many instances, however, available data are insufficient to perform subgroup analysis.

The overall goals of meta-analysis are to improve statistical power, provide guidance for the design of future trials, clarify conflicting data, and aid in therapeutic decision making (77). Thus, meta-analysis may be used to quantitate the statistical significance and extent of benefit from a proposed treatment (73). Additionally, meta-analysis can define areas of uncertainty where answers to key questions are likely to change medical practice. The importance of scientific rigor in published trials, of publication bias, and of data availability have been highlighted by meta-analysis.

Designing the Meta-analysis

The validity of conclusions drawn from a meta-analysis depends upon the work remaining free from bias, the identification of all important studies that deal with the subject, unbiased judgment of the quality of available studies, and the use of statistically valid methods of pooling (65–73). Meta-analysis has been used to investigate the value of a single drug, of a family of drugs, or of a class of interventions.

Before the meta-analysis is performed, the hypothesis should be stated and a protocol for testing the hypothesis should be developed in detail. New hypotheses may also be generated at the end of the analysis after viewing the results and may lead to future studies. However, to ensure statistical validity, hypotheses to be tested by the meta-analysis should be stated before the analysis is begun (66, 73). The protocol should define which outcomes are to be studied, how data will be obtained, how the quality of studies will be judged, how heterogeneity among clinical trials will be dealt with, and which statistical methods will be used to pool the data. Each of these steps is described in detail below.

Outcomes

Clinical trials have end points ranging from the definitive (i.e., death) to the less than definitive (i.e., quality of life, depression, agitation) (40, 78–84). Definitive end points are easily incorporated into a protocol, but often restrict the focus unnecessarily. It is certainly important to prevent death, but also important to prolong disease-free survival. The problem with the latter outcome is that the period of freedom from disease depends on how vigorously one looks for recurrence and at what stage the disease is actually recognized as recurrent. To perform a meta-analysis using a less than definitive outcome requires an established definition of that outcome. Care must be taken to avoid a definition so restrictive that a review of published trials will be unlikely to yield enough data to meet the criteria. Conversely, a vague definition will foster controversy when results evolve into conclusions.

Data Acquisition

Obtaining data for a meta-analysis is not as simple as it might seem in this era of computerized data bases (85). Procurement from such a data base is dependent upon the search criteria, which must be broad enough to encompass all likely articles and restricted enough to obviate review of thousands of irrelevant studies.

References used in articles identified through the computerized literature search are then reviewed to identify missed references. Other data bases such as *Current Contents* and data registries may be investigated. Multiple publications of the same data, although discouraged, do occur and should be identified so that the same trial is not counted twice (86–88).

As any investigator knows, not all trials are published. Trials remain unpublished because of methodological problems, failure to enroll a sufficient number of subjects, failure to reject the null hypothesis, or lack of time to draft them into manuscript form (89). Some never make it through peer review into a journal. The utility of including unpublished data has been a subject of controversy. A review limited to published data may be biased toward positive results, but may be more amenable to judgments of methodologic validity (69, 89–91). For example, the meta-analysis of adjuvant therapy for breast cancer included substantial amounts of unpublished data obtained through direct cooperation with the investigators responsible for the randomized trials, through governmental cancer agencies, and through tumor registries (76). In one instance, a major clinical trial that included a "no treatment arm" was halted when the preliminary results of the meta-analysis showed treatment to prolong disease-free survival (92). Although the results of the meta-analysis would have had less power if confined to published data, conflicts about conclusions based partially on unpublished data that was not universally available and that had not been subjected to formal peer review or independently verified underscore the drawbacks of unpublished data (93, 94). Finding unpublished data is also difficult. Abstracts of conference proceedings that have not been published in manuscript form may identify authors who could be contacted. Appeals for unpublished work may be published in journals or at conferences. The decision about whether or not to include unpublished data therefore depends on its availability and on its quality. An interesting approach has been to calculate the number of unpublished or future trials with results—contrary to that found by the meta-analysis—which would be required to negate the conclusions of the meta-analysis (90, 95). If only a small number of contradictory trials are required to overthrow the conclusions, then the results of the meta-analysis must be considered tentative.

Selecting Trials for Analysis

After all individual trials have been identified, the ones to be used in the meta-analysis must be selected. The selection protocol should be determined in advance. The initial selection process often is designed to exclude all but randomized clinical trials. One is then faced with the choice of pooling data from all these trials or including only those of high quality. In the latter case, an algorithm might be used to score the selected trials using the completeness of randomization, degree of blinding, design criteria, and internal quality control measures (96, 97).

At this point, personal bias on the part of the investigator becomes a real threat to contamination of the results. An unblinded investigator may harbor unwitting prejudices in favor of certain journals or investigators (or against certain journals or investigators) or against foreign publications regardless of quality. The investigator desires the meta-analysis to be published and may subconsciously be more likely to select articles with favorable outcomes. Blinding the investigator has been proposed to circumvent these difficulties. In a blinded selection process, an expert reviewer extracts the important aspects of the methods section including the type of population studied, eligibility criteria, type of randomization, and expected length of follow-up. The extract is then checked by a second reviewer for accuracy and completeness. The extract does not contain the name of the journal, the results of the trial, the name of the trial, or the names of the trial's authors. Two investigators who were not involved in data extraction then review the extracts and score the studies according to the protocol established prior to initiation of the meta-analysis. This elaborate procedure is designed to minimize selection bias, but cannot completely eliminate it (70). Thus, some investigators prefer that the analysis be performed both with all available trials and again with only selected trials to determine the importance of selection to the outcome of the analysis (73). When publishing a meta-analysis, the selection criteria should be detailed and the list of selected and rejected trials and reasons for rejection should be included.

Pooling Data

Once trials are selected and their data extracted, the results must be pooled. There is no consensus on the single best method for pooling data (98–101). Crude pooling methods, such as averaging *p* values or test statistics do not allow quantitative conclusions about the effects of treatment, and confidence limits cannot be calculated (66, 73, 102). In addition, such methods do not take into account the heterogeneity among trials.

A more common method of pooling data is to develop a 2 × 2 table for each trial detailing the outcomes in each treatment group. One of several pooling procedures is then used (40). The method detailed by Peto and co-workers (104) is based on a modification of the Mantel-Haenszel procedure (105). The expected number of events is calculated under the null hypothesis of no treatment effect. For example, if the event of interest is death, then the expected number of deaths in the treatment group would be equal to the proportion of the population randomized to the treatment group multiplied by the total number of deaths in the study. Thus, if half of the study population were randomized to the treatment group and 100 people died in the study, one would expect 50 deaths in the treatment group. The difference between the observed and expected number of deaths is used to derive an estimate of the pooled odds ratio. The standard error of the odds ratio may also be calculated to determine if the null hypothesis may be rejected (103). The Peto method assumes that the effects of the treatment itself are constant and do not vary among different trials. Recently, it has

been suggested that the Mantel-Haenszel method of calculating odds ratios may be more consistently accurate than the Peto modification, when the treatment effect is large (101, 105).

DerSimonian and Laird (106) have described an alternate method of pooling data based on differences in proportions of events between treatment and control groups. The proportion of events is defined as the number of events occurring in the group divided by the number of patients in the group. Thus, if 30% of the control group died, the proportion of events in that group would be 0.30. Variance is estimated using the binomial distribution. The result is used to calculate the pooled mean difference in proportions between treatment and control groups. Thus, the DerSimonian and Laird method results in a quantitative measure of the actual difference in outcomes due to treatment, and the Peto method results in calculation of the odds ratio for the occurrence of the outcome event.

Still another method of pooling data is based on a Bayesian analysis (107, 108). This method estimates the probability distribution of a treatment effect or outcome based on a chosen prior distribution. Each individual study is associated with its own probability distribution. The distributions may be combined to yield a pooled probability distribution describing the treatment effect. Bias in studies, failure to give patients the treatment to which they were assigned, and other methodological flaws may be incorporated if they can be estimated. Differences in outcome measures and in experimental design may be incorporated in calculating the individual probability distributions. Although sophisticated and not yet widely applied, this technique holds significant promise for the future.

A final method of pooling data is logistic modeling. A data base containing pertinent dependent and independent variables for each participant in every trial is required (107). This method requires access to detailed data on every patient enrolled in the selected trials and is therefore not often used.

Heterogeneity

The effect of a treatment depends not only on its inherent virtue, but also on patient-dependent factors and the method by which the effect is monitored. If the efficacy of a treatment varies widely among trials because of these factors, heterogeneity exists. Ideally, pooled studies should be so similar that the efficacy of the treatment remains constant. The hypothesis that the treatment effect is constant and therefore subject only to random variation around a central value may be tested. Both Peto and DerSimonian and Laird provide a method for deriving a test statistic based on observed and expected events and variance. The test statistic follows a χ^2 distribution. If the null hypothesis of constant treatment effect is accepted, the trials are said to be "homogeneous." If the hypothesis is rejected, there is "heterogeneity" among the trials. Heterogeneity implies that a single treatment has different effects on patients according to the design and manner of execution of the trial.

The DerSimonian and Laird method of pooling is more conservative than the Peto method and will in some instances fail to confirm a significant treatment effect found by the Peto method. A major reason for this is that the DerSimonian and Laird method does not assume that the treatment effect is constant among different trials, but rather may vary according to differences in the population studied, the time of the study, the duration of follow-up, etc. DerSimonian and Laird essentially incorporated variance among studies into their method. If all pooled trials are homogeneous and the variance among studies is small, the two methods seldom differ. However, if significant heterogeneity exists, the DerSimonian and Laird method would be preferred (103). In some cases, significant heterogeneity may preclude meta-analysis (109).

Shortcomings

Meta-analysis is a useful aid to clinical decision making when definitive answers from randomized prospective clinical trials are not available. The technique is not, however, a substitute for definitive trials. Meta-analyses are only as good as the trials used for pooling (110, 111). For example, a pooling of four trials investigating the effect of phenobarbital in preventing intraventricular hemorrhage in neonates concluded that the drug appeared beneficial even though none of the studies reached significance by themselves (112). However, a subsequent randomized trial showed that the drug actually was associated with a significantly increased risk of hemorrhage (113). This is not an indictment of the entire technique, but rather evidence that caution should be used in changing treatment recommendations based solely on meta-analyses if no clinical trial can statistically support the conclusion.

In addition to depending on the quality of the individual trials, meta-analyses must be as free from bias and performed as meticulously as possible. A recent review of published meta-analyses by Sacks and colleagues (77) revealed that only 28% addressed important issues in study design, ability to combine trials, control of bias, statistical analysis, and application of results. Occasionally, because of these problems, different meta-analyses dealing with the same topic will come to different conclusions (114). Published meta-analyses should contain enough detail to allow the reader to judge the methods and reproduce the results (75).

Controversies exist over inclusion of unpublished data, the need to blind reviewers who select studies for inclusion, the criteria for study selection, the importance of heterogeneity, and the selection of an appropriate statistical method for pooling. One way to address these issues is with sensitivity analysis (77). Essentially, this is a "what if" situation in which the investigator asks what would have happened if the methods used in the meta-analysis were changed. For example, if only published trials were included, the number of unpublished trials with contrary results required to overturn the conclusion may be calculated (90–95). Additionally, the analysis might be performed with all studies and again with only selected studies to determine the impact of selection on the robustness of the results. The analysis might be repeated using only homogeneous studies. Finally, more than one statistical method of pooling might be used to determine the dependence of the results on the statistical technique.

Despite these difficulties, meta-analysis, properly applied, can bring order and logic to a complex problem encumbered with multiple inconclusive studies. As O'Rourke and Detsky (71) have pointed out, the major difficulties encountered are not inherent in the technique of meta-analysis, but rather a result of flaws in clinical trials and inconsistent study designs.

Interpretation

Meta-analyses have been used by the Food and Drug Administration and others to aid in judging the value of a medication (73, 115, 116). Many important topics in cardiovascular medicine, oncology, and psychology have already been addressed. In the future, more emphasis on this quantitative technique and less emphasis on qualitative and subjective reviews may be expected.

As with all studies, the results of a meta-analysis should be clinically as well as statistically significant. Thus, a minimal or marginal benefit should not necessarily prompt changes in clinical therapeutics even if the p value is small.

Meta-analysis in Quality Assurance

One of the most common criticisms given by persons who voluntarily or involuntarily participate in quality assurance activities is that there is little proof that interventions actually prevent adverse occurrences. In fact, the literature is replete with small studies and suspiciously devoid of large randomized controlled trials. Meta-analysis is designed to fill such voids and point to areas where further investigation might prove fruitful.

Meta-analyses that apply to quality of care have been performed. For example, are prophylactic antibiotics in selected settings truly beneficial (117–120)? How toxic are aminoglycosides (121, 122)? What rate of venous thrombosis can be expected after general surgery (123)? Does contact with high risk infants place pediatric nurses at increased risk for cytomegalovirus infections (124)? Which sociodemographic characteristics predict satisfaction with medical care (125)? Is it really important to emphasize treatment in elderly patients with hypertension (126)? How important is perioperative parenteral nutrition (127)? Are preoperative educational interventions beneficial (128, 129)? How strongly should exercise be emphasized in persons with hyperlipidemia (130)? The ability to judge and utilize published meta-analyses is fundamental to the practice of quality assurance.

Meta-analysis may be used, therefore, to identify areas where the literature supports the benefit of an intervention or treatment. Conversely, the technique may be used to show that the literature is completely inadequate to support institution of a specific intervention. Because it can quantify the benefit of a treatment or intervention, meta-analysis may be used to compare the relative importance of several interventions in order to give priority to the most beneficial. Finally, meta-analysis may point to areas where the literature is suggestive but not definitive and where further study is likely to prove important.

In conclusion, clinicians use the techniques of meta-analysis daily by assimilating new data, pooling the data with previous knowledge, weighting according to personal judgment of relative importance, and drawing conclusions based on this subjective and intuitive review to alter their clinical practices. The results of meta-analyses supplement intuitive analysis by bringing the force of objective, statistical methods to bear on the extensive medical literature.

References

1. Hartley RM, Markowitz MA, Kamaroff AL. The expense of testing in a teaching hospital: The

predominant role of high-cost tests. Am J Public Health 1989;79:1389–1391.

2. Eddy DM. Clinical decision making: From theory to practice. What do we do about costs? JAMA 1990;264:1161–1170.
3. Fuchs VR. The health sector's share of the gross national product. Science 1990;247:534–538.
4. Leaf A. Cost effectiveness as a criterion for Medicare coverage. N Engl J Med 1989;321:898–901.
5. Nettleman MD. Decision analysis: A tool for infection control. Infect Control Hosp Epidemiol 1988;9:88–91.
6. Weinstein MC, Fineberg HV. Clinical decision analysis. Philadelphia: WB Saunders, 1980.
7. Pauker SG, Kassirer JP. Decision analysis. N Engl J Med 1987;316:250–258.
8. Kassirer JP, Moskowitz AJ, Lau J, Pauker SG. Decision analysis: A progress report. Ann Intern Med 1986;105:189–193.
9. Patton DD. Introduction to clinical decision making. Semin Nucl Med 1978;8:273–282.
10. McNeil BJ, Keeler E, Adelstein SJ. Primer on certain elements of medical decision making. N Engl J Med 1975;293:211–215.
11. Weinstein MC, Fineberg HV, Elstein AS, Frazier HS, Neuhauser D, Neutra RR, McNeil BJ, eds. The elements of clinical decision making. In: Clinical decision analysis. Philadelphia: WB Saunders, 1980: 1–11.
12. Greep JM, Siezenis LM. Methods of decision analysis: Protocols, decision trees, and algorithms in medicine. World J Surg 1989;13:240–244.
13. Diamond GA, Rozanski A, Steuer M. Playing doctor: Application of game theory to medical decision-making. J Chron Dis 1986;39:669–677.
14. Eckman MH, Pauker SG. Let's decide who's playing doctor! J Chron Dis 1986;39:679–680.
15. Nettleman MD. Game theory: For adults only. Infect Control Hosp Epidemiol 1989;10:222–224.
16. Bergman DA, Pantell RH. The art and science of medical decision making. J Pediatr 1984;104:653–656.
17. Glasziou P, Hilden J. Decision tables and logic in decision analysis. Med Decis Making 1986;6:154–160.
18. Benish WA. Graphic and tabular expressions of Bayes' theorem. Med Decis Making 1987;7:104–106.
19. Small RD, Schor SS. Bayesian and non-Bayesian methods of inference. Ann Intern Med 1983;99:857–859.
20. Rembold CM, Watson D. Posttest probability calculation by weights: A simple form of Bayes' theorem. Ann Intern Med 1988;108:115–120.
21. Schoenbaum SC, McNeil BJ, Kavet J. The swine influenza decision. N Engl J Med 1976;295:759–765.
22. Weinstein MC, Fineberg HV, Elstein AS, Frazier HS, Neuhauser D, Neutra RR, McNeil BJ, eds. Clinical decisions and limited resources. In: Clinical decision analysis. Philadelphia: WB Saunders, 1980: 240–241.
23. Eisenberg JM. Clinical economics: A guide to the economic analysis of clinical practices. JAMA 1989;262:2879–2886.
24. Rice DP, Hodgson TA. The value of human life revisited. Am J Public Health 1982;72:536–537.
25. Landefeld JS, Sesking EP. The economic value of life: Linking theory to practice. Am J Public Health 1982;72:555–566.
26. Rice DP, Hodgson TA, Kopstein AN. The economic costs of illness: A replication and update. Health Care Finan Rev 1985;7:61–80.
27. Avorn J. Benefit and cost analysis in geriatric care: Turning age discrimination into health policy. N Engl J Med 1984;310:1294–1301.
28. Finkler SA. The distinction between costs and charges. Ann Intern Med 1982;96:102–109.
29. Detsky AS, Naglie IG. A clinician's guide to cost-effectiveness analysis. Ann Intern Med 1990;113:147–154.
30. Sackett DL, Torrance GW. The utility of different health states as perceived by the general public. J Chronic Dis 1978;31:697–704.
31. Nettleman MD. Outcome measurements in decision analysis: Life versus quality of life. Infect Control Hosp Epidemiol 1989;10:521–524.
32. LaPuma J, Lawlor EF. Quality-adjusted life-years: Ethical implications for physicians and policymakers. JAMA 1990;263:2917–2921.
33. Sisk JE. Drummond's "Resource allocation decision in health care: A role for quality of life assessments?" J Chronic Dis 1987;40:617–619.
34. Mehrez A, Gafni A. Quality-adjusted life years, utility theory, and healthy-years equivalents. Med Decis Making 1989;9:142–149.
35. Drummond MF. Resource allocation decision in health care: A role for quality assessments? J Chronic Dis 1987;40:605–616.
36. McNeil BJ, Pauker SG, Sox HC, Tversky A. On the elicitation of preferences for alternative therapies. N Engl J Med 1982;306:1259–1262.
37. Guyatt GH, Veldhuyzen Van Zanten SJ, Feeny DH, Patrick DL. Measuring quality of life in clinical trials: A taxonomy and review. Can Med Assoc J 1989;140:1441–1448.
38. Froberg DG, Kane RL. Methodology for measuring health-state preferences II: Scaling methods. J Clin Epidemiol 1989;42:459–471.
39. Weinstein M. A QALY is a QALY is a QALY—Or is it? J Health Econ 1988;7:289–290.
40. Kassirer JP. Adding insult to injury: Usurping patients' prerogatives. N Engl J Med 1983;308:898–901.
41. Bulpitt CJ, Fletcher AE. Measuring costs and financial benefits in randomized controlled trials. Am Heart J 1990;119:766–771.
42. Boyd NF, Sutherland HJ, Heasman KZ, Tritchler DL, Cummings BJ. Whose utilities for decision analysis? Med Decis Making 1990;10:58–67.
43. Mulley AG. Assessing patients' utilities: Can the ends justify the means? Med Care 1989;27:S269–S281.
44. Longini IM, Clark WS, Byers RH, Ward JW, Darrow WW, Lemp GF, Hethcote HW. Statistical analysis of the stages of HIV infection using a Markov model. Stat Med 1989;8:831–843.
45. Beck JR, Pauker SG. The Markov process in

medical prognosis. Med Decis Making 1983;3: 419–458.

46. Lipscomb J. Time preference for health in cost-effectiveness analysis. Med Care 1989;27:S233–S253.

47. Roper WL, Winkenwerder W, Hackbarth GM, Krakauer H. Effectiveness in health care: An initiative to evaluate and improve medical practice. N Engl J Med 1988;319:1197–1202.

48. Wennberg JE. Improving the medical decision-making process. Health Affairs, Spring 1988:99–106.

49. Katz BP, Hui SL. Variance estimation for medical decision analysis. Stat Med 1989;8:229–241.

50. Schwartz WB. Decision analysis: A look at the chief complaints. N Engl J Med 1979;300:556–559.

51. Garland MJ, Crawshaw R. Oregon's decision to curtail funding for organ transplantation. N Engl J Med 1988;319:1420.

52. Welch HG, Larson EB. Dealing with limited resources: The Oregon decision to curtail funding for organ transplantation. N Engl J Med 1988; 319:171–173.

53. Hoffman JJ. A piece of my mind: Keeper of the gate. JAMA 1990;263:1825.

54. Nettleman MD, Jones RB. Proportional payment for pelvic inflammatory disease. Sex Transm Dis 1989;16:36–40.

55. Nettleman MD, Jones RB, Roberts S, Katz B, Washington E, Dittus R, Quinn T. Cost-effectiveness of culturing patients attending a sexually transmitted diseases clinic for *Chlamydia trachomatis*. Ann Intern Med 1986;105:189–196.

56. Fryback DG. Decision maker, quantify thyself! Med Decis Making 1985;5:51–60.

57. Sox HC. Decision analysis: A basic clinical skill? N Engl J Med 1987;316:271–272.

58. Williams S. The limit of quantitative ethics. Med Decis Making 1987;7:121–123.

59. Siegler M. Decision analysis and clinical medical ethics: Beginning the dialogue. Med Decis Making 1987;7:124–126.

60. Greenes RA. Interactive microcomputer-based graphical tools for physician decision support: Aids to test selection and interpretation in use of Bayes' theorem. Med Decis Making 1983;3:15–21.

61. Fagan TJ. Nomogram for Bayes' theorem. N Engl J Med 1075;293:257.

62. Silverstein MD. A clinician decision analysis program for the Apple computer. Med Decis Making 1983;3:29–37.

63. Lau J, Kassirer JP, Pauker SG. Decison Maker 3.0: Improved decision analysis by personal computer. Med Decis Making 1983;3:39–43.

64. Glass GV: Primary, secondary, and meta-analysis of research. Educ Res 1976;5:3–8.

65. Chalmers TC. Meta-analysis in clinical medicine. Trans Am Clin Climatol Assoc 1987;99:144–150.

66. Jenicek M. Meta-analysis in medicine. Where we are and where we want to go. J Clin Epidemiol 1989; 42:35–44.

67. L'Abbe KA, Detsky AS, O'Rourke K. Meta-analysis in clinical research. Ann Intern Med 1987;107:224–233.

68. Mulrow CD. The medical review article: State of the science. Ann Intern Med 1987;106:485–488.

69. Peto R. Why do we need systematic overviews of randomized trials? Stat Med 1987;6:233–240.

70. Ellenberg SS. Meta-analysis: The quantitative approach to research review. Sem Oncol 1988;15: 472–481.

71. O'Rourke K, Detsky AS. Meta-analysis in medical research: Strong encouragement for higher quality in individual research efforts. J Clin Epidemiol 1989;10:1021–1024.

72. Boissel JP, Sacks HS, Leizorovicz A, Blanchard J, Panak E, Peyrieux JC. Meta-analysis of clinical trials: Summary of an international conference. Eur J Clin Pharmacol 1988;34:535–538.

73. Boissel J-P, Blanchard J, Panak E, Peyrieux J-C, Sacks H. Consideration for the meta-analysis of randomized clinical trials. Controlled Clin Trials 1989;10:254–281.

74. Dickersin K, Higgins K, Meinert CL. Identification of meta-analyses: The need for standard terminology. Controlled Clin Trials 1990;11:52–66.

75. Meinert CL. Meta-analysis: Science or religion? Controlled Clin Trials 1989;10:257S–263S.

76. Early Breast Cancer Trialists' Collaborative Group. Effects of adjuvant tamoxifen and of cytotoxic therapy on mortality in early breast cancer. N Engl J Med 1988;319:1681–1692.

77. Sacks HS, Berrier J, Reitman D, Ancona-Berk VA, Chalmers TC. Meta-analysis of randomized controlled trials. N Engl J Med 1987;316:450–455.

78. Nettleman MD. Outcome measurements in decision analysis: Life versus quality of life. Infect Control Hosp Epidemiol 1989;10:521–524.

79. Sackett DL, Torrance GW. The utility of different health states as perceived by the general public. J Chronic Dis 1978;31:697–704.

80. Pliskin JS, Shephard DS, Weinstein MC. Utility functions for life years and health status. Operations Res 1980;28:206–210.

81. Wortman PM, Yeaton WH. Cumulating quality of life results in controlled trials of coronary bypass graft surgery. Controlled Clin Trials 1985;6:289–305.

82. Patten SB. Propranolol and depression: Evidence from the antihypertensive trials. Can J Psychiatry 1990;35:257–259.

83. Schneider LS, Pollock VE, Lyness SA. A meta-analysis of controlled trials of neuroleptic treatment in dementia. J Am Geriatr Soc 1990;38: 553–563.

84. Grossberg GT. The pitfalls of metaanalysis. J Am Geriatr Soc 1990;38:607.

85. Dickersin K, Hewitt P, Mutch L, Chalmers I, Chalmers T. Comparison of MEDLINE searching with a perinatal trials database. Controlled Clin Trials 1985;6:306–317.

86. Wenzel RP, Maki DG, Crow S, Schaffner W, McGown JE. Duplicate publication of a manuscript. Infect Control Hosp Epidemiol 1990; 11:341–342.

87. Angell M, Relman AS. Redundant publications. N Engl J Med 1989;320:1212–1214.

88. Editors. Policy on repetitive publications and copyright. Ann Intern Med 1990;112:662.

89. Dickersin K, Chan S, Chalmers TC, Sacks HS, Smith H Jr. Publication bias and clinical trials. Controlled Clin Trials 1987;8:343–353.

90. Rosenthal R. The "file drawer problem" and tolerance for null results. Psychol Bull 1979; 86:638–641.

91. Collins R, Gray R, Godwin J, Peto R. Avoidance of large biases and large random errors in the assessment of moderate treatment effects: The need for sytematic overviews. Stat Med 1987; 6:245–250.

92. Chlebowski RT, Blackburn GL, Nixon DW, Jochimsen P, Scanlon EF, Insull W, Buzzard IM, Wynder EL, Elashoff R. Unpublished data summaries and the design and conduct of clinical trials: The nutrition adjuvant study experience and commentary. Controlled Clin Trials 1989; 10:368–377.

93. Dickersin K, Chan SS, Chalmers TC, Sacks HS, Smith H. Publication bias and randomized control trials. Controlled Clin Trials 1987;8:343.

94. Chalmers TC, Levin H, Sacks HS, Reitman D, Berrier J, Nagalingam R. Meta-analysis of clinical trials as a scientific discipline. I: Control of bias and comparison with large co-operative trials. Stat Med 1987;6:315–325.

95. Orwin RG. A fail-safe N for effect size in meta-analysis. J Ed Stat 1983;8:157–159.

96. Lichtenstein JF, Mulrow CD, Elwood PC. Guidelines for reading case-control studies. J Chron Dis 1987;40:893–903.

97. Chalmers TC, Smith H Jr, Blackburn B, Silverman B, Schroeder B, Reitman D, Ambroz A. A method or assessing the quality of randomized control trials. Controlled Clin Trials 1981;2:31–49.

98. Goodman SN. Meta-analysis and evidence. Controlled Clin Trials 1989;10:188–204.

99. Zucker D, Yusuf S. The likelihood ratio versus the p value in meta-analysis: Where is the evidence? Controlled Clin Trials 1989;10:205–208.

100. Goodman SN. Response to commentary of Zucker and Yusuf. Controlled Clin Trials 1989; 10:209–210.

101. Greenland S, Salvan A. Bias in the one-step method for pooling study results. Stat Med 1990; 9:247–252.

102. Gaffey WR. A new statistical test for summarizing the results of independent epidemiologic studies. Public Health Rev 1988;16:153–162.

103. Berlin JA, Laird NM, Sacks HS, Chalmers TC. A comparison of statistical methods for combining event rates from clinical trials. Stat Med 1989; 8:141–151.

104. Yusuf S, Peto R, Lewis J, Collins R, Sleight P. Beta blockade during and after myocardial infarction: An overview of the randomized trials. Prog Cardiovasc Dis 1985;27:335–371.

105. Mantel N. Chi-square tests with one degree of freedom: Extensions of the Mantel-Haenszel procedure. J Am Stat Assoc 1963;58:690–700.

106. DerSimonian R, Laird N. Meta-analysis in clinical trials. Controlled Clin Trials 1986;7:177–188.

107. Detrano R. Optimal use of literature knowledge to improve the Bayesian diagnosis of coronary artery disease. J Clin Epidemiol 1989;42:1041–1047.

108. Eddy DM, Hasselblad V, Schachter R. An introduction to a Bayesian method for meta-analysis: The confidence profile method. Med Decis Making 1990;10:15–23.

109. Nicolucci A, Grilli R, Alexanian AA, Apolone G, Torri V, Liberati A. Quality, evolution, and clinical implications of randomized, controlled trials on the treatment of lung cancer: A lost opportunity for meta-analysis. JAMA 1989;262: 2101–2107.

110. Eysenck HJ. An exercise in mega-silliness. Am Psychol 1978;33:517.

111. Glass GV, Smith ML. Reply to Eysenck. Am Psychol 1978;33:517–519.

112. Chalmers I, Elbourne D, Grant A. Phenobarbitone to prevent periventricular haemorrhage in very-low-birthweight babies. Lancet 1984; 10:285–286.

113. Kuban KC, Leviton A, Krishnamoorthy KS, Brown E, Teele RL, Baglivo JA, Sullivan KF, Huff KR, White S, Cleveland RH, Allred EN, Spritzer KL, Skouteli HN, Cayea P, Eptin M. Neonatal intracranial hemorrhage and phenobarbital. Pediatrics 1986;4:443–450.

114. Chalmers TC, Berrier J, Sacks HS, Levin H, Reitman D, Nagalingam R. Meta-analysis of clinical trials as a scientific discipline. II: Replicate variability and comparison of studies that agree and disagree. Stat Med 1987;6:733–744.

115. King PR. Appraising the quality of drug-evaluation research: I. A method of meta-analysis for acute treatment medications. Can J Psychiatry 1990;35:316–319.

116. Holtzman JL, Weeks CE, Kvam DC, Berry DA, Mottonen L, Ekholm BP, Chang SF, Conard GJ. Identification of drug interactions by meta-analysis of premarketing trials: The effect of smoking on the pharmacokinetics and dosage requirements for flecainide acetate. Clin Pharmacol Ther 1989;46:1–8.

117. Baum ML, Anish DS, Chalmers TC, Sacks HS, Smith H, Fagerstrom RM. A survey of clinical trials of antibiotic prophylaxis in colon surgery: Evidence against further use of no-treatment controls. N Engl J Med 1981;305:795–799.

118. Chodak GW, Plaut ME. Use of systemic antibiotics for prophylaxis in surgery. A critical review. Arch Surg 1977;112:326–334.

119. Polk BF. Antimicrobial prophylaxis to prevent mixed bacterial infection. J Antimicrob Chemother 1981;8(Suppl D):115–129.

120. Meijer WS, Schmitz PIM, Jeekel J. Meta-analysis of randomized, controlled clinical trials of antibiotic prophylaxis in biliary tract surgery. Br J Surg 1990;77:283–290.

121. Kahlmeter G, Dahlager JI. Aminoglycoside toxicity—A review of clinical studies published between 1975 and 1982. J Antimicrob Chemother 1984;13(Suppl A):9–22.

122. Cone LA. A survey of prospective, controlled clinical trials of gentamicin, tobramycin, amikacin, and netilmicin. Clin Ther 1982;5:155–162.

123. Colditz GA, Tuden RL, Oster G. Rates of venous thrombosis after general surgery: Combined results of randomised clinical trials. Lancet 1986;2:143–146.

124. Flowers RH, Torner JC, Farr BM. Primary cytomegalovirus infection in pediatric nurses: A meta-analysis. Infect Control Hosp Epidemiol 1988;9:491–496.

125. Hall JA, Dornan MC. Patient sociodemographic characteristics as predictors of satisfaction with medical care: A meta-analysis. Soc Sci Med 1990; 30:811–818.

126. Davidson RA, Caranasos GJ. Should the elderly hypertensive be treated? Evidence from clinical trials. Arch Intern Med 1987;137:1933–1937.

127. Detsky AS, Baker JUP, O'Rourke K, Goel V. Perioperative parenteral nutrition: A meta-analysis. Ann Intern Med 1987;107:195–203.

128. Devine EC, Cook TD. Clinical and cost-saving effects of psychoeducational interventions with surgical patients: A meta-analysis. Res Nurs Health 1986;9:89–105.

129. Hathaway D. Effect of preoperative instruction on postoperative outcomes: A meta-analysis. Nurs Res 1986;35:269–275.

130. Tran ZV, Weltman A. Differential effects of exercise on serum lipid and lipoprotein levels seen with changes in body weight. A meta-analysis. JAMA 1985;254:919–924.

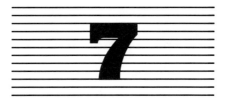

Severity of Illness and Other Confounders of Quality Measurement

Peter A. Gross, M.D.

In 1986 the Secretary of Health and Human Services was mandated by the Omnibus Budget Reconciliation Act (OBRA) to develop a legislative proposal to improve Medicare's DRGs-based prospective payment system (PPS). The mandated improvement was expected to occur when DRGs were adjusted for severity of illness and case complexity (1, 2).

Adjustments for costs used by Medicare included urban or rural location, labor costs, indirect teaching costs, the fraction of hospital patients eligible for Supplemental Security Income or Medicaid, the DRG at the time of discharge, and whether or not the case was an outlier. Only 67.4% of the variation in the average cost/case was explained by these adjustments (1).

Case-mix adjustment and severity of illness were thought to account for a large part of the remaining variation. Before examining these issues further, we need to define a glossary of critical terms (2–4).

Glossary

Case-mix a classification measure to characterize, literally, the precise mixture of cases.

Severity of illness the probability of an adverse outcome (e.g., organ failure or death) during the natural course of a disease or condition. The intent and definition of severity vary widely among the case-mix and severity measures.

Principal diagnosis the disease or condition responsible for the patient's hospital admission. The principal diagnosis is the key determinant for DRG selection.

Comorbidity a preexisting disease or condition present on hospital admission in addition to the principal diagnosis. There may be more than one per patient.

Complication a disease or condition that develops after admission. There may be more than one per patient.

ICD-9-CM the International Classification of Disease, ninth revision, Clinical Modification is a five-digit code that identifies the existence, but not the extent, of a disease or condition. (The tenth revision will be released soon.) The principal diagnosis, comorbidities, and complications are converted into ICD-9-CM codes.

UHDDS the Uniform Hospital Discharge Data Set includes the patient's age, sex, principal and other discharge diagnoses, procedures performed, the type and place where the patient is sent after discharge, and whether the patient was discharged alive, dead, or against medical advice. This data set is the basis for determining the DRG classification.

Outlier a case where the length of stay or hospital charges significantly exceed the cutoff value for the DRG.

The DRG system was developed by Thompson and Fetter at Yale University in the early 1970s as a tool for evaluating and comparing case-mix (2). In 1983 its use was greatly expanded when Medicare adopted it as the basis for its Prospective Payment System to pay hospitals under Part A.

DRG system uses the UHDDS available on most medical records. Assignment of a patient is first made to 1 of 23 major diagnostic categories (MDCs) using the principal diagnosis. Then the patient is assigned to 1 of 467 DRGs based on the principal diagnosis, age, procedures performed, presence of comorbidities, and the discharge status. The number of DRGs was expanded in later years.

While the resources consumed by individual patients within one DRG may vary widely, taken in the aggregate these resources should average out to the amount assigned for payment to that DRG. Moreover, because DRGs are based on the readily available UHDDS, the DRG methodology lends itself to computerization.

A number of major problems with the DRG system have been cited (5–13). The lack of severity of illness adjusters is just one of them. Errors in coding DRGs occur and may be intentional or unintentional. The intentional errors, also referred to as "gaming" or "DRG creep," may occur when a patient with more than one diagnosis has the most lucrative one selected as the principal diagnosis. Another objection concerns the imprecision in the ICD-9-CM classification system used to identify the diagnosis and conditions. Patients with diseases that vary significantly in severity or in resource consumption may be grouped within the same ICD-9-CM code. DRG coding categories have also been criticized for being too few in number and, hence, not sufficiently diverse to be representative. Comorbidities and complications are not adequately considered in the initial versions of the DRG system. For example, the development of a nosocomial infection may not be accounted for under DRGs. There was concern that hospitals would favor admissions for the better paying DRGs. Referral hospitals feared they would be paid inadequately because

their patients were more severely ill. Variations in the way physicians diagnose and treat the same disease are not adequately captured by DRGs. Such variations may significantly affect the resources used. The outlier is an anomaly that may result from an inadequate number of DRGs, incorrect coding, variation in physician practice, inappropriate patient management, or inadequate information abstracted from the medical record. Outliers probably need to be excluded when comparing DRGs to other case-mix systems because they are anomalies. Finally, DRGs do not distinguish appropriate from inappropriate care.

Of all the criticisms cast on the DRG system, the lack of severity of illness adjustment is the most common one cited, as analysis of this single criticism requires a careful examination of the major severity of illness indicators.

MEDISGROUPS

MedisGroups is the acronym for Medical Illness Severity Grouping System. It is a proprietary system, marketed by MediQual Systems, Inc. in Westborough, MA (14–16).

The system was developed by Alan Brewster and Bruce Karlin at St. Vincent's Hospital in Worcester, MA (17, 18). These two physicians were concerned that mortality data by itself did not give a complete view of the care rendered to patients. Adjusting for the severity of a patient's illness was required to paint a more accurate picture. They attacked the problem by developing a list of key clinical findings (KCFs) that they felt were indicative of the severity of a patient's illness. The KCFs were assigned a number from 0 to 3 to indicate illness severity. The numbers were originally assigned using clinical judgment based on the presence or likelihood of developing organ failure.

KCFs may be either present or absent (i.e., dichotomous) (Table 7.1) or represent part of a continuum (Table 7.2). The worst value in the continuum for that test or physical finding is chosen, and then assignment is made to a severity group.

Table 7.1.
Examples of Dichotomous KCFs and Severity Group Assignments[a]

Group 0 KCFs
  History of diabetes mellitus
  Murmur on physical examination
  Chronic obstructive pulmonary disease on
    chest x-ray
  Colonic polyp on barium enema
  Genitourinary stones on cystoscopy
Group 1 KCFs
  Lung perfusion defect on radionuclide scan
  Gastrointestinal hemorrhage on endoscopy
  Skin infection on physical examination,
    group 1
  Wheezing on physical examination
  Joint effusion on bone films
  Cardiac valve area <1.0 cm^2 on cardiac
    catheterization
  Urinary retention on cystometrogram
Group 2 KCFs
  Spinal cord obstruction on myelogram
  Obstruction on endoscopy
  Pancreatic pseudocyst on ultrasound
  Pulmonary embolism on arteriogram
Group 3 KCFs
  Coma or stupor on neurological examination
  Ventricular standstill on electrocardiogram
  Aortic dissection on arteriogram

[a]Adapted from Iezzoni, LI. A primer on MedisGroups. Penn Med 1989;92:28–33.

There are 260 KCFs; more than one-third of them belong to severity group 0.

Scoring is recorded on at least two occasions (14–16, 19). The first is on admission when the score derives from the KCFs. The data accumulated during the first 48 hours of admission as well as the 48 hours before admission are considered. The information is derived from the admission history and physical examination, as well as from the laboratory, radiology, and other reports. For surgical cases, the data gathered up to the time of surgery are considered. However, if surgery occurs on day 4 or later, then only the first 2 days are considered. A MedisGroups score is then determined on a scale from 0 to 4 as shown in Table 7.3. Assignment to a MedisGroup score is based on the number of KCFs with the highest severity scores.

Later during the hospital stay a second MedisGroups score is determined.

Whereas the assignment is also based on the number of KCFs with the highest severity scores, the second MedisGroups score has three instead of five groups and the terms "none", "morbid" and "major morbid" are used instead of numeric designations (Table 7.4).

The second score is taken from the data acquired between the 3rd and 7th day of the hospital stay. If the patient stay does not extend to the 7th day, then this second review is not performed. For surgical cases, the second score usually considers the data collected during the 5 days following surgery. Laboratory and other physiologic data are collected only during the last 48 hours of the review period to avoid consideration of transient abnormalities that occur immediately following surgery.

Only certain KCFs are eligible for consideration. And these KCFs are grouped into "acute" and "persistent" KCFs. Acute KCFs incorporate group 2 KCFs, such as ventricular tachycardia and exposed bone, and group 3 KCFs, such as hematocrit less than 20 and cardiac arrest. Persistent KCFs comprise only group 2 KCFs such as disoriented mental status and congestive heart failure.

The first MedisGroups score on admis-

Table 7.2.
Examples of Continuous KCFs and Severity Group Assignments[a,b]

Group 0 KCFs
  Heart rate >40 and <125 beats per minute
  Systolic blood pressure >80 mm Hg
  Potassium >2.4 and <5.4
Group 1 KCFs
  Hematocrit 25.0 to 29.9 or >55
  Temperature $>101°F$ orally
  Diastolic blood pressure 120 to 140 mm Hg
Group 2 KCFs
  Potassium >6.9
  Total bilirubin >3.0
  Respiratory rate >35
Group 3 KCFs
  Blood urea nitrogen >120
  Hematocrit <20.0
  Systolic blood pressure <60 mm Hg

[a]These examples relate to adult, nonobstetrical cases.
[b]Adapted from Iezzoni, LI. A primer on MedisGroups. Penn Med 1989;92:28–33.

Table 7.3.
Admission MedisGroups Score[a]

Score	Meaning of Score	Computation of Score
0	No significant findings	Cases with group 0 KCFs
1	Minimal findings, indicating a low potential for organ failure	One or two group 1 KCFs
2	Either acute findings connoting a short time course with an unclear potential for organ failure, or severe findings with high potential for future organ failure	One group 2 KCFs or three or more group 1 KCFs
3	Both acute and severe findings indicating a high potential for imminent organ failure	One group 3 KCF or two or more group 2 KCFs
4	Critical findings indicating the presence of organ failure	Two or more group 3 KCFs

[a]Adapted from Iezzoni, LI. A primer on MedisGroups. Penn Med 1989;92:28–33.

sion is designed to adjust for the likelihood of a poor outcome. It is intended to determine the severity of illness when the patient enters the medical care system before any medical intervention is interposed. The second score is intended to reflect the effect of iatrogenic occurrences, and as such, it could function as an outcome measure. For each scoring period, the most abnormal values are considered.

The data abstracted from the medical record are logged onto data sheets and then entered into a computer. An algorithm then determines the score.

In evaluating MedisGroups, several issues need to be considered. Nowhere in the MedisGroups score is the diagnosis considered as it is in the Computerized Severity Index (CSI) and Disease Staging (19, 20). The developers of MedisGroups felt that the precise determination of a diagnosis is often difficult and subject to too many variables, such as the manner in which a patient presents and the method that the physician uses to reach his or her diagnosis. Yet, despite the developers intent, some of the dichotomous KCFs are dependent on making specific diagnoses.

Age, sex, and the chief complaint are not considered. The relative unimportance of age as a factor is borne out by a few recent studies that suggest that prognosis is more dependent on the severity of the underlying illness than it is dependent on age.

The reviewer must look through the medical record for each patient for all of the 260 KCFs. Yet, the average case has only five to 10 KCFs. The requirement for thorough chart review unnecessarily lengthens the review time for most cases. In order for a KCF to be counted, it must be documented in the physician's admission note, progress notes, laboratory reports, radiology procedure notes, or the nurses' graphic sheet for temperature and other vital signs. Information available in the nurses' notes is omitted.

The patient's functional status is not considered in either of the two scoring periods. As a result, the patient's degree of dependency is not considered in the severity scoring. Bed ridden patients are more likely to develop decubitus ulcers, urinary tract infections, and aspiration pneumonia, yet this risk factor is not factored into the scoring method. Information on other chronic illnesses is also excluded from the scoring process.

Some abnormal values may not be considered significant unless they are very low. For example, in adults, only hematocrit values below 30 are recorded. More

Table 7.4.
MedisGroups Morbidity Score[a]

Score	Computation of Score
None	All other
Morbid	One group 2 ACUTE KCF or one or more group 2 PERSISTENT KCFs
Major morbid	One or more group 3 ACUTE KCFs or more than one group 2 ACUTE KCFs or one or more group 2 ACUTE KCF and one or more group 2 PERSISTENT KCF

[a]Adapted from Iezzoni, LI. A primer on MedisGroups. Penn Med 1989;92:28–33.

mild degrees of anemia are not recorded. Other severity measures based on physiologic values, such as APACHE II, include abnormal values omitted by MedisGroups in their scoring methodology.

Group 0 KCFs are not counted in the final score. Many of them would be considered significant in other severity scoring systems. Some of the group 0 KCFs, such as high systolic blood pressure and low respiratory rate, could have significant prognostic implications, but they are nevertheless omitted. In addition, during the scoring for the second "midstay" review, not all group 2 and 3 KCFs are counted when computing the score. And the assignment of congestive heart failure to the "persistent" rather than the "acute" category of KCFs is variable and will depend on the individual patient.

There is no method to assure the accuracy of information written in the medical record. A patient may have a friction rub or papilledema. If it is not observed or if it is observed and not entered into the medical record, the information will be lost.

Some KCFs are dependent on the use of advanced medical technologies. For example, hospitals where physicians perform endoscopy or cardiac catheterization may be unfairly compared to hospitals that do not.

If MedisGroups is shown to be effective in predicting outcome, it may not necessarily be as effective in predicting hospital costs. In Iezzoni et al.'s study of Medis-Groups, the authors found that the Medis-Group scoring method at admission was able to explain only 3% of costs that were not accounted for by DRGs alone. For individual DRGs, the range was 0 to 21%. Clearly then, the addition of an admission

MedisGroups Score to DRGs will not significantly increase the predictive value of hospital costs (15). We should not expect any one of these severity scoring methods to be useful for all clinical and administrative aspects of medical care.

Finally, normative scores or normative distributions of scores are not widely available for comparing the findings in one hospital with another. The same caveat applies when comparing scores among providers.

APACHE II

APACHE is the acronym for Acute Physiology and Chronic Health Evaluation. The "II" indicates that it is the second version. It is in the public domain, but a computerized version is available from APACHE Medical Systems, Inc., in Washington, D.C. (2).

William Knaus and Douglas Wagner developed Apache in the early 1980's at the ICU Research Unit in the Department of Anesthesiology at George Washington University Medical Center in Washington, D.C. (21). The scoring system was created to predict the intensity of service and the patients' risk of death in an intensive care unit (ICU). It uses objective data readily available for ICU patients. Like Medis-Groups, it is not disease-specific. Instead, its measurements reflect final common pathways for many illnesses.

There are two components to the APACHE score: a physiologic score that indicates the severity of the acute illness, and a chronic health score that measures health status prior to the acute illness.

The first version of APACHE used 34

measurements to assess the physiologic score. Assessment of the chronic health score incorporated the patient's functional status, productivity, and the type and frequency of medical encounters 6 months before admission. APACHE has been validated as an accurate method for predicting outcome and mortality in ICU patients (22).

The initial APACHE methodology has been refined and the number of scoring measurements reduced. The second version, APACHE II, was released in 1985 (23). It uses 12 instead of 34 physiologic measurements. The 12 measures can be grouped as follows:

Vital signs—heart rate, mean blood pressure, respiratory rate, temperature;
Venous blood tests—hematocrit, white blood cell count, serum potassium, sodium, and creatinine;
Arterial blood gases—pH and PaO_2; and
Glasgow coma scale, which includes scores for eye opening and verbal and motor responses.

The findings for each measure are converted to a score between 0 and 4, based on the degree of abnormality. Table 7.5 shows the conversion table, and Table 7.6 enumerates the Glasgow coma scale.

The final score is made up of three components. The first component is the acute physiologic score (APS), and it has a maximum of 60 points. The second component is age, and it contributes a maximum of six points (Table 7.7). The final component is the chronic illness score, and it adds a maximum of five points (Table 7.8). The total for all three components theoretically may reach 71 but most often is less than 30 (Table 7.9).

The APACHE score should be determined within 24 hours of admission to the ICU. The most abnormal value for each measurement is chosen. Scoring can also be done at other times during hospitalization, depending on the investigator's intention.

APACHE II is one of the most widely studied severity of illness indicators. It has been validated by its developers as well as by other investigators (24, 25). While it was originally designed to show the relationship between severity of illness and the risk of death in medical and surgical intensive care units, many additional applications have been studied.

Institutional differences in the accuracy of APACHE II as a predictor of mortality have been shown to be due to differences in the effective functioning of the ICU's staff (24). The degree of interaction and communications among the staff personnel within the ICU was directly correlated with a favorable outcome. Conversely, the lack of effective communication adversely affected outcome. Knaus et al. (24) felt that the coordination among the staff was more critical than the administrative structure of the unit, the specific therapies given, or the teaching status of the hospital.

Clinical assessment with APACHE II can facilitate appropriate utilization of an ICU (26). Patients with low APACHE II scores are unlikely to require admission to ICUs or can be discharged from ICUs.

The likelihood of a patient's receiving long-term benefit from hemodialysis in an ICU has been assessed (27). In conducting this study, Dobkin and Cutler used an equation to predict the risk of death. The equation was weighted with data from APACHE II, the presence of an emergency operation, and the diagnosis. The equation correctly predicted a patient's death with 100% specificity. The sensitivity and negative predictive value were low, however, showing that the equation did not consistently select the survivors. As medical care expenses increase nationally, similar types of analysis will be proposed to ration health care services.

Rubins and Moskowitz (28) showed that the acute physiologic score (APS) component of APACHE II, the presence of upper gastrointestinal bleeding, and age, were independent predictors of an unexpected death or a readmission to the ICU. They did not, however, use the information to discharge low risk patients from the ICU. The study shows how the major component of APACHE II, namely, the APS score, can be used.

The methodology of APACHE II score

Table 7.5.
Acute Physiology Score of APACHE II[a]

Physiologic Variable	High Abnormal Range				0	Low Abnormal Range				Score
	+4	+3	+2	+1		+1	+2	+3	+4	
Temperature—rectal (°C)	≥41°	39°–40.9°		38.5°–38.9°	36°–38.4°	34°–35.9°	32°–33.9°	30°–31.9°	≤29.9°	
Mean Arterial Pressure—mm Hg	≥160	130–159	110–129		70–109		50–69		≤49	
Heart Rate (ventricular response)	≥180	140–179	110–139		70–109		55–69	40–54	≤39	
Respiratory rate (nonventilated or ventilated)	≥50	35–49		25–34	12–24	10–11	6–9		≤5	
Oxygenation: A-aDO₂ or PaO₂ (mm Hg)[b] a. FiO₂ ≥ 0.5 record A-aDO₂	≥500	350–499	200–349		<200					
b. FiO₂ < 0.5 record only PaO₂					PO₂>70	PO₂61–70		PO₂55–60	PO₂<55	
Arterial pH	≥7.7	7.6–7.69		7.5–7.59	7.33–7.49		7.25–7.32	7.15–7.24	≤7.15	
Serum sodium (mmol/liter)	≥180	160–179	155–159	150–154	130–139		120–129	111–119	≤110	
Serum potassium (mmol/liter)	≥7	6–6.9		5.5–5.9	3.5–5.4	3–3.4	2.5–2.9		<2.5	
Serum creatinine (mg/100 ml) (Double point score for acute renal failure)	≥3.5	2–3.4	1.5–1.9		0.6–1.4		<0.6			
Hematocrit (%)	≥60	50–59.9		46–49.9	30–45.9		20–29.9		<20	
White blood count (total/mm³) in (1,000s)	≥40	20–39.9		15–19.9	3–14.9		1–2.9		<1	
Glasgow coma score (GCS): Score = 15 minus actual GCS										
Total acute physiology score (APS): Sum of the 12 individual variable points										
Serum HCO₂ (venous-mmol/liter) (Not preferred, use if no ABGs)	≥52	41–51.9		32–40.9	22–31.9		18–21.9	15–17.9	<15	

[a]Adapted from Knaus WA, Draper EA, Wagner DP, Zimmerman JE. APACHE II: A severity of disease classification system. Crit Care Med 1985;13:818–829.
[b]Oxygenation:
If FiO₂ > 0.5, then record alveolo-arterial oxygen pressure difference.
If FiO₂ < 0.5, then record PaO₂ only.

Table 7.6.
Glasgow Coma Scale

Eye opening	
Spontaneous	4
To voice	3
To pain	2
None	1
Verbal response	
Oriented	5
Confused	4
Inappropriate words	3
Incomprehensible sounds	2
None	1
Motor response	
Obeys command	6
Localizes pain	5
Withdraw (pain)	4
Flexion (pain)	3
Extension (pain)	2
None	1
Total score	

Table 7.7.
Age Points for APACHE II

Age	Points
<44	0
45–54	2
55–64	3
65–74	5
≥75	6

may not be uniformly applied. Jacobs and co-workers (29) used the best rather than the worst Glasgow coma score in a study done in Riyadh, Saudi Arabia. This methodologic difference, as well as certain host factor differences, resulted in higher than expected mortality rates in their ICU. The important host factors included the presence of a high proportion of patients with such chronic illnesses as end-stage liver cirrhosis from schistosomiasis or hepatitis B virus and metastatic malignancy as well as the inclusion of patients transferred from other hospitals who were victims of motor vehicle accidents.

Predictions of death improved when more than one APACHE II score was determined. These scores are best calculated on the day of admission and on day 3 (30).

In another study from Jacob's group (31), APACHE II scores were shown to be more accurate predictors of outcome when corrected for major organ system failure. The criteria for organ failure were actually developed by Knaus and his colleagues, who also developed APACHE II. The presence of acute renal failure, neurological failure, as well as cardiovascular and hematological failure, had the best predictive

values. Respiratory failure, while common, had no predictive value. The number of organ system failures correlated well with outcome. Counting the number of organ system failures is analogous to counting the number of comorbidities, which will be discussed in a later section. The authors propose that APACHE II scores, adjusted for the number of organ system failures, might be used to aid decisions on whether or not to proceed with aggressive medical therapy.

Echoing the above findings, Cerra et al. (32) found that APACHE II failed to predict the emergence of the multiple organ failure syndrome. They found the important factors that predicted the syndrome were time-dependent changes in PaO_2-to-fraction of inspired oxygen ratio, as well as serum lactate, bilirubin, and creatinine. Only one of these factors, namely, serum creatinine, is a component of the APACHE II score. The study was conducted in postoperative surgical patients.

The utility of APACHE II as an outcome predictor has also been questioned in certain other types of critically ill patients. Fedullo and colleagues (33) found that patients with respiratory failure from cardiogenic pulmonary edema was not accurately categorized for prognosis by APACHE II. They also found an inverse relationship between APACHE II scores and mortality rather than the direct one showed by Knaus et al. (23). When the case-mix is weighted toward cardiac pulmonary edema, APACHE II may not be a reliable prognostication.

The utility of APACHE II to predict who would benefit most from total parenteral nutrition has been studied and found lacking (34). While the indication was highly specific in predicting who would live, it

Table 7.8.
Chronic Health Points for APACHE II

If the patient has a history of severe organ system insufficiency or is immunocompromised, assign
  points as follows:
  a. For nonoperative or emergency postoperative patients: 5 points
     or
  b. For elective postoperative patients: 2 points

DEFINITIONS
Organ insufficiency or immunocompromised state must have been evident prior to this hospital
  admission and conform to the following criteria:
LIVER: Biopsy-proven cirrhosis and documented portal hypertension; episodes of past upper GI
  bleeding attributed to portal hypertension; or prior episodes of hepatic failure/encephalopathy/
  coma.
CARDIOVASCULAR: New York Heart Association Class IV.
RESPIRATORY: Chronic restrictive, obstructive, or vascular disease resulting in severe exercise
  restriction, i.e., unable to climb stairs or perform household duties; or documented chronic
  hypoxia, hypercapnia, secondary polycythemia, severe pulmonary hypertension (>40 mm Hg), or
  respirator dependency.
RENAL: Receiving chronic dialysis.
IMMUNOCOMPROMISED: The patient has received therapy that suppresses resistance to
  infection, e.g., immunosuppression, chemotherapy, radiation, long-term or recent high dose
  steroids, or has a disease that is sufficiently advanced to suppress resistance to infection, e.g.,
  leukemia, lymphoma, AIDS.

had a low sensitivity in predicting who
would die. It appears that APACHE II is
not better than clinical judgment in predicting who would live or die. This sentiment was also recorded by Kruse et al. (25)
in their study comparing physicians' and
nurses' predictions of mortality to
APACHE II in a medical ICU.

Modifications of APACHE II are common. Moreau and colleagues (35) compared an Acute Physiologic Score (APS), a
Simplified Acute Physiologic Score (SAPS),
Coronary Prognostic Index (CPI), and
APACHE II. APS is composed of the 34
physiologic measurements in the first version of APACHE. SAPS uses the 13 measurements from the APS component of
APACHE II and adds age as well as the
need for mechanical ventilation. They
found that for short-term prognosis in ICU
patients with acute myocardial infarctions
SAPS and APACHE II gave more accurate
information than APS.

Moreau et al. (35) also pointed out the
value of examining Receiver Operating
Characteristic (ROC) curves. The ROC
curve shows the relationship between the
proportion of true positives (i.e., sensitivity) and false positives (1-specificity). They

Table 7.9.
APACHE II Score

Sum of $A + B + C$	
A, APS points	_____
B, Age points	_____
C, Chronic health points	_____
Total APACHE II	_____

define true positives as the nonsurvivors.
Sensitivity of their severity indicators,
then, is defined as the ratio of the correctly
predicted number of nonsurvivors to the
total number of nonsurvivors, while specificity is defined as the ratio of the correctly
predicted number of survivors to the total
number of survivors. Parenthetically, the
reader should take note that these definitions vary by author. Moreau defines true
positives as nonsurvivors, whereas Hopefl
defines them as survivors.

Because of the above concerns with
APACHE II, a large-scale study is underway to develop an improved version,
which will be called APACHE III (36). The
methodologic approach for developing
APACHE III has been described, but the
final version of APACHE III has not yet
been determined.

The three areas for further development are the physiologic measures, the chronic health measures, and disease categorization (37).

More physiologic measures will be assessed in the research plan. In particular, six measures will be added: blood urea nitrogen (BUN), bilirubin, $PaCO_2$, serum glucose, urine output, and serum albumin.

The chronic health status will also be further developed. APACHE II captures only certain severe end-stage comorbidities. Less severe stages, which may represent significant functional limitations, will now be appraised.

The effect of the patient's primary life-threatening diagnosis will be evaluated. APACHE III will access 150 disease categories grouped by organ system and operative status. With the incorporation of disease-specific information, APACHE III will more closely resemble CSI and other disease-oriented severity indices.

The time of measurement will also be investigated. A patient's status often changes significantly over 5 days. How the patient spends his or her initial hospital stay is relevant. If the patient is in the emergency department and no scoring is performed until transfer to ICU, the result may be misleading. Other factors, such as whether the patient is continuously or intermittently monitored may also affect the measured values.

Finally, how the information can be used will be studied. What is its value in identifying low-risk patients who may not require ICU admission or who may be discharged from the ICU? How worthwhile will it be for predicting which high-risk patients are unlikely to respond to further treatment because of multiple organ failure (38)?

CSI

CSI is the acronym for the Computerized Severity Index and is the successor to the Manual Severity of Illness Index. It is available through Health Systems International, Inc. in Meriden, CT (39–42).

The Severity of Illness Index was developed in the mid-1980s by Susan Horn and her colleagues at the Center for Hospital Finance and Management, The Johns Hopkins University, in Baltimore, MD. A computerized version (CSI) was developed in the late 1980s. The index was designed to explain hospital-to-hospital variations in resource use not explained by the DRG system. Unlike MedisGroups and APACHE II, CSI is disease specific. Horn et al. attempt to capture and score the total burden of the patient's illness by considering the principal diagnosis, comorbid conditions and complications, disease severity, and the patient's response to the illness.

The original manual Severity of Illness Index was not disease specific and was based on seven dimensions designed to capture the total impact of the illness on the patient (Table 7.10). The first three dimensions were found to be the most important criteria for predicting the burden of illness. The principal diagnosis, the secondary diagnoses or comorbidities, and the complications of hospitalization have also been found by many investigators to be the critical components.

Dependency, the fourth dimension reflects care rendered by nurses, physical therapists, and other ancillary personnel. It correlates highly with the second and third dimensions, that is, with complications and comorbidities. For the fifth dimension, only life-support procedures, such as the decision to use dialysis and/or put a patient on a ventilator, are considered severity level 3 or 4. Other routine diagnostic and therapeutic procedures are scored at severity level 1 or 2. Both of these dimensions serve as internal monitors and were found not to be necessary in predicting overall severity. The fourth and fifth

Table 7.10.
Seven Dimensions of Manual Severity of Illness Index

1. Stage of principal diagnosis on admission
2. Complications related to principal diagnosis
3. Concurrent interacting conditions or comorbidities
4. Dependency on hospital staff
5. Non-operating room procedures
6. Response to treatment
7. Residual disease at discharge

dimensions show the patient's response to treatment and the extent of residual disease at the end of the hospital stay.

Scoring the manual Severity of Illness Index was difficult and time consuming. As a result, Dr. Horn and her colleagues developed the CSI.

CSI includes the first three dimensions of the original manual index, namely, the principal diagnoses, comorbidities, and complications. It omits the other four dimensions. The first three dimensions were able to predict 68–75% of the variation predicted by the complete seven dimension index.

One additional step was taken and that was to tie the severity index into the existing ICD-9-CM diagnostic coding system used by most hospitals in the United States. The ICD-9-CM diagnostic codes are codes for the principal diagnosis, comorbidities, and complications experienced by the patient. The codes contain up to five digits each and are routinely listed on the UHDDS at the time of discharge. The codes, however, do not contain a severity score, nor do they necessarily reflect the severity of the patient's principal diagnosis, or the comorbid conditions or complications that occur in the hospital.

Dr. Horn and her colleagues proposed that a sixth digit be added to the five-digit ICD-9-CM coding system. The sixth digit would be listed on a scale from 1 to 4 based on the severity of illness for the particular ICD-9-CM code. When fully developed, a fourth book would be added to the three-volume ICD-9-CM series. The fourth book would contain the criteria for assigning a score of 1 to 4 as the sixth digit.

The severity scale of 1 to 4 represents an ordinal not a linear progression. For example, the differences in clinical severity between level 1 and 2 may be slight, while the clinical differences between level 2 and 3 may be great.

Horn groups several ICD-9-CM codes that reflect a similar diagnosis. She uses one set of criteria to determine severity for all the codes in the group. For example, most types of pneumonia use one criteria set as shown in Table 7.11. The different types of acute myocardial infarction use another criteria set. There are approxi-

mately 700 criteria sets for over 10,000 ICD-9-CM codes.

The same sign or symptom may be assigned a different severity level in different criteria sets. For example, a fever of 102°F is severity level 2 in the pneumonia criteria set but is severity level 3 in the leukemia criteria set.

When the patient fails to meet any of the severity criteria, a level of 0 is assigned and the diagnosis may also be questioned. The diagnosis would have to be examined since the findings listed in the criteria set are also the criteria used to make the diagnosis on clinical grounds.

At least two criteria at a specific severity level or higher must be met to be assigned to a severity level. For example, level 2 fever and level 3 blood count results will be assigned a severity level 2 for the diagnosis. A single extreme criteria, therefore, will not bias the determination of the severity level.

Like the disease staging index, CSI eliminates secondary diseases that are directly related to the principal diagnosis. Also eliminated is the chance that a single patient characteristic will be used more than once in determining the severity level for different patient diagnoses.

An overall severity score is determined for each patient. The overall score utilizes the severity level of each diagnosis and weights them to reflect the interaction between the diagnoses (Table 7.12).

Dr. Horn and her colleagues have done numerous validation studies. In one early study (39), 106,000 discharges from 15 hospitals showed that DRGs adjusted with her Severity of Illness Index explained 61% of the variability in resource use per patient while unadjusted DRGs explained only 28% of the variation.

These researchers also explored the variations within DRGs. Using the same 15 hospitals, Horn et al. showed that for 24% of the patients, the Severity of Illness Index explained more than 50% of the variations in resource used. When they examined a larger group, or 94% of the patients, only 10% of the variations in resource use could be explained (43).

Other problems within DRGs have been pointed out by Dr. Horn. Cystic fibrosis

Table 7.11.
Pneumonia Criteria Set for Four Categories of Severity: Pneumonia with Associated
ICD-9-CM Codes[a]

	Pneumonia			
480.0–486 668.00–668.04	506.3 997.3	507.0–507.1 112.4	516.8 136.3 055.1	517.1 518.3 518.5
Category	1		2	3 4
Cardiovascular	•pulse rate <100; ST segment changes on ECG	•pulse rate 100–129; PACs, PAT, PVCs on ECG	•pulse rate ≥130	•life-threatening arrhythmias or hypotension
Fever	•≦100.4 and/or chills	•100.5–102.0	•102.1–103.9 and/or rigors	•≧104.0
LABS ABGS	•pH 7.35–7.45	•pH 7.46–7.50 7.34–7.25	•pH 7.51–7.60 7.24–7.10	•pH ≧7.61 ≦7.09; pO$_2$ ≦50
Hematology	•WBC × 1000 4.5–11.0/cu mm; Bands <10% WBC × 1000 11.0–4.5/cu mm	•WBC × 1000 11.1–20.0/cu mm; Bands 10–20% WBC × 1000 4.4–2.4/cu mm	•WBC × 1000 20.1–30.0/cu mm; Bands 21–40% WBC × 1000 2.3–1.0/cu mm	•WBC × 1000 ≧30.1/cu mm; Bands >40% WBC × 1000 <1.0/cu mm
Neurology		•chronic confusion	•acute confusion	•unresponsive
Radiology chest x-ray or CT scan		•infiltrate and/or consolidation in ≦1 lobe; pleural effusion	•infiltrate and/or consolidation in >1 lobe but ≦3 lobes; cavitation or necrosis lung •cyanosis	•infiltrate and/or consolidation in >3 lobes
Respiratory		•dyspnea on exertion; stridor; rales ≦50%/≦3 lobes; decreased breath sounds ≦50%/≦3 lobes; positive for fremitus over site of infiltrate	•dyspnea at rest •rales >50%/>3 lobes; decreased breath sounds >50%/>3 lobes	•apnea •absent breath sounds >50%/>3 lobes
	•white, thin mucoid sputum	•hemoptysis NOS	•frank hemoptysis	

(CF), for example, can be classified into one of 87 DRGs. Horn found that 1,763 patients with CF and 25,628 patients without CF could be classified within the same 87 DRGs. Using the eight DRGs where most patients with CF were grouped, she found significant discrepancies in the length of stay and the cost of treatment for the patients with CF compared to other patients classified within the same DRGs. The average length of stay in the CF group was 14.9 days compared to 8.3 days in the others. The average cost for the CF group was $7,262 per patient compared to $2,908 for the others. For the two groups, the ratio of costs was 2.5 while the ratio for lengths of stay was 1.8. The higher ratio for costs indicates the high resource use per patient day for the patients with CF (11).

With the clarion call for quality assessment ringing throughout the land, the desire to compare hospitals to one another or to compare physicians' quality of care is irresistible. A severity measure will be

Table 7.12.
Overall Severity Determinations: Interaction among Diagnoses on Two Patients with Pneumonia

| | | DRG 89—Simple Pneumonia | | |
	Age	Diagnoses	Disease Severity	Overall Severity
Patient 1	72	Pneumonia	3	2
Patient 2	71	Pneumonia	2	3
		CHF[a]	3	
		COPD	3	

[a]CHF, congestive heart failure; COPD, chronic obstructive pulmonary disease.

necessary to make these comparisons. Horn et al. examined health care expenditures by physician. They found large differences in physician expenditures for patients within the same DRGs. For 37% of the physicians, the differences were greater than $10,000. When the DRGs were adjusted for severity, many of the differences disappeared (44). Profiling physicians by unadjusted DRGs was clearly unwarranted.

Consistency of the raters who score any severity index is always a concern. Horn and Horn (45) have described their methods for training raters. In reliability testing from 18 hospitals, they found that raters with at least 2 months experience in scoring agreed with the original staff rater between 91 and 98% of the time.

Numerous ethical issues have been raised about the DRG system. A particularly perplexing one concerns the temptation of hospitals to admit primarily patients with higher paying DRGs. If hospitals are paid appropriately for severity-adjusted DRGs, this temptation will be less attractive (46).

Horn's Severity of Illness Index has been assessed in a non-medical-surgical setting. A specialized Psychiatric Severity of Illness (PSI) Index has been developed by Horn's group. In a 10-hospital study, they found that most of the psychiatric diagnoses fell within four severity of illness groups. In these groups, PSI explained the variations in length of stay better than the DRGs (47).

CSI is difficult to assess because most of the studies have been conducted by its developer. Furthermore, the literature lacks large scale studies of CSI, either examined alone or in comparison to other severity indices (48).

DISEASE STAGING

Disease Staging was developed by Joseph Gonnella and his colleagues at Jefferson Medical College in Philadelphia during the mid-1970s (49). It has undergone further development by Daniel Louis and his associates at Systemetrics, Inc. in Santa Barbara, CA (50–53). Their most recent product EQCEL (Evaluation of Quality, Costs and Effectiveness Levels) is an integrated, computerized package that can be used for severity and case-mix analysis, quality assurance, utilization review, and financial analysis.

The concept behind Disease Staging is based on the staging criteria developed by oncologists in the 1950s. They devised a staging system for the purpose of evaluating the efficacy of cancer treatment. Gonnella, Louis, and their colleagues applied this concept by stating that all diseases and disorders can be divided into four major stages of increasing severity (54):

Stage I   Conditions with no complications or problems of minimal severity.

Stage II   Problems limited to an organ or system; significantly increased risk of complications.

Stage III Multiple site involvement; generalized systemic involvement; poor prognosis.

Stage IV   Death.

Within each stage there are substages defined for most diseases, and they are designated by numbers to the right of the decimal point. With appendicitis, for example, the patient's presentation may fall into one of the following stages and substages:

1.0 Appendicitis
2.1 Appendicitis with perforation causing: localized peritonitis and/or peritoneal abscess
2.2 Appendicitis with perforation causing: generalized peritonitis
2.3 Intestinal obstruction
2.4 Pylephlebitis with or without liver abscess
3.1 Septicemia, bacteremia
3.2 Shock
4.0 Death

Patients can be staged at any time during their hospital course. Changes to higher stages may indicate a problem with the quality of care or the natural progression of the disease.

Complication and comorbid diseases are related and specified by classifying the patient in a higher stage or are unrelated and indicated by listing the patient in another disease category. For example, look at a patient with the following diagnostic ICD-9-CM codes:

402.11 Hypertensive heart disease with congestive heart failure
436 Cerebrovascular accident
303.9 Chronic alcoholism
571.2 Alcoholic cirrhosis of liver

This patient would be classified with the Disease Staging Unrelated Comorbidity Algorithm into the Staging Disease Categories of:

829 Essential hypertension, Stage 3.1
242 Alcoholism, Stage 3.4

Two different formats are available for using Disease Staging. The first one uses the medical record and is called Clinical Staging. The second format employs the automated medical record abstract and is called Coded Staging. The software package for Coded Staging is called Q-Stage. These two formats access different information in the medical record.

Clinical Staging assesses diagnostic, laboratory, and physical findings. It can be used at different times during the hospital course. It is best used when the application involves relatively few charts. The infor-

mation for classification is available in the latest edition of Gonnella's *Clinical Criteria to Disease Staging* available through SysteMetrics (53).

For large scale studies, the computerized Code Staging methodology is more appropriate. The software package, Q-Stage, can be used to examine all ICD-9-CM diagnostic codes, procedure codes, sex, and discharge status, which are found in the automated medical record discharge abstract or UHDDS. The output is a Q-Scale. The final determinations are affected by inaccuracies in ICD-9 coding. This method does not take into account all the physiologic information available for scoring that is used by the manual Clinical Staging method. Q-Scale is a linear or continuous scale rather than an ordinal scale, so it can be averaged across different patient populations.

Q-Scale produces three severity values. The first value, DRGSCALE, shows the patient's severity relative to the national mean severity for a particular DRG. For example, a value of 150 shows that the patient's severity level is 50% higher than the average national severity for that DRG.

The second Q-Scale value, TOTSCALE, represents the patient's severity level relative to all DRGs for the nation. It combines the within-DRG severity value, the DRG relative weight, disease stage, major surgical operations, age, and sex. TOTSCALE increases the predictive power of DRGs for resource utilization.

The third Q-Scale value, QSCALE, indicates the patient's severity level relative to the national level regardless of the DRGs. Surgery, age, and sex are omitted. It can be used when DRG information is not available. It does not predict resource use as well as TOTSCALE.

Q-Scale has been validated by SysteMetrics, using 50,000 randomly selected hospital discharges. An almost linear correlation was shown for charges per patient and Q-Scale score. The reviewers also showed that Q-Scale improves the predictive power of DRGs for hospital charge variation by 48.2%, that is, from 19.1 to 28.3% (54).

Coffey and Goldfarb (50) evaluated the length of stay variations among patients in

50 Maryland hospitals. They found that large hospitals were paid more under a DRG-based system than when Disease Staging (Code Staging) was the basis of payment. Since Disease Staging does not include all the procedures performed, the finding implies that the use of Disease Staging would promote disincentives for performing surgery.

Gonnella, Hornbrook, and Louis (52) scored a large group of patients with diabetes mellitus using Coded Staging. Length of stay increased for each of the four stages of Disease Staging. Other important factors were age, type of admission, surgical status, payment source, hospital ownership, number of beds, and teaching status.

McMahon and Newbold (55) examined the effect of physicians' practice patterns on length of stay. The severity of illness for each patient was adjusted by using Disease Staging. They showed that variability in resource use was better explained by physicians' practice patterns than by the patient's severity of illness.

PATIENT MANAGEMENT CATEGORIES

Patient Management Categories (PMCs) system was developed in the late 1970s and early 1980s by Wanda Young and her colleagues at the Health Care Research Department of Blue Cross of Western Pennsylvania (BCWP). In the mid-1980s, the staff of the research department was transferred to the Pittsburgh Research Institute, a not-for-profit affiliate of BCWP (56, 57).

PMCs were developed to create a case-mix measure that incorporated both severity of illness and comorbidity. The developers proposed PMCs as a replacement for DRGs rather than as a supplement.

The PMC system was created by defining approximately 50 disease or disorder groups. Each group requires a separate diagnostic and treatment plan. Within the disease groups, multiple Patient Management Categories were defined. A total of 800 PMCs were devised.

The Patient Management Categories that Young et al. developed describe illnesses most often found in an acute care hospital. The system is computerized, and severity of illness is factored into the PMCs classification system. The variables for each patient included age, sex, one to five diagnoses, and one to three procedures. The diagnoses and procedures are identified by ICD-9-CM codes. All of this information is available in the Uniform Hospital Discharge Data set (UHDDS). The order of the diagnoses does not affect the PMC selected. Although up to five PMCs are considered per patient, only one PMC per disease or disorder group is permitted. When more than one PMC occurs in a disease group, the most severe is selected.

A relative cost weight (RCW) is assigned to each PMC. Physicians determined RCWs to show the resources required for effective and efficient patient management. The RCW is independent of the actual resources used on a patient and is independent of hospital inefficiencies. Multiple PMCs for a patient are evaluated to give a single RCW.

Table 7.13 shows a patient with only one PMC. The software for PMC classification analyzes all ICD-9 diagnostic codes before assigning a PMC. Related ICD-9 codes are identified.

Table 7.14 illustrates a patient with more than one PMC. In this case, each diagnosis was associated with a procedure. The RCW for each PMC would have been 25.626 for the cardiac PMC and 14.137 for the proximal femoral fracture. A weightor computer routine selected the PMC with the highest cost. To arrive at a single RCW of 34.693, it combined overlaps between the two PMCs and added the cost of components of care.

A case-mix analyses package, based on the PMC classification system, is also available for the computer.

Multiple uses for PMCs have been proposed by the developers. Since DRGs do not adequately reflect severity of illness and comorbidity, the PMC classification system could substitute for DRGs. The relative cost weights (RCWs) derived for PMCs could be used as financial guidelines for more cost-efficient care. Utilization review and quality assurance coordinators

Table 7.13.
Example of PMC Classification for Patient with One PMC

A.	*Principal diagnosis*	41090	Myocardial infarction NOS[a]
	Diagnosis code	43800	Late effects of cerebrovascular disease
	Diagnosis code	42731	Atrial fibrillation
	Diagnosis code	00000	
	Diagnosis code	00000	
B.	*Principal procedure*	00000	
	Procedure code	00000	
	Procedure code	00000	
C.	*Age*: 68 years		
D.	*Sex*: Female		
PMC:	0302 Acute MI: Tachyarrythmia		
PMC:	0000		
PMC:	0000		
PMC:	0000		
PMC:	0000		
RCW:	12.800		

[a]Not otherwise specified.

Table 7.14.
Example of Patient with More Than One PMC

A.	*Principal diagnosis*	42613	Atrioventricular block, 2nd degree
	Diagnosis code	82022	Subtrochanteric fracture closed
	Diagnosis code	00000	
	Diagnosis code	00000	
	Diagnosis code	00000	
B.	*Principal procedure*	03774	Insertion permanent pacemaker ventricular-transvenous
	Procedure code	07935	Reduction, internal fixation of femur
	Procedure code	00000	
C.	*Age*: 73 years		
D.	*Sex*: Male		
PMC:	3914 Cardiac: bradycardia/heart block with operation		
PMC:	1901 Femur fracture proximal: operative repair		
PMC:	0000		
PMC:	0000		
PMC:	0000		
RCW:	34.693		

could use the RCWs to identify persistent problem areas in the delivery of care. The approach to utilization could then be extended to assess the need for facility alterations and to evaluate regional needs.

Unfortunately, little of the PMC developers experience has been published. Most of the published studies on the value of PMCs are available only in comparative studies, which we will consider later.

OTHER SEVERITY OF ILLNESS MEASURES

We have examined five of the major severity measures. There are other mea-sures that have been studied less extensively or that were designed for specific types of patients, such as those with trauma.

The following is a listing of other general severity measures (2). The completeness of evaluation for these indices is variable.

Prospective Individualized Reimbursement (PIR) (58)
Therapeutic Intervention Scoring System (TISS) (59)
Physiologic Stability Index (PSI) (60)
Mortality Prediction Models (MPM) (60)
Nursing Intensity (61)
Clinical Classification System (CCS) (62)

The following is a listing of the severity measures designed to evaluate patients with specific categories of illness:

Clinically Related Groups for psychiatric patients (63)
Trauma score (TS) (64)
Injury Severity Score (ISS) (64)
Acute Physiologic Score for Children (APSC) (59)
Pediatric Risk of Mortality (PRISM) (59)
Hanover Intensity System (HIS) (65)
Organ Failure System (66)
American Society of Anesthesiologists Classification (ASA) (68)

Many more references are available for these severity measures, but only one representative reference is listed. In addition, many other severity measures have been described that are not shown.

Some authors combine two or more severity scoring systems to make a new one. For example, Jordan et al. (67) combined TISS and APACHE II with a multiple organ failure scale to derive their own rating system, which they claim is a more effective indicator of the severity of sepsis than are the component parts. Some authors use different severity indicators separately but sequentially and have shown that the addition of one to another significantly improves the predictive power. For example, Rhee et al. (64) found that TS and ISS added to the predictive power of APACHE II.

Finally, an index based on the number of comorbidities should be considered (69–74). A comorbidity is usually defined as other conditions or diseases present on admission beyond the principal diagnosis. The score usually is determined by simply counting the number of comorbidities. The higher the number, the more severely ill the patient. Several studies have been conducted with this type of measure. However, no single definition of the measure has prevailed. The confusion lies in at least two areas. The first is the definition of comorbidities, namely, whether it should include complications that occur after hospitalization. The second is the activity of the condition or comorbidity at the time of scoring. The studies that count only active comorbidities confirm the value of a comorbidity index as a reliable measure of severity (69, 70). Few studies have been conducted to examine the comparability of a comorbidity index with the five major commercially available severity measures. In one study, the comorbidity index was comparable to APACHE II and CSI (74). With more extensive validation studies, a comorbidity index may become one of the major severity measures.

COMPARISONS OF SEVERITY SCORING SYSTEMS

To assess the value and validity of the major severity of illness scoring systems, one must carefully examine many factors (Table 7.15). Most reports on individual severity systems have been prepared by the developers or the commercial vendors. Consequently, the objectivity of the findings is a concern of some people. Comparative studies conducted by independent investigators are necessary for a thorough evaluation.

The severity scoring systems described have been compared in several studies. Comparison, however, is difficult because they were derived differently, their intended purposes were often dissimilar, and their data bases are disparate (2). *DRGs* were developed as a tool for evaluating hospitalwide case-mix and not as the

Table 7.15.
Considerations When Comparing Severity of Illness Indicators

Original premise and purpose
Makes clinical sense to physicians
Consistency among raters
System based on reliable information
Information is readily available at a reasonable cost
Manageable number of categories
Grouping of patients who consume equivalent resources
Freedom from manipulating final score
Method of scoring
Time of calculating score
Available in computerized format
Cost of purchasing, training, and maintaining

basis for Medicare's prospective payment system. It uses routinely collected data from the UHDDS. *APACHE II* was developed to predict intensity of service and risk of death in intensive care units. It uses physiologic measurements available in the ICU. *Disease Staging* is a patient classification system whereby researchers could measure interhospital differences in case-mix. It extrapolates the concept of staging used in oncology to score all disorders into stages of severity. *Computerized Severity Index* was created to explain variations in resource use that confounds data interpretation in the DRG system. CSI uses a combination of UHDDS information and physiologic data. *MedisGroups* was developed for quality assurance review, not to improve the prospective payment system. It uses physiologic as well as other clinical findings for scoring. *Patient Management Categories* was developed to predict resource utilization, as well as to assess appropriate diagnostic and treatment processes. It was also promoted as a substitute for the DRG system. It uses the UHDDS and is weighted for comorbidities.

All of the five major severity systems described—MedisGroups, APACHE II, CSI, PMCs, and Disease Staging—are computerized. They are all undergoing periodic revisions, which complicates attempts to compare one to another. In addition, the computer algorithms for assigning a severity category have not been published for all the severity scoring systems. The lack of access to this information prevents us from assessing the logic in the algorithms.

The costs of acquiring the software varies from inexpensive (in the $100s) for APACHE II to very expensive (in the $10,000s) for Disease Staging, CSI, Medis-Groups, and for mainframe versions of PMCs. The cost of training personnel is an additional expense that may cost $10,000 or more for some of the more elaborate systems. Finally, licenses, maintenance, and software update fees need to be considered for most of the systems.

Do the various scoring systems make clinical sense? All of them were developed with the help of physicians or other health care workers, so that they are credible to physicians. But the systems dependent on

ICD-9-CM codes, such as Disease Staging, CSI, and PMCs, are victims of the inherent subjectivity in diagnostic coding and the reduced accuracy of this classification system (9).

There is little agreement on the most appropriate time for scoring severity of illness. Should the patient's score be determined on admission before medical intervention, during the admission, or at the time of discharge? When scored early, readily reversible conditions, such as pulmonary edema, may result in an exceptionally high score. When the score is determined at discharge, complications of hospitalization, such as an adverse drug reaction or a procedure complication, may falsely elevate the severity score from that of admission. The timing will depend on the purpose of scoring, be it determining resource utilization or quality assurance evaluation.

The definition of severity will vary depending on the perspective of the end user (6). The direction of the severity scale also will be related to the intentions of the user. For example, a terminal cancer patient who requests only palliative measures and dies within a few days of admission will receive a high severity score from a physician because the patient is at the end-stage of the illness. A nurse may give the patient an intermediate score on a psychosocial adjustment scale if the patient is upset but accepting of the prognosis. An economist, on the other hand, may give the same patient a low score because the patient consumed few hospital resources during a short length of stay.

Reliability of information used in the severity scoring system is critical. An Institute of Medicine study indicated that the principal diagnosis was coded incorrectly 37% of the time when it was recorded (75). Doremus and Michenzi (76) found errors in the principal diagnosis 20% of the time. Recent studies indicate that the miscoding rate has declined (77). The ICD-9-CM was put into use in 1979. It has 10,171 possible diagnoses or codes. Yet no rules exist for determining whether a patient's diagnosis fits a particular code (12). The severity indices dependent on the ICD-9-CM classification system are DRGs, Disease Staging,

PMCs, and to some extent, CSI, whereas MedisGroups and APACHE II are not.

Interrater reliability is another critical factor in accessing severity systems. It concerns the consistency of rating between different raters when they apply a measure to the same medical records. Thomas and Ashcraft (78) compared APACHE II, MedisGroups, DRGs, PMCs, and Disease Staging Q-Scale. Cohen's κ and Interrater Reliability Coefficient (R_I) were used for reliability statistics because they adjust for the probability that the raters could agree upon purely by chance. γ and τ, which are ordinal statistical measures of association, were also used because they can better assess the noninterval scaled measures, namely PMCs, Disease Staging, and DRGs. They found, as expected, that severity scoring systems based on clinical data collected directly from the medical record MedisGroups and APACHE II had more interrater reliability. Severity measures based on diagnostic information found in the discharge abstract, such as PMCs and Disease Staging, were less reliable (Table 7.16). The differences occur because the diagnostic information in the poorer performing indices is based on ICD-9-CM codes. DRGs are also based on data from the discharged abstract, namely, ICD-9-CM codes. Yet, the reliability of DRGs was the highest of all five measures studied. DRGs' alleged shortcoming of clinical heterogeneity, that is, the grouping of several, not closely related, ICD-9-CM codes into a single DRG, is a strength that causes the DRG system to equal or outperform the other classification systems.

CSI was not examined in this study but would be expected to have a high degree of interrater reliability because, like APACHE II and MedisGroups, it is based on clinical data collected directly from the medical record. However, unlike APACHE II and MedisGroups, CSI also uses diagnostic information based on ICD-9-CM codes. CSI's predecessor, the manual severity of illness index, has been analyzed for interrater reliability. Horn and colleagues (79) found R_I scores in the 0.57 to 0.87 range for the manual SII. Soeken and Prescott (80), when studying Horn's manual SII, found R_I mean scores in the 0.360 to 0.469 range and κ averages of 0.065 to 0.26. Schumacher et al. (81) found averages for κ between 0.21 and 0.63. If these four studies using R_I and κ statistics are comparable, the manual SII shows less interrater reliability than expected and less than the other major severity classification systems.

How much can any of the severity systems improve the cost per case variation when using the DRG system for payment? Calore and Iezzoni (82) examined PMCs and Disease Staging to determine if either could replace DRGs or serve to modify DRGs effectively for severity. PMCs and Disease Staging were thought to be a significant improvement over DRGs. These two severity measures consider all diagnoses; the order in which diagnoses are listed is not critical. In contrast, the order of diagnoses determines the DRG assignment. DRGs, therefore, are subject to gaming by switching the order of the ICD-9-CM codes. PMCs and Disease Staging also use multiple diagnostic codes for more precise patient definition, and they separate complications of the principal diagnosis from comorbidities. Despite these theoretical advantages, the DRG system was not significantly inferior to the other two patient classification systems. Used alone, DRGs explained 33% of the variation, PMCs 26%,

Table 7.16.
Summary Statistics for Interrater Reliability

Measure	κ	R_I	γ	τ-B
APACHE II	0.726	0.874	0.925	0.837
MedisGroups	0.631	0.840	0.920	0.780
Disease Staging Q-Scale	0.461	0.708	0.736	0.621
PMC normative weights	0.446	0.524	0.596	0.496
DRG relative weights	0.879	0.892	0.922	0.872

and Disease Staging 17%. When PMCs or Disease Staging was used together with DRGs, only 1–2% more of the variation was accounted for.

Thomas, Ashcraft, and Zimmerman (20) presented one of the earliest comprehensive comparisons of several severity measures. They evaluated the measures by several criteria. *Construct validity* described how well the measure forecasted the probability of death or organ failure if appropriate care was not given. *Content validity* referred to whether the measure made clinical sense. *Predictive validity* showed how well the measure predicted variations in costs per patient. *Interrater reliability* tested whether the measure, when used by different raters and/or at different times, assigned the same score for the same patient. This criteria is also an indicator of unintentional manipulation. The *potential for intentional manipulation* of the measure was also assessed because of the temptation to increase hospital payment. The *cost of implementation and operation* varied widely among the measures and was the last criterion assessed.

PMCs and MedisGroups were the best in construct validity. APACHE II scored highest in content validity. Clinical Staging and PMC empirical cost weights were superior in predictive validity. APACHE II and MedisGroups performed best in interrater reliability. APACHE II was freest from manipulation. Finally, Coded Staging and PMCs were the least costly to implement and operate. The authors concluded that no one of the evaluated severity measures was clearly better than another for all criteria tested. CSI was not included in their study.

McMahon and Newbold (13), in their review of the Disease Staging severity measure, pointed out that severity of illness has had an undue amount of attention when attempting to explain variations in resource use within a particular DRG. Some of the other factors—such as the lack of clinical specificity of the ICD-9-CM coding system, the recording errors made when abstracting data for the UHDSS, and the constraints imposed when developing the DRG system—have been described previously. Physician practice variation is one critical factor that has received insufficient attention.

The study of variations in physician practices examines the different methods by which a physician makes a diagnosis and administers treatment to similar types of patients. Factors include the use of laboratory and radiology tests, admissions to the hospital, and the length of stay for admitted patients.

McMahon and Newbold (13) use length of stay as an indicator of physician practices and Disease Staging as an indicator of the severity of illness. They studied a limited number of DRGs. For all hospitals studied, the mean reduction in variance explained by the physician factor was 25.0% (range: 16.9 to 42.0%), whereas the severity factor accounted for only 0.4% (0.3 to 0.5%) of the mean reduction in variance.

It has been assumed that teaching hospitals have more severely ill patients than nonteaching hospitals, and that teaching hospitals, under the DRG system, are paid at a higher rate per patient. The validity of this assumption requires further examination. Goldfarb and Coffey (83) compared case-mix at teaching and nonteaching hospitals (83). They examined case-mix by two weighting methods. The first was the DRG system, where the weighting scheme is based on resource consumption in today's hospital. It assumes that current physician practices are the most clinically appropriate and economically efficient. The second case-mix methodology was Disease Staging. It is based primarily on clinical factors and is independent of treatment practices and, hence, free of resource consumption biases.

Goldfarb and Coffey found that teaching hospitals had a more serious case-mix than nonteaching hospitals when a resource consumption measure, such as DRGs, was used. But when the weighting system used was independent of resource consumption (i.e., Disease Staging), few case-mix differences between teaching and nonteaching hospitals were observed.

Finally, it has been suggested that, rather than adjust DRGs for severity, we should modify about 10% of the DRGs to reduce the heterogeneity (84). DRGs, in fact, are undergoing periodic modification to improve their efficiency in explaining variations in resource use.

In conclusion, severity of illness measures do not explain most of the variation in costs observed under the DRG system. No one severity measure is superior to another when examining validity, reliability, freedom from manipulation, and cost. Complex severity measures are often no better than less complex ones and may, in many situations, be no better than measures based on clinical judgment.

At this time, it appears unnecessary to add a severity measure to adjust for DRGs. A number of revisions have already been made to the DRG system, in response to concerns over severity (85). The refinements have increased the number of DRGs to 758, have separated patients with a major comorbidity or complications from less ill patients, and have revised the high and low trim points for outliers.

In conclusion, it would be more worthwhile to examine variations in physician practice patterns. Practice pattern differences appear to account for wider variations in resource consumption than does severity of illness. Perhaps the severity of illness indices would be useful in adjusting an individual physician's case-mix. This possibility needs to be studied with large numbers of different types of patients in a variety of hospitals. In addition, some of the severity of illness adjusters may prove useful in quality assurance programs, utilization review, and other data-monitoring evaluations. They may also be helpful in the analysis of resource utilization when making administrative decisions on staffing needs, product development, and other support issues (2). However, the use of severity adjusters in other settings requires the same type of assessment as previously described for DRGs.

References

1. Jenks SF, Dobson A. Refining case-mix adjustment: The research evidence. N Engl J Med 1987;317:679–686.
2. Gross P, Beyt E, Decker M, Garibaldi R, Hierholzer W, Jarvis BW, Larson E, Simmons B, Scheckler W, Harkavy L. Description of case-mix adjusters by the Severity of Illness Working Group of the Society of Hospital Epidemiologists of America (SHEA). Infect Control Hosp Epidemiol 1988;9:309–316.
3. Hornbrook MD. Hospital case mix: Its definition, measurement and use: Part II. A review of alternative measures. Med Care Rev 1982;39:75–123.
4. Shakno RJ, ed. Physician's Guide to DRGs. Chicago: Pluribus Press, 1984: 232.
5. Jenks SF, Dobson A, Willis P, et al. Evaluating and improving the measurement of hospital case mix. Health Care Financing Rev 1984;6(suppl): 1–11.
6. Gertman PM, Lowenstein S. A research paradigm for severity of illness: Issues for the diagnosis-related group system. Health Care Financing Rev 1984;6(suppl):79–90.
7. Horn SD, Bulkley G, Sharkey PD, et al. Interhospital differences in severity of illness. N Engl J Med 1985;131:220–224.
8. Kominski GE, Williams SV, May RB, et al. Unrecognized redistributions of revenue in diagnosis-related group-based prospective payment systems. Health Care Financing Rev 1984; 6(suppl):57–69.
9. Mullin RL. Diagnosis-related groups and severity. ICD-9-CM. The real problem. JAMA 1985; 254:1208–1210.
10. Smits HL, Fetter RB, McMahon LF. Variation in resource use within diagnosis-related groups. The severity issue. Health Care Financing Rev 1984;6(suppl):71–78.
11. Horn SD, Horn RA, Sharkey PD, Beall RJ, Hoff JS. Misclassification problems in diagnosis-related groups. Cystic fibrosis as an example. N Engl J Med 1986;314:484–487.
12. Rosko MD. DRGs and severity of illness measures: An analysis of patient classification systems. J Med Systems 1988;12:257–274.
13. McMahon L, Newbold MM. Variation in resource use within diagnosis-related groups. Med Care 1986;24:388–397.
14. Iezzoni LI, Moskowitz MA. A clinical assessment of MedisGroups. JAMA 1988;260:3159–3163.
15. Iezzoni LI, Ash AS, Cobb JL, Moskowitz MA. Admission MedisGroups score and the cost of hospitalizations. Med Care 1988;26:1068–1080.
16. Iezzoni LI. A primer on MedisGroups. Pen Med 1989;92:28–33.
17. Brewster AC, Jacobs CM, Bradbury RC. Classifying severity of illness by using clinical findings. Health Care Financing Rev 1984;6(suppl):107–108.
18. Brewster AC, Karlin BG, Hyde LA, et al. MedisGroups: A clinically based approach to classifying hospital patients at admission. Inquiry 1985; 12:377–387.
19. Iezzoni LI, Ash AS, Moskowitz MA. MEDISGROUPS: A clinical and analytic assessment. Research report. Section of General Internal Medicine, The University Hospital, Boston University School of Medicine, 1987:203.
20. Thomas JW, Ashcraft MLF, Zimmerman J. An evaluation of alternative severity of illness measures for use by university hospitals. In: Vol 1: Management Summary. Department of Health Services Management and Policy, School of Pub-

lic Health. Ann Arbor: The University of Michigan, 1986:1–13.

21. Knaus WA, Zimmerman FE, Wagner DP, Draper EA, Lawrence DE. APACHE—acute physiology and chronic health evaluation: A physiologically based classification system. Crit Care Med 1981;9:591–597.

22. Wagner DP, Knaus WA, Draper EA. Statistical validation of a severity of illness measure. Am J Public Health 1983;73:878–884.

23. Knaus WA, Draper EA, Wagner DP, Zimmerman JE. APACHE II: A severity of disease classification system. Crit Care Med 1985;9:591–597.

24. Knaus WA, Draper EA, Wagner P, Zimmerman JE. An evaluation of outcome from intensive care in major medical centers. Ann Intern Med 1986; 104:410–418.

25. Kruse JA, Thill-Baharozian MC, Carlson RW. Comparison of clinical assessment with APACHE II for predicting mortality risk in patients admitted to a medical intensive care unit. JAMA 1988;260:1739–1742.

26. Wagner DP, Knaus WA, Draper EA. Identification of low-risk monitor admissions to medical-surgical ICUs. Chest 1987;92:423–428.

27. Dobkin JE, Cutler RE. Use of APACHE II classification to evaluate outcome of patients receiving hemodialysis in an intensive care unit. West J Med 1988;149:547–550.

28. Rubins HB, Moskowitz MA. Discharge decision-making in a medical intensive care unit. Am J Med 1988;84:863–869.

29. Chang RWS, Jacobs S, Lee B. Predicting outcome among intensive care unit patients using computerized trend analysis of daily APACHE II scores corrected for organ system failure. Intensive Care Med 1988;14:558–566.

30. Jacobs S, Chang RWS, Lee B. One year's experience with the APACHE II severity of disease classification system in a general intensive care unit. Anesthesia 1987;42:738–744.

31. Jacobs S, Chang RWS, Lee B. Audit of intensive care: A 30 month experience using the APACHE II severity of disease classification system. Intensive Care Med 1988;14:567–574.

32. Cerra FB, Negro F, Abrams J. APACHE II score does not predict multiple organ failure or mortality in postoperative surgical patients. Arch Surg 1990;125:519–522.

33. Fedullo AJ, Swinburne AJ, Wahl GW, Bixby KR. APACHE II score and mortality in respiratory failure due to cardiogenic pulmonary edema. Crit Care Med 1988;16:1218–1221.

34. Hopefl AW, Taaffe C, Herrman VM. Failure of APACHE II alone as a predictor of mortality in patients receiving total parenteral nutrition. Crit Care Med 1989;17:414–417.

35. Moreau R, Soupison T, Vauquelin P, Derrida S, Beaucour H, Sicot C. Comparison of two simplified severity scores (SAPS and APACHE II) for patients with acute myocardial infarction. Crit Care Med 1989;17:409–413.

36. Zimmerman JE, ed. APACHE III study design: Analytic plan for evaluation of severity and outcome in intensive care units. Crit Care Med 1989;17(12 part 2):S169–221.

37. Wagner D, Draper E, Knaus W. APACHE III study design: Analytic plan for evaluation of severity and outcome in intensive care units. Development of APACHE III. Crit Care Med 1989;17(12 part 2):S199–203.

38. Knaus W, Mayner D. APACHE III study design: Analytic plan for evaluation of severity and outcome in intensive care units. Individual patient decisions. Crit Care Med 1989;17(12 part 2):S204–209.

39. Horn SD, Sharkey PD, Chambers AF, et al. Severity of illness within DRGs: Impact on prospective payment. Am J Public Health 1985;75: 1195–1199.

40. Horn SD, Horn RA. The computerized severity index: A new tool for case-mix management. J Med Syst 1986;10:73–78.

41. Muller C. Paying hospitals: How does a severity measure help? Am J Public Health 1983;73: 14–15.

42. Horn SD, Sharkey PD, Bertram DA. Measuring severity of illness: Homogeneous case mix groups. Med Care 1983;21:14–25.

43. Horn SD, Horn RA, Sharkey PD, Chambers AF. Severity of illness within DRGs. Homogeneity study. Med Care 1986;24:225–235.

44. Horn SD, Horn RA, Moses H. Profiles of physician practice and patient severity of illness. Am J Public Health 1986;76:532–535.

45. Horn SD, Horn RA. Reliability and validity of the Severity of Illness Index. Med Care 1986;24:159–178.

46. Horn SD, Backofen JE. Ethical issues in the use of a prospective payment system: The issue of a severity of illness adjustment. J Med Philos 1987;12:145–153.

47. Horn SD, Chambers AF, Sharkey PD, Horn RA. Psychiatric severity of illness. A case mix study. Med Care 1989;27:69–84.

48. Magni G, Schifano F, De Leo D. Low utility of the CSI in depressed elderly patients with medical disturbances [Letter]. J Clin Psychiatry 1988; 47:275.

49. Gonnella JS, Zeleznik C. Factors involved in comprehensive patient care evaluation. Med Care 1974;12:928–934.

50. Coffee RM, Goldfarb MKG. DRGs and disease staging for reimbursing medicare patients. Med Care 1986;24:814–829.

51. Conklin JE, Lieberman JV, Barnes CA, et al. Disease staging: Implications for hospital reimbursement and management. Health Care Financing Rev 1984;6(suppl):13–22.

52. Gonnella JS, Hornbrook MC, Louis DZ. Staging of disease. A case-mix measurement. JAMA 1984; 251:637–646.

53. Gonnella JS, ed. Disease staging clinical criteria. 3rd ed. Santa Barbara, CA: SysteMetrics, McGraw-Hill, 1986:624.

54. Disease Staging: Q-Scale. Santa Barbara, CA: SysteMetrics, McGraw-Hill, 1988:38.

55. McMahon LF Jr, Newbold R. Variation in resource use within diagnosis-related groups: The effect of severity of illness and physician practice. Med Care 1986;24:388–397.

56. Young WA. Incorporating severity of illness and

comorbidity in case-mix measurement. Health Care Financing Rev 1984;6(suppl):23–31.

57. Blue Cross of Western Pennsylvania: Patient management categories final report, Pittsburgh. The Pittsburgh Research Institute, Pittsburgh, PA, 1985:51.

58. Johansen S. Comparison of two prospective rates-setting models: The DRG and PIR models. Health Serv Res 1986;21:547–559.

59. Zobel G, Kutting M, Ring E, Grubbauer HM. Clinical scoring systems in children with continuous extracorporeal renal support. Child Nephrol Urol 1990;10:14–17.

60. Lemeshow S, Teres D, Ayrunin JS, Gage RW. Refining intensive care unit outcome prediction by using changing probabilities of mortality. Crit Care Med 1988;16:470–477.

61. Thompson JD. The measurement of nursing intensity. Health Care Financing Rev 1984; 6(suppl):47–55.

62. Yeh TS, Pollack MM, Holbrook PR, Fields AI, Ruttiman U. Assessment of pediatric intensive care—Application of the Therapeutic Intervention Scoring Systems. Crit Care Med 1982;10:497–500.

63. Mitchell JB, Dickey B, Liptzin B, Sederer LI. Bringing psychiatric patients into the medicare prospective payment system. Am J Psychiatry 1987;144:610–615.

64. Rhee KJ, Baxt WG, Mackenzie JR, Willits NH, Burney RE, O'Malley RJ, Reid N, Schwabe D, Storer DL, Weber R. APACHE II scoring in the injured patient. Crit Care Med 1990;18:827–830.

65. Lehmkuhl P, Jeck-Thole S, Pichlmayr I. A new scoring system for disease intensity in a surgical intensive care unit. World J Surg 1989;13:252–258.

66. Turner JS, Potgieter PD, Linton DM. Systems for scoring severity of illness in intensive care. S Afr Med J 1989;76:17–20.

67. Jordan DA, Miller DF, Kubos KL, Roger MC. Evaluation of sepsis in a critically ill surgical population. Crit Care Med 1987;15:897–904.

68. Tinker JM, Robert SL. Anesthesia risk. In: Miller RD, ed. Anesthesia. 2nd ed. New York: Churchill Livingstone, 1986;1:359–380.

69. Greenfield S, Aronow HU, Elashoff RM, Watanabe D. Flaws in mortality data: The hazards of ignoring comorbid disease. JAMA 1988; 260:2253–2255.

70. Jenks SF, Williams DK, Kay TL. Assessing hospital-associated deaths from discharge data. JAMA 1988;260:2240–2246.

71. Munoz E, Goldstein J, Benacquista T, Mulloy K, Wise L. Diagnosis related group "all payor" hospital payment and medical diseases: Financial risk and hospital cost in medical noncomplicating condition-stratified diagnosis related groups. Arch Intern Med 1989;149:417–420.

72. Kaplan MH, Feinstein AR. The importance of classifying initial comorbidity in evaluating the outcome of diabetes mellitus. J Chron Dis 1974; 27:387–404.

73. Pompei P, Charlson ME, Douglas RG Jr. Clinical assessments as predictors of one year survival after hospitalization: Implications for prognostic stratification. J Clin Epidemiol 1988;41:275–284.

74. Gross PA, Stein MR, Van Antwerpen C, DeMauro PJ, Boscamp J, Hess W. Comparison of severity of illness indicators in an intensive care unit. Arch Int Med, in press.

75. Reliability of National Hospital Discharge Survey data. Institute of Medicine Publication No. 10M80-02, Washington, D.C., 1980.

76. Doremus H, Michenzi E. Data quality: An illustration of its potential impact upon a diagnosis-related group's case-mix index and reimbursement. Med Care 1983;21:1001–1011.

77. Ginsburg P, Carter G. The Medicare case-mix index increase. Health Care Financing Rev 1986;7:51–66.

78. Thomas JW, Ashcraft MLF. Measuring severity of illness: A comparison of interrater reliability among several methodologies. Inquiry 1989; 26:483–492.

79. Horn SD, Chachich B, Clopton C. Measuring severity of illness: A reliability study. Med Care 1983;21:705–714.

80. Soeken RL, Prescott PA. Issues in the use of Kappa to estimate reliability. Med Care 1986; 24:733–741.

81. Schumaker DM, Parker B, Kofie V, Munns JM. Severity of Illness Index and the Adverse Patient Occurrence Index: A reliability study and policy implications. Med Care 1987;25:695–704.

82. Calore KA, Iezzoni L. Disease staging and PMCs: Can they improve DRGs? Med Care 1987;25:724–737.

83. Goldfarb MG, Coffey RM. Case-mix differences between teaching and nonteaching hospitals. Inquiry 1987;24:68–84.

84. McNeil B, Kominiski G, Williams-Ashman A. Modified DRGs as evidence for variability in patients' severity. Med Care 1988;26:53–61.

85. Amendment to the New Jersey DRG List Regulation, N.J.A.C. 1990;8:31B–5.3.

8

Evaluating Clinical Studies

Bradley N. Doebbeling, M.D., M.S.

Currently, 74,000 scientific and biomedical journals are published annually. Additionally, it has been estimated conservatively that the volume of medical knowledge doubles every 10 years. Obviously, no one can read every paper published. Thus, the clinician must develop an approach to the medical literature that identifies only those articles that are valid and relevant to one's own practice or that address a particular question or decision. This chapter will review basic principles of epidemiology and study design, as well as the available medical literature regarding the evaluation of clinical studies, particularly clinical trials. It will also suggest approaches to reading articles that may be of value to the clinician.

BASIC PRINCIPLES

A variety of important terms should be defined. Epidemiology is a research discipline concerned with the distribution and determinants of disease in populations (1). Populations are large groups of people in a particular setting, such as a population of smokers or of hospitalized patients. A sample is a group of individuals drawn from a specific population. Within populations and samples there are factors that are associated with an increased risk or probability of developing disease: these characteristics are referred to as risk factors.

Epidemiologists frequently study samples of populations and attempt to draw conclusions about the population based on their findings in the sample. In that quest epidemiologists make two basic assumptions: human disease does not occur at random, and further, causal and preventive factors can be identified through the systematic study of population samples.

The repertoire of epidemiological studies is vast. These studies may attempt to identify causes of disease, to gather information about the natural history and clinical course of a given disease, to collect information on disease frequency in populations, or to assess the impact of diseases on human populations. An epidemiologic study requires the development of a hypothesis. The hypothesis is then tested by comparing an exposed sample group representing the population at risk to an unexposed, appropriate control group. The null hypothesis of no difference between groups is assumed. Data are collected systematically and analyzed statistically to determine the strength of an association between the risk factor and disease (2). The validity of any observed association must be evaluated and alternative explanations eliminated, such as chance, bias, and confounding (1–3). Finally, one must judge whether an observed association actually represents a cause and effect relationship between an exposure and subsequent disease. Such causal associations are more likely to be accepted when similar relationships are noted in several studies.

Chance

Epidemiologic studies evaluating disease frequency assume that one may draw an inference about an entire population based upon evaluation of a sample. However, characteristics of a sample group are likely to differ from the true value in the population due to random variation. Random variation is just as likely to result in sample values above the true population value as below it. As larger samples are taken, the mean of the samples draws closer to the true population value. Chance may affect every aspect of a study, from the selection of subjects to the evaluation of the dependent (or outcome) variable(s). Importantly, random variation cannot be totally eliminated and should be considered in evaluating the results of any study (1). Statistical tests allow one to estimate the probability that random variation or chance may account for the differences between study groups.

The p value represents the probability that an effect at least as extreme as that observed may have occurred by chance alone (assuming that the null hypothesis of no difference between groups is true). In a clinical trial, the p value is the probability that one would incorrectly conclude that a treatment was effective if in truth it was not effective. The p value is typically considered "statistically significant" if the probability of observing a difference as extreme as that observed in the clinical trial is less than or equal to 1/20, or 0.05. This threshold level of significance, or α, was arbitrarily selected by Fisher in evaluating his experiments with field crops. A number of authors report the exact p value in a study, since there is some disagreement about the appropriate level of α to accept. Some authors have arbitrarily required an α level of 0.01, often referred to as "highly significant." Levels of α greater than one in five (20%) are sometimes reported as $p >$ 0.20, since the probability of an α error

greater than one in five is generally considered unacceptably high (1).

Although the differences between two groups may be highly statistically significant, the p value does not provide information regarding the magnitude of the difference or its clinical importance. Similarly, a considerable difference may be observed in a given trial but not achieve statistical significance, due to the small number of subjects in the trial. In evaluating a study, the reader must always consider the size of the difference between groups and whether the difference observed is clinically important. For example, a new antihypertensive in a large clinical trial may significantly ($p < 0.001$) lower systolic blood pressure compared to standard therapy. However, if the magnitude of the difference between the two treatments is only 5 mm Hg, the difference is not likely to be clinically meaningful (i.e., probably does not substantially reduce the consequences of untreated hypertension, such as stroke frequency or early death).

Bias

Bias is a systematic error in the design, conduct, or analysis of a study that distorts the true differences (or risk of outcome after exposure) between two study groups. Bias is a nonrandom error and is impossible to eliminate once the study is complete. Clinical research is more prone to bias than laboratory-based research because of the complexities inherent in working with human subjects (1). Although a variety of different types of bias have been identified, most fit within the following categories. Design or selection bias is of concern when two groups are compared that differ systematically on the basis of determinants of disease other than those under study. An example would be if there were a design that insured that only men received the new drug and women received the placebo. Conduct or measurement bias is evident when a systematic error occurs in measurement between two groups. If a small arm blood pressure cuff were used to measure blood pressure in both thin and obese patients, there would be a systematic distortion of the recordings in the obese subjects. Analysis bias occurs when the relationship between two variables in a study with regard to disease cannot be separated. For example, if in a case-control study all smokers were drinkers and all nonsmokers were nondrinkers, one might falsely conclude that alcohol is a risk factor for lung cancer. Figure 8.1 demonstrates the relationship between bias and chance in the measurement of blood pressure.

Types of Studies

Descriptive epidemiology estimates the rates and distribution of disease or health within a population. Most descriptive epidemiologic studies are preliminary investigations, undertaken when little is known of the epidemiology of a disease. Such descriptive studies provide data on the patterns of disease and occurrence within populations according to demographic characteristics, such as age, race, gender, marital status, occupation, etc. Descriptive epidemiologic studies are primarily useful for the formulation of hypotheses that can be tested subsequently in analytic studies.

Descriptive studies may be performed either in individuals (i.e., case reports and case series), or in populations (i.e., aggregate or correlational studies).

Analytic epidemiology evaluates the determinants of disease and/or the causes of increased or decreased frequency in different groups. Most analytic studies are designed to test causal hypotheses and often allow more definitive conclusions to be reached about causation than are possible in descriptive studies. Analytic studies can involve careful observation or the institution of a specific intervention. Analytic studies include cross-sectional surveys, case-control studies, and cohort studies.

Cross-sectional surveys evaluate exposure and disease in groups of subjects at one point in time. Disease rates are compared among those with and without exposure or at different levels of exposure. Cross-sectional studies are frequently based on a sample of the general population and are often used for public health planning and occasionally for testing epidemiologic hypotheses.

Case-control studies are retrospective studies that compare the exposure of indi-

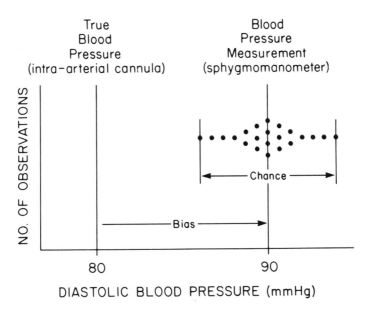

Figure 8.1. The relationship between bias and chance. Blood pressure measurements by intraarterial cannula and sphygmomanometer. (From Fletcher RH, Fletcher SW, Wagner EH. Clinical epidemiology: The essentials. 2nd ed. Baltimore: Williams & Wilkins, 1988:11.)

viduals with disease (cases) and those without disease (controls) to one or more potential risk factors. Case-control studies are extremely efficient and are particularly well suited to studying rare diseases or those with long latent periods. Additionally, they are particularly useful in evaluating questions of risk or cause. However, they are more prone to bias (i.e., selection and recall bias) than other analytic designs.

A cohort is a group of people assembled and observed over time for the development of disease. Cohort studies may be either retrospective or prospective, and further evaluate any association between exposure and disease. A prospective cohort study divides a group of individuals apparently free of disease into those exposed and those unexposed to a particular risk factor. Both subgroups are followed into the future to determine the incidence of disease in each group. A retrospective cohort study uses existing records to assemble groups of individuals who are followed from a defined starting point in their past to some point in their more recent past for the development of disease. Cohort studies may be particularly helpful in evaluating questions of incidence, risk, cause, and prognosis.

Intervention studies are a special type of cohort study, also referred to as clinical trials. Ideally, these are prospective, blinded (masked), randomized comparisons of outcome between a particular intervention and a standard therapy (or placebo).

STUDIES OF TREATMENT

Many forms of therapy are based upon clinical experience. Few would argue the need for surgery in major trauma, or the utility of nitroglycerine in the treatment of angina. However, other types of intervention are less clearly beneficial. In such a setting, it is important to compare treatments formally. Indeed, although certain treatments seem likely to be beneficial based upon knowledge of the pathophysiology of a disease, such therapy may actually be harmful. For example, carotid bypass surgery in patients with cerebral ischemia and obstructed internal carotid

arteries would seem to be a reasonable therapy. However, a randomized, controlled trial of medical versus surgical therapy demonstrated that, although patients undergoing surgery had similar rates of mortality and stroke to those treated medically, they actually died *earlier* than the medically treated patients (4).

OBSERVATIONAL TRIALS

Observational studies evaluate outcomes associated with different therapeutic approaches already in place. However, since treatment groups often differ considerably with respect to a variety of baseline characteristics, it is difficult to determine whether the outcome results observed are related to different therapy or to differences in underlying disease or other risk factors. Because systematic differences between groups frequently occur in observational studies of therapy, it is usually helpful to compare treatments in a more controlled fashion. For example, a widely cited observational study of the treatment of Kawasaki disease (mucocutaneous lymph node syndrome) concluded that steroids are contraindicated in this disease (5). However, the study compared the effect of five therapeutic regimens already in use on the development of coronary aneurysms in patients with Kawasaki disease. Different combinations of the five regimens were used in the five study hospitals. In fact, three of the hospitals used only a single regimen. Since subjects were not randomized and the baseline characteristics of the groups were not examined and compared, it is impossible to conclude from this study that patients deteriorated *after* being placed on steroids and that steroids are contraindicated for this disease.

CLINICAL TRIALS

A clinical trial is a unique type of cohort study in which the conditions of the study are controlled by the investigator in order to obtain an unbiased estimate of the effects of treatment (1). Clinical trials are also referred to as experimental or intervention studies.

In a clinical trial, a cohort of individuals with a particular disorder is randomly divided into two groups, an experimental and a control group. The experimental or treatment group receives a new or unproven treatment, while the control group is managed similarly except for receipt of a placebo or a standard therapy. The outcomes of the two groups are then compared. A clinical trial thus comes closer than any other analytic study design to eliminating bias or systematic error in the evaluation of different treatments (1, 6).

A number of important methodological issues (Table 8.1) should be evident in a clinical trial (7). The purpose of the study should be clearly stated in the introduction or methods section of a paper and the dependent or outcome variables precisely identified. Similarly, the sampling strategy used is important and should also be well described. The exclusion criteria used in a particular study are often designed to ensure the homogeneity of the groups and the completion of the trial by most subjects, as well as to prevent adverse occurrences. The exclusion criteria should be explained, as well as the number or proportion of subjects excluded. Clinical trials that enroll only a small proportion of potential subjects may have internal validity but, because of strict inclusion criteria, may not be generalizable to the population at large (external validity). The relationships between internal and external valid-

Table 8.1.
Important Factors to Be Considered in the Evaluation of a Clinical Trial

Comparison (control) group adequate
Allocation of patients blinded and random
Assessment of compliance in treatment and control groups
Blinding of both study subjects and investigators
Assessment of outcomes by individuals unaware of experimental group
All clinically relevant outcomes reported
Clinically important differences (δ) observed
Statistically important differences (α) observed
Negative trials require an evaluation of the study power
Important confounders considered and controlled

ity are demonstrated in Figure 8.2. The clinician reading the paper must not only attempt to determine if a particular study is internally valid, but also decide if the study applies to his or her patient population.

Comparison Groups

The choice of a control group is critically important in a clinical trial or any other type of analytic study. A carefully selected control group is especially important if the outcome of a given disease is unpredictable. Uncontrolled trials may demonstrate apparently favorable outcomes for a variety of reasons: unpredictable outcomes, regression to the mean, predictable improvement, or the Hawthorne effect (1). Since most disease states have unpredictable outcomes, the appropriate selection of a comparison group is mandatory to determine whether the improvement observed with a new treatment is actually due to the intervention itself. Similarly, patients are frequently selected for therapy on the basis of markedly abnormal test values, such as elevated serum cholesterol or glucose levels. The random variation in such values, however, tends to move each patient's results closer to normal with subsequent measurements. This phenomenon is referred to as regression to the mean. Additionally, a number of disorders such as headaches or "colds" have predictable improvement (i.e., tend to improve with time). Evaluation of the treatment of such a disorder is difficult unless an appropriate comparison group is provided.

Finally, the Hawthorne effect must also be considered. Subjects in a study typically alter their behavior by virtue of the attention they receive during the study, a response entirely separate from the effect of a given treatment (8). This effect was first described in a study by the Western Electric Company at its Hawthorne Works plant in Chicago in the 1920s. Experiments were performed to determine the effect of lighting on worker efficiency. Illumination was either increased, decreased, or held constant, but surprisingly the productivity increased regardless of the level of illumination, apparently because of the attention received.

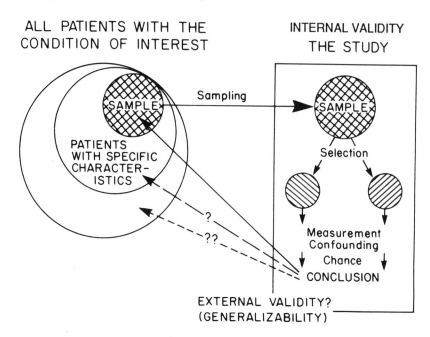

Figure 8.2. The relationships among internal and external validity, bias, and chance. (From Fletcher RH, Fletcher SW, Wagner EH. Clinical epidemiology: The essentials. 2nd ed. Baltimore: Williams & Wilkins, 1988:14.)

Comparisons across time or place are difficult to perform adequately (1). Many studies, particularly those of new chemotherapy or antibiotics, compare the results of a current regimen with the results from a regimen used in the past. Sacks et al. (9) reported that studies with historical controls were approximately four times more likely to report a significant improvement with a new therapy than were studies with concurrent randomized controls. Selection of concurrent controls eliminates an apparent bias in favor of new treatment regimens. Different clinical settings, however, often have a very different patient mix, referral base, and therapeutic approach, frequently resulting in very different patient outcomes. Comparing therapeutic responses of patients treated in different centers is problematic, unless the distribution of treatment and control groups is similar geographically.

Comparison Treatments

The selection of an appropriate comparison treatment for a clinical trial is clearly important. The control group simply may

be observed, may receive a placebo (inactive agent), or may receive the current or standard therapy for a given disorder. As mentioned previously, observation alone is associated with important changes in behavior. A number of studies have shown that when a placebo is given with assurance to a patient, a measurable improvement in symptoms is often seen. For example, severe postoperative pain, angina, or cough may be relieved by placebo in up to 40% of patients (10). The "placebo effect" is an important, measurable dimension of the doctor-patient relationship and must be considered if the true effects of a therapeutic intervention are to be evaluated. Treating the control group with a placebo helps ensure that any difference between the treatment and control groups is due to the active drug, rather than a nonspecific effect of receiving treatment (11). When no known efficacious treatment is available, a placebo treatment may be beneficial. Finally, the appropriate comparison treatment may be the standard therapy for a given disorder. For example, following the demonstration of prolonged survival and decreased frequency of opportunistic infections in patients with the acquired immune deficiency syndrome (AIDS) treated with zidovudine, the drug became the standard therapy against which other agents must be compared (12).

Treatment Allocation

Allocation of patients to treatment arms of a study is another important aspect of a clinical trial. If performed appropriately, the effects of bias on study results can be limited. Whenever an investigator makes a decision to allocate patients to different treatments, he or she does so based on some criteria (13). Although the investigator may have every intention of assigning subjects equally to treatment groups, it is difficult to avoid selection bias.

In a clinical trial, randomization is the "assignment of treatments to patients using a chance procedure" (14). Randomization eliminates bias due to patient allocation, makes the treatment groups equal in most important respects, ensures that the statistical results are valid, and improves the acceptance of the study by clinicians (11). Random allocation of patients to treatments is clearly an important requirement of a clinical trial. Failure to assign patients randomly to treatment arms of a study can have profound effects on study results. For example, the allocation of treatments could be performed based on the day of enrollment, hospital number, or any of a variety of other factors (8). In a study of the use of anticoagulants versus standard care as treatment of acute myocardial infarction, patients admitted on even days were allocated to the control group, while those admitted on odd days received anticoagulants (15). Patients receiving anticoagulants had a better outcome than those in the control group. However, this method of patient allocation did not result in random assignment of patients to the two groups. Considerably more patients were admitted on odd days. Apparently, some participating physicians referring patients for the trial favored anticoagulation and, therefore, postponed admitting the less seriously ill patients until the odd days. The difference in allocation of patients resulted in proportionately more seriously ill patients receiving the control treatment (referral bias), thus causing an error in the outcome of analysis.

There are disadvantages to randomization, however. Randomization may lead to unequal numbers in each group due to chance alone, particularly in a small study. Similarly, randomization may occasionally result in groups that differ with respect to some important determinant of outcome due to the vagaries of chance. Finally, it may be less efficient than matching (11). Randomization should occur immediately after it is determined that the subject is eligible for a trial, before the subject or investigator is aware which treatment is about to be allocated.

Blinding (Masking)

Both the subjects and the investigator should remain unaware of the actual intervention received to avoid measurement bias (11). As noted above, an adequate control group is necessary to account for improvement due to the natural history of the disease and eliminate the placebo effect. If only the subjects are unaware of which treatment they are receiving, the study is referred to as single-blind or single-masked. If both the investigator and subjects are unaware of the treatment received, the study is double-blind or double-masked. Blinding is particularly important when subjective symptoms such as pain or nausea are being measured.

Chalmers and colleagues (13) evaluated 145 controlled clinical trials of the treatment of acute myocardial infarction to determine if bias in treatment assignment had a potential influence on outcome. At least one prognostic variable was maldistributed in 14% of blinded randomization trials, in 27% of unblinded randomization trials, and in 58% of nonrandomized trials. Similarly, differences in the case-fatality rates between treatment and control groups were found in 9% of the blinded randomization trials, 24% of the unblinded randomization studies, and 58% of the nonrandomized studies. These data underscore the importance of randomly assigning treatment in a blinded fashion.

The individual assessing outcome in a clinical trial should remain unaware of the treatment received. As Fletcher notes, "Both in initial assessment of the patients and the subsequent assessment of their progress the tests should be applied by observers who remain unaware of which patient is undergoing treatment and which is a control" (16). Otherwise, subjectivity may affect the results. Generally, the more clear-cut the outcomes are, the less opportunity there is for bias (1).

Compliance

The failure of subjects to follow therapeutic advice (noncompliance) can bias the results of a study. Compliance may differ between the treatment and control groups, making comparison of outcomes problematic. Noncompliance in a treatment group could cause the effect of an intervention to be smaller than expected (11). Subjects in the control group may be noncompliant or they may use the experimental treatment or intervention on their own, leading to a smaller treatment effect than expected.

TYPE I AND TYPE II ERROR

The probability that an observed difference between two sample groups is due to chance alone is measured by a significance test (11). A type I error occurs by rejecting the null hypothesis when it is true (i.e., accepting that a difference is significant when, in fact, no true difference exists between the two treatment groups). The probability of a type I (or false-positive) error is defined by the p value, and the threshold for significance is called the α level.

A type II error occurs by accepting the null hypothesis when it is false, i.e., concluding that no difference exists between two treatments when one actually does. The probability of a type II (or false-negative) error is referred to as β. The optimal study is one with a low probability of a type II error, and such a study is said to have a great deal of statistical "power." More specifically, the power of a trial is the probability of avoiding a type II error, or $1 - \beta$.

Confidence limits should be reported for results in negative clinical trials, i.e., those that demonstrate no difference, since they are more easily understood than the power of a study (11). For example, estimates of the 90% confidence intervals for the true improvement in a large series of "negative" clinical trials demonstrated that in two-thirds (68%) of the studies whose power was less than 90% to detect a 50% difference in response rate, a potential 50% improvement was possible. In other words, the 90% confidence interval about the difference observed included a potential 50% treatment effect (17).

To perform a clinical trial adequately, planning must include estimation of the size of the trial in order to be able to detect a meaningful therapeutic effect if it exists (17). Determination of sample size requires selecting acceptable levels of type I and type II errors, as well as the size of the clinically important therapeutic effect (or meaningful difference, δ). δ may define a clinically important drop in diastolic blood measure of 15 mm Hg or a decrease in toxicity due to a therapeutic agent, e.g., a 25% reduction.

Freiman et al. (17) reviewed randomized controlled clinical trials published in the 20 major medical journals from 1960 to 1977 to determine whether the "negative" trials, i.e., $p > 0.05$, had included enough patients to allow detection of a clinically meaningful difference (δ). One-half of the 71 trials concluding that there was no significant difference between study arms had βs in excess of 74% to detect a true 25% therapeutic improvement, i.e., a power of $\leq$ 0.26! Only 6% of the trials had enough subjects to ensure a $\beta \leq 0.10$ (power ≥ 0.90). If a 50% difference between treatment groups (δ) is considered important, one-half of the trials had βs greater than 40% (power < 0.60). This is an important type II error. Clearly, further attention is needed in the planning and analysis of clinical trials to avoid missing a clinically important therapeutic difference because of small sample size. One need not memorize formulas for calculating sample size, since a series of sample size nomograms are available for evaluating negative clinical trials (18).

CONFOUNDING

A confounding variable is one that is causally related to the disease under study and is also associated with the exposure under study in the study population, but is not a consequence of the exposure. In a clinical trial, the effect of such a variable is to modify the influence of treatment. For example, coffee drinking has been identified as a potential risk factor in the development of atherosclerotic coronary disease. However, coffee drinkers are also more likely to smoke cigarettes than the general population. Any investigation of the association between coffee drinking and coronary disease would need to evaluate the independent role of smoking as a potential confounder.

To assure an equal distribution of subjects according to several different variables related to prognosis, the process of stratification may be used. Stratification is the randomization of subjects within certain defined levels such as age, underlying disease, or severity of illness. Subjects can also be matched prospectively for important confounding variables. Finally, confounding may be accounted for in the analysis of the study.

READING JOURNALS

The clinician must take an active role in assessing both the validity of clinical research and its generalizability to his or her own patients. Fletcher and colleagues (1) have suggested that a hierarchy exists in the utility of different types of articles to clinical decision making. Reviews and editorials are useful summaries of information that may be clinically relevant; however, they do not contain entirely original information and are prone to bias. Basic or bench research is important in generating and testing hypotheses of illness; however, they usually have little direct relevance to the clinical decision-making process. Clinical research on intact humans is more useful, but often poorly performed. Just a small number of studies are methodologically strong and well performed. Only these studies should have a major

impact on clinical practice. It is the responsibility of the reader (and of editors) to identify such papers and examine them carefully.

The process of identifying useful articles entails the development of a careful strategy to search through the large number of articles on a given topic and recover the most relevant. First, the question to be answered must be defined as precisely as possible. Often it may be useful to generate a list of related terms or topics that further define the question of interest. For example, to determine the incidence of anaphylaxis to penicillin, one might select the terms antibiotics, anaphylaxis, adverse effects, and cohort study. The Medical Subject Headings—Annotated Alphabetic List is a useful reference in generating such a list (19).

Next, the titles of a large number of articles must be screened for the search terms to identify potentially useful papers. One of the most efficient methods of screening many articles is to use a computerized data base, such as MEDLINE, which can be accessed via a personal computer from the office, library, clinic, or home (20). Other sources of potentially useful article titles include *Index Medicus,* review articles, textbooks, or colleagues knowledgeable in the specific area. Fletcher et al. (1) suggest three major criteria for identification of appropriate papers: (*a*) an article addressing the specific question raised; (*b*) original research; and (*c*) strong methodology. The list can usually be narrowed easily based on the titles of the articles. If a computerized data base is used, the abstracts of many articles can be reviewed on-line to eliminate additional papers that are not clinically relevant. Once a limited number of papers is identified, the methods section of each should be reviewed and a decision made regarding their methodological strength (21). If the paper is both relevant to the question at hand and methodologically strong, the entire paper should be reviewed.

The McMaster's approach (22) to reading clinical journals suggests a series of six guides to learn about the quality of clinical care. First, the study should "focus on what clinicians actually do." In other words, the article should deal with the process of clinical care of a profile of patients cared for in one's own hospital. Second, the study should evaluate clinical actions shown to "do more good than harm." As a corollary to this point, if the clinical action under study has not been shown to do more good than harm, it should attempt to determine if a particular clinical action is linked to clinical outcome. To do so, an inception cohort should have been assembled, high compliance rates ensured, all relevant outcomes included in the study, and the prognosis considered (22). Third, the type of clinical practice, patients, and clinicians should be similar to those of the reader. Fourth, clinical actions need to have been measured in a "clinically sensible fashion." Similarly, clinical actions also must have been measured in a "scientifically credible fashion." Finally, one must ask if both clinical and statistical significance were evaluated (22).

Other authors have suggested guidelines for keeping up with the medical literature (21–24) and how to read articles critically (25–30). The reader is referred to these articles, as well as several important, well-written texts of interest (1, 11, 31).

The elements of good study design and important aspects of clinical trials have been reviewed to invite the reader to develop and improve his or her skills in evaluating clinical studies. One must invest considerable time and effort in the evaluation of clinical studies to find the few articles that are both methodologically strong and generalizable to one's own clinical practice. Although an evaluation of the literature is occasionally a struggle, the potential rewards of being able to read critically the articles that will assist in clinical decision making are worth the challenge.

References

1. Fletcher RH, Fletcher SW, Wagner EH. Clinical epidemiology: The essentials. Baltimore: Williams & Wilkins, 2nd ed., 1988.
2. Moses LE. Statistical concepts fundamental to investigations. N Engl J Med 1985;312:890–897.
3. Research Development Committee, Society for Research and Education in Primary Care Internal Medicine. Clinical research methods: An annotated bibliography. Ann Intern Med 1983;99:419–424.
4. The EC/IC Bypass Study Group. Failure of extracranial-intracranial arterial bypass to reduce the risk of ischemic stroke. N Engl J Med 1985;313:1191–1200.
5. Kato H, Koike S, Yokoyama T. Kawasaki disease: Effect of treatment on coronary artery involvement. Pediatrics 1979;63:175–179.
6. Lavori PW, Louis TA, Bailar JC III, Polansky M. Designs for experiments—Parallel comparisons of treatment. N Engl J Med 1983;309:1291–1298.
7. DerSimonian R, Charette LJ, McPeek B, Mosteller F. Reporting on methods in clinical trials. N Engl J Med 1982;306:1332–1337.
8. Roethlisberges FG, Dickson WJ, Wright HA. Management and the worker. An account of a research program conducted by the Western Electric Company, Hawthorne Works, Chicago. Cambridge, MA: Harvard University Press, 1946.
9. Sacks H, Chalmers TC, Smith H Jr. Randomized versus historical controls for clinical trials. Am J Med 1982;72:233–240.
10. Beecher HK. The powerful placebo. JAMA 1955;159:1602–1606.
11. Bulpitt CJ. Randomized controlled clinical trials. The Hague: Martinus Nijhoff, 1983.
12. Hirsch MS. Antiviral drug development for the treatment of human immunodeficiency virus infections: An overview. Am J Med 1988;85(Suppl 2A):182–185.
13. Chalmers TC, Celano P, Sacks HS, Smith H Jr. Bias in treatment assignment in controlled clinical trials. N Engl J Med 1983;309:1358–1361.
14. Zelen M. The randomization and stratification of patients to clinical trials. J Chron Dis 1974;27:365–375.
15. Wright IS, Marple CD, Beck DF. Myocardial infarction. Its clinical manifestations and treatment with anticoagulants. New York, Grune & Stratton, l954;8–10.
16. Fletcher CM. Criteria for diagnosis and assessment in clinical trials. In Hill AB, ed. Controlled clinical trials. Springfield, IL: Charles C Thomas, 1960.
17. Freiman JA, Chalmers TC, Smith H Jr, Kuebler RR. The importance of Beta, the Type II error, and sample size in the design and interpretation of the randomized controlled trial. N Engl J Med 1978;299:690–694.
18. Young MJ, Bresnitz EA, Strom BL. Sample size nomograms for interpreting negative clinical studies. Ann Intern Med 1983;99:248–251.
19. National Library of Medicine. Medical subject headings—Annotated alphabetic list, 1991. Bethesda, MD: National Library of Medicine, 1990.
20. Haynes RB, McKibbon KA, Walker CJ, Mousseau J, Baker LM, Fitzgerald D, Guyatt G, Norman GR. Computer searching of the medical literature: An evaluation of MEDLINE searching systems. Ann Intern Med 1985;103:812–816.
21. Haynes RB, McKibbon KA, Fitzgerald D, Guyatt GH, Walker CJ, Sackett DL. How to keep up with the medical literature: I. Why try to keep up and

how to get started. Ann Intern Med 1986;105:149–153.

22. Department of Clinical Epidemiology and Biostatistics, McMaster University. How to read clinical journals: VI. To learn about the quality of clinical care. Can Med Assoc J 1984;130:377–380.

23. Haynes RB, McKibbon KA, Fitzgerald D, Guyatt GH, Walker CJ, Sackett DL. How to keep up with the medical literature: II. Deciding which journals to read regularly. Ann Intern Med 1986;105:309–312.

24. Haynes RB, McKibbon KA, Fitzgerald D, Guyatt GH, Walker CJ, Sackett DL. How to keep up with the medical literature: III. Expanding the number of journals you read regularly. Ann Intern Med 1986;105:474–478.

25. Haynes RB, McKibbon KA, Fitzgerald D, Guyatt GH, Walker CJ, Sackett DL. How to keep up with the medical literature: IV. Using the literature to solve clinical problems. Ann Intern Med 1986; 105:636–640.

26. Department of Clinical Epidemiology and Biostatistics, McMaster University. How to read clinical journals: I. Why to read them and how to start reading them critically. Can Med Assoc J 1981; 124:555–558.

27. Department of Clinical Epidemiology and Biostatistics, McMaster University. How to read clinical journals: II. To learn about a diagnostic test. Can Med Assoc J 1981;124:703–708.

28. Department of Clinical Epidemiology and Biostatistics, McMaster University. How to read clinical journals: III. To learn the clinical course and prognosis of disease. Can Med Assoc J 1981; 124:869–872.

29. Department of Clinical Epidemiology and Biostatistics, McMaster University. How to read clinical journals: IV. To determine etiology or causation. Can Med Assoc J 1981;124:985–990.

30. Department of Clinical Epidemiology and Biostatistics, McMaster University. How to read clinical journals: V. To distinguish useful from useless or even harmful therapy. Can Med Assoc J 1981;124: 1156–1162.

31. Sackett DL, Haynes RB, Tugwell P. Clinical epidemiology: A basic science for clinical medicine. Boston: Little, Brown & Co, 1985.

Section III

Quality Issues

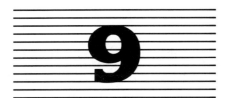

Access to Health Care

Robert L. Schiff, M.D., M.S., David Goldberg, M.D., and David A. Ansell, M.D.

Access to health care is a growing problem in the United States. Access may be defined as how well the health needs of the person fit with the dimensions of the health care system (1). The dimensions of access to health care include at least five key components: availability, accessibility, accommodation, affordability, and acceptability (1). A 1986 report by the Robert Wood Johnson Foundation stated that: ". . . as many as 38.8 million persons needed health care during the previous year but had difficulty obtaining it" (2). Groups who most often encounter obstacles to access include the medically indigent, residents of rural areas, undocumented workers, minorities, the mentally handicapped, and children and young adults.

Recent studies indicate that 37 million people in the United States are medically uninsured, representing 15.5% of the population (3). This has increased from 25 million uninsured, or 12.3% of the population in 1977 (3, 4). Minorities are more likely to be uninsured with 22.0% of African-Americans and 31.5% of Latinos uninsured, as compared with 12.4% of whites (3). Young adults are more often uninsured with 30.2% of those aged 19–24 lacking insurance (3). In addition, many of those who have insurance have inadequate coverage, with an estimated 25–30 million Americans being underinsured (2).

The uninsured have lower rates of hospitalization and physician visits and are less likely to receive preventive care and adequate prenatal care (5). A study from a California clinic devoted to indigent health care found that many patients could not afford the medical care that was recommended (6). One million United States families are actually denied care annually for financial reasons (7). Another study reported that 16.7% of uninsured adults reported not receiving health care for economic reasons, more than two and one half times the 6.5% reported by those with insurance (8). One of the most dramatic examples of denial of care is the practice of patient dumping by hospitals who deny care to emergency patients and transfer them to another hospital because they are medically indigent.

Access problems occur in spite of an affluent health care economy. The United States spent an estimated $600 billion in 1989 on health care services, increased from $75 billion in 1970 (2). The United States spends a greater percent of its gross national product (GNP) on health care than any other industrialized country, and the United States rate of spending has rapidly increased in the past two decades from 7.4% of the GNP in 1970 to 12.0% in 1989 (2). Despite present levels of spending and advanced technology, the problems of access remain, and the United States ranks below many other countries in health statistic indicators. The United

States infant mortality rate ranks 17th among nations with a rate of 10.6 (7, 9). Mean life expectancy at birth is 75.0 years in the United States, which ranks 17th among developed countries (10). Problems in access to care and inequitable distribution of resources likely account for a significant part of these inferior statistical indicators.

FINANCIAL ASPECTS OF ACCESS TO HEALTH CARE

Medicaid and the Medically Indigent

Those who lack medical insurance are disproportionately the poor and near poor. Of those whose family income is less than 100% of the poverty line, 35% are uninsured, and 29% of families with income at 100–199% of the poverty line are uninsured (5). Many of the working poor do not receive employee health benefits, and 54% of the uninsured live in families headed by a full-time worker (7). Medicaid legislation was enacted by the United States in 1965 to meet the health needs of the country's medically indigent. Medicaid programs are financed by the federal and state governments and are administered by the states. In 1988 Medicaid covered 24.2 million people (11). For many, it did improve access to care, particularly during the first 15 years of the program. Hospital care and outpatient care became more accessible for many. A number of significant improvements in health statistics coincided with the institution of Medicaid. These improvements include improved life expectancy, decreased mortality among blacks, and decreased deaths during childbirth (12). For example, "In the fifteen years before Medicaid, black infant mortality in this country declined 10%. In the ten years after Medicaid passed, it declined 50%" (13).

However, the Medicaid program has frequently been criticized. The cost of the program rose much faster than anticipated, in part, paralleling the skyrocketing rate of inflation for the financing of health services. This inflationary trend was great-

est in the years following the passage of Medicare and Medicaid legislation in 1964. Beginning in 1981, under the administration of President Reagan, the federal government made cutbacks in the extent and level of funding of many Medicaid programs, in an attempt to curtail Medicaid spending. From 1981 to 1985 more than one million people lost their Medicaid coverage because of changes in eligibility requirements (14). More than half of the poor are not receiving any Medicaid benefits. In 1987 only 40% of the poor qualified for Medicaid, as compared with 63% in 1975 (15, 16).

Cuts in the Medicaid program have been clearly shown to have deleterious effects on health, as illustrated by a recent study from California (17). In 1982 California eliminated Medicaid coverage for 270,000 adults. A follow-up study of 186 patients showed that 6 months after the program was eliminated the general health of the patients studied was significantly worse (17). Among hypertensive patients, diastolic blood pressure was significantly higher, rising a mean of 10 mm Hg. And at the 6-month follow-up only 50% of patients who lost their Medicaid coverage were able to identify a usual source of care, whereas 96% of the group still receiving Medicaid could identify a usual source of care (17).

Low reimbursement rates for hospital care and outpatient care are often a disincentive to caring for Medicaid patients. Medicaid pays only $0.50–0.75 per dollar of cost for hospital care (18). And Medicaid fees average just 53% of the charges for a follow-up office visit (19). As a result, many physicians refuse to care for Medicaid patients, and many others limit the number they will care for (20). In addition, many hospitals have a variety of restrictions on the admission of Medicaid patients.

A 1989 survey of pediatricians found that 44% of them limited access for Medicaid patients to their practice (21). Some pediatricians refuse to care for Medicaid patients and others limit the number they will see. The survey also found that pediatricians were significantly more likely to refuse Medicaid patients in 1989 than in

1978 (21). The most frequent reasons cited for limiting their Medicaid participation were low payments by Medicaid (reported to be about one-half of their usual fees) and the unpredictability of Medicaid payments (21).

Because Medicaid is administered by the states, there are 50 separate sets of programs, with multiple different categories and eligibility criteria in each state. This results in a complex, often confusing, system for the public, health care providers, and social service agencies. In addition, income eligibility levels vary widely among states, with some states having extremely low levels of income required to qualify for Medicaid. For example, in 1989 the maximum allowable annual income for a family of three ranged from $1416 in Alabama to $8328 in California (2). In 1989 the federal poverty level was $10,060 for a family of three, and 30 states set the maximum income eligibility level for Medicaid at less than half of that poverty level (2). These low limits exclude many of the poor from the program.

Medicare

Medicare legislation was passed in 1965 to provide medical insurance for the elderly and disabled. As the population in the United States has grown older, an increasing percentage of the population depends of Medicare. In 1988, 32 million people were covered by Medicare (22). Although Medicare does cover virtually all of the elderly, the percentage of health care costs covered has steadily fallen in the past 25 years. In 1984 the mean total spending on health care was $4202 per aged person (23), and less than 49% of that was covered by Medicare (24).

For some, costs not paid by Medicare are covered by supplemental private insurance or by Medicaid. But for other people these become out-of-pocket costs. Some of the costs not covered by Medicare include prescription drugs, routine physical examinations, eyeglasses, hearing aids, and most dental care (24). Medicare covers very little nursing home care, a fact not known by most Medicare recipients (24). The financial burden of these out-of-pocket costs falls particularly on those without supplemental coverage and those with serious health problems (23). About 20% of the elderly have no other health insurance, and 32% of the elderly who are poor lack supplemental coverage (25).

Changes in Fiscal Policy and Access to Hospital Care

In the past decade, forces in the economics of health care have caused many hospitals to change their corporate policies and business practices. These forces include health care competition and cost containment efforts by third party payers, Medicare, and Medicaid. A more competitive environment has resulted in many institutions adopting policies to restrict the number of indigent patients that they care for. Examples of these practices include institutions that require large preadmission deposits, premature discharges, selective admission of Medicaid patients and the medically indigent, and the dumping of uninsured emergency patients. A stark portrayal of this process of dumping undesirable patients and the simultaneous skimming of more profitable ones was depicted by one author's description: "Nobody wants the indigent, nonpaying patient. No one wants the intensely ill patient whose treatment consumes more hospital resources than the payment covers. The name of the game is skimming, and this is no longer frowned upon. All providers are involved in this process . . ." (26). As a result, access to hospital care has become increasingly more difficult for the medically indigent, during the past decade.

Some health policy analysts have argued that there are safety nets in our health care system to protect the medically indigent. These safety nets include public hospitals and uncompensated care provided by private hospitals. But, public hospitals have increasingly been plagued by problems of their own such as underfunding and overcrowding. Some communities have lost their public hospitals because of closure, often caused by competitive disadvantages and fiscal pressures. In recent years, 70 public hospitals have closed (5). In addition, many private hospitals, particularly those in inner city areas, have closed because of financial distress. Between 1985 and 1988, 10 hospitals in Chicago closed (27), and these were located predominantly in poor, underserved, inner city areas. Many private hospitals have responded to competitive pressures by further restricting the amount of uncompensated care that they provide.

United States hospitals provided an estimated $7.5 billion of uncompensated care in 1987, approximately 4.9% of expenses (18). This includes bad debt and charity care, which are usually lumped together in hospital financial reports. Bad debt accounts for more than two-thirds of this total and includes uncollected and uncollectible bills, some from patients who are able to pay. Charity care is care provided to uninsured patients who are at the time of admission knowingly unable to pay. The burden of uncompensated care is borne disproportionately by public hospitals, and in particular for charity care. In 1982 public hospitals represented 21% of all hospital beds, but provided 55% of all charity care (28). The growing numbers and health needs of the medically indigent far outstrip the ability of these institutions to fill all the gaps in providing care to the indigent.

ACCESS ISSUES FOR SPECIAL POPULATIONS

Access and Minorities

Minority groups face unique obstacles in obtaining health care. Studies have demonstrated that African-Americans and Latinos are more likely to be uninsured than whites (5). Financial barriers to care are more common for African-Americans as illustrated by a study that found 9.1% of African-Americans reported not receiving health care for economic reasons as compared with 5.0% of whites (29). Nonwhites are also more likely than whites to use hospital emergency rooms for care and not to have a regular family physician (30).

The widening of the gap between uninsured minorities and uninsured whites is a disturbing trend. The 1977 and 1987, National Medical Expenditure Surveys included data on the percentages of whites, Latinos, and African-Americans that lacked medical insurance (3, 4). In 1977, African-Americans were 66% more likely than whites to be uninsured, and in 1987 were 77% more likely. In 1977, Latinos were 74% more likely to be uninsured than whites, and in 1987 a striking 154% more likely.

A 1986 study showed significant problems in access to health care for African-Americans in the United States, and this gap was demonstrated for all income levels of African-Americans (29). A national survey found that 37% of African-Americans and 38% of Latinos had not seen a physician in the previous 12 months, as compared with 32% of whites (31). African-Americans apparently have significantly less access to care for cardiovascular disease, as they are much less likely to be evaluated by a cardiologist, to undergo coronary angioplasty, and to have coronary artery bypass surgery (32). And for patients with kidney disease, their race has been shown to correlate with the likelihood that they will be given long-term hemodialysis or a kidney transplant (33).

Many studies have demonstrated that there is a large gap in adult mortality rates between blacks and whites in the United States for all age groups (34). In particular, "Vital statistics from the National Center for Health Statistics show that the all-cause mortality rate for blacks exceeds that for whites in the United States by 149% and 97%, respectively, for 35- to 44-year olds and 45- to 54-year olds" (34). The largest contributions to excess deaths include cancer, heart disease, strokes, cirrhosis, and diabetes (34).

Life expectancy at birth remains significantly lower for African-Americans than whites in the United States. Life expectancy for African-American women is 73.5 compared with 78.7 for white women, and 65.3 for African-American men compared with 71.9 for white men (35). The infant mortality rate for African-Americans at 18.2 is twice the 9.3 rate for whites (35). African-Americans are more likely to have low birth weight infants; in 1987 African-Americans had a 12.7% rate of low birth weight as compared with the rate of 5.7% among whites (36). Differences in access to health care contributes to the differential in African-American and white mortality rates.

Rural Health Care

Residents of rural areas have been shown to have poorer access to health care than urban residents. In the 1986 Robert Wood Johnson Foundation survey of access to care, 9.4% of rural residents were uninsured whereas 8.8% of urban residents were uninsured. Rural residents were more likely to be in fair or poor health and were more likely to have a serious or chronic illness than urban residents (31). The 1982 survey by the Center for Health Administration Studies showed nonurban residents to have been more likely to use emergency rooms or hospital outpatient departments as a regular source of care than urban residents. They were less likely to have had a blood pressure measurement during the preceding year or, in the case of women, to have had a Pap smear or a breast examination (30). These indicators reflect that there are obstacles to access to care for rural residents.

Factors that contribute to poorer access for rural residents include their greater likelihood of being impoverished compared with that of urban residents. Among the nonelderly, 18% of rural residents had incomes below the poverty line, whereas 13% of urban residents had income below the poverty level (37). Thirty-seven to 43% of rural African-Americans and 33% of rural Latinos are impoverished (37, 38), rates that are higher than those for urban minorities. There is a high proportion of jobs in rural America that are agricultural or in a small business, and these jobs are less likely to offer health insurance as a benefit (37). In states with higher proportions of rural residents, Medicaid eligibility limits are set at lower income levels (39). Thus, whereas 44% of the urban poor are covered by Medicaid, only 36% of the rural poor have Medicaid coverage (37).

There is also a shortage of physicians in rural areas. Rural areas constitute 24–29% of the population (31, 40), but only 13–20% of physicians are located in rural areas (39, 40). Although doctors in rural areas are more likely to be in family and general practice and are less likely to be specialists (41), there are shortages of both primary care physicians and specialists in rural areas. These trends become worse as the size of the town decreases. There is evidence that these urban-rural disparities may be increasing (39). For example, in Minnesota the primary care physician-to-population ratio decreased by 2% in rural areas between 1965 and 1985 while it increased by 63% in urban areas (42). Moreover, rural access has been impaired by the disproportionate number of rural hospitals that have closed. In 1988, 53% of all hospital closures occurred in rural areas (40). A 1989 survey found that there were no hospitals or clinics that provided prenatal care in 799 counties across the country. These counties accounted for 215,000 births (43). Rural residents may also face long travel times to reach health care services, involving expenses that can be prohibitive for the rural poor (44). The travel distances can make specialty care virtually unobtainable.

There is evidence that rural access problems have an impact on patient outcomes. A study of pregnant women in the state of Washington demonstrated that women who resided in counties with high rates of patients leaving the county for prenatal care had poorer outcomes. Women in those counties were more likely to have complicated deliveries, they delivered more premature babies, and their babies had more costly neonatal care (45). Furthermore, a demonstration project showed that, when access to prenatal care in rural areas was improved, infant mortality declined dramatically, by 2.6 per 1000. There were steeper declines among African-Americans (46). The study concluded that infant mortality rates in poor, isolated rural areas with large minority populations can be improved to levels experienced elsewhere in the United States. These changes occurred rather rapidly in that demonstration project by improving access to prenatal care (46).

ACCESS TO OUTPATIENT CARE

Ambulatory Care

The uninsured receive less ambulatory care with a mean of 3.2 physician visits per year, whereas those with insurance have a mean of 4.4 visits (47). Indigent patients actually have greater health needs, as they are more likely to be in fair or poor health. For those who are in fair or poor health, uninsured patients have 5.6 mean annual ambulatory visits compared with 11.9 for insured patients (8).

The medically indigent are less likely to obtain appropriate ambulatory care in their community. A lack of access to primary care often forces indigent patients to use emergency departments for nonemergency care (48). 17.5% of the uninsured reported that a hospital ambulatory clinic or an emergency room was their usual source of care, in comparison with only 8.3% of those with insurance (8). The uninsured are also more likely not to have a regular source of care, as 24.8% of the uninsured lack a regular source of care and 12.6% of the insured lack one (49). "Having a regular or usual source of care has frequently been identified as a facilitator of access and as an indicator that the individual is not alienated from the health care system" (50). Having a regular source of care is also important for access to preventive care.

Uninsured pregnant women are less likely to get first trimester prenatal care (8), which has been shown to be beneficial and highly cost-effective for preventing perinatal morbidity and mortality. In fact, every $1 spent on prenatal care and nutrition can save $2–$11 in care otherwise needed for babies of mothers denied such services (51). Poor women are also more likely to have low birth weight babies (52). A recent Institute of Medicine study on preventing low birth weight concluded that the best method for preventing the problems of low birth weight was to provide prenatal care for all women, particularly for women at higher risk for poor pregnancy outcomes (52). A 1989 survey reported that 24% of all women and 39% of African-Americans and Latinos fail to receive first trimester prenatal care in the United States (43).

A study of low birth weight infants in California showed that 4% of women who received prenatal care had a low birth weight infant and 14% of those without prenatal care did (53). And among low birth weight babies, those from mothers who had received prenatal care had ". . . significantly better perinatal survival as well as less frequent respiratory distress and intraventricular hemorrhage" (53). The mean hospital charge was almost 50% greater for those infants born to mothers without prenatal care. Unfortunately, in recent years there has been a trend toward fewer women receiving early prenatal care in some states (52). During 1985, the infant mortality rate actually increased in 17 states in the United States (54).

Preventive Care

Access to preventive care services is inadequate for many Americans. The mortality rates from heart disease, cancer, and cerebrovascular disease, the major causes of death in the United States (55), could be significantly reduced if greater emphasis were placed on preventive care. It has been estimated that a moderately effective preventive program could save 400,000 lives yearly in the United States (56). For example, the decline in mortality from coronary artery disease and stroke since 1965 has been temporally related to modification of risk factors for coronary artery disease among the United States population. Risk factors that have been modified include smoking, hypertension, dietary fat, and blood cholesterol (57, 58). However, smoking alone remains responsible for 390,000 United States deaths annually, more than one of every six deaths (59). Yet, few insurance plans in the United States pay for preventive services (56). Only 2.3% of the total United States spending on health care is directed toward prevention (56). Numerous studies have shown that many physicians fail to practice accepted preventive medicine guidelines (60, 61).

Meanwhile, countering what meager prevention services that are available in the United States are groups such as the tobacco industry, which in 1988 spent $3.27 billion on cigarette advertising and promotions, a 27% increase over 1987 expenditures. These advertising campaigns are increasingly targeting minorities, women, and blue collar workers (62).

While access to preventive care is limited for all Americans, it is more problematic for the uninsured, the poor, and minorities. A study of factors related to the receipt of preventive examinations among women found that lack of insurance was the strongest predictor of failure to receive a screening test (63). Individuals without a regular source of care are less likely to make a preventive health visit of any kind than those who have regular sources of health care. Fifty percent of adults with a regular source of care had made a preventive visit in the previous year as compared with 28% of adults without a regular source of care (64).

These racial and income disparities in access to preventive care exist for many medical conditions. There is a strong association between race, lack of insurance, and inadequate blood pressure control. Among known hypertensives, 30% of African-Americans had not had an annual blood pressure check compared with 19% of whites (29). Likewise, women who lack insurance have a greater likelihood of not being screened for hypertension than women with insurance (63).

Poor and minority children face major obstacles in obtaining vaccinations. For example, there was a decline in the immunization rates for children in the United States in the 1980s (56). Forty percent of children in the United States have not received a full set of vaccinations (7). Eighty percent of minority children have not been adequately immunized (7), rates that are worse than most developing countries. Recent outbreaks and deaths from measles in the United States are directly a result of inadequate immunization practice. During a measles epidemic in Chicago in 1989, 75% of the cases occurred in unvaccinated individuals. The proportion of children who were adequately vaccinated by the age of 2 years was only 26% in areas that had high measles attack rates. School surveys noted marked racial differ-

ences in measles vaccination rates with minorities having significantly lower rates than whites (65).

Access to cancer prevention and control services is often limited to those who can afford them. Low-income Americans have lower cancer survival rates than higher income groups. And, African-Americans have the highest cancer mortality rates of any ethnic group in the United States (66). Yet access to cancer screening services is frequently limited for these high risk groups. A recent study reported that 27% of United States women had inadequate screening for cervical cancer, and 38% had inadequate breast screening examinations (63). Those without insurance were significantly less likely to be screened (63).

While the general awareness regarding the importance of screening mammograms has increased in the United States over the past few years (67), African-American women are less likely to have heard about mammography and less likely to have received a mammogram (68) than whites. The Illinois Division of the American Cancer Society conducted a survey of all health facilities in the state of Illinois and was able to identify only one hospital in the state that offered free mammography services and only a handful that offered charity care for any cancer prevention, screening, or diagnostic services (69).

The high correlation between insurance status, income, race, and the receipt of preventive services is particularly disturbing because low income individuals and minorities are at the highest risk for a preventible illness and the least likely to receive preventive services.

ACCESS TO EMERGENCY CARE: PATIENT DUMPING

The denial or limitation of the provision of medical care to a patient for economic reasons and the referral of that patient elsewhere has been called patient dumping. The transfer of patients in need of emergency care from one hospital emergency department to another for economic reasons is among the most widely reported and studied categories of patient dumping

(70). Other forms of patient dumping include the transfer of hospitalized patients for economic reasons and the referral of ambulatory patients to other health facilities (71, 72). Emergency department dumping, although a long-standing practice in many areas of the United States, increased dramatically during the 1980s from approximately 50,000 transfers in 1980 to 250,000 in 1988 (73). The most common reasons for patient dumping are absent or inadequate insurance coverage (70).

Patient dumping has been reported from urban and rural areas, and a number of studies have documented the medical, social, and fiscal implications of this practice (74–78). The patients involved are generally uninsured or underinsured. A study at Highland General Hospital in Oakland found that of 458 patients transferred to its emergency department from other hospitals 63% were uninsured, 21% had Medicaid, and only 3% had private insurance (75). In a study at Chicago's Cook County Hospital, 87% of patients transferred were uninsured (74). The reason for transfer was "no insurance" for 87% of these patients. In studies from Oakland, Chicago, and Memphis, the majority of transferred patients were minorities (74–76).

Patient dumping has serious medical implications. The foremost is that patients in need of emergency care are being denied appropriate treatment and being transferred for economic reasons. Many of these patients have been found to be in an unstable condition at the time of transfer. For example, in one study 24% of transferred patients were in an unstable condition at the transferring hospital (74). Similarly, 27% of transfers in another study were found to be unstable (76). Also, emergency patients may suffer harm by having their treatment delayed (74). In one study, the treatment delay caused by the transfer of patients ranged from 1 to 18 hours with an average delay of 5.1 hours (74). There have been reports of patient disability or even death resulting from patient dumping (79, 80).

The interhospital transfer of individuals in need of emergency care for economic reasons is but one facet of patient dumping. Hospitals may avoid treating indigents by diverting patients during ambulance transport or they may turn indigents away prior to emergency department treatment and refer them to the nearest public facility. Finally, they may render some evaluation and treatment, and then discharge a patient who might otherwise need hospitalization (80). These individuals may be referred to the public hospital or clinic for further care, often without prior authorization and without accompanying medical records (81).

Some hospitals have closed specialty services such as trauma units and obstetric units to avoid taking care of indigent patients. For example, in Los Angeles 10 of 23 trauma centers dropped out of the regionalized trauma system (18). In Chicago, 4 of 10 trauma centers dropped out of the system between 1988 and 1990, citing financial reasons (82). In addition, physicians in community hospitals have reported difficulties in getting individuals with medical problems requiring tertiary care transferred to appropriate facilities when the patient lacks adequate coverage (83).

In 1986 the federal government passed antidumping legislation as part of the Consolidated Omnibus Budget Reconciliation Act (COBRA) of 1986 (84). This legislation required that all emergency patients coming to a hospital that receives Medicare funding receive a medical screening examination and that they be stabilized prior to transfer to another facility. This law also provided for civil and administrative penalties against physicians and hospitals who knowingly violated its provisions. The law was amended in 1989 (85) in response to widespread criticism (70, 80). These amendments require that a hospital's responsibility for initial treatment of emergency patients must include services and treatments available within the hospital's entire capabilities not just that of the emergency department. It also stipulates that, for all emergency patients, necessary treatment may not be delayed in order to assess financial status of the patient. The hospital is prohibited from transferring unstable patients without their written request coupled with informed consent regarding the hospital's COBRA obligations and the potential risks of transfer (85).

Hospitals and physicians are subject to sanctions under the law's provisions. The sanctions include a fine of up to $50,000 and exclusion from Medicare/Medicaid programs. Finally, any hospital with specialized facilities such as burn, trauma, and neonatal intensive care units are required to accept all patients who require these services regardless of insurance status (85).

The federal antidumping legislation has several weaknesses that compromise its ability to resolve this access problem. The definition of what constitutes an emergency is vague and quite narrowly defined. The law also allows patients to be transferred once stabilized, a concept that is subject to conflicting interpretation and potential abuse (70, 80). The editor of the *New England Journal of Medicine* has stated that " 'stabilization' of emergency cases is a notion used by hospital managers to justify transfers for economic reasons, but it is an elusive and dangerous concept" (86).

As of the end of 1988, only 243 investigations of COBRA violations had been completed. Only six institutions had been fined and only two had lost their Medicare contracts, one of which had it reinstated (86). The number of actual penalties levied pales in light of the more than 500,000 economic transfers that occurred between 1986 and 1988. There is no evidence that COBRA has been a deterrent to the practice of patient dumping. Studies from Chicago and Memphis, both completed after COBRA, show that patients continue to be transferred for economic reasons despite being in unstable medical conditions (87, 88).

HIV, AIDS, AND ACCESS TO CARE

No single health care problem is stimulating such a vigorous debate on access to care as human immunodeficiency virus type I (HIV) infection. This debate is occurring in the context of expanding needs for HIV-related care in the United States. HIV seroconversion and the number of new AIDS cases continues to increase with an ever-widening geographic distribution. There is a shifting pattern of epidemiology from its starting point among largely gay men and recipients of blood products (89–92) to the population of intravenous drug users, with women and children representing rapidly growing demographic groups (93). Heterosexual transmission, especially from men to women, has increased, and there has been a shift from a largely white population to a disproportionately African-American and Latino population (93–97). There are pressing needs for far-reaching preventive programs that involve culturally relevant health education, together with strategies to alter sexual and drug using practices (98). Costly new therapies are available that prolong healthful survival (99, 100), but require screening and follow-up in the asymptomatic period. Although HIV is a new health care concern requiring dramatic responses both nationally and in the specific regions of the country with the highest rates of infection, the issues it raises, recapitulate many of the access issues we have discussed.

There is evidence that the insurance status of people with AIDS (PWAs) differs from the national mean. Table 9.1 compares the insurance status of hospital discharges of PWAs with all hospital discharges for 1985 (101, 102). The striking features of the data include: *(a)* the very low rate of Medicare coverage for AIDS, *(b)* the high percentage of AIDS patients covered by Medicaid, *(c)* the extremely low rate of private insurance in the public sector for AIDS patients, *(d)* the high percentage of AIDS patients who are medically indigent, and *(e)* the relatively high burden for AIDS care from the prison system. More recently (103), a dramatic trend has unfolded with a further decline in the proportion of AIDS care covered by private insurance and concomitant increases in the proportion of care covered by Medicaid. This trend has been called the "Medicaidization" of AIDS (103).

The skewed distribution of insurance coverage has the greatest impact on hospi-

Table 9.1.
Health Insurance Status of AIDS Hospital Discharges and All Hospital Discharges

	AIDS (101)			All (102)		
	Total	Public	Private	Total	Public	Private
	%			%		
Medicare	2	1	3	30	26	30
Medicaid	54	62	35	11	13	9
Private	17	7	45	46	44	48
Self-pay	17	18	13	8	10	7
Prison	3	4	1	NA	NA	NA
Other	7	8	3	6	7	6

[a]NA, not available.

tals with high volumes of AIDS care. It threatens the financial stability of these hospitals due to the high rates of uncompensated and undercompensated care. Patient dumping from the private sector to the public sector may increasingly occur as a means for private hospitals to minimize uncompensated care. Moreover, public hospital services are at risk of further overcrowding, which can and has led to deterioration of services, for both PWAs and other patients (104). Local governments are being pressured to provide additional funds for public hospital care due to the failure of private, federal, and state funding sources to adequately insure AIDS patients. The epidemic threatens to overwhelm the prison health care system, as well. These factors pose a threat to access to hospital care for AIDS and are likely to have a similar impact on outpatient care (103, 105).

A 1987 study from New York analyzed factors accounting for differences in survival for PWAs (106). The group of white, gay men who had Kaposi's sarcoma at presentation had the most favorable survival and served as the reference group. Other patient groups had as much as a threefold higher mortality rate. Although manifestations of AIDS at diagnosis was the single most important influence on excessive risk, ethnicity (African-American and Latino), risk group (drug using), and sex (women) contributed to nearly 30% of the increased mortality in that study (106). Whereas the study did not specifically evaluate whether access to care contributed to the differences in survival, these

variables are well documented to confer poorer overall access to health care.

Another marker of access to AIDS care is the initial mode of detection of HIV infection and whether therapy is begun in the asymptomatic period. The current standard of care is early detection of HIV by screening for the purpose of instituting zidovudine (AZT) in the asymptomatic period (99, 100, 107). It also includes delivery of aerosolized pentamidine for prophylaxis of *Pneumocystis carinii* pneumonia (108, 109), a common cause of pneumonia in AIDS with a high mortality rate. A study from Maryland showed that minorities and intravenous drug users as compared with other groups were significantly less likely to receive AZT and aerosolized pentamidine (110). As of 1990, at urban public hospitals, HIV infection continued to be discovered most frequently when late manifestations of the disease occurred. Screening programs, including regular patient follow-up and AZT prophylaxis, had not yet consistently reached the urban poor and minorities (111).

Financing of Care for HIV Infection

There are several reasons that HIV-positive persons are disproportionately medically indigent. The insured or potentially insurable person with HIV infection is at risk of becoming medically indigent as the disease progresses. The poor and already medically indigent have an increased likelihood of acquiring HIV disease. In addition, Medicare and Medicaid have failed to cover those with AIDS adequately.

HIV-infected persons who are privately insured have difficulty maintaining their insurance (112). The progressive nature of the disease forces many to leave their jobs. Debilitated individuals may thus lose their private insurance coverage prior to needing their most costly care. There are mechanisms for some people to maintain private insurance coverage despite losing their job. However, these options involve considerable out-of-pocket costs. They frequently become unaffordable, causing eventual loss of insurance. One author has called this a "two-tier care system for AIDS patients," with care beginning in the private sector covered by private insurance and later in the disease falling to the public sector (113).

HIV-infected persons or high risk groups for HIV infection have difficulty obtaining individual insurance policies (112). These difficulties result from insurance company practices of testing for HIV and including questions on sexual orientation and intravenous drug use on insurance applications. Insurance carriers sometimes redline entire areas of cities and/or occupations with higher than average prevalence rates of HIV infection (112). There is evidence that these practices achieve their goals. Data from the Health Insurance Association of America and the American Council of Life Insurance found that, while group policy expenditures for claims more than doubled for AIDS-related care between 1986 and 1987, those expenditures for individual policies were nearly unchanged (112).

There are barriers, as well, for PWAs to qualify for Medicare and Medicaid. PWAs are eligible for Medicare based on disability. However, there is a minimum 29-month waiting period from the onset of disability to the time of qualifying for Medicare benefits. These 29 months are usually crucial months for health care needs. Medicaid eligibility requirements exclude many people despite their medical need. There are also vast state-by-state differences in the benefits Medicaid confers for PWAs (112). The result of financial barriers for HIV care is the high rate of

Medicaid covered and medically indigent PWAs. As the number of people requiring care increases, the financial implications for HIV care could worsen.

Health Service Needs for HIV Care

Aside from the inpatient demands for HIV-related care, there is a growing need for outpatient services. The demonstration that antiretroviral therapy with AZT can prolong life when given in the asymptomatic period (99, 100) underlines the need for early identification and care of HIV seropositive persons in the outpatient setting. For the estimated one million seropositive individuals in the United States, providing comprehensive primary care will ". . . radically increase demands on the health care system" (114). In addition to general medical, gynecological, obstetrical, and pediatric care, a comprehensive ambulatory program would require screening, health education, access to abortion services, dental services, and antiretroviral therapy. There are large needs for psychological and social support services for PWAs and their families (115, 116). Furthermore, this care needs to be well-coordinated (117). Skilled workers in each of these areas have to be trained. A comprehensive ambulatory care system for HIV care is unlikely to be developed quickly enough to meet the projected need (114).

Substance abuse poses an unique problem for AIDS care because of the risk of acquiring HIV infection, continued transmission of HIV by infected intravenous drug users, and the difficulty of complying with therapy while using drugs. Yet there is inadequate access to substance abuse programs. Nationally, approximately 20% of intravenous drug users are in drug treatment programs (118). In New York City there are 35,000 treatment slots for an estimated 200,000 addicts (119). In San Francisco, there are more than 4,500 people on waiting lists for drug treatment, with waiting lists as long as 6 months (120). Many of those on waiting lists will be lost to follow-up. Furthermore, publicly funded substance abuse programs are not linked with public general medical programs because of different sources of funding. Additionally, as many as one-quarter of New York's addicted population enter the prison system yearly, further complicating their general medical and substance abuse care (119).

Prevention programs have been successful in gay communities of some cities, reducing the rates of new seroconversion (121). Generalizing these successes to other populations may be difficult because of lack of access to primary care for high risk adolescents and young adults (3, 122), inadequate HIV risk assessment and education by health care providers (123), and the failure of school and other health education programs to provide explicit substance abuse and sex education (97, 124, 125). For social and political reasons, AIDS prevention has not been placed prominently on national and many community agendas (97, 126–129).

For persons with advanced AIDS, there is a scarcity of programs to deliver appropriate chronic care. Needed programs include home care, day care, nursing home care, and hospice care (117). These problems are revealed by figures from New York that showed that 13% of the 420 PWAs in the public hospitals during November 1987 had prolonged hospital stays because of difficulties with discharge planning (130). In the state of Illinois, there were only 4 designated nursing home beds for AIDS patients as of late 1989, while the estimated need for Chicago alone was 85 to 100 beds (131). The chronic care problems are more difficult for drug users and children (132). In addition, homelessness is a problem facing a disproportionate number of HIV-infected persons.

Discrimination and AIDS

Health care is a very human endeavor with attitudes playing an important role together with service availability and clinical skill. HIV-related care has been impaired by discrimination at both the level of providing care and the level of social policy and attitudes. Attitudes projected by health care institutions and the individuals who work within them may create barriers to access.

HIV-related care has been hampered by fear of contagion (133). There is a decided bias among some health care workers against treating HIV-infected patients. Survey data show that many health care workers fear that AIDS can be passed by casual contact, by examining the patient, or by entering the room of an AIDS patient. Many health care workers would like to have the right to choose not to work with HIV-infected patients (133).

Health care workers have expressed bias against caring for AIDS patients who are gay, substance users, ethnic and racial minorities, or women. Canadian physicians and nurses showed preferences in caring for AIDS patients who contracted the disease by blood transfusion rather than homosexual transmission or intravenous drug use (133). A survey of internal medicine residents in the United States showed a tendency to blame AIDS patients for their disease, a trend that was stronger when the particular risk of being a racial minority, gay, or an intravenous drug user was identified (134, 135). Women face sex-based discrimination, being blamed for the transmission of HIV to children or men (129, 136). While the impact of discrimination is difficult to measure, institutional and health care worker attitudes may pose additional obstacles to obtaining HIV-related information and care.

Currently, there is a myriad of federal, state, local, private, and voluntary programs for the multiple needs for HIV-related health care. These programs have not been able to ensure access for HIV care. Ultimately, the solutions to the problems of accessible, comprehensive, and nondiscriminatory health programs for HIV care will require commitment to a national system of care rather than incremental patches for aspects of HIV care grafted onto the current health care system (117).

SOLUTIONS

We have discussed some of the many serious problems in access to health care in the United States that have been identified. These include access for the medically indigent, minorities, persons with AIDS, and for those in rural areas. Access is an obstacle for hospital care, ambulatory care, and for preventive health services. A multitude of short- and long-term solutions for these problems has been proposed and recently reviewed (2). Solutions to the access problem will have to address the crisis in financing for health care services, as well as the availability, distribution and coordination of health services. There is broad-based public support for solving the access problem, as repeatedly shown in public opinion polls in the United States. Eighty-two percent of the public believe that everyone has a right to adequate health care, and 76% believe it is the responsibility of the federal government to guarantee it (137).

Proposals that have been most widely advocated include expanding the number of those with private insurance by either encouraging or requiring employers to provide private insurance to their employees. Expansion of Medicaid eligibility is another proposed solution to improve access to health care. Health insurance risk pools for high risk people (who may otherwise be uninsurable) funded by state governments have been considered; some states have recently implemented such programs (2). Although these proposals may have some short-term merit for addressing subsets of individuals in a piecemeal fashion, they do not resolve the larger issue of providing equitable access to comprehensive health care for all.

Long-term solutions will require sweeping changes in health policy to reorient the health care system to guaranteeing equal access to health care for all. As of 1990, the United States and South Africa were the only two industrialized countries in the world without a national health plan program. Many individuals and organizations have argued that such a program is a necessary component to solving the access problems in the United States. Some of the groups that have advocated a national health plan for the United States that would guarantee access to comprehensive care for all include the Physicians for a National Health Program (138), The American College of Physicians (2), the Coalition for a National Health Service, and the Gray Panthers.

The Physicians for a National Health Program proposal borrows many features from the Canadian national health program. It would provide universal coverage for all persons in a single public health plan (138). Comprehensive coverage would be provided for all health services including hospital care, ambulatory care, preventive services, prescription drugs, dental services, and long-term care (138). Funding for the program would be based on a system of progressive taxation at the federal level (138). Although the expanded access to services would increase costs, these costs would be offset by savings of 10% or more on administration and billing (138). A national health plan such as this would establish a right to accessible, comprehensive health care in the United States.

References

1. Penchansky R, Thomas JW. The concept of access: Definition and relationship to consumer satisfaction. Med Care 1981;19:127–141
2. American College of Physicians. Access to health care (position paper). Ann Intern Med 1990;112:641–661.
3. Short P, Monheit A, Beauregard K. A profile of uninsured Americans. National Medical Expenditure Survey Research Findings 1, National Center for Health Services Research and Health Care Technology Assessment. Department of Health and Human Services Publication No. (PHS) 89-3443. Rockville, MD: Public Health Service, September 1989:1–18.
4. Davis K, Rowland D. Uninsured and underserved: Inequities in health care in the United States. Milbank Q 1983;61:149–176.
5. Bazzoli GJ. Health care for the indigent: Overview of critical issues. Health Serv Res 1986;21:353–393.
6. Hubbell FA, Waitzkin H, Rucker L, Akin BV, Heide MG. Financial barriers to medical care: A prospective study in a university-affiliated community clinic. Am J Med Sci 1989;297:158–162.
7. Woolhandler S, Himmelstein DU. Resolving the cost/access conflict: The case for a national health program. J Gen Intern Med 1989;4:54–60.
8. Freeman HE, Aiken LH, Blendon RJ, Corey CR. Uninsured working-age adults: Characteristics and consequences. Health Serv Res 1990;24:811–823.
9. McGoldrick KE. Prenatal care: Investing in the future. J Am Med Wom Assoc 1990;45(2):35.
10. Centers for Disease Control. Mortality in developed countries. MMWR 1990;39:205–209.
11. Brown ER. State approaches to financing health care for the poor. Annu Rev Public Health 1990;11:377–400.

12. Rogers DE, Blendon RJ, Moloney TW. Who needs Medicaid? N Engl J Med 1982;307:13–18
13. Weill JD, Rosenbaum S. Reflections on twenty years of Medicare and Medicaid. Health Advocate (Newsletter of the National Health Law Program, Los Angeles, CA) Summer 1985; 145:5.
14. Kotulak R. Poor patients given the silent treatment. *The Chicago Tribune*. July 14, 1986;Section 1:1,4.
15. Akin BV, Rucker L, Hubbell FA, Cygan RW, Waitzkin H. Access to medical care in a medically indigent population. J Gen Intern Med 1989;4: 216–220.
16. Iglehart J. Views of a health policy activist: A conversation with Henry Waxman. Health Aff (Millwood) 1987;6(4):20–29.
17. Lurie N, Ward NB, Shapiro MF, Brook RH. Termination from Medi-Cal—Does it affect health? N Engl J Med 1984;311:480–484.
18. Friedman E. Hospital uncompensated care: Crisis? JAMA 1989;262:2975–2977.
19. Curtis R. The role of state governments in assuring access to care. Inquiry 1986;23:277–285.
20. Oswalt CE. Expensive health care: A solvable problem? Arch Intern Med 1990;150:1165–1166.
21. Yudkowsky BK, Cartland JDC, Flint SS. Pediatrician participation in Medicaid: 1978–1989. Pediatrics 1990;85:567–577.
22. Gerety MB, Winograd CH. Public financing of Medicare. J Am Geriatr Soc 1988;36:1061–1066.
23. Davis K. Medicare financing and beneficiary income. Inquiry 1987;24:309–323.
24. Rice T, Gabel J. Protecting the elderly against high health care costs. Health Aff (Millwood) 1986; 5(3):5–21.
25. Christensen S, Long SH, Rodgers J. Acute health care costs for the aged Medicare population: Overview and policy options. Milbank Q 1987;65:397–425.
26. Anonymous. The future of the MIO in a price-competitive, price-driven market. Top Health Care Financ 1984(Winter);11(2):84–92.
27. Anonymous. More hospitals close as costs rise, income drops: Fifteen Illinois hospitals closed since 1985. Illinois Medicine (published by the Illinois State Medical Society) 1988(September);1:7.
28. Friedman E. Public hospitals often face unmet capital needs, underfunding, uncompensated patient-care costs. JAMA 1987;257:1698–1701.
29. Blendon RJ, Aiken LH, Freeman HE, Corey CR. Access to medical care for black and white Americans: A matter of continuing concern. JAMA 1989;261:278–281.
30. Aday LA, Andersen RM. The national profile of access to medical care: Where do we stand? Am J Public Health 1984;74:1331–1339.
31. Weisfeld VD, ed. Access to health care in the United States: Results of a 1986 survey. Princeton, NJ: Robert Wood Johnson Foundation;1987: special report no. 2.
32. Strogatz DS. Use of medical care for chest pain: Differences between blacks and whites. Am J Public Health 1990;80:290–294.
33. AMA Council on Ethical and Judicial Affairs. Black-white disparities in health care. JAMA 1990;263:2344–2346.
34. Otten MW, Teutsch SM, Williamson DF, Marks JS. The effect of known risk factors on the excess mortality of black adults in the United States. JAMA 1990;263:845–850.
35. Rice MF, Winn M. Black health care in America: A political perspective. J Natl Med Assoc 1990; 82:429–437.
36. U.S.: Grim health scene for blacks. *The Chicago Tribune*. March 23, 1990;Section 1:5.
37. Rowland D, Lyons B. Triple jeopardy: Rural, poor, and uninsured. Health Serv Res 1989;23: 975–1004.
38. Norton CH, McManus MA. Background tables on demographic characteristics, health status, and health service utilization. Health Serv Res 1989; 23:725–756.
39. McManus MA, Newacheck PW. Rural maternal, child, and adolescent health. Health Serv Res 1989;23:807–848.
40. Burke M. Policymakers struggle to define essential access. Hospitals 1990;64:(Feb 5):38–42.
41. Newhouse JP. Geographic access to physicians' services. Annu Rev Public Health 1990;11:207–230.
42. Dennis T. Changes in the distribution of physicians in rural areas of Minnesota, 1965–1985. Am J Public Health 1988;78:1577–1579.
43. Witwer MB. Prenatal care in the United States: Reports call for improvements in quality and accessibility. Family Plann Perspect 1990;22:31–35.
44. Freeman HP. Barriers to cancer control: Findings and challenges of regional hearings. In: Proceedings from the national conference on cancer in the poor: Bridging the gaps in health care. Atlanta: American Cancer Society, 1989:34–43.
45. Nesbitt TS, Connell FA, Hart LG, Rosenblatt RA. Access to obstetrical care in rural areas: Effect on birth outcomes. Am J Public Health 1990;80:814–818.
46. Gortmaker SC, Clark CJG, Graven SN, Sobol AM, Geronimus A. Reducing infant mortality in rural America: Evaluation of the Rural Infant Care Program. Health Serv Res 1987;22:91–116.
47. Freeman HE, Blendon RJ, Aiken LH, Sudman S, Mullinix CF, Corey CR. Americans report on their access to health care. Health Aff (Millwood) 1987;6(1):6–18.
48. Koska MT. Indigent care and overcrowding threaten EDs. Hospitals 1989;63(14):66, 68, 70.
49. Howell EM. Low-income persons' access to health care: NMCUES Medicaid data. Public Health Rep 1988;103:507–514.
50. Kuder JM, Levitz GS. Visits to the physician: An evaluation of the usual-source effect. Health Serv Res 1985;20:579–596.
51. Mundinger MO. Health service funding cuts and the declining health of the poor. N Engl J Med 1985;313:44–47.
52. Cagle CS. Access to prenatal care and prevention of low birth weight. MCN 1987;12:235–238.
53. Leveno KJ, Cunningham FG, Roark ML, Nelson SD, Williams ML. Prenatal care and the low birth weight infant. Obstet Gynecol 1985;66:599–605.

54. Braveman P, Oliva G, Miller MG, Schaaf VM, Reiter R. Women without health insurance: Links between access, poverty, ethnicity, and health. West J Med 1988;149:708–711.
55. Center for Disease Control. Mortality trends. United States 1986–1988, MMWR 1989;38:117–118.
56. Himmelstein DV, Woolhandler S. Pitfalls of private medicine: Health Care in the USA. Lancet 1984;391–393.
57. Levy RI. Declining mortality in coronary heart disease. Arteriosclerosis 1981;1:312–325.
58. Stamler J. Coronary artery disease: Doing the "right things". N Engl J Med 1985;312:1053–1055.
59. Fiore ML, Pierce JP. Cigarette smoking: The clinician's role in cessation, prevention and public health. Dis Mon April 1990. 185–241.
60. McGinnis JM, Woolf SH. Background and objectives of the U.S. Preventive Services Task Force. J Gen Intern Med 1990;4(suppl):11–13.
61. Lurie N, Manning WG, Peterson C, Goldberg GA, Phelps CA, Lillard L. Preventive care: Do we practice what we preach? Am J Public Health 1987;77:801–804.
62. Centers for Disease Control. Cigarette advertising—United States—1988. MMWR 1990;39:261–265.
63. Woolhandler S, Himmelstein DU. Reverse targeting of preventive care due to lack of health insurance. JAMA 1988;259:2872–2874.
64. Lave JR, Lave LB, Leinhardt S, Nagin D. Characteristics of individuals who identify a regular source of care. Am J Public Health 69;1979:261–267.
65. Centers for Disease Control. Update: Measles outbreak—Chicago, 1989. MMWR 1990;39:317–319, 325–326.
66. Freeman H. Cancer in the economically disadvantaged. Cancer 1989;64(suppl):324–334.
67. Centers for Disease Control. Trends in screening mammograms for women 50 years of age and older—Behavior risk factors surveillance system, 1987. MMWR 1989;38:137–140.
68. Centers for Disease Control. Provisional estimates for the national health interview survey supplement on cancer control—United States, Jan–Mar 1987. MMWR 1988;37:417–420, 425.
69. Report of the Ad-Hoc Committee on Cancer in the Poor. Illinois Division of the American Cancer Society, March 3, 1990. Available from the Illinois Division of the American Cancer Society, Chicago, IL.
70. Ansell DA, Schiff RL. Patient dumping: Status, implications and policy recommendations. JAMA 1987;207:1500–1502.
71. Kerr HD, Byrd JC. Community hospital transfers to a VA medical center. JAMA 1989;262:70–73.
72. Schiff G, Angus K, Razafinariuo S. The base of the iceberg: Outpatient dumping in Chicago. Health/PAC Bull 1984;15:14–16.
73. Wolinsky H. Fivefold rise in "patient dumping" found. Chicago Sun-Times. Friday, March 20, 1987:24.
74. Schiff RL, Ansell DA, Schlosser JE, Idris A. Transfers to a public Hospital. N Engl J Med 1986; 314:552–557.
75. Himmelstein DU, Woolhandler S, Harnly M, et al. Patient transfers: Medical practice as social triage. Am J Public Health 1984;74:494–497.
76. Kellerman AL, Hackman BB. Emergency department patient "dumping": An analysis of interhospital transfers to the regional medical center of Memphis, Tennessee. Am J Public Health 1988; 78:1287–1292.
77. Anderson RJ, Cawley KA, Andrulis DP. The evolution of a public hospital transfer policy. Metropolitan Hospital. 1985;2(winter):1–2 (available from the American Hospital Association, Chicago, IL).
78. Lebow M, MacMillan W. Patient transfers to a public hospital. J Emerg Med 1988;6:447–450.
79. Curran WJ. Economic and legal considerations in emergency care. N Engl J Med 1985;312:374–375.
80. Equal access to health care: Patient dumping. Hearing before a subcommittee of the Committee on Operations, United States House of Representatives. One hundredth Congress, First Session, July 22, 1987. Washington, D.C.: Government Printing Office, 1988.
81. Uzych L. Patient dumping. J Fla Med Assoc 1990;77:97–100.
82. Merriner J. Health care gap widens: Insurance inadequate for 3 in 10 here. Chicago Sun-Times. 1990 Jun 18:1(col 3), 48(col 1–3).
83. Wrenn K. No insurance, no admission. N Engl J Med 1985;312:373–374.
84. Examination and treatment for emergency medical conditions and women in active labor. Congressional Record. 1985;131(Oct 23):S13902–S13904.
85. Anonymous. New dumping law amendments proposed. Health Advocate. Spring 1989;160:14–15.
86. Relman AS. Economic considerations in emergency care: What are hospitals for? N Engl J Med 1985;312:372–373.
87. Kellerman AC, Hackman BB. Patient dumping post-COBRA. Am J Public Health 1990;80:864–867.
88. Handler A, Driscol M, Rosenberg D, Mullner R, Cohen M. Regional perinatal care in crisis: maternal transfers to a public hospital. Presented at the American Public Health Association Annual Meeting, Boston, MA. November 15–17, 1988.
89. Centers for Disease Control. Pneumocystis pneumonia—Los Angeles. MMWR 1981;30:250–252.
90. Durack DT. Opportunistic infections and Kaposi's sarcoma in homosexual men. N Engl J Med 1981;30:1465–1467.
91. Centers for Disease Control. Update on acquired immune deficiency syndrome (AIDS) among patients with Hemophilia A. MMWR 1982;31:644–652.
92. Centers for Disease Control. Possible transfusion-associated acquired immune deficiency syndrome (AIDS)—California. MMWR 1982;31:652–654.
93. Centers for Disease Control. Update: Acquired immunodeficiency syndrome—United States, 1989. MMWR 1990;39:81–86.
94. Guinan ME, Hardy A. Epidemiology of AIDS in women in the United States: 1981 through 1986. JAMA 1987;257:2039–2042.

95. Gayle JA, Selik RM, Chu SY. Surveillance for AIDS and HIV infection among black and Hispanic children and women of childbearing age, 1981–1989. MMWR 1990;39(suppl. 3):23–30.

96. Selik RM, Castro KG, Pappaioanou M. Racial/ethnic differences in the risk of AIDS in the United States. Am J Public Health 1988;78:1539–1545.

97. Friedman SR, Sotheran JL, Abdul-Quader A, et al. The AIDS epidemic among blacks and Hispanics. Milbank Q 1987;(suppl. 2):455–499.

98. Fineberg HV. Education to prevent AIDS: Prospects and obstacles. Science 1988;239:592–596.

99. Fischl MA, Richman DD, Grieco MH, et al. The efficacy of azidothymidine (AZT) in the treatment of patients with AIDS and AIDS-related complex: A double-blind, placebo-controlled trial. N Engl J Med 1987;317:185–191.

100. Volberding PA, Lagakos SW, Koch MA, et al. Zidovudine in asymptomatic human immunodeficiency virus infection: A controlled trial in persons with fewer than 500 CD4-positive cells per cubic millimeter. N Engl J Med 1990;322:941–949.

101. Andrulis DP, Beers VS, Bentley JD, Gage LS. The provision and financing of medical care for AIDS patients in US public and private teaching hospitals. JAMA 1987;258:1343–1346.

102. Sloan FA, Morrisey MA, Valvona J. Case shifting and the Medicare prospective payment system. Am J Public Health 1988;78:553–556.

103. Green J, Arno PS. The "Medicaidization" of AIDS: Trends in the financing of HIV-related medical care. JAMA 1990;264:1261–1266.

104. Levi J. Access to care issues and AIDS. American Public Health Association Annual Meeting, New Orleans, October, 1987.

105. Andrulis DP, Weslowski VB, Gage LS. The 1987 US hospital AIDS survey. JAMA 1989;262:784–794.

106. Rothenberg R, Woelfel M, Stoneburner R, Milberg J, Parker R, Truman B. Survival with the acquired immunodeficiency syndrome: Experience with 5833 cases in New York City. N Engl J Med 1987;317:1297–1302.

107. Friedland GH. Early treatment for HIV: The time has come. N Engl J Med 1990;332:1000–1002.

108. Girard PM, Gaudebout C, Lottin P. Prevention of *Pneumocystis carinii* pneumonia relapse by pentamidine aerosol in zidovudine-treated AIDS patients. Lancet 1989;1:1348–1353.

109. Centers for Disease Control. Guidelines for prophylaxis against *Pneumocystis carinii* pneumonia for persons infected with human immunodeficiency virus. MMWR 1989;38(suppl. 5):1–9.

110. Hidalgo J, Sugland B, Moore R, Chaisson RE. Access, equity, and survival: Use of ZVD and pentamidine by persons with AIDS. VI International Conference on AIDS, San Francisco, June, 1990 (abstract Th.D.59).

111. Anonymous. AIDS unchanging among certain populations. AIDS Alert 1990;5:143–144.

112. Bartlett L. Financing health care for persons with AIDS: Balancing public and private responsibilities. In: Gostin LO, ed. AIDS and the health care system. New Haven: Yale University Press, 1990:211–220.

113. Mansell PWA. M. D. Anderson Hospital and Tumor Institute. In: Griggs J, ed. AIDS: Public policy dimensions. New York: United Hospital Fund of New York, 1987:131–137.

114. Arno PS, Shenson D, Siegel NF, Franks P. Lee PR. Economic and policy implications of early intervention in HIV disease. JAMA 1989; 2262:1493–1498.

115. Tross S, Hirsch DA. Psychological distress and neuropsychological complications of HIV infection and AIDS. Am Psychol 1988;43:929–934.

116. Mail PD, Matheny SC. Social services for people with AIDS: Needs and approaches. AIDS 1989; 3(suppl. 1)S273–S277.

117. Levine C. In and out of the hospital. In: Gostlin LO, ed. AIDS and the health care system. New Haven: Yale University Press, 1990:45–61.

118. Centers for Disease Control. Update: Reducing HIV transmission in intravenous-drug users not in drug treatment—United States. MMWR 1990; 39:529–538.

119. Joseph SC. Combating IV drug use. In: Rogers DE, Ginzberg E, eds. The AIDS patient: An action agenda. Boulder: Westview Press, 1988: 78–83.

120. Gottlieb MS, Hutman S. The case for methadone. AIDS Patient Care 1990;4(Apr):15–18.

121. Winkelstein W, Samuel M, Padian NS. The San Francisco Men's Health Study: III. reduction in human immunodeficiency virus transmission among homosexual/bisexual men, 1982–1986. Am J Public Health 1987;77:685–689.

122. Newacheck PW, McManus MA, Brindis C. Financing health care for adolescents: Problems, prospects, and proposals. J Adolesc Health Care 1990;11:398–403.

123. Gerbert B, Maguire BT, Coates TJ. Are patients talking to their physicians about AIDS? Am J Public Health 1990;80:467–468.

124. Peterson JL, Marin G. Issues in prevention of AIDS among black and Hispanic men. Am Psychol 1988;43:871–877.

125. Brooks-Gunn J, Boyer CB, Hein K. Preventing HIV infection and AIDS in children and adolescents: Behavioral research and intervention strategies. Am Psychol 1988;43:958–964.

126. Kramer L. A "Manhattan Project" for AIDS. *The New York Times* 1990 Jul 16:15(col 1).

127. Dalton HL. AIDS in blackface. Daedalus. 1989; 118(3):205–227.

128. Mays VM, Cochran SD. Issues in the perception of AIDS risk and risk reduction activities by black and Hispanic/Latina Women. Am Psychol 1988;43:949–957.

129. Treichler PA. AIDS, gender and biomedical discourse: Current contests for meaning. In: Fee E, Fox DM, eds. AIDS: The burden of history. Berkeley: University of California Press, 1988: 190–266.

130. Keegan ME. Financing the AIDS epidemic in New York City: Past, present, future. In: Rogers DE, Ginzberg E, eds. The AIDS patient: An

action agenda. Boulder: Westview Press, 1988: 127–135.

131. Anonymous. AIDS strategic plan. Chicago, IL: Chicago Department of Health, 1989.

132. Weinberg DS, Murray HW. Coping with AIDS: The special problems of New York City. N Engl J Med 1987;317:1469–1473.

133. Kegeles SM, Coates TJ, Christopher TA, Lazarus JL. Perceptions of AIDS: The continuing saga of AIDS-related stigma. AIDS 1989;3(suppl.1): S253–258.

134. Cooke M, Koenig B, Beery N, Folkman S. Which physicians will provide AIDS care? VI Interna-tional Conference on AIDS, San Francisco, June, 1990 (abstract S.D.50)

135. Anonymous. Many plan to avoid AIDS care in practice. Internal Medicine News 1990;23(Aug): 1, 22.

136. Anastot K, Marte C. Women—The missing persons in the AIDS epidemic. Health/PAC Bull 1989;19(4):6–13 and 1990;20(1):11–18.

137. Blendon RJ. What should be done about the uninsured poor? JAMA 1988;260:3176–3177.

138. Himmelstein DU, Woolhandler S. A national health program for the United States: A physi-cians' proposal. N Engl J Med 1989;320:102–108.

10

Hospitalwide Surveillance Activities

Michael D. Decker, M.D., M.P.H., and
Mitzi W. Sprouse, R.N., C.P.Q.A.

A fundamental component of the concept of a learned profession is that the profession must ensure its own quality, as the performance of a professional can be evaluated properly only by another professional. The health of our patients and of our professions depends on the continued active participation of individual clinicians and their professional communities in the assessment and improvement of the quality of medical care (1).

In this chapter, we will provide a practical guide to the organization and operation of a comprehensive hospitalwide quality assessment (QA) program. This hospitalwide component can be augmented with the specialty-specific material presented in subsequent chapters in order to create a complete program appropriate to the local circumstances.

We will briefly recount the evolution of medical QA and then thoroughly review key aspects of current requirements. We will describe the new approaches to QA that are vigorously challenging the status quo and anticipate the changes they will bring. Finally, we will detail the organization of a hospitalwide QA program.

A QA program is expected to respond to the demands of many external organizations, of which two dominate: the Joint Commission on the Accreditation of Healthcare Organizations (JCAHO) and Medicare. In large measure, the history of medical QA is found in the history of these two entities.

THE PAST: HISTORICAL DEVELOPMENT
The Early Years

Organized attempts to assure the quality of health care provided in United States hospitals can be traced to the Third Clinical Congress of Surgeons of North America, which in 1912 resolved "that some system of standardization of hospital equipment and hospital work should be developed, to the end that those institutions having the highest ideals may have proper recognition before the profession, and that those of inferior equipment and standards should be stimulated to raise the quality of their work" (2).

A committee was formed under the leadership of Boston surgeon Dr. Ernest Codman to develop a program for hospital standardization, in order to improve both the quality of care provided to patients and the quality of training provided to neophyte surgeons. These efforts were intensified with the formation in 1913 of the American College of Surgeons and its adoption in 1914 of a requirement that each candidate for fellowship submit detailed reports of at least 50 major operations, a requirement that many found difficult to meet due to disorganized or nonexistent hospital medical records. In 1917 the College published the Minimum Standard (Table 10.1), which formed the basis for the voluntary Hospital Standardization Program launched in 1918.

The first surveys under this program were conducted by fellows of the College in 1919. The Hospital Review Committee met at a New York hotel to review the results from the first 692 large hospitals seeking accreditation, and found to their dismay that only 89 met the standards. Rather than subject the remaining 603 hospitals and medical staffs to the embarrassment that would accompany report of such findings, the Committee elected to consign all records and reports of the surveys to the hotel's furnace (3). Despite this shaky beginning, the accreditation program grew in impor-

tance and sophistication to the point that, in 1952, the College could no longer carry the burden alone and was joined by the American College of Physicians, the American Medical Association, the Canadian Medical Association, (since replaced by the American Dental Association), and the American Hospital Association in the formation of the Joint Commission.

Modern JCAHO standards date from the 1966 decision to devise standards that no longer defined the minimum considered essential, but rather the optimum achievable, and the appearance in 1969 of the first *Accreditation Manual for Hospitals (AMH)*, which placed further responsibility on the medical staff to "assist in promoting and maintaining high quality care" (4).

Government as Purchaser: New Demands

An important influence on the JCAHO and on QA in general has been the grow-

Table 10.1.
The Minimum Standard of 1917

1. That physicians and surgeons privileged to practice in the hospital be organized as a definite group or staff. Such organization has nothing to do with the question as to whether the hospital is "open" or "closed", nor need it affect the various existing types of staff organization. The word STAFF is here defined as the group of doctors who practice in the hospital inclusive of all groups such as the "regular staff", "the visiting staff", and the "associate staff".
2. That membership upon the staff be restricted to physicians and surgeons who are (a) full graduates of medicine in good standing and legally licensed to practice in their respective state or provinces, (b) competent in their respective fields, and (c) worthy in character and in matters of professional ethics; that in this latter connection the practice of the division of fees, under any guise whatever, be prohibited.
3. That the staff initiate and, with the approval of the governing board of the hospital, adopt rules, regulations, and policies governing the professional work of the hospital; that these rules, regulations and policies specifically provide:
   (a) That staff meetings be held at least once each month. (In large hospitals the departments may choose to meet separately.)
   (b) That the staff review and analyze at regular intervals their clinical experience in the various departments of the hospital, such as medicine, surgery, obstetrics, and the other specialties; the clinical records of patients, free and pay, to be the basis for such review and analyses.
4. That accurate and complete records be written for all patients and filed in an accessible manner in the hospital—a complete case record being one which includes identification data; complaint; personal and family history; history of present illness; physical examination; special examinations, such as consultations, clinical laboratory, X-ray and other examinations; provision or working diagnosis; medical or surgical treatment; gross and microscopical pathological finding; progress notes; final diagnosis; condition on discharge; follow-up and, in case of death, autopsy findings.
5. That diagnostic and therapeutic facilities under competent supervision be available for the study, diagnosis, and treatment of patients, these to include, at least (a) a clinical laboratory providing chemical, bacteriological, serological, and pathological services; (b) an X-ray department providing radiographic and fluoroscopic services.

ing role of government as purchaser and auditor of medical care services. When the Medicare program was established in 1965, the Conditions of Participation stipulated that any hospital accredited by the Joint Commission would be deemed to have met the Conditions. This "deemed status" provision made the program more acceptable to the profession by recognizing its historical role in assuring quality and by permitting JCAHO accreditation as an alternative to Federal inspection. In return, however, the government is able to profoundly influence the JCAHO through the threat of loss of deemed status.

Federal regulation soon followed federal dollars; in 1972, Congress mandated programs of utilization review and quality assessment. In response, new Joint Commission policies culminated in the 1975 Quality of Professional Services standard calling for retrospective quality audits (5). Experience showed, though, that audits often targeted topics of no great importance and generated meaningless statistics. Accordingly, in 1980 the Joint Commission devised a new quality assurance standard requiring a hospitalwide quality program with emphasis on areas where problem resolution was possible. However, Joint Commission surveys still noted only the existence of audit activity, with no regard to the quality, pertinence, or effect of the studies. The targeting of audits at areas of suspected problems had two conceptual failings: since a problem had to be suspected to be evaluated, unknown problems were unlikely to be identified; and since the focus was on resolvable problems rather than the important aspects of care, effort often was expended on minor issues. Most seriously, there was no clear requirement for the development or implementation of corrective measures based on the findings of the audits (6).

In 1985, the JCAHO responded to these concerns by requiring the ongoing and systematic monitoring, evaluation, and improvement of the quality and appropriateness of patient care (7). Although individual case review and the identification of aberrant cases remained important, an emphasis was placed on the identification of potentially problematic patterns or

trends of care. These requirements remain in effect.

THE PRESENT: KEY STANDARDS AND REQUIREMENTS, 1991–1992
JCAHO Monitoring and Evaluation Standards

The 1991 *AMH* encompasses 283 pages of standards (8); clearly, most will not be reviewed here. Guidance regarding many requirements is available in JCAHO publications (6, 9). However, a few concepts are so fundamental to satisfaction of JCAHO standards that they deserve a detailed presentation. Chief among these is the process known as "Monitoring and Evaluation."

Current and proposed JCAHO standards require a monitoring and evaluation process that should include:

1. Identifying important aspects of care,
2. Identifying indicators,
3. Collecting and organizing data,
4. Evaluating care, and
5. Taking corrective action.

The Joint Commission has promoted for several years a 10-step process for the accomplishment of the monitoring and evaluation function; the 10 steps are detailed in a preamble to standard QA.3 in editions of the *AMH* through 1991. However, contrary to the common impression, use of the 10-step process is not required; the standards require the components listed above, whether implemented in five steps or 15 steps. The 1992 *AMH* is expected to contain a revised QA preamble that will not include the 10-step process. Nonetheless, the 10-step process remains an excellent model for implementing the required monitoring and evaluation process; those who have explicitly implemented it certainly have no reason to change their procedures.

Monitoring and evaluation must be undertaken housewide, including both medical staff functions (Table 10.2) and hospital

Table 10.2.
Areas of Required Medical Staff Monitoring and Evaluation

Medical staff units or functions
  Each department, division, or clinical service
  Surgical/invasive procedure case review
  Drug usage (medication) evaluation
  Medical record review
  Blood/blood component usage review
  Pharmacy and therapeutics function
Hospitalwide
  Infection control
  Utilization review
  Safety
  Risk management (must link with rest of
    program)

Table 10.3.
Examples of Hospital Services within Which Monitoring and Evaluation Should Occur

Alcoholism and drug dependence
Anesthesia
Ambulatory care
Diagnostic radiology
Dietary
Emergency
Laboratory
Nuclear medicine
Nursing
Pathology
Pharmacy
Radiation oncology
Rehabilitation
Respiratory care
Social work
Special care units
Surgery

service functions (Table 10.3). Monitoring and evaluation for diagnostic radiology, nuclear medicine, pathology, the laboratory, anesthesia, and surgical services is often conducted as part of the appropriate medical staff departmental monitoring and evaluation.

With respect to medical staff departmental review, the organization must decide how it will subdivide itself for quality review purposes; monitoring and evaluation must be conducted within each subdivision. Large hospitals may choose to organize at the division level; intermediate hospitals, at the department level; and very small hospitals or those with a narrow focus, without subdivisions. The choice should correspond with the manner in which the medical staff is organized for purposes of credentialing privileges and holding monthly or quarterly meetings.

Identifying Important Aspects of Care

Within each organizational unit whose services are being monitored and evaluated, the staff must consider the care they provide and the procedures they perform and identify the most important aspects of that care; that is, those that pose the highest risk, are of the greatest volume, or are prone to problems, so that monitoring and evaluation can be focused on areas with the greatest potential impact on quality. Consideration should be given to whether care is provided when indicated, not provided when not indicated, and performed properly when provided.

Identifying Indicators

The organization is expected to develop "clinical indicators" to monitor aspects of care that it has identified as important. According to JCAHO, a clinical indicator is "a quantitative measure that can be used as a guide to monitor and evaluate the quality of important patient care and support service activities. An indicator is not a direct measure of quality. Rather, it is a screen or flag that identifies or directs attention to specific performance issues that should be the subject of more intense review" (10).

Types of Indicators. Indicators should be able to be expressed as rates of events. As always, the calculations of the rates will involve defining a time interval of surveillance, collecting the count of events of interest during the interval, and tabulating the total number of patients (or other pertinent item) at risk of appearing in the numerator during the interval. For some indicators the monitored event is expected to always occur (for example, recording of an admitting physical examination) or never occur (for example, postpartum maternal death); such indicators are termed *sentinel event indicators.* For indicators that do not monitor sentinel events, the rate is expected to fall between 0 and 100%; these indicators are termed *rate-based.*

An indicator measures a structure, process, or outcome of care (see Figure 10.1).

The concepts of structure, process, and outcome as determinants of quality of care were articulated by Avedis Donabedian in a series of influential papers and books first appearing in 1966 (11–13). *Structure* refers to the "relatively stable characteristics of the providers of care, of the tools and resources they have at their disposal, and of the physical and organizational settings in which they work" (12, p. 81). *Process* is "the set of activities that go on within and between practitioners and patients" (12, p. 79); it concerns itself with what is done to and for the patient. *Outcomes* are the end results of health care and were understood by Donabedian to include changes in patients' current and future physical, social, and psychological health attributable to prior health care as well as patient satisfaction and changes in knowledge and behavior. The availability of processes and the likelihood of their success without complications are influenced by institutional and organizational structure and by the availability of human and material resources. In turn, outcomes are influenced (often, determined) by the appropriateness and success of the processes by which medical care is delivered. Schematically, this relationship is: structure → process → outcome.

Structure.   Evaluations of structure are the most straightforward and formed the basis for the profession's earliest attempts at quality assurance; the Minimum Standard (Table 10.1) was almost exclusively concerned with structure. Theoreticians of quality have urged greater reliance on evaluation of process and outcome than structure. However, the JCAHO has been unable to convince the government to revise the conditions of participation (which were originally constructed from the then-existing Joint Commission standards) to reflect modern understandings of the determinants of quality (14). Nonetheless, some degree of structural standards remain desirable to ensure, at a minimum, the existence of an effective institutional governing body committed to the continuous improvement of quality and dedicating the authority and resources necessary to ensure institutional adherence to that commitment.

Process.   Process measurements are extremely attractive for a number of theoretical and practical reasons. By law and tradition, the physician's duty is to act in accord with the profession's current best understanding of medical science and art; process is under the control of the physician, whereas outcome is in the hands of God. Compared to outcomes, processes are readily observed and evaluated. Evaluations of processes are relatively easy to interpret and explain and can point directly to areas needing improvement. Process can be evaluated and modified at the level of the physician, the department, or the hospital. Almost invariably, steps taken to improve quality of care involve alterations in process. For these reasons, Donabedian considered process to be the "primary object of assessment" (12, p. 79). The vast majority of clinical quality indicators in current use are process measures ("blood pressure will be measured every five minutes during the procedure"; "every surgical procedure for excision of cancer will be supported by a pathologic specimen positive for malignancy").

Outcome.   Although the purpose of controlling quality of medical care is to influence outcome positively, evaluating that care solely by outcome measurements can be difficult and contentious. The difficulty arises in selecting an appropriate outcome to evaluate (death? disability? days lost from work? functional status? satisfaction?); devising a method to measure the outcome while controlling for biologic variability, confounding variables, and chance; and allocating the resources to collect and analyze the measure. Contention can be introduced by disagreements as to the meaning of an outcome (for example, even death may be viewed as a positive or negative outcome, depending on the circumstances) and by uncertainty as to the assignment of responsibility for an adverse outcome (a postoperative death might be the result of inappropriate referral for surgery, poorly performed surgery, unnecessarily prolonged surgery, inadequate postoperative care, and so on). Nonetheless, the point of medical care is the outcome, not the process, and appropriate, useful, and efficient measures of outcome should be sought and analyzed (15–17).

Figure 10.1.   Structure, process, and outcome.

Structural indicators may help assess whether the organization has the resources to provide quality care (example: "The head nurse on each unit shall be a registered nurse with at least five years experience."). Process indicators often incorporate standards of practice or care, either externally or internally developed (18) (examples: "An appropriate culture shall be obtained before initiating antibiotic therapy for a suspected postoperative wound infection involving drainage." "A cholecystectomy should be supported by the following clinical, radiologic, or historical indications (list)."). Outcome indicators typically measure the frequency of desired or undesired events following care (example: "The proportion of patients returned to OR within 24 hours following surgery.").

Attributes of Indicators. Indicators should be well defined and objective. It is desirable that they be sensitive, so that they will detect most cases in which quality problems exist, and specific, so that they flag few cases in which quality problems do not exist. Indicators should be valid; that is, they should detect circumstances that represent true quality problems. At least initially, few indicators will have been demonstrated in a research environment to be valid; lacking such demonstration, one relies on "face validity"—that is, the extent to which the measure appears to experienced viewers to be reasonable.

The Joint Commission offers a number of publications that contain examples of indicators and describe their development (6, 9, 10). However useful these may be, they remain examples; it is important that indicators be developed, selected, and/or modified by the staff of the individual institution and approved prior to use by the group whose activities they will be used to survey. For example, the above cholecystectomy indicator would be developed or approved by the division of general surgery; the wound infection culture indicator might be approved by the pharmacy and therapeutics committee or, perhaps, the infection control committee. Indicators should be developed by those knowledgeable in the pertinent clinical and quality assessment fields, rest

on the published literature, and be recognized as derived from authoritative sources (19).

Thresholds. Each indicator should be coupled with a criterion for triggering more intensive review, termed a threshold. For sentinel event indicators, of course, the threshold is crossed with any deviation from 0 or 100% (the choice depending on whether the event is supposed to never occur or always occur). For the more general types of rate-based indicators, thresholds may be derived in a variety of ways. Thresholds might be based on normative rates derived from the literature (for example, "25% of cardiac catheterizations demonstrate normal coronary anatomy"). Thresholds might be defined by statistical criteria either implicitly (example: "Class I wound infection rate > 2.0%") or explicitly (example: "Class I wound infection rate deviating more than two standard deviations above the mean"). Another illustration of a threshold would be the identification of a usual pattern (such as "More patient falls occur at night than the daytime.") which , when altered, triggers review ("But now, more patients fall in the day than the night on the weekends.").

How are thresholds set? They are set by consensus of the professional staffs responsible for the development and application of the indicator, based on the literature, the best clinical judgment of the involved parties, and most importantly, on an ongoing review of the results of surveillance. Thresholds need to be individualized to the indicator and the institution. Thresholds for rate-based indicators should neither be set so close to the mean that they trigger an inappropriate review due to meaningless fluctuations in the monitored rate, nor set so far from the mean that deviations highly unlikely to occur by chance alone fail to trigger appropriate review. As may be apparent, the development of indicators and thresholds is greatly benefitted by the participation of an experienced epidemiologist.

Indicators Do Not Define Quality. It must be clearly understood by all involved that an indicator is *not* a measure of quality. It is a monitoring and screening tool that can perform one or both of two functions. First, it can provide a numerical measure of performance that can be serially evaluated to detect patterns and trends in performance and, when indicated, trigger more intensive review (for example, surgical wound infection rate). Second, it can reduce the large volume of cases potentially available for review by screening out those unlikely to reveal a quality problem, leaving a smaller number of cases within which more intensive review has a higher likelihood of producing useful findings (for example, a surgical indications screening system). The fact that a case may have fallen out of such a screen produces no presumption of a quality problem; it merely selects the case as one in which more focused review may be useful. Most such cases will be found to represent acceptable care.

In a surgical indications screening system, for example, nurses performing preliminary review might be guided by criteria developed by the surgeons that call for every cholecystectomy to be supported by compatible symptoms and an imaging procedure demonstrating cholelithiasis. As cholecystectomy is generally considered indicated in a symptomatic patient with radiologically demonstrated gallstones, removing such cases from the pool presented for physician review preserves physician time with a negligible loss of sensitivity. Clearly, however, this indicator does not define a standard of care; many other appropriate indications for cholecystectomy exist, and it is entirely likely that all the remaining cases will be found to be equally appropriate when reviewed.

If these precepts are kept in mind, one can avoid the common tendency to try to incorporate into the indicators every rare or unusual possibility that could justify a particular intervention or component of care. Such efforts are self-defeating; if the indicators are defined so that cases rarely or never fall out for further review, then the system has failed.

Joint Commission Indicators. In 1988, the Joint Commission began developing clinical indicators for obstetrics and anesthesiology, which have now been published as an appendix to the 1991 *AMH* (8).

A total of nine indicator sets are planned for development; the next five, covering oncology, trauma, cardiovascular care, infection control, and medication use, are undergoing testing. The 1992 *AMH* scoring guidelines are expected to require that the organization document that it has reviewed the JCAHO indicators and considered their use, and may in fact require use of the obstetrics indicators (20).

Collecting and Organizing Data

In order to collect and organize the data needed for quality assessment, five questions need to be addressed. Where are the data located? How are they collected? Are they collected in their entirety or by sample? How often are they collected? Once collected, how are they compared with the thresholds that have been set; that is, how are they analyzed?

Data Sources. The indicator itself will substantially define the range of data sources capable of providing the data. Existing data sources to consider include patient charts, indices and tabulations maintained by medical records departments, emergency room records, laboratory reports, medication sheets, pharmacy records, respiratory care department records, nursing flow sheets, surgical logs, incident reports, customer satisfaction surveys or complaints, and so on (21). Data may also be collected directly for the purpose of the indicator, rather than harvested from other records. The decision as to who will collect the data is complex and must be made by those responsible for the monitoring and evaluation function being performed and, especially, those who will be responsible for analysis of the data. Some data may be sufficiently unambiguous that clerical staff can collect them; others may require trained abstractors or clinically astute professionals. Regardless, it is essential that the data collection be reliable and conducted with appropriate safeguards for confidentiality. It is prudent to perform periodic audits of the data collection process to assure the accuracy and validity of data collected.

Automated Data Collection. Information is a precious institutional asset and not to be wasted; systems must be organized so that data, once collected, are available to all appropriate users. However, in most hospitals evaluation of the indicator "unplanned return to surgery" would require labor-intensive methods to collect instances of such returns and generate counts of all surgical cases that could have returned to surgery in order to calculate rates. But in virtually every hospital, the billing computer carefully records each patient's use of the operating room (OR) and each procedure performed. Why not simply generate for further evaluation a periodic report by division, physician, and/or procedure, listing salient facts concerning each patient having a second OR visit within a predefined period following a prior visit, along with a count of all patients having surgery during the surveillance period (again, by division, physician, and/or procedure)? Alas, although conceptually simple, in most hospitals such efficiency is only a dream. Almost universally, hospital information systems departments are unequipped for (and usually uninterested in) providing direct electronic transfer of data from existing computer records in a manner that permits their use for quality assessment purposes.

This inefficiency is intolerable. Hospital information systems managers must recognize that providing the data necessary for assuring and improving the quality of medical care is a function no less important than is providing the data necessary for billing. Indeed, the need for numerical data and statistical evaluation in quality assessment programs will increase dramatically in the next few years, increasing the demand for electronic data management. Fortunately, the Joint Commission has recognized the essential role sophisticated data management will play in the future of quality assessment activities and is preparing standards and supporting materials designed to help hospitals and their information systems departments to move in the needed direction.

Sampling. The JCAHO recognizes that sampling is an appropriate way to monitor common elements of care, permitting finite resources to be allocated so as to broaden the scope of monitoring rather than monitoring intensively only a few indicators. For example, if hundreds of cholecystectomies are performed annually, it may be appropriate to review a 10 or 20% sample, stratified by surgeon to ensure that even infrequent operators receive some minimal level of monitoring. Understandably, sampling is considered inappropriate for rare procedures or for rare but serious complications, which might fail to be included in the sample. Future standards are expected to ease existing restrictions and further support epidemiologically sound sampling schemes.

Frequency of Data Collection. It is neither necessary nor possible to monitor all conceivable indicators at all times. Some aspects of care will be considered so critical to quality (highest risk, known problem areas, and so on) that they warrant continuous monitoring; most will merit periodic monitoring, at an interval and according to a sequence that assures balanced and appropriate surveillance, while some may be monitored once and then not again for an indefinite period. Such judgments are properly the province of the professional staff, based on the institution's individual needs, the volume of various services, and any history of identified or potential problem areas.

For indicators undergoing continual monitoring, a second question concerns the length of the collect/evaluate cycle. Are data tabulated and analyzed daily, weekly, monthly, quarterly, or annually? For rate-based data, the averaging period should be chosen in light of the volume and stability of the data, so that the interval is neither so brief that random fluctuation dominates the pattern nor so long that important problems are not detected in a timely manner. The averaging period used to aggregate the data for the purpose of calculating periodic means and standard deviations will not necessarily correlate with the frequency of meeting of the body reviewing the data. For example, the infection control committee might meet quarterly, yet be presented with monthly rates to review.

Organization of Data. As indicated previously, there is growing emphasis by JCAHO and others on devising indicators that can be expressed numerically as rates of events and then establishing thresholds to trigger more intensive evaluation of care. Readers of this volume are likely to be quite familiar with these concepts and with the methods of statistical analysis that permit discrimination between fluctuations likely to represent chance variation and those likely to represent true differences.

It is important to display findings in a manner that permits the evaluators to see the pertinent results and to understand the patterns present. The clinicians who will be asked to review the surveillance data and evaluate possible quality problems will have little patience for data that are complex, poorly organized, and inconsistent from meeting to meeting. For rate-based indicators, graphical displays can prove valuable. A standardized case summary form prepared by the reviewing nurse may facilitate subsequent physician review for sentinel indicators or for the case review required when a rate-based indicator has crossed its threshold.

Evaluating Care

Once the accumulated data reach the defined threshold for more intensive review, staff members with appropriate clinical expertise should evaluate the care to determine if a problem exists. This evaluation may involve a more detailed review of the individual case, consideration of patterns of care by (for example) unit, shift, practitioner, patient group, procedure, diagnosis, and so on, and consideration of historical patterns or trends within any such subgroups. This more intensive review may be conducted by designated physicians, by a committee, or by trained QA staff. Once more intensive review is triggered, however, the process generally would be expected to result in formal presentation of the findings to a QA committee or other entity responsible for the monitoring and evaluation process.

Beginning with the 1992 *AMH*, the Joint Commission will increasingly stress the importance of looking for explanations for variation in care not only in the independent actions of individuals, but also (and preferably, first) in the constraints and effects of the systems within which the individuals operate. Such systems problems might include barriers to effective communication, poor staffing levels or inappropriate assignments, inventory or equipment problems, problems in policies and procedures, defects in organizational structure, and so on.

Questions of individual performance will invariably require more focused investigation, the nature of which will depend on the specific circumstances. All findings of quality problems relating to individual performance must ultimately rest on peer review, often (though not always) involving review of individual charts. Chart review is a laborious process that can rapidly consume the time and good will of the physician reviewers. Careful attention to the devising of indicators and setting of thresholds can pay great dividends by permitting QA staff to screen out those cases unlikely to benefit from physician review, thereby ensuring that the time of busy clinicians is most productively used.

If the accumulating data do not reach the defined thresholds for further evaluation, or if further evaluation is indicated but, when performed, fails to identify any quality problem, then the monitoring and evaluation process should continue according to the overall plan established. However, if evaluation identified a quality problem (or opportunity for quality improvement), then action needs to be taken.

Taking Action

The group responsible for the monitoring and evaluation process (division staff, committee members, etc.) must decide on a plan of corrective action if a quality problem is identified. The plan should specify the problem identified and the change desired, the action(s) felt appropriate in response to the problem, the person or group responsible for implementing and overseeing the action, and the time frame in which the action should occur. The process may be iterative; for example, an initial intervention may be designed to gather more data or may reveal a new aspect to the problem that results in a new plan of action. The action plan might incorporate components designed to correct knowledge deficiencies among one or all staff members, to address behavior or judgment problems, or to address systems problems that are preventing individuals from performing at their highest level.

Once action is taken, monitoring and evaluation must proceed in order to evaluate the effects of the action. This cycle should continue until the problem is solved or the desired improvement accomplished, justifying a decision to forego further action and, perhaps, to redirect monitoring and evaluation efforts at other indicators.

It is vital that the results of the process (conclusions, recommendations, and actions) be communicated to all appropriate groups and individuals. This will enhance the ability of others to identify and respond to similar situations or to detect problems that involve more than one division or service area. In addition, pertinent results must be shared with those responsible for performance evaluation, credentialing, and so on.

1992 Revisions to JCAHO QA Standards

The Joint Commission expects to replace the existing Quality Assurance standard with an entirely new chapter in the 1994 *AMH* (22). It is likely that the QA chapter in the 1992 *AMH* will foreshadow a number of the changes planned for 1994, beginning with a change in chapter title from "Quality Assurance" to "Quality Assessment and Improvement" (QA&I). This name change manifests the concept that quality is not a static goal whose accomplishment one can assure, but rather, a process of continuous assessment and improvement.

The QA processes defined in earlier versions of the *AMH* focus on the identification of "problems"; if no problem were identified, then implicitly, no change was necessary. For several reasons, this has been an unsatisfying approach. First, the absence of a "problem" (transient worsening) does not imply that the "normal" (baseline) performance is acceptable; a hospital or a practitioner might be providing consistently awful care. Second, the

state of the art constantly advances; the best hospital of 1970, absent continuous improvement, might be the worst hospital in 2000. Just as medicine itself seeks continuous improvement, so must those who guide and monitor the processes by which medical care is delivered.

The existing preamble to *AMH* standard QA.3, which now concerns itself with monitoring and evaluation and the 10-step plan, will note the necessity for management to be trained for and active in quality improvement activities and will introduce a shift from the current *AMH*'s departmental orientation to one based on key patient care functions. The preamble will emphasize that the ability of individuals to deliver quality care is substantially determined by the available systems and processes, and that improvements in care often depend upon improvements in those processes.

Most of the QA&I standards in the 1992 *AMH* will be substantially similar to the QA standards of prior years. However, it is planned that the chapter will lead off with an entirely new standard concerned with the involvement of the organization's leaders (governing board, top management, medical staff leaders, clinical chiefs, senior nursing personnel, department heads, and so on) in the development and implementation of procedures to assess and improve quality (22). These leaders will be expected to obtain personal training in the concepts and techniques of continuous quality improvement; to set priorities and allocate adequate time, personnel, and information systems resources for assessment and improvement activities; to assure the training of staff in assessing and improving quality; and to evaluate their own performance in accomplishing these objectives. It is expected that the first of these requirements (personal training) will be a surveyed standard in 1992, with the remainder phased in thereafter.

Utilization Review

We will conclude our review of current JCAHO standards with a brief mention of the utilization review (UR) standard, which requires the hospital to monitor the appropriate allocation of its resources through a written plan that includes a focus on known or suspected UR problems and an early and active discharge planning process. There should be written criteria and length of stay norms that are specific to diagnoses, problems, or procedures and that are approved by the medical staff. The UR program should avail itself of pertinent findings of the QA program and is one of the hospitalwide components for which monitoring and evaluation is required.

In our opinion, such a UR program is an inherent component of, and should be completely integrated with, a comprehensive QA program. In this regard, it is pertinent that Medicare considers many "UR issues" to be quality issues; for example, failure to provide appropriate discharge planning services is a Level 1 quality problem.

A separate consideration, however, is the burgeoning demand by third-party payers for detailed data to support preadmission certification and subsequent recertification. Collection and telephonic reporting of these data are increasingly burdensome tasks that can consume personnel resources while making a negligible contribution to the quality of care or the proper utilization of resources. In response, some institutions are refusing to provide recertification data more often than a minimum interval, are charging a flat fee for each recertification interaction, or taking other steps to respond to those private payer activities that smack of cost containment through harassment (23). The most promising approach to such problems would appear to be regional negotiations between hospital associations and major payers to reach accord on standard intervals and methods for precertification and recertification, so that the legitimate interests of the payers are protected while repetitive, wasteful effort is reduced for both parties.

Medicare

The Health Care Financing Administration (HCFA) acts to enforce the requirements of the various federal legislative acts defining and regulating the Medicare program through its contracted Peer Review Organizations (PROs) and fiscal intermediaries. The PROs are to act to ensure the necessity of care, the appropriateness of care, and the quality of care through review of admissions, outliers, and invasive procedures, validation of diagnosis-related groups (DRGs), and quality reviews. Quality review objectives include reductions in unnecessary readmissions, invasive procedures, complications and deaths, and verification that all necessary services are provided.

HCFA's most recent (1989) mandate to the PROs provided for review of 3% of all discharges, 50% of all transfers, 25% of all readmissions within 30 days (including, for 20%, any intervening care), 100% of cases in DRGs 468 (unrelated OR procedure), 474 (tracheostomy), and 475 (mechanical ventilation with endotracheal tube), 25% each of day and cost outliers, and 5% of ambulatory surgeries.

The review process involves the application by nurse reviewers of "generic screens," so called because they are not specific to the diagnosis, procedure, or DRG in question but apply generally. The current inpatient generic screens review for the adequacy of discharge planning; stability of the patient at discharge with respect to blood pressure, pulse, or temperature; abnormal diagnostic results that are not adequately addressed; IV therapy on day of discharge; purulent or bloody drainage within 24 hours of discharge; postoperative death; death following return within 24 hours to a special care unit; unexpected death; hospital-acquired infection (this screen was withdrawn after reevaluation by HCFA in 1991 (24)); unscheduled return to surgery; unplanned surgery; fall; complications or errors of anesthesia, medication, or transfusion; decubitus ulcer acquired or worsened in hospital; or care/lack of care resulting in potentially serious complications. Generic screens for ambulatory surgery are similar in concept and focus on the adequacy of preoperative assessment, adequacy of response to problems, adequacy of postoperative care, and documented discharge planning including adequacy of patient education.

Incidents discovered by the generic screens are categorized into one of three severity levels: no potential for significant adverse effects (level 1), potential for significant adverse effects (level 2), or significant adverse effects (level 3). A scale of interventions determines the PRO's response, based on awarding the following scores for each confirmed quality problem: level 1, 1 point; level 2, 5 points; level 3, 25 points. Interventions begin with as few as 3 points in a quarter, and a single level 3 event (25 points) triggers consideration of sanctions.

One can have no complaint with HCFA's generic screens; they encompass issues properly of interest to any competent QA program. However, the punitive orientation, lack of uniform standards (25, 26), and the significant latitude for subjective interpretation are justifiable concerns for the hospital. Clearly, it is essential that the hospital's QA program be alert to issues considered pertinent by HCFA. We shall discuss turning the PRO's activities to the advantage of the hospital QA program later in this chapter.

THE FUTURE: 1993 AND BEYOND

The first era of medical quality assurance in the United States, from the early 1900s through the end of the 1960s, was typified by the Minimum Standard: simple, predominantly structural standards that helped to assure that hospitals were capable of providing quality care. The second era, incorporating the 1970s and 1980s, has been marked by the proliferation of complex standards stimulated at least as much by the government, other insurers, and industry as by the medical profession. The third era is now beginning, and over the next 5–10 years there likely will be considerable change in our approach to, and understanding of, QA. Why? What's wrong with the current system?

In the second era, quality was viewed as a static goal satisfied by meeting defined minimum standards. If no problem was found, no action was indicated. Such an approach is not commensurate with the remarkable and continuous improvement throughout the century in the science of

medicine or with the traditional dedication among individual physicians to continual personal improvement (which existed long before requirements to document continuing medical education).

Moreover, when a standard was not met, the first order of business often seemed to be to identify a person or organization to blame and punish. In addition, the focus was predominantly on the performance of physicians, with little attention paid to the contributions of other participants in the process or to the organization of the process itself. The concept of quality of care was narrowly restricted to technical patient outcomes; there was little concern for patient satisfaction or responsiveness to the legitimate needs of other parties such as families, employers, or other health care providers.

There is an alternative approach to attaining quality that has been extensively developed over the past 50 years and whose use is widespread. This alternative approach is generally termed the model of *continuous quality improvement*.

Continuous Quality Improvement

Statistical Process Control

Continuous quality improvement (CQI; also known as total quality management, total quality control, or industrial quality control), a general model for quality in any organized activity, is based on concepts developed in the 1930s by Dr. Walter A. Shewhart, a statistician at Western Electric (Bell Laboratories), and refined by physicist Dr. W. Edwards Deming and engineer Dr. Joseph M. Juran. The fundamental concept of statistical process control (SPC) developed by Shewhart was that the limits of random variation in any task or product could be charted and control limits established. Processes that remained within their control limits were under control and could be allowed to continue uninterrupted. Processes that transgressed their control limits were out of statistical control, and adjustments were needed to return the process to control. The workers themselves could make the needed measurements and maintain the control charts, giving them more meaningful responsibility for, and personal investment in, the quality of product and permitting the rapid detection and correction of unacceptable variation. Two types of variation were described: that due to *assignable* or *special* causes, marked by an acute deviation of the measurement outside its control limits (or a run of measurements progressively deviating from the mean); and *common* causes, which are the effects of chance variation and the inherent design of the system. The elimination of special causes of variation is the primary responsibility of those operating the processes, who detect the variation and study its causes in order to find and correct the source of variation (equipment out of adjustment, deviation from policy, etc.). The improvement of common causes of variation is the responsibility of management, as the workers are constrained to operate within the processes handed them by management and cannot independently affect the common causes.

As an example, consider a control chart representing the monthly clean surgical wound infection rate; the selected control limits have been placed 2 standard deviations from the mean. Imagine that a persistent violation of the upper control limit is noted in the spring of 1991. A cause is sought, and it is discovered that preoperative antibiotics are being given too soon, resulting in suboptimal antibiotic blood levels during surgery. Once the problem is corrected, the rate declines.

Apart from the springtime deviation, the monthly rate fluctuates within the control limits. These month-to-month variations represent chance events, not correctable sources of variation. The long-term mean is determined by common causes of variation and, if it is to be improved, requires improvements by management (which might mean the physicians, the administration, or medical science) in the underlying determinants of wound infections (choice and use of prophylaxis, patient preparation, surgical scrub techniques, methods of cautery and closing, and so on).

The key concept of SPC is that, through the control chart, the process itself is speaking to its operators and alerting them to any unacceptable deviation. Traditional postproduction inspection is unnecessary and, indeed, is viewed as a wasteful technique for most processes. Quality should be designed into the process, rather than having failures inspected out at the end; one cannot inspect quality into a product. When inspection finds a defective product, the defectives can be discarded (scrap waste) or redone (rework waste); improved process quality eliminates both forms of quality waste, permitting improved quality at lower cost. Even the overhead of inspection is reduced, as SPC techniques permit a random sample to be measured, allowing sensitive detection of loss of process control while conserving resources.

Adoption of CQI

In the late 1930s, Deming was charged with developing the statistical sampling program for the 1940 United States Census. During the same period, he demonstrated that SPC could be applied to clerical and service operations as well as industrial operations. With the outbreak of war, he was asked to teach the techniques of SPC to key staff at war industries; some 31,000 engineers and inspectors were trained. After the war, undamaged American industry produced a flood of goods for the eager consumers of the world; quality was of little importance in such a seller's market, with European and Japanese industry devastated, and by 1950 all the companies that had adopted SPC during wartime abandoned it as unnecessary.

Deming was detailed to Japan in 1947 by the United States government to assist in organizing a census. While there, he was asked by the Japanese Union of Scientists and Engineers to teach them how to produce quality goods. His influence was so rapid and profound that in 1951 the Japanese established the Deming Prize, awarded annually for outstanding implementation of CQI. Juran also began to consult with the Japanese during the 1950s and contributed an emphasis on organizing for quality that, combined with Deming's statistical and management teachings, revolutionized industry.

Many readers can recall the early 1950s,

when the label "Made in Japan" was a joke—a sign of a cheap product of poor quality. Many can recall the event that perhaps most profoundly altered that impression: the marketing of the first pocket transistor radio, produced by an unknown little company called Sony. Within a decade, Japanese production quality was universally respected; within another decade, United States industries and their inferior products were being driven from the marketplace. In 1979, Xerox engineers visiting Japan found copiers being produced at half of Xerox's cost, with one-thirtieth the defects (27). Today no United States manufacturer produces videocassette recorders or single lens reflex cameras; only one still produces televisions.

These events finally prompted American industry to rediscover and embrace the teachings of Deming, Juran, Philip Crosby, and other exponents of CQI. The precepts of CQI are now widely accepted in United States industry and have had profound results (consider, for example, the remarkable resurgence of Ford Motors in the 1980s). In 1987, Congress established the United States equivalent of the Deming Prize, the Malcolm Baldrige National Quality Award (Xerox, having learned its lesson well, won the Baldrige award in 1990). Health care may well be the largest United States industry that has not yet implemented CQI (27, 28); to stimulate and recognize such activity, the Commerce Department is currently considering establishing a specific Baldrige Award category for hospitals and other health care organizations (29).

Management Concepts

Although CQI rests on the ongoing objective data provided by the techniques of statistical process control, it is a complete management method that incorporates a number of distinct differences from past practices. The most crucial concept is that quality is defined as "a continuous effort by all members of the organization to meet the needs and expectations of the customer" (28). The concept of customer is deliberately broad; it includes not only the external end purchaser but also all persons or entities, internal or external, who de-

pend on the efforts or outputs of workers within the organization. "A customer is any organization or individual who makes quality judgments about, or has expectations regarding, an output" (30, p. 10). (When applied to health care, it might be best to refer to "patients and other customers," to emphasize that the term "customer" is not intended as a deprofessionalizing substitute for "patient," but rather is intended to explicitly acknowledge the dependence of each group of health care workers on the efforts of others and on the processes within which they work. For example, it is reasonably evident that physicians are customers of the pharmacy and the laboratory. It is less obvious that the laboratory and pharmacy are also customers of the physicians; but in order to produce their outputs, they depend on inputs from the physician and cannot begin their tasks until those inputs (orders) are properly produced (legible) and delivered.

Quality must flow from the top down, in the sense that top management must set an unwavering commitment to the continuous improvement of quality, understand how to pursue quality, and ensure that the enterprise is organized for quality. Management must recognize that it alone controls the important aspects of quality through its control of organization and processes. Processes, not individuals, are the focus of CQI: ". . . health care professionals are already deeply committed to the highest-quality work. Quality depends more on good system design, consistent long-term direction, adequate training, leadership, and follow-up—all management functions—than on individual motivation" (30, p. 7). Failures to achieve quality are generally not due to the personal failures of employees, but rather to the failures and shortcomings of the processes those employees must function within.

It is a precept of CQI that workers at all levels want to perform to the best of their ability and with rare exception will do so when given the appropriate support. "Physicians . . . and health care workers . . . must be assumed to be trying hard, acting in good faith, and not willfully failing to do what they know to be correct. When they are caught in complex systems and performing complex tasks, of course clinicians make mistakes; these are unintentional, and the people involved cannot be frightened into doing better" (27). On the other hand, every worker must be dedicated to quality and trained in achieving quality. All workers in the organization must "understand the same quality terms, speak the same quality language, and share the same quality vision" (30, p. 39). The best way to improve performance is to imbue in the employee a sense of ownership in and responsibility for the success of the enterprise. Management systems that set arbitrary objectives, that do not encourage worker involvement in process improvement, and, worse, that reward based on factors beyond the control of the worker (such as common-source variation) are anathema.

Applying the Principles

The pursuit of quality involves a continuous process of evaluating performance in order to identify opportunities to improve, a philosophy the Japanese call *kaizen* and whose spirit is captured in their concept that "every defect is a treasure"; that is, every identified defect is another opportunity to improve (31). How are the defects identified and the processes improved? In the broadest terms, special causes of variation are first sought, identified, and eliminated. Once the process is in control and consistently producing output of the highest quality possible with the existing process, effort can be directed at the more difficult task of improving the process itself so that common-cause variation is reduced.

First, find a process to evaluate and improve. Second, organize a team that is intimately familiar with the process and contains persons who perform the process, that understands the principles of CQI and SPC, and that has the authority (or access to authority) to implement change. The team then analyzes the process to identify its inputs, outputs, customers, and the intermediate steps in the process. The expectations of all identified classes of customers are explicitly measured (surveyed), to avoid perpetuating errors of

assumption (Detroit *knew* that Americans cared more about chrome and tail fins than reliability and mileage). The process and all internal subprocesses are documented; flow charts are often helpful in order to schematically reveal the interrelations of complex processes. Key process factors are identified; these are process steps that causally determine whether an output will meet quality expectations (30, p. 27). Specifications are generated that permit objective measurements of key output features and process steps and that reflect customer expectations (18). As understanding of the process improves or customer desires change, specifications should be adjusted. Measurements are then obtained, and the techniques of SPC are used to eliminate inappropriate variation. (Note that indicators with thresholds, as defined by the JCAHO, are *not* necessarily the same as specifications. Unlike thresholds, specifications contain no arbitrary level of acceptable performance. For example, an indicator with threshold might be "clean surgical wound infection rate of 2% or less." The comparable CQI specification might be, "the patient experiences no surgical wound infection.")

Once the process is stable (in statistical control), efforts can begin to reduce common cause variation—that is, to improve the process itself to establish new standards of quality. In the 1930s, Shewhart described a plan for the improvement of a stable process or the investigation of special causes in a process out of control (32, p. 88; 33, p. 5). This Shewhart Cycle is also known as the Plan—Do—Check—Act or PDCA cycle for its four components: *plan* a change or test; carry out (*do*) the change or test; *check* the effects of the change or test; study the results and *act* to adopt or modify the change or test. The cycle continues until no further improvement can be obtained.

The Hospital Corporation of America has popularized an acronym to describe and teach CQI: FOCUS-PDCA (30, p. 33; 34). By this, they mean:

Find a process to improve;
Organize a team that knows the process;
Clarify current knowledge of the process (PDCA);

Understand causes of process variation (PDCA);
Select the process improvement; then Plan—Do—Check—Act.

Practitioners of CQI have developed or emphasized a number of graphical tools that facilitate the FOCUS-PDCA cycle. Flow charts can be invaluable for displaying the inputs, sequences, functional relationships, subprocesses, and outputs in any complex process. Another useful graphic tool is the Ishikawa or "fishbone" cause-and-effect diagram (35). Ishikawa diagrams can be useful for stimulating and focusing thought, demonstrating the level of understanding, and identifying areas for data collection.

Special Considerations in Applying CQI to Health Care

The techniques of statistical process control and continuous quality improvement initially were developed for use in manufacturing industries. However, CQI and SPC are considered to be general systems of project management, applicable to any organized endeavor. The application of CQI and SPC to health care does, however, involve a number of unique considerations.

First, institutions responsible for delivering health care range from small, rural hospitals or clinics to university medical centers. The complex organizational structures and multiple missions of the latter can pose a considerable challenge for hospital management wishing to introduce a new approach, particularly in light of the medical center's organization into somewhat autonomous academic divisions whose chiefs are selected and retained based predominantly on factors unrelated to the administration of their hospital services. Clearly, no one model of CQI will fit this entire spectrum of organizations; nonetheless, the principles have been successfully applied throughout the spectrum (31, 36–38).

Another barrier to implementation of CQI and SPC in health care is the terminology; not only is it unfamiliar to health care workers, but some of it may arouse hostility because it appears to echo phrases used by those who wish to deprofessionalize medicine. Such a concern is unfounded; indeed, the precepts of CQI are quite congenial to the universal desire of clinicians that their professionalism, dedication to the highest level of care, and devotion to their patients be recognized. Clinicians are likely to be receptive to the CQI principles that the ability of even the most conscientious clinician to deliver quality care is constrained by the performance of the systems within which the clinician must operate, that the pursuit of quality involves the continuous improvement of those systems so that clinicians can deliver the very best care, and that problems are more often due to defects in systems than in people.

Another consideration is the unique role of the patient in health care. The organization exists to serve the patient's needs; but unlike the situation in other industries, the primary customer, the patient, is rarely the purchaser of the services, and rarely is an appropriate judge of the quality of the services. The first issue is easily managed by keeping in mind CQI's broad definition of customer: the patient is the primary customer, but third party payers also are customers (as are the employer, the family, and many others external to the hospital). The second issue is managed by differentiating "content quality" from "delivery quality." In industry, content quality refers to whether the product meets the customer's expectations; in medicine, it is understood to refer to the technical component of medical care. The content quality of medical care cannot be evaluated properly by the patient; it must be evaluated by the professional staff. Remember that "a customer is any organization or individual who makes quality judgments about, or has expectations regarding, an output" (30, p. 10). Because of the unique characteristics of a profession, the profession itself is a customer of each of its members; the content quality of a professional's work is evaluated by the profession. Delivery quality, on the other hand, refers to the organization's interaction with the customer in delivering the output. Patients can independently evaluate delivery quality; for example, the cardiac bypass patient may not be qualified to critique the choice of graft, but surely can judge the clarity of education regarding convalescence or the courtesy of the staff (39).

A further consideration involves the unique role of the physician in health care. In the industrial model of CQI, the worker works within processes designed and organized by management. In health care, the physician, neither an employee nor management, takes on the characteristics of each. In some respects the physician, like the factory worker, is entirely constrained to work within the processes provided by hospital management (laboratory support, nursing support, equipment availability, etc.). However, the physician's broad control over the diagnostic and therapeutic processes and exceptional discretion to select from available processes are generally outside the experience of industrial CQI. For these reasons, applications of CQI to health care stress the key role of the profession in evaluating the content quality of each professional's work and include explicit mechanisms for managing unacceptable variation attributable to the individual physician.

Within industry, there generally is a single corporate leadership that, once committed to CQI, can ensure the adoption of CQI throughout the organization. Successful adoption of CQI in health care usually requires the coordinated action of two leadership structures that do not always agree on tactics or goals: the hospital administration and the medical staff. Although one group or the other may be more involved in driving the process to implement CQI, both must be willing participants if the effort is to succeed. Fortunately, there are a number of factors that will promote the needed cooperation.

CQI offers the hospital the opportunity to improve its reputation, enhance its competitive position, obtain greater understanding and control of its key internal processes, reduce costs, and increase employee satisfaction. CQI offers the medical staff the opportunity to participate in the evaluation and improvement of key internal hospital processes on which the physi-

cians depend to accomplish their tasks. CQI explicitly reorients the hospital away from a "find the bad apple" approach to QA, toward a process that assumes (until proven otherwise) that quality failures are process failures, not personal failures. With its recognition that the profession itself is the principle knowledgeable customer of, and thus evaluator of, the content quality of medical care, CQI appropriately ensures the profession's continued leadership role in the evaluation of its own performance. In addition to these intrinsic attractions of CQI for the medical staff and administration, there will be external incentives for adoption of CQI (40), the most compelling being the progressive revision of JCAHO standards in accord with the concepts of CQI (41, 42).

The Joint Commission and CQI

Agenda for Change

Many readers are familiar with the "Agenda for Change" that the JCAHO announced in 1986, intended to move accreditation from the question *"can* the organization provide quality care" to *"does* the organization provide quality care." The objectives of the Agenda for Change were to reduce the number and complexity of standards, refocus the standards on key functions, promote continual improvement, stimulate development of performance indicators related to key functions, develop methods for data collection and establish a national comparative database, and improve the survey process to support these goals (41). The JCAHO has stated that the "philosophical context for the Agenda for Change is set by the theories of Continual Quality Improvement. . . ." (42). In order to implement this agenda, the JCAHO has convened many expert panels to review current standards, suggest new approaches, and develop the necessary tools (clinical indicators, data management, and analysis schemes, etc.).

Initial Implementation

The results of some of these efforts are now, or soon will be, apparent. Clinical indicators are in various stages of development and implementation. Clinical indicators for infection control, medication use, cardiovascular care, trauma, and oncology are in various stages of development. The 1991 *AMH* contains a new nursing care chapter, which has been extensively revised to emphasize leadership responsibility and an orientation toward processes (termed "key functions" by the JCAHO) rather than structures (8). The 1992 *AMH* will begin the QA&I chapter with the new leadership responsibility standards (22). The 1993 *AMH* is expected to be considerably more lean than the current manual, as efforts continue to rid the manual of a structural orientation and to eliminate standards that are redundant or of marginal relevance to patient care (22, 43). The 1993 *AMH* is likely to contain as appendices the most prominent of the changes expected for 1994, including the completely revised QA&I chapter; some of these changes may, indeed, be implemented in 1993.

1994 *AMH*

The Joint Commission expects that most of the changes set in place by the Agenda for Change will appear together for the first time in the 1994 *AMH* (22). The *AMH* will be considerably reduced in size and will be organized by key functions, rather than by departments. It is expected to present a coherent, integrated vision of CQI that will contain, in the form of standards, the expectations expressed in the "Principles of Organizational and Management Effectiveness" promulgated in 1989:

Total organizational commitment to continuously improve the quality of patient care is the central concern. . . . This commitment is woven throughout the fabric of the organization, appearing in strategic planning, allocation of resources, role expectations, reward structures, (and) performance evaluations. . . . An ongoing, comprehensive self-assessment system supports and promotes continuous improvement. (44)

In the fall of 1988, the JCAHO formed a Quality Improvement Task Force to de-

velop new standards, which are expected to take effect in the 1994 *AMH* (45). Based on work to date, the 1994 QA&I standards are expected to cover five distinct areas. The first consists of the leadership standards that will appear in the 1992 *AMH*. The second area includes the techniques of CQI, including ongoing monitoring, surveying of customers, setting of priorities, assessment and improvement of processes, and the assignment of responsibility for CQI.

The third area given attention will be education and training. The organization will be expected to educate personnel in the techniques of CQI, specifically including the developing of measures, collection of data, performing of analyses, evaluation of processes, and development of conclusions and proposals for change. Continuing education, using internal and external resources, should be provided and guided by evaluation of needs. In addition, personnel should be educated regarding the ways in which patients from other cultural backgrounds might have differing health care expectations, values, and goals than do the workers.

The organization will be expected to provide two types of information support: reference literature, and database management. The traditional requirement for a medical library will be extended to include literature pertinent to CQI, management, and medical ethics. In addition, the organization will be expected to maintain or have access to a database that describes the hospital's own performance and that of comparable institutions, and to make use of the data to evaluate and improve its processes.

The remaining areas of attention involve the existence of mechanisms to ensure appropriate communication and collaboration between various individuals and components of the institution, and the ongoing evaluation of the effectiveness of CQI activities.

To those only familiar with traditional medical quality assurance activities, accreditation standards based upon modern theories of CQI may represent a change so dramatic as to be shocking. However, the JCAHO has been actively publicizing since

1987 its intent to promote a more pertinent and effective program for quality assessment and improvement and its plans for the complete reorganization of the accreditation process. Some changes are already in effect; most will be evident no later than the 1994 *AMH*. Those responsible for guiding QA programs should begin immediately to educate themselves, their colleagues, and their administrative and medical leadership in the principles and processes of CQI. The preceding material and the suggested readings provide the guidance necessary to (re)organize for the new agenda with confidence that the institution will be well prepared for an accreditation survey under the new standards.

ORGANIZATION OF A HOSPITALWIDE QA PROGRAM

The preceding sections described standards and principles pertinent to the hospitalwide QA program. This section will address how to organize to accomplish the required tasks. The optimum QA program for each institution will be unique, and the following material is not intended as a blueprint. Rather, we have sought to identify some of the important alternatives and to illustrate those structural and functional components we consider most important for an effective QA program.

Institutional Support

Administrative Support

Consider two hospitals. In one, the QA staff members are told, "Organize a program that will pass accreditation. Minimize expenses and be as unobtrusive as possible." In the other, the staff is told, "Organize a program that can provide a valid and comprehensive assessment of the quality of care we provide and can assist us in continually improving that quality." Although few institutions would acknowledge electing the first approach, it comes to describe the reality in many. If the second approach is to be maintained, it must be institutionalized.

The commitment to quality should be reflected in the organization's mission statement and clearly expressed by the governing board through its oversight of the QA process. The administrative leadership must demonstrate support for the concept and goals of the program and be willing to provide it with the resources necessary to accomplish those goals (46, 47). These resources include not only staff and equipment but, most importantly, the time and attention of senior management.

Medical Staff Support

Even when administrators recognize that a comprehensive QA program is in the best long-term interests of the institution, their ability to implement such a program may be limited by medical staff resistance. That there might be resistance is unsurprising; given the approach to QA shown by Medicare and many insurers, physicians often associate QA/UR with uninformed second-guessing, an eagerness to find fault and assign blame, and a desire to control expenditures with no true concern for the impact on the patient. Because the active support and participation of the medical staff is essential to a successful QA program, this response must be anticipated and countered. The medical staff must be shown that the QA program serves their interests by helping to protect them from the erratic and potentially punitive actions of outside entities and by improving the systems within which they work, thus enhancing their ability to provide quality care.

In our experience, the most successful programs are those in which the medical staff has a sense of ownership: although the administration provides the resources, and the administration and the medical staff collaboratively determine the goals and procedures, the medical staff is largely in control of the operation of those components of the QA program pertinent to the JCAHO medical staff QA standards. They explicitly set the criteria by which judgments are made; they vigorously participate in and usually control decisions regarding QA projects or emphases; they compose the committees to which QA reports are made. They make all decisions regarding the quality of care provided by their peers and determine the appropriate response to any deficiencies.

In order to further this investment of the medical staff in the QA process, the QA program should be substantially subject to the control of a senior physician who commands the respect of the medical staff and who has been selected on the basis of support for QA. It is important that the chosen physician be paid for this activity. In small institutions, the position may be part-time and pay nominal; but the relationship demonstrates the commitment of the hospital to quality. In larger institutions, this responsibility is often a component of a full-time salaried position.

In addition, the officers of the organized medical staff need to provide consistent leadership and support to the QA program. Our medical staff president chairs the top-level QA committee, and the president-elect chairs the next-highest committee. Not only does each spend 2 years in each position, but candidates for president-elect must have chaired lower-level QA committees. Thus, the medical staff president has spent at least 4 to 6 years chairing a variety of QA committees. This lends the prestige of the medical staff leadership to the QA process, ensures an appropriate understanding of and support for the QA program by the senior clinicians, and demonstrates to younger staff that meaningful involvement in the QA program is a prerequisite for advancement in the medical staff hierarchy.

Data Support

A failure to provide adequate tools for the acquisition, storage, and manipulation of data can throttle the QA program. The QA staff will directly generate some of the needed data, but much will reside in other records. Consideration should be given to converting from paper to electronic storage for data regularly used in analyses (48, 49) and devising ways to make use of data collected for administrative or financial purposes. Once data are in the hands of the QA program, they must be stored and analyzed. Although some institutions use custom mainframe programs for these purposes, most find greater efficiency and economy using personal computers and standard commercial software with such programming support as may be necessary to customize databases and reports. It is well to remember that the purchase price of a personal computer typically is less than 10% of the annual cost of salary and benefits for the employee whose productivity the device is intended to increase.

Epidemiologic Support

We cannot fail to note the important role that a qualified epidemiologist can play in a QA program. The assistance that epidemiologists can provide in study design, sampling techniques, data management, and statistically sound analysis can be critical to the success of the program. In the process of providing consultation, the epidemiologist provides valuable training for the QA staff in the effective collection, analysis, and presentation of data. In addition, a physician epidemiologist can provide another link between the QA program and the medical staff, thereby enhancing the confidence of the medical staff in the pertinence and accuracy of data collection and analysis. The time to be devoted by the epidemiologist to the QA program will depend on local circumstances, but likely would be comparable to, or somewhat more than, the time a physician epidemiologist would give to the infection control program in the same institution.

QA Department Organization

Centralization

An issue that must be decided early is the degree to which the QA program should be centralized. There are certain theoretical advantages to a decentralized program. First, every member of the organization should be equally responsible for quality; the existence of a "quality department" implies that concerns about quality can be left to that department. Second, when each area of expertise evaluates its own work, the work is being evaluated by those most expert in the area. Furthermore, performing QA within the department may make it more likely that the results of surveillance are immediately available to influence activities.

We believe, however, that the arguments

for a predominantly centralized program are far more compelling. Even if substantial components of the QA program can successfully be decentralized, there is need for a central resource that coordinates overall QA activities, assures institutional compliance with external requirements, provides training and technical support, and ensures the appropriate communication of identified quality problems and effective interventions. In addition, a program with a strong centralized component is likely to be the most efficient. Unlike industry, where records required for the evaluation of different processes are likely recorded in disparate locations, in health care the activities of many processes are recorded in a single location: the patient chart. To have one reviewer harvest from that record the data necessary to evaluate multiple processes is usually more efficient than having a representative from each process visit the chart to collect data.

If medical QA activities are decentralized to each clinical area under the direction of the service chief, there is a much greater risk of variation in the diligence accorded QA activities. Even if the commitment to QA within each department is secure, it nonetheless may be more difficult for those who perform the work to be entirely objective in the evaluation of the work; a central QA department is more likely to apply uniform criteria throughout the institution in the evaluation of performance. In addition, those who work daily within the department being reviewed may be so accustomed to departmental routines that they fail to recognize as a problem something that would be apparent quickly to a trained outside observer.

Health care rarely follows the simple linear flow that might characterize an industrial process. In the hospital, many processes are operating simultaneously and interact in their effects on each other and on the patient. Centralized QA programs are better able to identify or manage problems arising from the coordination or interactions of diverse departments, and the centralized QA database that may be needed to evaluate complex or interrelated processes is more readily generated and managed by a centralized QA system.

In our experience, the medical staff members are most receptive to the QA process if there is a limited cadre of QA workers whose procedures they understand and whose judgment they have come to trust. Although this consideration may seem to favor decentralized QA, in practice the activities of each medical staff division are interrelated with so many disparate processes (respiratory care, laboratory, pharmacy, physical therapy, etc.) that decentralization of QA actually increases the number of persons reviewing activities pertinent to a given division.

Therefore, we favor establishing a department that has plenary responsibility for the QA activities of the organization. This group will coordinate and oversee all QA functions and perform a substantial proportion of the monitoring and evaluation. It will guide the various divisions and clinical departments in establishing indicators and defining thresholds and will assist them in evaluating their data and identifying problems or opportunities to improve. Although the opportunity and responsibility for process improvement will rest primarily with those who perform the process, QA department staff will remain involved as facilitators, coordinators, and reporters.

Concurrent or Retrospective Review

Another issue that is fundamental in determining the organization of the QA process concerns the extent to which the organization will attempt to perform concurrent review. The term "concurrent review" generally refers to review performed while the patient is still in the hospital; more pertinently, we consider review concurrent when the results of review are able to influence the care of the patient whose management is being reviewed.

A number of considerations have favored retrospective review. The historical focus of QA programs on surgical outcome and medical records (Table 10.1) have conditioned a retrospective approach that remains dominant in many institutions. Retrospective review is often more efficient, as the chart is complete and can provide most needed data in one review.

There are some problems or indicators for which retrospective review is the only reasonable way to perform monitoring and evaluation. Typically, these are studies or surveillance systems that depend on the medical records staff having completed coding or on reports that do not reliably appear in the chart prior to discharge. Exploratory studies are often most efficiently performed by retrospective review of an appropriate sample of charts. Finally, the JCAHO medical staff and QA standards thus far have no requirement for concurrent review (although its performance is implied in the UR standard). Despite these considerations, we believe strongly that the QA program should be built around a comprehensive system of concurrent review, reserving retrospective review for those circumstances where it is particularly indicated.

Only with concurrent review is there the opportunity to intervene so as to benefit the patient whose care is being reviewed. If our goal is care of the highest quality, then we should organize our QA system to detect problems in time to correct them.

Only concurrent review offers the opportunity to help the physician avoid situations that might precipitate adverse action by external regulatory agencies. Indeed, this benefit of concurrent review is a major contributor to the strong medical staff support enjoyed by our QA program. On those occasions when circumstances have caused the proportion of patients receiving concurrent review to be reduced, there has been vigorous protest by the medical staff and a demand for more complete concurrent review.

Only concurrent review can permit a QA committee to review each month the care given the prior month, as aspect appealing to the physicians. Retrospective review rarely is performed so promptly. Furthermore, retrospective review generally means postdischarge review, which is most delayed for those with the longest stay; these are often the cases most in need of review.

A comprehensive concurrent review program facilitates studies that are difficult or impossible to perform retrospectively. Any study requiring data not otherwise routinely collected, or requiring data that often are incomplete or inaccurate in the medical record (for example, management of IV catheters) is best performed concurrently. For such studies, the data collection is merely appended to the routine concurrent surveillance. Finally, the concurrent review staff can simultaneously review for UR, reaping the same benefits and permitting incidents of inappropriate utilization to be corrected rather than merely tabulated.

Severity of Illness Systems

Systems designed to control for severity of illness (SOI), so that differences in outcomes more likely reflect differences in care, have proliferated in the past decade (50, 51). SOI systems are discussed in Chapter 8, and we will make only a few comments.

An SOI system that could generate reliable results based on automated review (without manual data collection) would be most attractive. Unfortunately, the uniform hospital data discharge set, as currently specified, is marginally useful for these purposes. Most of the SOI systems are labor intensive and can require as many personnel to operate as would a comprehensive concurrent review system. Unless the hospital is willing to support both, it must choose; and we believe concurrent review offers more benefits.

Some specialized systems can provide concurrent results (for example, APACHE (52)), but most depend on a completed chart (and many on completion of medical records coding); results typically are presented to the medical staff many months after the fact. In addition, some of the systems are complex and nonintuitive, requiring considerable time and education to overcome physician skepticism.

Although the ability to stratify by patient severity was on occasion quite helpful, we found that results from the SOI system generally mirrored those derived from our existing program of concurrent and retrospective review. It may be that variations in patient acuity are less extreme within a single institution than is found when comparing disparate institutions, where the need for SOI correction may be greater.

Perhaps the most compelling reason to move slowly with respect to SOI systems is that the market remains unsettled. A number of regulatory agencies or insurers have already required the adoption of one system or another, and there is speculation that HCFA may, within the decade, impose a nationwide system. Furthermore, the JCAHO will likely impose their own requirements for data collection and transmittal. Until these issues are resolved, it might be best to invest resources in developing the QA and data management infrastructure within the hospital rather than in an SOI system.

The QA Staff

Number and Qualifications. The number of staff necessary for the QA department will depend on the degree to which the QA program is centralized, the duties assigned to the staff, the extent to which concurrent review is desired (comprehensive concurrent review generally requires more staff than a minimal program based on retrospective review), and of course the size and nature of the hospital involved. As an example, our own institution is a 572-bed private referral hospital with a very high Medicare case-mix index. The care of cardiac and vascular illness is prominent; there is no obstetrics or pediatric service. In order to provide concurrent and retrospective review for 22,000 admissions per year and provide staff support to 23 medical staff divisions and 10 QA committees, we employ one QA director, one assistant director, eight QA nurses (who staff the committees and perform the reviews), three data technicians (who enter data, perform analyses, and generate reports), and two secretaries.

Careful selection of the QA staff is essential (53). To the medical staff, the QA nurses *are* the QA program; medical staff support for the program will depend in large measure on the extent to which the physicians trust these nurses and enjoy working with them. Our QA nurses must be registered nurses with a BS degree and a minimum of 5 years nursing experience with at least 2 years supervisory experience; critical care experience is preferred. The positions are highly sought. Criteria for staff selection include reliability and integrity, the ability to work independently, oral and written communications skills, and the ability to work courteously and confidently with the medical staff. The QA nurses are expected to have or seek QA board certification and to participate in continuing education activities.

Duties. There are a number of ways in which nurses might be assigned specific duties; we favor a case management approach. The nurses receive a daily assignment sheet generated by a computer program that tracks current assignments, discharges, new admissions, and room changes based on the overnight census. Automated assignment of new patients is guided by existing workload and current nurse specializations. (For example, the nurse currently staffing the Cardiovascular Division will preferentially be given cardiovascular patients to review). Once assigned a patient, a nurse follows that patient from admission to discharge, a practice that enhances both professional responsibility and efficiency. The nurse is reponsible for determining the frequency and intensity of review for each patient. Review generally does not involve significant patient contact, but occasionally it is necessary to look in on the patient or to ask a few simple questions in order to clarify an issue. It is expected that, on average, charts are reviewed three times a week; but this might represent daily visits for those recently admitted and biweekly visits for stable long-term patients. Each nurse typically carries a service of 50 to 70 patients being followed concurrently.

There are two important sets of activities that we do *not* recommend delegating to the QA nurses: infection control and precertification/recertification. Although infection control is at heart a form of QA, the technical body of knowledge required to perform fully the infection control function is sufficiently large that it is not reasonable to expect every QA nurse to be up to the standards of a certified practitioner in infection control. In institutions of sufficient size, it is more effective to assign the primary responsibility for infection control to a specialist. However, the concurrent review performed by the QA nurse should include surveillance for suspected noso-comial infections, which would be referred for follow-up to the infection control practitioner.

We have found a number of problems with having the QA nurses who are already performing concurrent surveillance manage recertification. First, reviews required for recertification do not follow the pattern that is most effective for concurrent QA review. They frequently are demanded on short notice, disrupting the nurse's schedule. Although in theory recertification should require only the same type of review already required for a competent UR program, in fact unpredictable requests for minor clinical details often require a return to the chart. Thus, despite first impression, there is actually little efficiency gained by combining recertification with QA.

Worse yet, the payers typically require telephonic consultation with the reviewing nurse, but keep the nurses facing busy signals, waiting on hold, or awaiting callback for unconscionable periods. This may be tolerble in a program based on retrospective review, where the nurses work in the office, but it can severely disrupt a concurrent review program. In addition, although the personnel best suited to each task may be equally capable, they are likely to differ in their preferences, personalities, and specific talents. QA nurses chosen on the basis of their ability to handle complex tasks independently are likely to resent being tied to a telephone awaiting the chance to give report.

Finally, and most importantly, involvement in the recertification process can erode the good relationship the QA department has struggled to establish with the medical staff by converting the QA nurses into agents of a very unpopular regulatory process.

Committee Organization and Medical Staff Participation

The optimal committee structure will differ for every institution and its complexity will be determined by the size and needs of the institution. Many institutions will find suitable a more simple structure than we describe below. We recommend, however, that the program not be based solely on the traditional medical staff divisions or departments. Whether the institution is so small that the medical staff meets as a whole, or so large the medical staff is organized into dozens of divisions, there should be oversight of the medical QA process by hospitalwide committees that include physicians from various clinical specialties. There are four major benefits from this approach.

First, this structure reduces the risk that an entrenched service chief hostile to QA activities can undermine or frustrate the QA process within his or her domain. Second, it ensures that important quality issues are considered by persons with a variety of perspectives and interests, rather than solely by those invested in the process being reviewed. Third, it avoids the possibility that the only persons available to review care are the partners or associates of the physician whose care is being reviewed, a situation that can stymie critical review. Fourth, it markedly diminishes the risk of a successful antitrust suit grounded in the allegation that review was performed solely by the reviewed physician's economic competitors.

The QA program interfaces with the medical staff and administration through committees and key individuals. The senior element responsible for assessing and improving quality in our program is the professional affairs committee of the board of trust. This body, chaired alternately by the president of the medical staff and the chairperson of the board, receives reports from the medical executive and operations committees. These committees, in turn, oversee the medical and hospital QA programs.

Separation of the overall QA program into medical and hospital components has been important in gaining the trust and participation of the medical staff in the QA process. It preferentially lays before the physicians those issues most clearly requiring their expertise and attention. It facilitates the participation of the physicians in the frank evaluation of physician performance that is necessary for a vigorous QA program, something that is difficult or impossible to achieve in a committee not substantially composed of physicians. However, it requires special effort to ensure appropriate communication and coordination between the hospital and medical QA components and the proper evaluation of problems that involve the interaction of physicians with hospital systems.

A number of mechanisms are used to address these concerns. First, the centralized QA department participates in the activities of all components of the QA program and is responsible for integrating their activities, coordinating efforts, and communicating findings and decisions. Second, physicians are represented on all hospital committees, one or more senior administrators attend each medical staff committee, and QA staff are involved in the activities of both. The chief executive officer attends meetings of the medical executive; the chief operating officer attends meetings of the medical QA committee; and the chief medical officer attends operations committee. Finally, task forces that include appropriate medical, administrative, and staff members are formed as needed to address problems that might benefit from such an approach. As we move to implement more fully the precepts of CQI, we likely will make increasing use of these multidisciplinary task forces.

The medical QA program, under the leadership of the chief medical officer (a full-time salaried physician), is responsible for all QA activities that involve the evaluation of the performance of physicians. Examples of medical QA committees include mortality review and clinical risk, patient care monitoring, utilization review, and pharmacy and therapeutics. These committees are chaired by and composed primarily of physicians and contain only those administrative personnel necessary for pertinent data submission or liaison. Evaluation of the care rendered by individual physicians occurs in executive session. Certain committees receive reports from the various medical staff divisions regarding the divisions' QA activities, and all send pertinent reports to the divisions for their consideration. These committees report to the medical QA committee (chaired by the president-elect), which reports to the medical executive committee (chaired by the president). Each committee's functions and authority are detailed in the hospitalwide QA plan; as an example, the actions available to the medical QA committee are shown in Table 10.4.

The medical staff departments and divisions also play an important role in the QA

Table 10.4.
Actions Available to the Medical Quality Assurance Committee

General actions
  Request action by the medical executive committee, the bylaws committee, another medical staff
    QA committee, or a department/division of the medical staff
  Request action by the hospital QA committee, the operations committee, the chief operating
    officer, another appropriate hospital committee, or from an administrative or nursing
    representative
  Request action by the chief medical officer, chief of department, division head, or designee
  Request action by the continuing medical education committee or conduct an educational program
  Request more data or conduct a study
Physician-specific actions
  Request emergency action from the chief medical officer, in accord with the bylaws
  Request the executive committee to initiate an investigation or corrective action, in accord with the
    bylaws
  Request review by another medical staff QA committee or by hospital epidemiology
  Request review by the chief of department or division head
  Request physician interview, counseling, or education by the chief medical officer, chief of
    department, division head, or designee
  Request placement of a report in the credentials file
  Request placement of a report or data in the QA file

process. The divisions remain the source of expertise regarding specific clinical issues and the locus for many corrective actions. The division meetings are an important vehicle for communicating the findings and actions of the hospitalwide QA committees, and their responsibilities and agenda (Table 10.5) are mandated by the QA plan. The actions available to the divisions are included in those shown in Table 10.4.

In addition to the medical staff QA committees and the divisions, there is a third mechanism linking the QA program with the medical staff. Whenever a QA nurse performing concurrent review encounters a QA or UR issue that might merit immediate intervention or whose categorization requires additional clinical expertise, that issue is promptly presented (without identifying involved individuals) to an appropriate physician reviewer. If the physician reviewer feels that further intervention is indicated (for example, positive blood cultures with sepsis syndrome but no effective antibiotics), the issue is referred immediately to the chief of the appropriate department or the chief medical officer for review and action (without identifying the physician reviewer). All members of the active medical staff are solicited to serve as physician reviewers.

The hospital QA program is responsible for all QA activities involving the evaluation of hospital services and staff. The various hospital departments and hospital QA committees such as safety, nursing QA, and disaster report to the hospital QA committee, which reports to the operations committee. The hospital QA program is under the leadership of the chief operating officer, who chairs the hospital QA and the operations committees. (A few committees such as infection control are plenary and report both to the hospital and the medical components.)

Data Management

A vigorous QA program collects considerable data, the management of which can be challenging. As noted, the costs and capabilities of personal computer systems are such that even the smallest program should use these tools. However, not all data are appropriate for electronic storage, and it is a common error to enter unsuitable data in the computer. Material that will be mathematically manipulated (counted, summed, averaged, graphed, etc.) or rearranged and printed out (tables, line listings, etc.) is appropriate for entry into a database system. On the other hand, it is rarely productive to enter narrative material or data that will simply be stored and not further manipulated.

Modern systems of quality control emphasize the establishing of numerical indicators, tracking measurements of these indicators serially over time, establishing thresholds or control limits for the indicators, and analyzing the data for trends and patterns. Such rate-based material is generated, for example, by review of generic screens, by the UR program, and by procedure monitoring. Recording and evaluating such data can be markedly facilitated by thoughtful use of computer tools. Some customized software is available; for example, several companies offer packages specialized for infection control.

For the QA program in general, however, the variety of data to be collected and analyzed and the certainty that new data storage needs will constantly arise argue strongly for selecting a few powerful software tools (for example, a database manager, a statistical package, a graphing package, and a word processor) and securing the training or programming support necessary to ensure their effective employment.

Data management is another area in which the support of a trained epidemiologist can be critical. Decisions as to which data to store electronically, how to organize the data systems, how to analyze the data, and how to report the data so that they are meaningful and understandable are not trivial. We have found that the involvement of an epidemiologist in these matters can do much to enhance the acceptance of QA program reports by an audience of critical physicians.

The QA program gives rise both to raw surveillance data and to quality assessments based on those data. Data such as are produced by generic screens or infec-

Table 10.5.
Responsibilities and Agenda of Medical Staff Division, as Mandated by QA Plan

The division:
1. Is accountable for all professional, clinical, and administrative activities within the division/ department related to the effective delivery of quality patient care.
2. Reviews data submitted from the medical staff QA committees and data obtained from divisional monitoring activities.
3. Provides for the ongoing, planned, and systematic monitoring and evaluation of the quality and appropriateness of patient care through review and evaluation of QA data and by adherence to the following prioritized, mandated agenda:
   A. QA/risk indicators and studies
   B. Mortality review report
   C. Blood/blood products report
   D. Drug utilization report
   E. Infection control report
   F. Surgical and procedural case review report
   G. Utilization review report
   H. Medical records report
      (1) Delinquent charts
      (2) Attestation statements
      (3) Clinical pertinence
   I. Appointments/reappointments
   J. Medical staff cost containment reports
   K. Other reports
4. Responds to requests for corrective action or specific recommendations from the medical staff QA committees.
5. Develops valid screens, criteria, and other monitoring tools for use in the ongoing monitoring and evaluation process; identifies high risk, high/low volume or specific problem areas within the speciality in order to resolve important patient care problems and/or identify opportunities to improve care.
6. Documents and reports semiannually (or more often, if indicated) to the patient care monitoring committee the actions taken to resolve problems and improve patient care and reports information about the impact of the action taken; requests assistance from the committee if unable to appropriately resolve problems.
7. Assists in development and analysis of appropriateness data regarding pertinent aspects of specific and related hospital departments/services.
8. Participates in continuing education activities that relate, in part, to the privileges granted, the findings of QA activities, and the expressed needs of the constituency.
9. Provides for continuing surveillance and peer review of the professional performance of all individuals with delineated clinical privileges within the division/department; evaluates scope of privileges data from the QA department to assure that all services provided are within the scope of clinical privileges granted.
10. Establishes qualifications, provides for peer review, and develops valid criteria for use in recommending clinical privileges to the appropriate credentialing committee for each member of the division.
11. Uses QA information to support the reappraisal and the resulting reappointment recommendation.
12. Participates in other review functions, as delegated, including internal and external disaster plans, hospital safety, infection control, and utilization review.
13. Reviews and approves standardized formats for the medical record.
14. Maintains a system for follow-up to determine if action taken results in problem resolution (problem tracking forms).
15. Maintains accurate and timely records, minutes, and problem tracking forms of all division/ department meetings and activities.
16. Enforces the strict observance of and adherence to the confidentiality policy.
17. Meets monthly.

tion surveillance have no meaning until they are subjected to analysis and reviewed by an appropriate entity. If the data in question are pertinent to the practice of individual physicians, peer review (perhaps involving chart review) is then required. Only after this process is complete are the data suitable for use in consideration of privileges, sanctions, etc. In recognition of this dichotomy, we maintain two sets of records that are kept conceptually and physically distinct: the raw QA files and the credentialing files. All data collected by QA are kept in the QA files. The credentialing file contains only material that has been the subject of review and final judgment by an individual or committee acting within their role in the QA process. We have written policies (as illustrated in Tables 10.4 and 10.5) that define the function and scope of authority of each entity involved in the QA process, and data enters the credentialing file only in accord with those policies. Data in the raw QA files may not be used to support action specific to any individual; only data in the credentialing file can be so used.

The maintenance of confidentiality of the QA data is of paramount importance. Lapses in confidentiality can destroy the credibility of the program, erase years of effort in building the trust of the medical staff, and open QA records to discovery by opposing attorneys. Written confidentiality policies should define the storage of data, the access to data, and the release of data, analyses, or reports. Legal guidance should be sought to ensure that the fruits of the QA process are protected from outside discovery or review. For example, minutes from our mortality committee are printed on red-bordered paper emblazoned with the citation and text of the state law protecting such material from discovery, are uniquely identified on every page to be able to trace any photocopies, and are personally distributed and collected by the QA nurse staffing that committee.

In addition to maintaining databases reflecting its own activities, it is important (and, later in the decade, will be required by the JCAHO) that the institution maintain or have access to databases that can be used to compare the performance of the institution with that of others (15). Without such comparative data, it is all too easy for an institution to take comfort in its stable or slowly declining rate of nosocomial pneumonia (for example), when the rate in fact is three times that found in comparable institutions.

At present, such comparative data can be difficult to obtain. Some vendors of SOI systems maintain comparative databases for the use of their customers. The Joint Commission intends to provide comparative databases for the indicators it is developing, but it likely will take some years for these to be available. HCFA provides its well known annual release of Medicare mortality data (54–56); but the problems and limitations of these data are equally well known (57, 58). It likely will be several years before HCFA provides more comprehensive comparative data.

Other sources for comparative data include: associated or sister institutions; other institutions in the community willing to trade data; Blue Cross or other private insurers; and hospital associations or similar groups (for example, the Maryland Hospital Association's Indicator Project).

Key Program Functions

Staff Support

One of the most important functions of the QA nurses is to provide staff support to the medical QA committees. Although it absorbs a substantial portion of the QA nurses' time, we believe this activity to be essential in winning the trust and support of the medical staff and in ensuring the effective coordination of the QA program. Every medical QA committee, division, or department meeting is staffed by a QA nurse who is responsible for preparing the agenda and any QA materials to be presented, supervising the taking and preparing of minutes, and generating any required memos or reports. Between meetings, the QA nurse works with the physician chairperson to coordinate the activities of the committee.

The assignment of committees and divisions to the various nurses is revised every

2 to 3 years, thus ensuring substantial continuity and development of expertise while avoiding stagnation. The director of QA staffs the medical QA committee, assists in staffing the medical executive committee, and staffs the professional affairs committee of the board. The hospital QA committee is staffed by the assistant director of QA. Subsidiary hospital QA committees contain QA department representation but are staffed by personnel from the involved hospital services.

Concurrent Review and Notification

A comprehensive program of concurrent review is the bedrock of our hospitalwide QA and UR surveillance. Concurrent review is used as the vehicle to accomplish a number of functions.

One of the most important components of the review process is the application of a series of generic screens (Table 10.6). Although these should be developed by each institution and specific to its needs, it is essential that the Medicare generic screens

Table 10.6.
Generic QA Screens Performed During Concurrent Review

1. Patient injury incurred at the hospital, or patient/family complaint[a]
2. Inadvertent laceration, puncture, occurrence of hematoma, or other injury of an organ or body part during a medical or minor surgery procedure not performed in OR; or major complication following such procedure[a]
3. Inadvertent injury during an operative procedure[a]
   a. Partial or complete removal of an organ or body part (unplanned), or wrong procedure
   b. Laceration, puncture or other injury of an organ or body part (other than those routine in the intended surgical procedure)
4. Surgery for removal of inadvertently retained foreign body[a]
5. Other unplanned return to OR, same admission (specify related or unrelated cause)[b]
6. Acute MI or CVA during/within 48 hours of operative, major diagnostic, or therapeutic procedure[a,c]
7. Other adverse clinical issue[b,d]
   a. Delays in treatment or diagnosis, or missed treatments
   b. Clinical misjudgment or misdiagnosis
   c. Inappropriate indications for surgery/procedure
   d. Risk management concerns (refer to risk management department)
8. Organ failure or other complication not present on admission (cardiovascular, hematological, infectious, renal, respiratory, endocrine, MI, CVA, etc.)[b]
9. Unplanned readmission within 31 days of discharge
   a. For recurrence of prior condition(s)
   b. For complication of prior therapy
   c. Correct diagnosis not made on prior admission
   d. Nosocomial infection (also refer to hospital epidemiology department)
   e. Apparently unrelated to prior admission
   f. For complications following ambulatory surgery or procedure
   g. Within 48 hours following treatment in the ER
10a. Unplanned transfer to special/critical care (not previously in specified unit)
10b. Unplanned return to special or critical care
11. Inadequate or inappropriate documentation in the medical record (clinical pertinence)[a]
12. Life-threatening complications of anesthesia[a]
13. Failure to obtain informed consent[a]
14. Inappropriate personal interactions[a,d]
15. Drug or blood reaction or inappropriate utilization[d]
16. Formation or worsening of decubitus ulcer during hospitalization[a]
17. Possible nosocomial infection (refer to hospital epidemiology department)
18. Other (incident not categorized above; please describe thoroughly)

[a]Notify director of QA immediately.
[b]Notify director of QA if critical/urgent.
[c]MI, myocardial infarction; CVA, cerebrovascular accident; ER, emergency room.
[d]Consider presenting to physician reviewer.

be incorporated. We immediately communicate any finding pertinent to one of the Medicare PRO screens to the attending physician via a "concurrent notification letter." This nonjudgmental letter enables the attending physician to review the circumstances and take whatever action appears appropriate (this mechanism is used for issues that are not clinically urgent, in contrast to referrals via a physician reviewer to a department chief for immediate intervention). For example, suppose the QA nurse noted that the physician apparently had not responded to the radiologist's report of a pulmonary mass. Once notified, the attending physician can take appropriate action or document why no action was needed (for example, known pulmonary sequestration); in either case, the risk of PRO sanction is averted. This ability to alert physicians to issues that might, if uncorrected, pose problems with outside QA or UR reviewers has done much to generate support among the medical staff for the QA program and for concurrent review. At the same time, it is an effective educational tool that sensitizes the medical staff to the referred issues and improves the quality of care.

In addition to the PRO's screens, the generic screens include review for locally defined indicators and may be supplemented by service-specific or other special screens as needed. In addition, there usually will be one or more special studies undergoing data collection through concurrent review.

In the process of reviewing the charts, the QA nurses evaluate the medical record for the timeliness and adequacy of the entries (similar review is also performed by medical records) and to detect any activity that is outside the scope of privileges granted the practitioner. The activities of the ancillary clinical services (respiratory care, cardiac and other rehabilitation, physical and occupational therapy, etc.) can be reviewed during concurrent review if the QA nurses are trained to evaluate these disciplines. Similarly, the QA nurse can review and abstract data regarding nursing tasks and functions: documentation, patient assessment and monitoring, proper implementation of the patient's

plan of care, medication errors, technique errors, urinary catheter care, IV care, procedures to prevent falls and the occurrence of falls, and so on.

At the same time the chart is being reviewed for these quality issues, the QA nurse can be collecting data for the UR program and evaluating the appropriateness of the admission, of continued hospitalization, and of the current level of care (regular, telemetry, critical care, and so on); noting any inappropriate delays in providing necessary services; and verifying the presence of appropriate indications for procedures performed. Each institution will wish to target its UR program in light of its own specific needs and circumstances; the scheme for our bed utilization review is shown in Table 10.7. The assessment of the propriety of a specific utilization is based on criteria for intensity of service and severity of illness that have been reviewed, modified, and adopted by the appropriate medical staff. There are generic criteria applicable to all patients for intensity (example: receiving intravenous antibiotics) and severity (example: pulse above 140 beats/minute), as well as criteria that are specific to the unit (critical care, telemetry, etc.) or service (orthopedics, urology, etc.) of interest.

In addition to its use for QA issues, the concurrent notification program is used to notify physicians of UR findings. Typically, notified physicians will either make the indicated change in level of service or, more often, place in the chart the documentation needed to justify the current utilization.

Finally, whenever indicated, the QA nurse will request that social services commence discharge planning for the patient. This helps to ensure the timely availability of services needed in order to discharge the patient and is particularly important to the hospital and the attending physician in light of the current PRO emphasis on detecting and punishing any failure to provide discharge planning.

Although desirable, it is not necessary that concurrent review be applied to 100% of patients. First, unless there are QA nurses working nights and weekends, some patients will come and go without

Table 10.7.
Checklist for Review of Bed Utilization

1. Should not have been admitted
   A. Not receiving hospital level of care on admission
   B. Studies/procedures could have been performed on an outpatient basis
2. Delay in hospital providing services
   C. Unnecessary delay in providing or ordering services:
      (1) Due to physician
      (2) Due to hospital
      (3) Patient refused procedure or treatment
   D. Awaiting surgery; inpatient status not medically necessary
3. Should have been discharged
   E. Not receiving hospital level of care
   F. Studies/services/procedures could be provided on an outpatient basis
   G. Services could be delivered by home health service
   H. Days waiting transfer to nursing home
   I. Days waiting transfer to rehabilitation unit
   J. Days waiting transfer to long-term psychiatric unit
   K. Patient refuses to be discharged
4. Level of care
   L. Admitted via ER but not an emergency
   M. Could have been in a motel unit
   N. Should not have been in:
      (1) Critical care unit—met discharge screens, bed available
      (2) Special care unit—met discharge screens, bed available
      (3) Critical care unit—met discharge screens, no special care bed available
      (4) Special care—met discharge screens, no regular bed available
      (5) Telemetry unit—did not meet admission criteria
      (6) Telemetry unit—should have been in special care
      (7) Telemetry unit—should have been in critical care
      (8) Telemetry unit—should have been in regular bed
      (9) Special care—should have been in recovery room
      (10) Critical care—should have been in recovery room
      (11) Recovery room—should have been in critical care, but no beds
   O. Should have been in:
      (1) Diabetic unit
      (2) Critical care unit
      (3) Special care unit
      (4) Psychiatric unit
      (5) Ventilator only unit
      (6) Regular bed
      (7) Telemetry unit—patient in critical care
      (8) Telemetry unit—patient in special care
      (9) Telemetry unit—patient in medical-surgical unit
      (10) Telemetry unit—bed not available
   P. Left against medical advice
   Q. Left before medical advice

review. In addition, important projects on occasion may make demands of the QA staff that cannot be met while performing 100% review. Finally, illness or other unexpected staff shortages may make it impossible to maintain 100% surveillance. In these circumstances, one can elect to perform surveillance on a sample of all admissions; if desired, the sample can be stratified to give greater weight to certain subgroups. If the distribution and tracking of QA nurse assignments is handled by computer, provisions for random sampling can easily be incorporated into the program handling the assignments. However, there are two drawbacks to sampling that must be kept in mind. First, indicators for which universal review is required must be captured by retrospective review if concurrent review is based on sampling. Second, if the QA program has been successful in convincing the medical staff of the benefits of concurrent review, they will object to prolonged periods during which substantial numbers of patients are not reviewed concurrently.

If your institution has not yet developed intensity and severity criteria, there are a number of commercial suppliers who can provide these and other materials useful to your QA program. Among the vendors known to us are InterQual in Westborough, MA and Medical Management Analysis International in Auburn, CA. American Health Consultants in Atlanta and Bader and Associates in Rockville, MD publish pertinent newsletters. (In addition to these commercial sources, the American Hospital Association in Chicago offers a wealth of materials useful in the development of a QA program.) Finally, be sure to seek the intensity and severity criteria used by your local Medicare intermediary and by any private insurers important to your local situation.

Retrospective Review

In addition to the comprehensive program of concurrent review, the QA staff routinely performs retrospective review of selected medical charts or of pertinent indicators. Mortality review is a good example of a QA function best handled retrospectively: deaths are few, scattered throughout the hospital, often occur at hours during which concurrent review is not being performed, and are targeted for special review not routinely applied to all cases. The completed chart of every patient who died in the hospital is reviewed by a QA nurse according to a protocol developed and approved by the medical staff (Table 10.8). If the review suggests a potential problem, or if there is an actual or anticipated risk management issue, the chart is assigned by the mortality committee chairman to a member of the committee for review. At the monthly meeting, cases are presented by the reviewing committee member, without identifying involved physicians, and the care given (or not given) is vigorously debated.

The committee then refers the matter for any appropriate further action (as in Table 10.4).

A number of retrospective review systems are used to supplement the concurrent review of surgical and other invasive procedures. Tissue review and review for uniformity of preoperative and postoperative diagnoses are conducted monthly for the prior month's cases. Procedures are sampled for audit of indications, according to criteria developed by each division for the procedures it performs. All results are presented for discussion to appropriate committees and divisions.

Housewide and targeted infection control surveillance is performed according to guidelines of the Centers for Disease Control's National Nosocomial Infection Surveillance System and reported monthly to the infection control committee and then to the medical and hospital QA committees and any involved medical staff divisions or clinical services.

Many special studies commissioned by QA committees, medical staff divisions, hospital departments, or ad hoc task forces are performed retrospectively by the QA staff. Finally, all incident reports filed within the hospital are routinely reviewed for referral to the QA department, and pertinent findings are presented to the appropriate committee.

Credentialing

It is imperative that the granting of privileges to admit patients or perform procedures be closely integrated with the QA program. We accomplish this in a number of ways.

Authorized entities following established policy can direct the placement of pertinent quality evaluations (adverse or commendatory) in the permanent credentials file. In addition, the separately maintained raw data files of the QA department are reviewed for each physician undergoing recredentialing, and at that time material may be referred for review by an appropriate QA entity and subsequently added to the credentialing file (for example, a series of findings each individually minor but which, in aggregate, form a troubling pattern). Of course, the credentials file also contains all the records of education, licenses, recommendations, evaluations, data bank searches, and other material customarily required.

Prior to reappointment, a data sheet is completed for each individual incorporating relevant adverse or laudatory findings regarding generic screens, blood product utilization, drug audits or adverse reactions, medical records, infection control,

mortality, special studies, procedural review, utilization review, PRO reviews, and information from the National Practitioner Data Bank. The form is completed by QA staff in coordination with risk management, infection control, and others; reviewed by the chief of department and the chief medical officer; and sent to the appropriate credentialing committee for review and action.

Table 10.8.
Mortality Review Worksheet

Date of Death: _____	SS #: _____
Division: _____	Admitted: _____
Physician Number: _____	Principal Diagnosis/Procedure: _____
Medical Record Number: _____	_____
Incident Severity Code: _____	_____
Profiled: _____	_____
Referred CMO: _____	_____
Referred to a Committee: _____	Reviewed by: _____
Referred to Chief of Service: _____	Review Date: _____
Credentials File: _____	Patient's Age: _____
Comment: _____	Committee Review Date: _____

A. Is the documentation adequate to properly evaluate the case?
   Comments:

B. Was the patient's condition at admission such that death was likely, irrespective of treatment?
   IF NO: Go to section C. If YES, continue here.

   Even though death was likely at admission, are there other quality of care issues present in this case?

   IF NO: STOP. IF YES, go to section C.
   Comments:

C. Were diagnostic efforts appropriate, adequate, and timely?
   Were therapeutic efforts appropriate, adequate, and timely?
   Was there any failure to respond in a timely and appropriate manner to relevant and available information?
   Comments:

   Were actions or interventions taken that should not have been?
   Were actions or interventions not taken that should have been?
   Comments:

1. Did patient die in OR or within 48 hours of surgery?
2. Did patient die following any surgery performed during this admission?
3. Was Pre-op anesthesia evaluation done?
4. Surgical deaths: ASA Class _____   Anesthesiologist # _____
5. Did death occur within 24 hours of admission through ER?
6. Did death occur following a return to critical care or special care within 24 hours of having been transferred out of critical or special care?

A FINAL THOUGHT

We have sought to provide in this chapter an outline of the past, the present, and the future of medical quality assurance in the United States and a guide to satisfying present and future requirements. To this end, our approach has been more practical than academic; but let us briefly consider scholarly matters.

The literature of health care delivery and of medical quality assurance is burgeoning. Long and careful thought has been given to these issues by eminent scholars, some of whose work graces this volume. Medical journals are replete with studies demonstrating differences among physicians, institutions, regions, or societies in health care resource consumption or in patient outcome, differences that do not appear to be justified by differing circumstances. Such studies bolster the common sense understanding that medical care is not always as good as it can be, ought to be, or will be. Nonetheless, choices regarding the organization and activities of QA programs are not guided by a body of rigorous scientific evidence such as we customarily rely on in our other endeavors (59). Particularly lacking are studies that compare the benefits and costs of alternative approaches to quality assessment. The incredible difficulty of devising adequate controls for such studies, particularly when most changes in QA activities are mandated throughout the region or nation, makes their scarcity understandable but no less regrettable.

A few decades ago, the field of infection control similarly was guided more by common sense and good intentions than by rigorous science. However, the need was clear; and as the matter generally involved microbes and epidemics, workers in infectious diseases and in epidemiology took the subject matter as their own and gradually developed a robust body of knowledge, comprising the discipline now known as hospital epidemiology.

Although many workers publish in the field of quality assessment, it is not seen as the natural domain of any particular medical discipline. However, the skills and interests of those engaged in hospital epidemiology are well suited to these research possibilities (19, 21, 60–65), and we urge our readers to be alert not only to the practical needs of their programs but also to opportunities to build the epidemiologic literature of quality assessment.

References

1. Council on Medical Service. Quality of care. JAMA 1986;256:1032–1034.
2. Davis L. Fellowship of surgeons. A history of the American College of Surgeons. Chicago: Charles C Thomas, 1960:476.
3. Roberts JS, Coale JG, Redman RR. A history of the Joint Commission on Accreditation of Hospitals. JAMA 1987;258:936–940.
4. Joint Commission on Accreditation of Hospitals. Accreditation manual for hospitals. Chicago: Joint Commission on Accreditation of Hospitals, 1969.
5. Joint Commission on Accreditation of Hospitals. Supplement to the accreditation manual for hospitals. Chicago: Joint Commission on Accreditation of Hospitals, 1975.
6. Fromberg R. The Joint Commission guide to quality assurance. Chicago: Joint Commission on the Accreditation of Healthcare Institutions, 1988.
7. Joint Commission on the Accreditation of Healthcare Institutions. 1985 accreditation manual for hospitals. Oakbrook Terrace, IL: Joint Commission on the Accreditation of Healthcare Institutions, 1984.
8. Joint Commission on the Accreditation of Healthcare Institutions. 1991 accreditation manual for hospitals. Oakbrook Terrace, IL: Joint Commission on the Accreditation of Healthcare Institutions, 1990.
9. Joint Commission on Accreditation of Healthcare Institutions. Primer on indicator development and application. Chicago: Joint Commission on Accreditation of Healthcare Institutions, 1990.
10. Anonymous. Characteristics of clinical indicators. QRB 1989;15:330–339.
11. Donabedian A. Evaluating the quality of medical care. Milbank Memorial Fund Q 1966;44:166–203.
12. Donabedian A. Explorations in quality assessment and monitoring. Vol. I: The definition of quality and approaches to its assessment. Ann Arbor: Health Administration Press, 1980.
13. Donabedian A. The quality of care: How can it be assessed? JAMA 1988;260:1743–1748.
14. O'Leary DS. Deemed status continues to evolve. Joint Commission Perspectives 1990;10(5):2–3.
15. Luft HS, Hunt SS. Evaluating individual hospital quality through outcome statistics. JAMA 1986;255:2780–2784.
16. Schroeder SA. Outcome assessment 70 years later: Are we ready? N Engl J Med 1987;316:160–162.
17. Tarlov AR, Ware JE, Greenfield S, Nelson EC, Perrin E, Zubkoff M. The medical outcomes study: An application of methods for monitoring

the results of medical care. JAMA 1989;262:925–930.

18. Gottlieb LK, Margolis CZ, Schoenbaum SC. Clinical practice guidelines at an HMO: Development and implementation in a quality improvement model. QRB 1990;16:80–86.

19. Crede WB, Hierholzer WJ. Surveillance for quality assessment: III. The critical assessment of quality indicators. Infect Control Hosp Epidemiol 1990;11:197–201.

20. Koska MT. Pilot hospitals' input updates Agenda for Change. Hospitals 1990;64(1):50–54.

21. McGeer A, Crede W, Hierholzer WJ. Surveillance for quality assessment: II. Surveillance for noninfectious processes: Back to basics. Infect Control Hosp Epidemiol 1990;11:36–41.

22. O'Leary DS. Joint Commission begins shrinking *AMH*. Joint Commission Perspectives 1990; 10(4):2–3.

23. Grumet GW. Health care rationing through inconvenience: The third party's secret weapon. N Engl J Med 1989;321:607–611.

24. Weinstein R. SHEA Newsletter. Infect Control Hosp Epidemiol 1990;11:674.

25. Kellie SE, Kelly JT. Medicare peer review organization preprocedure review criteria: An analysis of criteria for three procedures. JAMA 1991; 265:1265–1270.

26. Wennberg JE. Unwanted variations in the rules of practice. JAMA 1991;265:1306–1307.

27. Berwick DM. Continuous improvement as an ideal in health care. N Engl J Med 1989;320:53–56.

28. Laffel G, Blumenthal D. The case for using industrial quality management science in health care organizations. JAMA 1989;262:2869–2873.

29. Fuchsberg G. Managing. *Wall Street Journal*, March 14, 1991:B1.

30. James BC. Quality management for health care delivery. Chicago: The Hospital Research and Education Trust of the American Hospital Association, 1989.

31. Berwick DM. Measuring and maintaining quality in a health maintenance organization. In: Lohr KN, Rettig RA, eds. Quality of Care and Technology Assessment: Report of a forum of the Council on Health Care Technology of the Institute of Medicine. Washington, D.C.: National Academy Press, 1988:34.

32. Deming WE. Out of the crisis. Cambridge, MA: MIT Center for Advanced Engineering Studies, 1982.

33. Lohr KN. Medical practice assessment report: Quality assessment for the health insurance industry. Washington, D.C.: Health Insurance Association of America, 1989.

34. Quality Improvement in Health Care, a Newsletter of the National Demonstration Project on Quality Improvement in Health Care. Brookline, MA: Harvard Community Health Plan, 1989 (premier issue).

35. Ishikawa K. Guide to quality control. White Plains, NY: Kraus International Publications, 1982.

36. McLaughlin CP, Kaluzny AD. Total quality management in health: Making it work. Health Care Manage Rev 1990;15(3):7–14.

37. Koska MT. Case study: Quality improvement in a diversified health center. Hospitals 1990; 64(23):38–39.

38. Re RN, Krousel-Wood MA. How to use continuous quality improvement theory and statistical quality control tools in a multispecialty clinic. QRB 1990;16:391–397.

39. Cleary PD, McNeil BJ. Patient satisfaction as an indicator of quality care. Inquiry 1988;25:25–36.

40. Lohr KN, Schroeder SA. A strategy for quality assurance in Medicare. N Engl J Med 1990;322: 707–712.

41. Joint Commission on Accreditation of Healthcare Organizations. The Joint Commission's Agenda for Change: Stimulating continual improvement in the quality of care, February 1990. Chicago: Joint Commission on Accreditation of Healthcare Organizations, 1990.

42. Joint Commission on Accreditation of Healthcare Organizations. A brief overview of the Joint Commission's "Agenda for Change." Chicago: Joint Commission on Accreditation of Healthcare Organizations, 1987.

43. Anonymous. A leaner *AMH* expected in 1992. Joint Commission Perspectives 1990;10(5):6–7.

44. Joint Commission on Accreditation of Healthcare Organizations. Principles of Organizational and Management Effectiveness for Health Care Organizations, March 1989. Chicago: Joint Commission on Accreditation of Healthcare Organizations, 1989.

45. Carroll JG. Continuous quality improvement and its implications for accreditation standards. Top Health Rec Manag 1991;11(3):27–37.

46. Sabin P. The cost of quality assurance: An exploratory study. Hosp Top 1989;67(6):28–34.

47. Jones L. The cost of a quality assurance program in a university hospital. J Qual Assur 1990; 12(1):26–30.

48. Barnett GO, Winickoff RN, Dorsey JL, Morgan MM, Lurie RS. Quality assurance through automated monitoring and concurrent feedback using a computer-based medical information system. Med Care 1978;16:962–970.

49. Pollack, VE. Computerized medical information system enhances quality assurance: A 10-year experience in chronic maintenance hemodialysis patients. Nephron 1990;54:109–116.

50. Gross PA, Beyt EB, Decker MD, et al. Description of case-mix adjusters by the Severity of Illness Working Group of the Society of Hospital Epidemiologists of America (SHEA). Infect Control Hosp Epidemiol 1988;9:309–316.

51. O'Brien JL. The Hospital Administrator's Guide to Severity Measurement Systems. Chicago: The Hospital Research and Education Trust of the American Hospital Association, 1989.

52. Knaus WA, Zimmerman JE, Wagner DP, et al. APACHE—Acute physiology and chronic health evaluation: A physiologically based classification system. Crit Care Med 1981;9:591–597.

53. Sprouse, MW. A realistic approach for gaining physician support of QA. J Qual Assur 1989; 12(4):12–17.

54. Jencks SF, Daley J, Draper D, Thomas N, Lenhart G, Walker J. Interpreting hospital mortality data:

The role of clinical risk adjustment. JAMA 1988;
260:3611–3616.

55. Daley J, Jencks S, Draper D, Lenhart G, Thomas
N, Walker J. Predicting hospital-associated mortality for Medicare patients: A method for patients with stroke, pneumonia, acute myocardial
infarction, and congestive heart failure. JAMA
1988;260:3617–3624.

56. Kahn KL, Brook RH, Draper D, et al. Interpreting
hospital mortality data: How can we proceed?
JAMA 1988;260:3625–3628.

57. Park RE, Brook RH, Kosecoff J, et al. Explaining
variations in hospital death rates: Randomness,
severity of illness, quality of care. JAMA 1990;
264:484–490.

58. Knauss WA, Wagner DP. Interpretation of hospital mortality rates: The current state of the art.
Mayo Clin Proc 1990;65:1627–1629.

59. Jaffe B. Does quality assurance assure quality?
Surgical Rounds 1990;12(11):13–14.

60. Crede W, Hierholzer WJ. Linking hospital epidemiology and quality assurance: Seasoned concepts in a new role. Infect Control Hosp Epidemiol 1988;9:42–44.

61. Crede W, Hierholzer WJ. Surveillance for quality
assessment: I. Surveillance in infection control:
Success reviewed. Infect Control Hosp Epidemiol
1989;10:470–474.

62. Nettleman MD. Using decision analysis to assess
the quality of quality assurance. Infect Control
Hosp Epidemiol 1990;11:260–262.

63. Caper P. The epidemiologic surveillance of medical care. Am J Public Health 1987;77:669–670.

64. Wenzel RP, Schaffner W. A new affiliation, a new
name, and new directions. Infect Control Hosp
Epidemiol 1988;9:7.

65. Decker MD. Novel applications for hospital epidemiology. Infect Control Hosp Epidemiol 1991;
12:101–102.

Suggested Readings

Berwick DM. Continuous improvement as an ideal in
health care. N Engl J Med 1989;320:53–56.

Deming WE. Out of the crisis. Cambridge, MA: MIT
Center for Advanced Engineering Study, 1982.

Donabedian A. Explorations in Quality Assessment
and Monitoring. Vol. III: The methods and findings
of quality assessment: An illustrated analysis. Ann
Arbor: Health Administration Press, 1980:80–125.

Fromberg R. The Joint Commission guide to quality
assurance. Chicago: The Joint Commission on the
Accreditation of Healthcare Institutions, 1988.

Ishikawa K. Guide to quality control. White Plains,
NY: Kraus International Publications, 1982.

James BC. Quality management for health care delivery. Chicago: The Hospital Research and Education
Trust of the American Hospital Association,
1989.

Joint Commission on Accreditation of Healthcare
Institutions. Primer on Indicator Development and
Application. Chicago: Joint Commission on Ac-
creditation of Healthcare Institutions, 1990.

Juran JM. Juran on planning for quality. New York:
The Free Press (Macmillan), 1988.

Laffel G, Blumenthal D. The case for using industrial
quality management science in health care organizations. JAMA 1989;262:2869–2873.

Spath PL, ed. Innovations in health care quality
measurement. Chicago: American Hospital Association, 1989.

Walton M. ed. The Deming management method.
New York: Dodd, Mead, and Co., 1986.

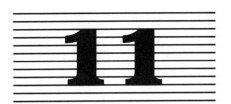

Quality Improvement

Controlling the Risk of Adverse Events

R. Michael Massanari, M.D., M.S.

"It is not a sign of weakness . . . to rise to the level of self-criticism."
Martin Luther King, Jr.

The practice of modern medicine utilizes sophisticated technologies to diagnose and treat disease. Although accomplishments in the ability to cure or palliate both acute and chronic diseases have been remarkable, new technologies are associated with an array of potential complications and adverse outcomes. When making clinical decisions, the physician is obligated to weigh, with the patient, potential risks and benefits of these technological interventions and to select options that maximize benefits and minimize risks. Unfortunately, quantitative estimates of benefits and risks are not readily accessible in the medical literature. Even more elusive, though more pertinent for this decision-making process, are provider-specific estimates of risks and benefits (1). Provider-specific data are almost never available because the practice and methods for producing this information are unfamiliar. Rather, risks and benefits are estimated from "our experience" (heuristic), a method subject to significant bias.

Meanwhile the national agenda for health care in the United States has called for constraints on expenditures for medical care while simultaneously insisting that the quality of care be improved. In the setting of these seemingly divergent objectives, it becomes ever more important to measure the process and outcome of medical care. Objective, provider-specific information describing the benefits and risks of health care would provide monitors for improving the quality of care and provide more objective information for patient-physician decision making.

The purpose of this chapter is to provide an overview of risks associated with medical care and to discuss methods that have been used to assess and prevent these untoward events. The discussion will begin with an overview of adverse outcomes associated with medical care followed by a discussion of ways in which causation for complications of care is assigned or derived. This will be followed by a discussion and critique of methods that have been used to evaluate and control risks associated with medical care. Special emphasis will be devoted to the application of epidemiological techniques to the analysis and prevention of adverse outcomes of care.

THE PROBLEM: ADVERSE OUTCOMES ASSOCIATED WITH MEDICAL CARE

The purpose of this section is to provide a brief overview of the spectrum and frequency of complications and adverse outcomes that are associated with the delivery of acute medical care. For this discussion, the terms complications and adverse outcomes will be used synonymously. There will be no attempt to distinguish iatrogenic from noniatrogenic adverse events. The rationale for this comprehensive approach to the problem will be elaborated later in the discussion.

Summary Estimates of the Risk of Adverse Outcomes Associated with Medical Care

What is the average risk or probability that a patient entering an "average" hospital will experience an untoward event or complication that was not anticipated on admission? Information addressing this question is scant. The most extensive information describes a relatively small subset

of complications of care, nosocomial infections. The SENIC study, completed in 1975, suggested that five of every 100 patients entering a hospital will experience a nosocomial infection (2). Death was directly attributable to this adverse outcome in 1% of patients with nosocomial infections. An extensive literature has been generated during the past three decades that identifies a variety of host, environmental, and provider factors that directly contribute to variation in the patient's risk of nosocomial infection.

Patients may experience a variety of adverse outcomes unrelated to infectious agents. Summary estimates for the risk of noninfectious events are not readily available, however. Table 11.1 provides a synopsis of six articles that report adverse outcomes for hospitalized patients (3–9). Some studies include data from multiple institutions whereas others focused on specific hospitals and specific subspecialty services. Therefore, the sample selection and methods of analysis were different. Except for the study from the Stanford Center for Health Care Research (5) and the New York State Study of Hospitalized Patients (8, 9), study objectives were to

Table 11.1.
Estimates of the Frequency of Adverse Events Associated with Hospitalization

References	Description of Study	Patient Episodes Examined	Description of Event	No. Events	Frequency per 100 Episodes	Associated Mortality[a]
California Medical Association (3)	23 California hospitals	20,864	Iatrogenic injuries	970	4.6	0.4
Stanford Center for Health Care Research	17 hospitals	8,593	Postoperative morbidity and mortality	411	4.8	NA[b]
Brennan et al. (8)	51 New York hospitals	30,121	Adverse events	1,133	3.7	13.6
Schimmel (4)	Medicine service in teaching hospital	1,252	Hazards of hospitalization	240	19.2	1.3
Steel et al. (6)	Medicine service in teaching hospital	815	Iatrogenic illness—major complication	76	9.3	2.0
Couch et al. (7)	Surgical service in teaching hospital	5,612	Errors in surgical care	36	0.6	0.2

[a]Mortality = "case fatality" rate, i.e., number of deaths per 100 events.
[b]Data unavailable.

identify "iatrogenic" disease. It is probable, therefore, that the reported frequency for iatrogenic complications underestimated the overall frequency of adverse events. Nevertheless, these articles suggest that from one to 20 of every 100 hospitalized patients experienced an adverse outcome. Death was associated with the complication in as many as 13% of patients who experienced an untoward event. Finally, the studies described adverse outcomes that were associated with almost every facet of medical care including diagnostic studies, surgical procedures, administration of medications, and nursing care.

A study of a random sample of 31,000 medical records of patients hospitalized in New York State during 1984 provides the most recent and comprehensive analysis of adverse outcomes associated with medical care (8, 9). The definition of adverse events in this study was limited to injuries resulting from medical care, and surveillance was limited to the medical record and its contents. Adverse events occurred in 3.7 per 100 hospitalizations. Substandard medical care was identified in 27.6% of patients who experienced adverse events. The untoward outcomes were associated with permanent disability in 2.6% of cases and with death in 13.6% of cases.

Using concurrent surveillance methods for identifying and analyzing adverse events associated with medical care (program described in detail below), the risk of complications can be estimated across a full compliment of subspecialty services in a 900-bed tertiary care hospital from data gathered over a 1.5-year period. The University of Iowa Hospital and Clinics has approximately 23,000 admissions per year.

During 1989, the overall rate of adverse events was 42.4 per 1000 patient days. This aggregate rate comprised a broad spectrum of events including expressions of dissatisfaction with care. During that same period, the following estimates of risk were noted for major subgroups of adverse events: adverse outcomes associated with medications: 11.0 (range 9–12) events per 1000 patient days: adverse outcomes associated with specific diagnostic or therapeutic procedures: 16.9 (range 16–18) per 1000 patient days; accidents: 3.0 (range 2.5–3.0) per 1000 patient days; and new conditions not present on admission, i.e., pulmonary embolus, stroke: 8.1 (range 7.5–9) per 1000 patient days. Adverse events associated with medications and procedures occurred at rates comparable to institutional rates for nosocomial infections. The incidence of adverse events was greater than that reported in the New York study. This disparity may in part be accounted for by broader definitions for adverse events and by use of concurrent surveillance that included the gathering of information from sources outside the medical record.

Analytical Studies of Specific Adverse Outcomes Associated with Multiple Technologies

Unlike nosocomial infections that have been systematically studied for causation and for effective preventive interventions, noninfectious complications of medical care have received less attention. In several recent studies (10–13), authors have identified a specific adverse outcome for analysis and conducted a retrospective study for these occurrences during hospitalization (Table 11.2). Fisher et al. (11)

Table 11.2.
Illustrative Publications That Describe Specific Adverse Events Associated with Acute Medical Care

Reference	Adverse Occurence	Estimated Frequency
Young and Blass (10)	Nutritional deficiency after gastric surgery	Vitamin B_{12} deficiency, 14–57%; osteomalacia, 5–41%
Fisher et al. (11)	Hypoglycemia	1.8 episodes per 100 admissions
Shusterman et al. (12)	Renal failure	2.0 episodes per 100 admissions
Landefeld et al. (13)	Hemorrhage on anticoagulant therapy	6.0 episodes per 100 treated

examined hypoglycemic events that occurred during hospitalization. As anticipated, hypoglycemia was associated with management of diabetes mellitus; however, hypoglycemia was also associated with treatment of renal failure and/or liver disease. Hospital-acquired acute renal failure was associated with the administration of aminoglycosides, treatment of congestive heart failure, exposure radiocontrast, and shock (12). In addition to describing the frequency of specific complications of medical care, these studies offered insight into the multiple factors that predispose to the adverse outcomes.

Multiple Complications Associated with Specific Medical Technologies

The medical literature is replete with reports of complications associated with specific technologies. For example, in a recent comprehensive review of extracapsular cataract extraction, 89 articles describing more than 50 different complications were published between 1975 and 1990 (14). Similar data exist for a variety of diagnostic and therapeutic technologies. The following selected literature reviews are cited simply to illustrate the magnitude of published information that addresses complications of specific technologies: carotid endarterectomy (15), coronary artery bypass surgery (16), permanent transvenous pacing (17), angiography (18), and anesthesia (19). In addition, there is a large body of literature describing adverse outcomes associated with the administration of specific pharmacologic agents. Two examples are halothane (21) and contrast materials (20). Finally, even routine interventions used to prevent accidents may contribute to adverse outcomes and attendant morbidity and mortality: death has been associated with the use of vest restraints (22); and falls have been associated with the use of bed rails (23).

The extensive literature describing complications of specific procedures and technologies of medical care provide a poignant reminder of the risks to which patients are exposed. However, applica-

tion of these data to specific clinical settings may be limited in several ways. First, the causal relationship between the technology and specific adverse outcomes is not always definitive. For example, clinical trials of new pharmacologic agents not infrequently describe an association between drug and leukopenia or thrombocytopenia without ever establishing clear causal relationships. Second, while clinical data provide estimates of the frequency of complications for specific technologies, the information may not be directly applicable to the practice of the "average" physician in the average hospital. Estimates of the expected frequency of specific adverse outcomes may be derived from controlled studies using a highly selected group of patients (studies of efficacy). These studies may underestimate the risk of adverse outcomes when a technology is practiced in a less selective clinical practice (effectiveness) (1).

Conclusions

Adverse outcomes of medical care are not rare events. Indeed, what information is available describing the overall frequency of noninfectious complications of medical care suggest that, in the aggregate, these events occur at least as frequently as nosocomial infections. Except for nosocomial infections, there have been only a few studies that described and systematically analyzed these events. Most of these studies have focused on events that are associated with potential errors of commission or omission. These data suggest therefore that at least some of the adverse outcomes are preventable. If this assumption is correct, programs dedicated to improving the quality of medical care should include efforts to quantify, monitor, and evaluate adverse outcomes of medical care.

ESTABLISHING CAUSATION FOR ADVERSE OUTCOMES OF MEDICAL CARE

Whether the purpose for evaluating adverse outcomes of medical care is to develop effective interventions and improve the quality of care or to exact retribution and recover losses due to personal injury, causation must be established. There is no universally accepted method for establishing causation. The courts, industry, and scientific communities have employed different methods for determining causation for events or phenomena of interest. The purpose of this section is to discuss methods that have been used to assign causation for adverse events in the medical care environment.

Judicial Methods for Assigning Causation

In ancient Babylon the cause for adverse outcomes following care by a physician was simply ascribed to the operator or physician. Hammurabi's codes established a mechanism whereby patients who were injured or died as a result of a physician's care could exact retribution through remuneration or punishment by amputation of the physician's arm. The codes assume that the injured party's adverse outcome was a direct consequence of errors of commission or omission on the part of the physician.

In the United States and United Kingdom, medical malpractice is assigned to tort rather than to criminal law. Therefore, when negligence is established, the physician is not subject to punishment for the injury. On the other hand, the injured party is entitled to compensation for the injury. Under tort law, responsibility for negligence, i.e., causation, is ascribed in at least two ways.

1. Establishing a Breach in the Standard of Care. The plaintiff, i.e., the injured patient is responsible for establishing that the defendant, i.e., the physician or other provider, was negligent in rendering care. The following steps are necessary to establish causation. First, the plaintiff must establish that a standard of care exists. Second, the plaintiff must prove that there was a breach in the standard of care. Third, the plaintiff must show that the breach in standard of care resulted in the injury. Finally, it must be established that the

plaintiff did, in fact, sustain damages as a result of negligence. Establishing proof for the existence of a standard of care and proof of the defendant's breach of standards requires more than the opinion of the defendant or other lay advocates. Proof for causation is accomplished by obtaining the support of expert witnesses—usually physicians—who render opinions based on implicit evaluations of the case.

2. Res Ipsa Loquitur. To ease the burden of the plaintiff to obtain expert witnesses, the courts may apply the doctrine of *res ipsa loquitur*—"the thing speaks for itself." An example would be surgical amputation of the wrong limb. In this instance, cause of the adverse outcome seems so readily apparent that expert witnesses are unnecessary to establish breach of standards.

But is causation necessarily apparent utilizing court doctrine? Even in the extreme case of res ipsa loquitur, are the causes for an egregious error such as amputation of the wrong limb the independent responsibility of a surgeon's negligence? Perhaps the surgeon was operating unrelieved for 36 hours and was mentally fatigued because of inadequate staffing by the Health Maintenance Organization for whom he worked. This is not stated to excuse this unacceptable outcome. Rather it is to focus attention on all factors that contributed to the adverse outcome. Failure to do so may impugn the surgeon's practice without improving the quality of medical care.

Much of the medical literature describing adverse outcomes of medical care assigns causation based on principles used in tort law. The articles summarized in Table 11.2 report on adverse outcomes that were judged to be consequences of negligence on the part of the provider (3–7). Causation was assigned using the implicit judgment of experts to evaluate the cases, a process not unlike that used in court proceedings. Many "quality assurance" programs continue to use implicit peer review to evaluate the quality of care and assign causation for complications and adverse outcomes (24). The primary objective of these programs is identification of adverse outcomes associated with provider errors and negligence. Recent reports suggest that using explicit methods to review medical records retrospectively one can reliably identify negligent practices (25). However, if the objective is to improve the quality of medical care, is it effective to begin by searching for adverse events that result from negligence? Do these implicit methods provide sufficient objective data to discern the multiple processes that contributed to the adverse outcome? If the focus is only on proximate cause, can one expect to improve the quality of medical care based on these data? Does the threat of punitive action that is associated with these methods inhibit the discovery of information that would facilitate identification of multiple factors that contribute to the adverse outcome?

Scientific Methods for Establishing Causation

An objective, systematic examination of causal factors for events of interest, whether disease or complications of medical care, usually reveals multiple factors that contribute to the outcome. Some factors are directly responsible for the outcome whereas others are indirectly associated with the event of interest. The infectious disease tuberculosis is caused, directly, by the microorganism *Mycobacterium tuberculosis*; however, socioeconomic factors, leading to malnutrition and crowded living conditions, and environmental conditions, such as ventilation systems, contribute indirectly to the probability of acquiring the disease (indirect factors). In addition, there are factors that, by virtue of their simultaneous association with the outcome of interest and with the known causal factors, are inappropriately implicated in causation when, in reality, the factors are unrelated. These factors are designated as confounders. In short, establishing causation for events such as adverse outcomes or complications of medical care may be complex and require sophisticated analyses not afforded by the traditional judicial implicit approach to causation.

The epidemiological method uses scientific principles to analyze diseases in populations in order to determine causal factors and to evaluate the efficacy of interventions (26). The epidemiological technique provides investigators with tools to sort through the multifarious factors associated with diseases such as infections, cancer, and cardiovascular diseases. These same tools have been applied, albeit less vigorously, to issues related to medical care such as adverse outcomes and complications of care.

Because the epidemiological method uses quantitative methods to study and analyze causation, the events of interest must be quantitated. In the case of adverse events or complications of care, one can estimate the "risk" of an event. Epidemiologists measure risks in a variety of ways. Often the risk of an adverse event or complication is described as a proportion (27). The risk of mortality related to a specific surgical procedure is defined as the number of deaths associated with the procedure divided by the total number of persons at risk or the number of persons undergoing the procedure.

$$\frac{\text{Number of operative deaths related to procedure X}}{\text{Total number of patients undergoing procedure X}}$$

A proportion is useful when analyzing the likelihood of adverse outcomes associated with a single, isolated event such as a surgical procedure; however, risk often accrues over time. Therefore, time must be included in estimating the risk of an event (26). The probability of an event occurring over a given period of time may be estimated from the following.

Probability of outcome =
$$1 - e^{(-[\text{mean per person incidence rate} \times \text{time}])}$$

The value in assigning numerical estimates of risk to events such as complications of medical care is to facilitate application of sophisticated statistical tools to sort out the direct causes, indirect causes, and confounders associated with the adverse events of interest.

In the next section, several methods that have been used to study "risks" associated with medical care will be reviewed. The strengths and weaknesses of these methodologies will be discussed in relation to the methodologies used to assign causation that were discussed above.

METHODS FOR EVALUATING AND PREVENTING ADVERSE OUTCOMES ASSOCIATED WITH MEDICAL CARE
Tort Law and Risk Management Programs

Historically, consumers of medical care have had to presume that rendering quality medical care was part of the conscious decision making of all properly trained and licensed professionals. When clinical negligence culminated in severe and permanent injuries, patients could resort to tort law for retribution and recovery of losses. Tort law pertains to rules that govern personal injuries that are not covered under laws of crime or contract.

Under tort law the plaintiff (patient or consumer) recovers for their injury or adverse outcome when they establish that the defendant (the physician or other provider) was negligent in rendering care. Thus, tort law provides the consumer with a legal check against negligent or improper medical care.

Danzon (28) suggests that tort law serves two purposes. First, it provides a form of insurance against losses sustained from medical care. Second, the threat of malpractice serves as a deterrent against future negligence by the medical care provider. As insurance against losses resulting from adverse outcomes, the existing malpractice policies are inefficient and ineffective. Only a small proportion of patients (4%) who sustain injuries as a result of medical care recovered losses through claims under tort law (3). Furthermore, plaintiffs who recover money through the tort system often receive rewards out of proportion to their willingness to purchase insurance. Danzon argues, therefore, that the principal rationale for the malpractice system is as a deterrent to negligence and, thereby, a method for improving the qual-

ity of medical care. The effectiveness of malpractice as a deterrent against negligence depends on establishing that the cost of the adverse outcomes prevented exceeds the overall cost of the existing malpractice system. To date, the effectiveness of the system has never been established. Even if the malpractice system can be shown to pay for itself relative to the adverse events prevented, is a punitive system necessarily the best method for identifying and controlling causes of adverse events? The disincentives created by the malpractice system impede discovery of adverse outcomes, particularly when the provider perceives that error may have contributed to the adverse outcome (29).

Risk management programs were conceived in industry in response to increasing financial losses due to claims of negligence under tort law. The primary objective of the risk management program is to safeguard the financial assets of the institution by reducing the risk of financial loss in matters of negligence (30). This management model for dealing with "risk" was adapted to the health care industry in response to increasing claims of negligence against the profession.

Pursuant to this objective, the traditional risk manager attempted to diffuse ill will that provided the catalyst for ever increasing claims against the profession. This post hoc assessment and management of the incident was often superficial and focused on issues of consent and documentation. Systematic analyses of causal relationships among multiple or recurring incidents was the exception.

To improve discovery and case finding by the risk manager, Craddick (24) developed a method of screening medical records using "indicators of quality." Variations on this methodology have been promoted commercially throughout the United States and, more recently, in the United Kingdom (31). Among the indicators used to identify adverse outcomes are the following: (a) readmissions to the hospital within 15–30 days of discharge from a previous hospitalization, (b) unplanned returns to the operating room, or (c) organ system failure. The underlying assumption is that quality of care contributes directly to the indicator occurrences. However, the utility of the indicators as screening tools for quality of care has never been validated.

In a recent study of readmissions to the University of Iowa Hospital and Clinics, "readmissions within 30 days of discharge" appeared to be an inefficient method for identifying issues related to quality of care. During a 6-month period, 1,965 admissions to surgical services were monitored for adverse outcomes using an epidemiology based program for monitoring adverse outcomes of medical care (32). During this same period, readmissions to the hospital within 30 days of discharge were also monitored. There were 87 readmissions (4.4 per 100 admissions) within 30 days of discharge. Twenty readmissions (23%) were planned, 11 (12.6%) were for reasons unrelated to the index admission, and 47 (54.9%) were associated with the disease that precipitated the initial admission. Only 9 readmissions (10.3%) were associated with issues of quality of care. Concurrent surveillance for adverse outcomes of care identified 221 occurrences among the 1,965 admissions (11.2 occurrences per 100 admissions). Table 11.3 summarizes the findings from this study and describes the utility of the indicator "readmissions within 30 days of dis-

Table 11.3.
Utility of the Indicator "Readmission within 30 Days" for Identifying Adverse Occurrences in Surgical Admissions[a]

		Adverse Occurrences Identified by Surveillance		
		Yes	No	Total
Readmit	Yes	9	78	87
within 30	No	212	1666	1878
days of	Total	221	1744	1965
discharge				

Sensitivity of the indicator = 4.1%
Specificity of the indicator = 95.5%
Positive predictive value = 10.3%

[a]From concurrent surveillance of all admissions (1,965) to a surgical service during a 6-month period.

charge" in terms of sensitivity, specificity, and predictive value positive. With a sensitivity of only 4.1% and predictive value positive of only 10.3%, this indicator was an inefficient tool for identifying issues of quality on surgical services at this 900-bed referral center.

Because considerable resource is expended to support this methodologic approach to risk assessment, these widely accepted indicators should be subjected to similar scrutiny before adopting this method. If other indicators are as inefficient as the foregoing data suggest, considerable resource will be wasted to produce information of limited utility.

Relying on standard risk management methodologies to identify and control risks of adverse outcomes may be subject to other limitations. A primary objective of risk management is to identify "errors" or negligence attributable to the provider. However, only a proportion of all adverse outcomes are directly related to provider negligence (8, 9). To distinguish iatrogenic from noniatrogenic adverse occurrences requires peer review by physicians, a step that is labor intensive and expensive. Furthermore, by excluding adverse outcomes in which there was no apparent provider error precludes a systematic analysis of the multiple factors that contribute to these outcomes and may overlook effective interventions for preventable problems. Although objectives and methodologies in risk management programs continue to evolve, prevention of adverse events has not been a primary concern. The case-by-case retrospective analysis of problems has focused on "damage control." When recommendations for prevention emerged from this process, interventions often focused on factors that contributed to the adverse outcome of a specific case. These interventions were often implemented with little regard to cost and without regard for the multifarious factors that contribute to similar adverse outcomes in other cases. Finally, there has been no documentation to support the efficacy of risk management programs for identifying and/or preventing adverse outcomes of medical care.

Epidemiologic Approach to Adverse Outcomes of Medical Care

Chance and Occurrence of Complications of Medical Care

Adverse outcomes of medical care occur stochastically. That is, when a patient is subjected to a certain procedure or is administered a specific pharmacologic agent, there is a chance that the outcome will not be what the physician and patient anticipated. Rather the patient may experience one or more untoward events. Observing a population of patients undergoing the procedure of interest, one can classify outcomes into one of two simple dichotomies: Patients who experience an adverse outcome vis-à-vis patients who have no untoward effects. By calculating a simple proportion,

$$\frac{\text{Patients experiencing adverse occurrences with treatment X}}{\text{Total number of patients receiving treatment X}}$$

one can estimate the chance or probability or risk of experiencing an adverse occurrence in that population of patients.

The magnitude of the risk of adverse occurrences associated with any specific procedure or technology may vary across populations, i.e., hospitals, physicians' practices, etc. The probability of complications varies because of random (common) variation or because of systematic (special) influences on variation. Random variation describes the usually low level of risk that is inherent in the use or application of any medical technology. For example, the intravenous administration of contrast dyes prior to radiologic studies may be complicated by acute tubular necrosis and renal failure. Even under optimum circumstances, there is a probability, albeit low, that the patient will experience the untoward event. These events appear to occur randomly and, given present state of the art, are unavoidable.

The magnitude of the risk of renal failure following administration of radiocontrast dyes may also vary among different patient groups because of systematic factors. Because of intrinsic renal disease, patients with diabetes mellitus or multiple myeloma are at greater risk for renal failure following administration of contrast dyes. Similarly, the inadvertent administration of excessive quantities of contrast agent, or the concomitant administration of other nephrotoxic agents, or a physician's inappropriate overuse of the procedure may all systematically influence the variation in the magnitude of risk for these respective groups of patients. Some of these factors that systematically increase the probability of renal failure are preventable.

The utility of measuring and quantitating the risk of adverse outcomes is to identify systematic factors that increase the risk of adverse outcomes and to monitor the efficacy of intervention strategies for reducing and controlling these systematic influences. The epidemiologic method provides the tools with which to examine and evaluate these stochastic events among populations of patients.

Nosocomial Infection Control: A Model of the Epidemiologic Approach

The application of population-based analytical techniques to the study of nosocomial infections illustrates the utility of this methodology. Nosocomial infections occur stochastically. Using epidemiological methods to monitor and analyze nosocomial infections, it is possible to estimate the probability that patients will acquire a nosocomial infection. Evidence suggests that at least 33% of infections are preventable (33). On the other hand, a substantial proportion of these untoward events are unpreventable. The latter constitute the random or common variation in risk of nosocomial infections associated with state-of-the-art medical care. Using techniques to monitor rates of nosocomial infection over time and compare observed against expected rates provides a concurrent indicator of potential problems that require further analysis (34). Not only has this methodologic approach to adverse occurrences been remarkably effective in reducing the risk of nosocomial infections, it is also cost-effective (33).

Industrial Models of Quality Improvement

The manufacturing industry has employed similar statistical methods for monitoring manufacturing processes to improve production and the quality of the product. This systematic approach to the study of work has provided the foundation for new models of industrial management (35). Berwick (36) has introduced these industrial technologies to the health care industry. Although the efficacy of this approach for improving the quality of care has not yet been confirmed, it utilizes a methodologic approach that will facilitate ongoing self-appraisals. This methodologic approach to improving the quality of care is discussed in greater detail elsewhere in this text.

Hospital-Specific Mortality Statistics as a Model for Monitoring Quality of Care

In the pursuit of "indicators" of quality of care, health care providers, third party payors, and purchasers of medical care have attempted to identify a small number of outcomes of care that, like nosocomial infections, provide monitors of the quality of care rendered by specific institutions and providers. The outcomes proposed as indicators of quality of care have routinely focused on negative outcomes of medical care. Hospital mortality, readmissions within 15–30 days of discharge, unplanned returns to the operating room, organ system failure, and others have been proposed as outcomes that reflect quality of care.

Hospital mortality, including death within 30 days of discharge, has received the most critical attention as an indicator of quality because of the Health Care Financing Administration's annual publication of hospital mortality rates (37). Based on the stochastic model, it was assumed that mortality rates should be similar across comparable institutions. When mortality rates exceeded expected rates for a specific hospital, systematic or special factors may have contributed to the high rates of complications. Furthermore, it was assumed that where the quality of care was substandard, it would be reflected in higher than expected hospital-specific mortality rates. There are many factors, however, that contribute to (or cause) mortality. To use hospital mortality as a monitor for quality, one must account for these multiple factors that are not subject to management by the provider (38). Otherwise it will be assumed that providers render poor quality care when, in fact, the high mortality rate resulted from variations in case-mix, proportion of patients admitted as emergencies, or proportion of patients over age 70 admitted to the hospital. Unfortunately, even when hospital mortality rates were controlled for multiple factors, quality of care accounted for little of the variation in mortality rates between hospitals (39, 40). In short, to date there is little evidence to validate mortality as a useful monitor of quality of care.

In face of the evidence that mortality rates are relatively poor monitors for quality of care across hospitals, it should not be inferred that mortality does not result from substandard care or that the population-based methodologic approach to evaluating quality is not equal to the task. Mortality as an outcome of poor quality care is probably a rare event, and therefore, systematic variation across hospitals may be insufficient to reflect variations in the quality of care. It may be more productive when monitoring quality of care to focus on morbidity rather than mortality.

Risk Control Program Based on the Epidemiologic Model

The University of Iowa Hospitals and Clinics (UIHC) has a long history of supporting programs dedicated to improving the quality of medical care. As part of its quality assurance program, UIHC supported the development and implementation of a Risk Control Program based on the model of Infection Control Programs.[a]

---

[a]The following individuals participated in the development of the Risk Control Program at University of Iowa Hospitals and Clinics: R. M. Massanari, M.D.; A. Streed, M.S.; K. Wilkerson, M.R.T.; I. E. Curto, M.S.; and S. Powers, R.N.

Based on evidence for the effectiveness of infection control programs, we designed a surveillance program to monitor non-infectious complications and adverse outcomes of medical care using epidemiological techniques (32). This systematic approach to the identification, analysis, and prevention of adverse outcomes of medical care was conceived as one component of a broader program designed to improve the quality of medical care. The following discussion will outline the components of this program.

Purpose and Objectives of the Program

The purpose of this component of the quality improvement program was to improve patient care by minimizing the risks of complications and adverse outcomes associated with acute medical care. Several objectives guided the design and development of the program.

1. Under the assumption that complications (risk of adverse outcomes) occur stochastically and that variation in the frequency of events of interest would provide useful information for studying causation and prevention, epidemiological methods provide the theoretical basis for the program.
2. Distinguishing iatrogenic from noniatrogenic complications of care was purposely avoided. We assumed that for most adverse outcomes there were multiple factors that contributed to the outcome. Avoiding this distinction also improved access to pertinent information required for the analysis of complications and reduced costly implicit analyses by physician peers.
3. The methodologic approach was designed so that a critical analysis of the program itself could be accomplished over time. The surveillance methodology will enable measurement of the efficacy of interventions to prevent adverse outcomes of interest.

Development of Criteria and Definitions of Adverse Outcomes

Apart from the "indicators" of quality cited above (24), there are few standard-ized, explicit definitions for adverse outcomes of care. Therefore, a lexicon of events of interest was developed using definitions derived from the medical literature or developed by the program's authors. The goal was to develop definitions that (a) were explicit, (b) relied on information readily accessible in the medical record, (c) required no additional radiological or laboratory testing, and (d) required a minimum of implicit judgment on the part of the technician.[b]

The events of interest were classified under one of five subsets of adverse outcomes: events associated with the administration of medications, events associated with diagnostic and/or therapeutic procedures, new conditions not present on admission unrelated to medications or procedures, accidents, and patient dissatisfaction.

After drafting the lexicon of adverse outcomes, the document was reviewed, revised, and approved by physician leaders in the institution. This step in the development was important in order to obtain physician ownership in the program.

Surveillance and Data Gathering

Standardized data abstraction forms were developed for use by epidemiology technicians. The abstraction forms included information regarding the specific adverse event along with pertinent demographic descriptive information regarding the patient, time, location, personnel, and circumstances associated with the event. The abstraction form was completed by trained epidemiology technicians when adverse events (defined in the lexicon) were identified. The surveillance was conducted simultaneous with surveillance for nosocomial infections, utilization review, and other quality of care parameters. Data from completed abstract forms were entered into a software program especially designed to support the Risk Control Program (32).

Epidemiology technicians obtained data

---

[b]Copies of the lexicon may be obtained by writing the author.

from three primary sources: (*a*) the clinical nursing specialist in charge of the patient care unit, (*b*) the medical record, and (*c*) incident reports. Although the ultimate objective was to eliminate passive reporting of adverse events via incident reports, for some units the incident report was the best source of information regarding adverse occurrences associated with the administration of medications.

Data Analysis and Reporting

Information describing complications and adverse outcomes of medical care were reported in the aggregate by clinical service and by patient care unit. Future goals include reporting selected information by specific procedure and by specific practitioner. Several different descriptive statistics expressed as rates, proportions, or ratios were used to report information to medical care providers and managers (see Table 11.4). In order to facilitate interpretation of these reports, confidence intervals based on data from the previous 12 months was included in tables or figures (see Figures 11.1–11.3). Thus, the individual reviewing these reports could quickly determine whether the risk of events for a specific time period was above, below, or consistent with previous experience.

An optional report that listed specific adverse events and pertinent descriptive

Table 11.4.
Descriptive Statistics for Estimating Risks of Complications and Adverse Occurrences

Procedure-related occurrences:

$$\frac{\text{No. specific procedure-related occurrences}}{\text{Total no. procedures performed}}$$

Medication-related occurrences:

$$\frac{\text{No. medication-related occurrences}}{10,000 \text{ doses administered}}$$

Accidents or new conditions acquired during hospitalization:

$$\frac{\text{No. occurrences}}{1,000 \text{ patient days}}$$

$$\frac{\text{No. occurrences}}{100 \text{ admissions}}$$

data can be provided on request. The goal of the periodic report was to provide clinicians and managerial personnel with pertinent trended information (run charts) that would be useful for developing and evaluating policies related to quality improvement. Figures 11.1–11.3 illustrate anonymous data describing rates of adverse outcomes associated with surgical procedures, medications, and accidents. Each figure illustrates the variation in adverse events that was observed over time or across patient care units. Further analysis of the procedure-related events in Figure 11.1 resulted in the identification of a specific complication associated with a specific surgical procedure. The contributing factor responsible for the complication was identified, and the operative procedure was changed to eliminate the factor responsible for the complication. Without surveillance for this specific adverse event among multiple patients, it is unlikely that this problem would have been identified and corrected.

Figure 11.2 summarizes data on patient falls for 1 year and illustrates striking variation in the frequency of falls across different patient care units. Comparing variations in frequencies of occurrences across patient care units must be done with caution since differences may reflect intrinsic predisposing factors among patient populations rather than differences in practice or quality of care. Further analysis of these data revealed that patients on unit F were at higher risk for falls because of underlying illnesses and use of central nervous system depressants. Nevertheless, a review of these aggregate data by nursing services focused attention on this potentially preventable problem and provided a catalyst for developing intervention strategies on units where rates were high. Follow-up unit-specific trended data will enable the providers to evaluate the efficacy of the interventions to prevent falls.

Evaluation of the Program

The Risk Control Program has been operational at the University of Iowa for 2 years. Because it is a new model without precedent, the program has required refinements during this developmental phase. It is too early to draw inferences regarding the effi-

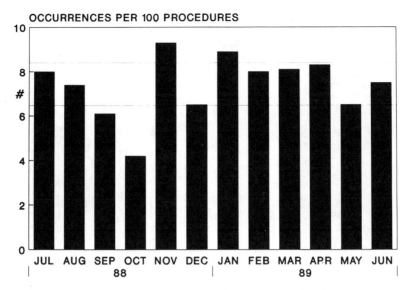

Figure 11.1.   Illustration of the variation in rates of procedure-related adverse occurrences over time on a subspecialty surgical service. The data summarize 196 occurrences in 2655 patients. #, 95% confidence intervals (6.4, 8.4).

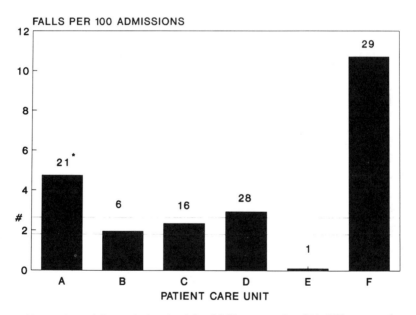

Figure 11.2.   Illustration of the variation in risk of falls across six of 39 different patient care units. The data are derived from surveillance over 8 months during which 354 falls occurred among 16,091 admissions to the institution. *, number of falls; #, 95% confidence intervals (1.97, 2.42).

cacy of this program for improving quality of care. However, several preliminary observations suggest that the model may prove effective and be applicable to other institutions. First, the surveillance program has identified several preventable complica-

tions associated with medical care. Second, the data base has facilitated analytical studies that have been helpful in identifying causal relationships. Third, the program has provided long-term follow-up for one moderately expensive intervention and provid-

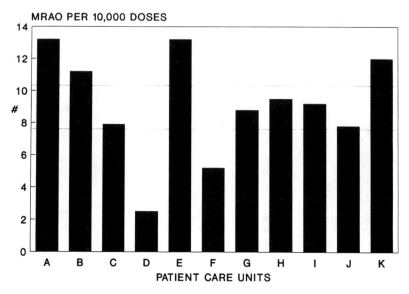

Figure 11.3.   Illustration of the variation in risk of medication-related adverse occurrences across 11 separate patient care units. The data are derived from surveillance over 3 months during which 204,502 doses were administered in 14,627 days at risk. MRAO, medication-related adverse occurrences; #, 95% confidence intervals (7.8, 10.2).

ed evidence for the efficacy of that intervention. Finally, the information that has been generated by the program will facilitate compliance with external mandates for monitoring clinical indicators. Monitoring and reporting hospital-specific data on selected indicators is part of the Joint Commission for Accreditation of Health Care Organizations' new program for quality improvement.

Methods for Investigating Rare Adverse Events Associated with Medical Care

There are some adverse events associated with medical care that occur only rarely but with disastrous results. Massive hemolytic blood reactions following transfusion of whole blood products are now rare events due to sophisticated laboratory techniques for typing blood products and to elaborate protocols assuring proper identification of donor blood and recipients. Preventable mortality as an adverse outcome of medical care probably falls into the category of rare events or accidents also.

To await the accumulation of sufficient data from multiple events before analysis and implementation of preventive strategies would be indefensible. On the other hand, simple assignment of proximate cause using customary risk management techniques may overlook important events that contributed to these rare but disastrous outcomes.

Investigators of fatal accidents such as airline accidents and industrial accidents have developed systematic processes for analyses of single events. Early approaches to investigations of accidents are illustrated by the aviation industry's "fly-fix-fly" approach. The investigative process was basically retrospective in that experts attempted to identify specific causes for that accident, intervene, and await the next accident to identify additional causal factors. With the recognition that accidents are processes and not the result of single events, new analytic approaches have been developed for evaluating these untoward events (41). Since an accident is a culmination of multiple prior events, the investigator attempts to identify causal factors (actors) responsible for each of the linear events preceding the accident. The individual linear processes are then arranged in chronological sequence. This stepwise reconstruction of events leading to the accident facilitates a more thorough analysis of the multiple factors that contributed to the adverse outcome.

It is not apparent that this systematic analysis of rare events has been applied to the health care profession. Surveillance for "sentinel events" or adverse outcomes associated with significant morbidity or mortality has been advocated. However, processes for analyzing these untoward outcomes and methods for generating useful information with which to develop intervention strategies are not routinely provided. This engineering approach to process analysis may provide a useful tool for health care providers charged with evaluating and improving the quality of medical care.

CONCLUSIONS

Despite remarkable advances in modern medical care, a patient entering the health care system is exposed to significant risks of complications and adverse occurrences. Recent studies suggest that adverse events occurred in 3.7% of hospitalizations and that 27% were related to negligence on the part of the provider. Apart from nosocomial infections, adverse events associated with medical care have received little systematic attention from health care providers.

The consumer's only recourse to assure quality and minimize risks in the system was through tort law and claims of malpractice. Although there is little evidence to substantiate the effectiveness of tort law for assuring quality medical care, a burgeoning legal and insurance industry has emerged in support of these policies. In response to increasing numbers and costs of malpractice claims and in response to external mandates to improve quality of medical care, the health care industry has committed resources to evaluating quality of care. However, many existing "quality assurance" programs utilize methods that have evolved from tort theories of causa-

tion and have been based on individual case analyses. There is no evidence that traditional quality assurance/risk management programs have positively influenced quality of care.

Under the assumption that complications or adverse outcomes of medical care occur stochastically, it is possible to estimate probabilities or risks of occurrences of interest and to study variations in risk for causal relationships with established scientific methods. Application of epidemiologic methods to the study of nosocomial infections provides a well-established model for improving the quality of medical care that is both effective and cost-effective. Preliminary observations from one institution in which epidemiologic methods have been used to monitor and evaluate noninfectious adverse occurrences suggest that this model may be applicable to other facets of quality improvement.

References

1. Brook RH, Park RE, Chassin MR, Kosecoff J, Keesey J, Solomon DH. Carotid endarterectomy for elderly patients: Predicting complications. Ann Intern Med 1990;113:747–753.
2. Haley RW, Culver DH, White JW, et al. The nationwide nosocomial infection rate: A new need for vital statistics. Am J Epidemiol 1985; 121:159–167.
3. California Medical Association. Report of the medical insurance feasibility study. San Francisco: California Medical Association, 1977.
4. Schimmel EM. The hazards of hospitalization. Ann Intern Med 1964;60:100–110.
5. Stanford Center for Health Care Research. Comparison of hospitals with regard to outcomes of surgery. Health Serv Res 1976;11:112–127.
6. Steel K, Gertman PM, Crescenzi C, Anderson J. Iatrogenic illness on a general medical service at a university hospital. N Engl J Med 1981;304:638–642.
7. Couch NP, Tilney NL, Rayner AA, Moore FD. The high cost of low-frequency events: The anatomy and economics of surgical mishaps. N Engl J Med 1981;304:634–637.
8. Brennan TA, Leape LL, Laird NM, Hebert L, Localio AR, Lawthers AG, et al. Incidence of adverse events and negligence in hospitalized patients. N Engl J Med 1991;324:370–376.
9. Leape LL, Brennan TA, Laird N, Lawthers AG, Localio AR, Barnes BA, et al. The nature of adverse events in hospitalized patients. N Engl J Med 1991;324:377–384.
10. Young RC, Blass JP. Iatrogenic nutritional deficiencies. Annu Rev Nutr 1982;2:201–227.

11. Fisher KF, Lees JA, Newman JH. Hypoglycemia in hospitalized patients. N Engl J Med 1986; 315:1245–1250.

12. Shusterman N, Strom BL, Murray TG, Morrison G, West SL, Maislin G. Risk factors and outcome of hospital-acquired acute renal failure. Am J Med 1987;83:65–71.

13. Landefeld CF, McGuire E, Rosenblatt MW.. A bleeding risk index for estimating the probability of major bleeding in hospitalized patients starting anticoagulant therapy. Am J Med 1990;89:569–578.

14. Massanari RM, Hilborne L, Wakefield DS, Carter C, Tobacman J. Cataract surgery: A review of the literature regarding efficacy and risks. RAND, 1991, in press.

15. Merrick NF, Fink A, Brook RH, Park RE, Kosecoff J, Roth CP, et al. Indications for selected medical and surgical procedures—A literature review and ratings of appropriateness: Carotid endarterectomy. RAND (R-3204) 1986.

16. Chassin MR, Park RE, Fink A, Rauchman S, Keesey J, Brook RH. Indications for selected medical and surgical procedures—A literature review and ratings of appropriateness: Coronary artery bypass graft surgery. RAND (R-3204) 1986.

17. Phibbs B, Marriott HJL. Complications of permanent transvenous pacing. N Engl J Med 1985; 312:1428–1431.

18. Hessel SJ, Adams DF, Abrams HL. Complications of angiography. Radiology 1981;138:273–281.

19. ECRI Technology Assessment. Deaths during general anesthesia. J Health Care Technol 1985; 1:155–175.

20. Parfey PS, Griffiths SM, Barrett BJ, Paul MD, Genge M, Withers J, et al. Contrast material-induced renal failure in patients with diabetes mellitus, renal insufficiency, or both. N Engl J Med 1989;320:143–149.

21. Farrell G, Prendergast D, Murray M. Halothane hepatitis. N Engl J Med 1985;313:1310–1314.

22. Dube AH, Mitchell EK. Accidental strangulation from vest restraints. JAMA 1986;256:2725–2726.

23. Rubenstein HF, Miller FH, Postel S, Evans HB. Standards of medical care based on consensus rather than evidence: The case of routine bed rail use for elderly. Law, Medicine and Health Care 1983;11:271–276.

24. Craddick JW. The medical management analysis system. QRB 1979;5:2–8.

25. Brennan TA, Localio AR, Leape LL, Laird N, Peterson L, Hiatt HH, Barnes BA. Identification of adverse events occurring during hospitalization. Ann Intern Med 1990;112:221–226.

26. Kelsey JL, Thompson WD, Evans AS. Methods in observational epidemiology. New York: Oxford University Press, 1986.

27. Feinstein AR. Clinical epidemiology. Philadelphia: WB Saunders, 1985.

28. Danzon PM. Medical malpractice. Cambridge, MA: Harvard University Press, 1985.

29. Fagerhaugh SY, Strauss A, Wiener CL. Hazards in hospital care. San Francisco: Jossey-Bass Publishers, 1987.

30. Rail R. Financial and risk management in hospitals. In: Troyer GT, Salman SL. Handbook of healthcare risk management. Rockville, MD: Aspen, 1986.

31. Bennett J, Walshe K. Occurrence screening as a method of audit. Br Med J 1990;300:1248–1251.

32. Streed SA, Massanari RM. Data management system for evaluating complications of health care. Proceedings of the Twelfth Annual Symposium on Computer Applications in Medical Care. 1988 (November):874–876.

33. Haley RW, Culver DH, White JW, Morgan WM, Emori TG, Munn VP, Hooton TM. The efficacy of infection surveillance and control programs in preventing nosocomial infections in U.S. hospitals. Am J Epidemiol 1985;121:182–203.

34. Morrison AJ, Kaiser DL, Wenzel RP. A measurement of the efficacy of nosocomial infection control using the 95 per cent confidence interval for infection rates. Am J Epidemiol 1987;126:292–297.

35. Deming WE. Out of crisis. Boston: Massachussetts Institute of Technology Center for Advanced Engineering Study, 1986.

36. Berwick DM. Continuous improvement as an ideal in health care. N Engl J Med 1989;320:53–56.

37. Medicare Hospital Mortality Information 1986. Washington, D.C.: United States Department of Health and Human Services, 1987.

38. Dubois RW, Rogers WH, Moxley JH, et al. Hospital inpatient mortality: Is it a predictor of quality? N Engl J Med 1987;317:1674–1680.

39. Park RE, Brook RH, Kosecoff J, Keesey J, Rubenstein L, Keeler E, et al. Explaining variations in hospital death rates. JAMA 1990;264:484–490.

40. Jessee WF, Schranz CM. Medicare mortality rates and hospital quality: Are they related? Quality Assurance Health Care 1990;2:137–144.

41. Hendrick K, Benner L. Investigating accidents with STEP. New York: Marcel Dekker, 1987.

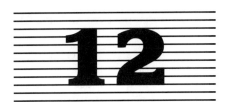

Ethical Issues in Measuring Quality Care

Robert F. Weir, Ph.D.

Concern over the ethical issues involved in measuring quality care has greatly increased in recent years. As medical science has become more specialized and medical technology more complicated, many persons inside and outside medicine have raised questions about the ethical costs of these advances. Indicative of this concern has been the development over the past 20 years of the field of biomedical ethics and the practice of clinical ethics consultations in many hospitals.

Likewise, as journalists, attorneys, judges, and politicians have increasingly focused the public's attention on problematic hospital cases and practices, many persons inside and outside hospitals have become skeptical about the quality of care that is available in hospitals. They have also raised questions about the multiple factors that influence the decisions that physicians, patients, and hospital administrators make about medical care in these institutional settings. Indicative of this concern has been the rapid growth of the fields of health law and health care economics over the past two decades.

The first three parts of this chapter will describe a number of the efforts in recent years to address ethical issues in measuring and ensuring quality medical care, with those efforts being made at the federal, state, and institutional levels. The last part of the chapter will focus on the ethical aspects of measuring quality care in indi-

vidual hospital cases. Along the way it will become clear that the ethical issues involved are of fundamental importance, because medical care delivered at a suboptimal level of ethical quality in hospitals means that crucial patient-care decisions are being made for the wrong reasons or by the wrong people with the wrong results, namely the prolonged illnesses or deaths of patients who would otherwise live healthier and longer lives.

ETHICS OF QUALITY CARE AT THE FEDERAL LEVEL

Several efforts have been made over the past two decades at the federal level to address ethical issues in quality care. Some of the efforts have focused on quality care for the subjects of medical research, with special attention being given to the ethical aspects of experimentation with fetuses, young children, prisoners, and mentally ill patients. Other efforts have centered on quality care for patients in hospital settings, especially for patients who are nonautonomous and thus unable to make their own health care decisions.

The National Commission (1974–1978)

For many years after World War II, Americans could feel self-righteous when thinking about the medical experiments performed in the German concentration camps. Even if the Nazis had been willing to perform a wide range of unethical experiments on human subjects, it was comforting to believe that harmful experiments would not be performed on unknowing and unconsenting humans by American researchers.

These feelings of moral superiority began to be challenged in the mid-1960s. Henry Beecher (1), among others, clearly demonstrated that in the post-Nuremberg era blatantly unethical research had been done and was continuing to be done by medical researchers in this country. An influential book by Jay Katz in the early 1970s (2) confirmed the extent of the problem. Perhaps most influential of all were the journalistic accounts of the infamous Tuskegee experiment, a research project conducted by the United States Public Health Service from 1932 to 1972 to track the course of untreated syphilis among approximately 600 poor, uneducated black men in Tuskegee, AL. The absence of quality care in this experiment is best illustrated by the fact that the men were neither informed about nor given penicillin after it became available in the 1940s.

In response to the growing ethical concern about research subjects, the Department of Health, Education, and Welfare (DHEW) published its first set of proposed regulations for DHEW grants in 1973 and its final set of regulations for research with human subjects in 1974. In July 1974, Congress responded to the continuing ethical concern by passing the National Research Act, which established the National Commission for the Protection of Human Subjects of Biomedical and Behavioral Research. The Congressional mandate to the Commission was threefold: (*a*) to identify the basic ethical principles that should underlie research involving human subjects, (*b*) to develop ethical guidelines for the research, and (*c*) to make recommendations to the DHEW Secretary regarding appropriate administrative action (3).

Formation of the National Commission was an unprecedented step by the federal government to examine the ethical aspects

of measuring quality care in the context of medical research with human subjects. In most respects, the Commission's work was monumental. Comprised of 11 commissioners from diverse professional backgrounds, the Commission's most obvious contributions to the improvement of quality care in research contexts were through its analysis of the basic ethical principles for medical research with human subjects, its published reports on research with children and other vulnerable patient groups, and its recommendation that institutional review boards (IRBs) be established to review all research proposals seeking federal funds for biomedical or behavioral research with human subjects (4–9).

Less obvious contributions of the Commission are also important for an understanding of the ethical issues involved in measuring and ensuring quality care. First, the Commission described at some length three of the fundamental ethical principles that apply to medical research and medical practice: respect for personal autonomy, beneficence, and justice (10). In the years since the Commission's work concluded in 1978, these ethical principles—along with the principle of nonmaleficence—have dominated discussions in this country about the ethical conduct of medical research and medical practice. Simply put, these principles help to define what quality care is.

Second, the Commission established new parameters around quality care by describing what quality care is not. In contrast to many earlier research practices, the Commission described quality care in the research context as not performing experiments apart from those for which a human subject's informed and voluntary consent was obtained, not doing research on human subjects apart from an assessment of the possible harms of the research to the experimental subject, and not doing funded research apart from an objective review by an IRB. As a consequence of the Commission's work, many types of research with human subjects done in earlier years are no longer done in this country, because they violate our Commission-influenced standards of quality care for research subjects.

The President's Commission (1980–1983)

Numerous ethical problems in medical practice during the late-1960s and 1970s required serious, sustained thought on the part of physicians, other health professionals, and reflective persons outside medical and health care fields. Unprecedented ethical problems having to do with organ transplantation, kidney dialysis, and mechanical ventilation forced health professionals working in hospitals to raise questions about how the advances of medical technology were to be managed, how scarce medical resources were to be allocated, and how death was to be defined in the age of modern medicine. Outside hospital settings, the news media carried stories (e.g., the Karen Ann Quinlan case) about the life-and-death decisions made in hospitals, and many state legislatures passed new statutes that attempted to build neurological criteria into updated definitions of death.

Given these developments, considerable uncertainty was created about what quality care meant in medical cases involving critically ill or terminally ill patients. For example, did quality care mean that ventilator-dependent patients could not be removed from the ventilators, or did quality care mean that mechanical ventilation could be discontinued in certain types of clinical cases? Did quality care mean that patients were to be defined as being alive or dead based on traditional cardiopulmonary criteria, or on criteria for neocortical function, or on criteria for whole-brain activity?

In terms of legal developments, the efforts by many state legislatures to update their definition-of-death statutes resulted in a patchwork assortment of state laws. Model statutes were proposed by individual authors, the American Bar Association, the American Medical Association, and the National Conference of Commissioners on Uniform State Laws. Some states retained their traditional definitions of death based on the absence of spontaneous cardiopulmonary activity, other states passed significantly different brain-death statutes, and others passed such idiosyncratic laws that

their application to clinical cases was difficult to fathom (11).

In response to these medical, ethical, and legal problems, another federal commission was created, this one being established in 1978 during the Carter administration. The President's Commission for the Study of Ethical Problems in Medicine and Biomedical and Behavioral Research began its work in 1980 and continued until early in 1983. The Commission was chaired by Morris Abrams, a law professor, and it consisted of 10 persons representing multiple professional fields. The Commission's staff was directed by Alexander Capron, also a law professor, and it consisted of physicians, attorneys in health law, philosophers, and professionals from other appropriate fields.

The President's Commission was another effort by the federal government to examine the ethical aspects of measuring and ensuring quality care, this time with the focus more on clinical practice than on medical research. If anything, the work of the President's Commission surpassed the earlier work of the National Commission in design, organization, and influence. The President's Commission held public hearings throughout the country, commissioned a number of research studies and reports, and published nine reports on some of the most pressing medical, ethical, and legal issues of the early 1980s.

Four of the reports of the President's Commission are particularly important for their emphasis on ethical issues related to quality care. In *Defining Death*, the Commission examined differing philosophical perspectives on the meaning of death, published medical guidelines for the clinical determination of death, and recommended nationwide adoption of the Uniform Determination of Death Act (12). In *Securing Access to Health Care*, the Commission emphasized that society has an ethical obligation to ensure all of its citizens equitable access to health care (13). In *Screening and Counseling for Genetic Conditions*, the Commission argued that genetic screening and counseling programs should be assessed in terms of their promotion of patient autonomy, confidentiality, and equity (14). In its most controversial and influential report, *Deciding to Forgo Life-Sustaining Treatment*, the Commission emphasized the importance of placing ethical and legal limits on the medical prolongation of life, recommended that hospitals establish institutional ethics committees as advisory groups for especially difficult cases, and set forth an ethical framework for limiting life-sustaining treatment in some cases involving disabled neonates and patients with permanent loss of consciousness (15).

In addition to the importance of these reports, the President's Commission itself represented an important, even if time-limited, commitment by the federal government to try to provide guidance on some of the tough ethical problems in medical practice. By its very existence, the Commission symbolized a recognition on the part of the federal government that some of the ethical issues involved in providing quality care are national in scope and are best addressed through a process of consensus decision making by a multidisciplinary body. Unfortunately, the politicization of some of the issues in recent years has made the establishment of a similar group for the late-1980s and 1990s an elusive goal.

Regulations for Neonatal Medicine (1983, 1985)

Ethical concern at the federal level over quality care in the nation's hospitals took a different turn during the Reagan administration. With the leadership of Surgeon General C. Everett Koop, a pediatric surgeon, the administration took unprecedented steps to define, measure, and ensure quality care for premature and disabled newborns in neonatal intensive care units (NICUs).

Although concern had been expressed by many persons for years about decisions not to treat some babies with life-threatening conditions, most of the debate about quality care for premature and disabled neonates had been restricted to hospitals and the professional literature. Only a few cases (e.g., the Johns Hopkins Hospital case of an infant with Down syndrome) had received publicity, and only a few

others (e.g., the Baby Boy Houle case in Maine) had involved court decisions (16).

The birth of a baby in Bloomington, IN, in April 1982, changed this situation dramatically. Known publicly only as "Baby Doe," the infant had Down syndrome plus esophageal atresia with tracheoesophageal fistula. When the national media gave the case wide publicity, the parents' decision to allow the baby to die without surgical and medical treatment struck many persons, including some persons in the Reagan administration, as being an egregious denial of quality care. Surgeon General Koop and the Department of Health and Human Services (DHHS) decided to take steps that would mandate the provision of life-sustaining treatment in virtually all neonatal cases, thus preventing the unnecessary deaths of other mentally retarded or physically disabled infants in any of the nation's hospitals.

The result was the publication of three successive versions of federal regulations in March 1983, July 1983, and January 1984. Known as the "Baby Doe" regulations, these rules for defining and ensuring quality care for neonates were an enactment into federal policy of a very conservative ethical position, namely that all newborns who are neither dying nor permanently unconscious should have their lives sustained with medical treatment without considerations being given to the extremity of their prematurity, the severity of their medical conditions, or the projected future quality of their lives.

The "final rules" of January 1984 had a straightforward measurement of quality care for neonates: quality care meant life-sustaining treatment for virtually all newborns, and decisions to abate life-sustaining treatment in cases of nondying neonates were interpreted as acts of discrimination against handicapped infants that were prohibited by law (based on an interpretation of the 1973 Rehabilitation Act that was subsequently ruled invalid by the United States Supreme Court). The final version of these regulations stated that hospitals receiving federal funds were obligated to post warning signs in public places regarding the selective nontreatment of infants and to provide immediate federal access to patient records (17).

A second set of federal regulations for quality care in NICUs was published in April 1985. Known as the ''child abuse'' regulations, these rules represent a policy implementation of the Child Abuse Amendments signed into law in October 1984. The core of the regulations is a legal definition of quality care in the specific circumstances of decisions to provide life-sustaining treatment or to abate life-sustaining treatment while caring for premature or disabled neonates. The regulations state the following:

The term ''withholding of medically indicated treatment'' means the failure to respond to the infant's life-threatening conditions by providing treatment (including appropriate nutrition, hydration, and medication) which, in the treating physician's (or physicians') reasonable medical judgment, will be most likely to be effective in ameliorating or correcting all such conditions, except that the term does not include the failure to provide treatment (other than appropriate nutrition, hydration, or medication) to an infant when, in the treating physician's (or physicians') reasonable medical judgment, any of the following circumstances apply: (1) The infant is chronically and irreversibly comatose. (2) The provision of such treatment would merely prolong dying, not be effective in ameliorating or correcting all of the infant's life-threatening conditions, or otherwise be futile in terms of the survival of the infant. (3) The provision of such treatment would be virtually futile in terms of the survival of the infant and the treatment itself under such circumstances would be inhumane (18).

Again, quality care is defined as providing life-sustaining treatment for all neonates who are neither dying nor permanently unconscious, with no considerations being given to whether that treatment is wanted by a baby's parents or is in the baby's best interests. Variations from this standard of quality care are interpreted as forms of child abuse instead of discrimination, with the possibility that physicians and parents who make decisions to abate life-sustaining treatment in a manner contrary to this policy

may be reported to state child protection agencies for further investigation.

ETHICS OF QUALITY CARE AT THE STATE LEVEL

Efforts have also been made at the state level to measure and ensure quality medical care, especially when that medical care concerns critically or terminally ill patients, the allocation of scarce medical resources, surrogate decision making for nonautonomous patients, and patients who have contracted infectious diseases that pose unusually serious threats to other persons inside and outside medical settings. In a few states, concern over ethical issues in the delivery of quality care has resulted in state-funded, multidisciplinary commissions and task forces, such as the New Jersey Bioethics Commission, the New York State Task Force on Life and the Law, the Massachusetts Task Force on Organ Transplantation, the Oregon Health Services Commission, and the Cook County (Illinois) State's Attorney's Task Force on the Foregoing of Life-Sustaining Treatment.

More commonly, states have addressed some of the ethical issues in controversial areas of medical care through their judicial systems and legislative bodies. In this manner, some of the ethical issues have been interpreted as matters of state law, with the result that many state courts have made decisions and many legislatures passed laws that now significantly influence how quality care from a legal perspective can be practiced in hospitals.

State Courts and Quality Care

The dramatic changes in medical technology and medical practice in the last two decades have been paralleled by a significant growth in the importance of the legal aspects of medicine. Although most of the media attention has been given to medical malpractice cases and the increasing animosity between the medical and legal professions, many of the medical cases that have gone to court in recent years have concerned matters other than malpractice. Often the medical cases that have been litigated have pertained to ethical and legal questions about quality care in hospitals. Does quality care, in some cases, include decisions to abate life-sustaining treatment by discontinuing mechanical ventilation or stopping technologically supplied nutrition and hydration? Does quality care, in some cases, involve supporting a pregnant woman's refusal of medical treatment for herself, even if that treatment is also necessary to preserve the life or health of her fetus? Does quality care, in some cases, mean treating a disabled neonate or critically ill child over the parents' objections? Does quality care, in some cases, require courses of action that are contrary to hospital policy?

The largest body of court decisions at the state level has involved the ethical issue of abating life-sustaining treatment with critically ill patients (19). The early cases in this body of case law confronted the ethical and legal aspects of providing life-sustaining treatment to adult Jehovah's Witness patients who refused the treatment on the basis of their religious beliefs (20–23). Other cases have dealt with other autonomous patients who refused surgery, chemotherapy, kidney dialysis, mechanical ventilation, and technological feeding (24–30). Most of the cases in this series have concerned difficult ethical and legal questions about discontinuing mechanical ventilation or technological feeding (31–49). One of these cases, the Missouri case of Nancy Cruzan, was appealed to the United States Supreme Court and became the first right-to-die case decided at the highest federal level (50).

The clear trends in these state court decisions provide helpful guidance regarding the ethics of quality care, as well as the legal parameters for quality care in hospitals. These courts are unanimous in saying that quality care includes the recognition by physicians and others that autonomous patients have a moral and legal right to refuse medical treatment, including medical treatment that is life-sustaining in nature. With the notable exception of the Cruzan decision in Missouri (49), the courts are in agreement that the surrogate of a nonautonomous patient is the most

qualified person to make a decision on the patient's behalf either to consent to or to refuse recommended medical treatment. Again, with the exception of the Missouri court, the courts are convinced that technological feeding is neither morally nor legally different from other life-sustaining technologies, that surrogates of nonautonomous patients should base their decisions on the known preferences of the patients or on an assessment of the patients' best interests, and that withdrawing life-sustaining treatment is neither morally nor legally different from withholding such treatment. In addition, the courts agree that physicians who abate life-sustaining treatment in accordance with a patient's preferences or best interests are not guilty of assisting a suicide or any other legally prohibited action.

State Legislatures and Quality Care

Most state legislatures have enacted numerous statutes that have bearing on both the ethical and legal aspects of quality care: abortion laws, homicide laws, informed consent laws, assisted-suicide laws, confidentiality laws, required reporting laws, and so forth. In recent years, however, two new areas of legislative action that impact on quality care have received unusual attention. Both of the areas of legislative action so markedly help to define and measure quality care in medical settings that they have elicited considerable lobbying activity on the part of state medical societies and activist groups of concerned citizens.

One of these areas of statutory law is commonly called natural death legislation. The first natural death act was passed in California in 1976 (51). Since that time, 41 other states and the District of Columbia have passed such legislation, with the individual laws being titled "Natural Death Acts," "Living Will Acts," "Death with Dignity Acts," and so on. No two of these legislative statutes are exactly alike, but they have many similar features, such as a definition of the medical circumstances (usually diagnosis of a terminal condition by two physicians) necessary for a person to qualify under the law, a declaration form that may be signed to indicate a person's preferences about medical treatment, a provision of immunity from civil or criminal liability for physicians who comply with a patient's stated wishes, and a requirement that a physician unable to follow those wishes transfer the care of the patient to another physician who will. The common theme to these various statutes is the ethical and legal view that autonomous persons should have the final word in defining and measuring what quality care means for them, especially during the terminal phase of their lives.

The second important area of statutory law is legislation concerning quality care for persons with human immunodeficiency virus (HIV) infection. All 50 states and the District of Columbia have passed legislation requiring physicians to report new cases of acquired immunodeficiency syndrome (AIDS), and over half of the states require the reporting of persons (by name, in many states) who have positive HIV antibody tests (52).

Given the undeniable seriousness of the disease, the risk of infection by health professionals and others, and the problem of discrimination against persons having AIDS, state legislatures have collectively considered hundreds of AIDS-related bills in recent years (53). Many, though certainly not all, of the resulting AIDS-related statutes have pertained to ethical issues in providing quality care for patients who are HIV positive or have AIDS, for the health professionals who give them medical and nursing care, and for other persons who may unknowingly be at risk for AIDS because of sexual activity or intravenous drug use (54).

ETHICS OF QUALITY CARE IN HOSPITALS

As discussed at some length by the authors of other chapters, federal and state regulations influence on a daily basis how quality care is defined and measured in hospitals. Many of these regulations con-

cern ethical aspects of quality care, especially those having to do with the moral and legal rights of hospital patients, patient-physician relationships, standards of medical care, payment and referral policies, informed consent, confidentiality and privacy, the limits placed on medical research with patients, the roles of surrogate decision makers, and so on (55).

At times the ethics of quality care in hospitals is directly influenced and changed by the policies and recommendations put forth by agencies of the federal government. Several relatively recent practices in hospitals provide examples: the use of consent documents for surgical procedures and many medical interventions, the use of diagnosis-related groups (DRGs) for accounting purposes, and the use of do-not-resuscitate (DNR) policies for decisions made by patients or their surrogates to forgo efforts at resuscitation. In a similar manner, the ethics of quality care in hospitals can be and sometimes is directly influenced by changes in state laws and policies, as illustrated by recent controversies in some hospitals over the impact of AIDS-related legislation on the confidentiality of patient information and the occasional need to breach confidentiality to protect other persons at risk of infection.

The ethics of quality care in hospitals is also being changed by actions taken by an increasing number of hospital administrators and hospital boards, with no federal or state agency requiring that the changes be made. Recognizing that ethical issues pertaining to quality care need to be addressed in a regular, systematic manner, many hospitals have in recent years established hospital ethics committees and/or begun to use ethics consultants for help with problematic cases.

Hospital Ethics Committees

The roots of the movement in the 1980s to establish hospital ethics committees (HECs) involve earlier efforts during the 1960s and 1970s to deal with especially difficult medical cases. The first such committee was established in a Seattle hospital in the 1960s to make allocation decisions regarding the use of kidney dialysis machines by patients with chronic kidney disease. This committee, called the "God committee" by the media, was composed of physicians, members of the hospital staff, and persons not affiliated with the hospital. With the scarcity of dialysis machines in the 1960s, the committee's task was to select the few patients who would actually receive hemodialysis from the much larger group of medically qualified persons in need of the treatment.

Given the negative publicity engendered by the committee and the subsequent decision by the federal government in 1972 to fund all treatment for end-stage renal disease, few if any hospitals followed the Seattle model of a multidisciplinary, decision-making committee connected with a dialysis program. Then in 1975, Karen Teel, a pediatrician, proposed in a law review article that a multidisciplinary committee—which she called an "ethics committee"—might have other purposes. She suggested that such committees might occasionally help physicians in a number of clinical areas to make "ethical judgments which we are sometimes ill-equipped to make." In her view, a committee "composed of physicians, social workers, attorneys, and theologians" would, in an advisory role, provide a "regular forum" for dialogue on difficult cases and thereby provide "safeguards for patients and their medical caretakers" (56).

This proposal received unusual attention the following year when the New Jersey Supreme Court adopted portions of the proposal in the court's landmark decision in the Karen Ann Quinlan case. In an attempt to have an appropriate procedure that would protect the interests of the permanently unconscious patient in the case, the court mandated the concurrence of four parties—Quinlan's family, her father in his role as guardian, her attending physicians, and a hospital "ethics committee"—before she could be removed from the ventilator believed to be sustaining her life. The court noted that the most appealing factor in the suggestion of a committee "seems to us to be the diffusion of professional responsibility for decision, comparable in a way to the value of multi-judge courts in finally resolving on appeal difficult questions of law" (31).

Some hospitals, especially in New Jersey and later in Washington, adopted the *Quinlan* court's model for an ethics committee, at least in cases involving the termination of life-sustaining treatment. In so doing, however, these hospitals did not actually establish *ethics* committees. Instead, following the court's recommendation, what they really established were *prognosis* committees, composed exclusively of physicians whose single purpose was that of confirming a prognosis made earlier by physicians in a particular case.

In 1983 the President's Commission included an analysis of ethics committees in its report on the termination of life-sustaining treatment. It had previously sponsored a national study of HECs, a 1981 study that found such committees in less than 1% of all hospitals and in 4% of hospitals having over 200 beds (57). Even with that meager number of committees in place, the President's Commission regarded multidisciplinary HECs as being potentially important—precisely because they might help to define, measure, and ensure quality care.

While emphasizing that "the responsibility for ensuring that decisionmaking practices of high quality falls first to the attending physician," the Commission suggested that hospitals consider establishing multidisciplinary ethics committees that could function in an advisory role to promote more effective decision making, especially in cases involving patients who lack the capacity to make health care decisions themselves. To the Commission, such committees, even if problematic in several ways, seemed a reasonable way of promoting quality care in hospitals through educational efforts, policy recommendations, and consultation on problematic cases (15).

That same year the American Academy of Pediatrics (AAP), in response to the first version of the Baby Doe regulations, proposed that hospitals establish Infant Bioethics Committees (IBCs). Submitted to the DHHS in July 1983, the AAP proposal specified that an IBC should be composed of at least eight members: a physician, a hospital administrator, an ethicist, an attorney, a disability specialist, a nurse, a member of the hospital's medical staff, and a lay community member. The establishment of pediatrics ethics committees would, according to the AAP, help to ensure quality care and make unnecessary the intrusive governmental steps proposed in the DHHS regulations (58).

The final version of the Baby Doe regulations (January 1984) contained the federal government's proposal for pediatrics ethics committees. Specifically responding to the AAP proposal, the DHHS recommended that hospitals establish Infant Care Review Committees (ICRCs). The following year the DHHS repeated its recommendation, in the child abuse regulations, that hospitals establish ICRCs to help define, measure, and ensure quality care for premature and disabled infants.

As a consequence of these widely publicized cases, reports, and recommendations, many hospitals established HECs during the 1980s to carry out educational activities, propose hospital policies for problematic aspects of patient care, and consult on difficult cases. Some hospitals also established more specialized ethics committees for particular clinical areas, such as NICUs. A survey in 1985 indicated that approximately 50% of the nation's hospitals had established HECs (59). Another survey, conducted by the AAP in 1986, suggested that approximately 60% of hospitals had HECs (60).

In addition, an extensive body of literature has been produced on HECs (61–66). So many hospitals were establishing HECs and so much was being published on HECs that the Hastings Center, a center for the study of ethical issues in medicine, put together a "core resources" collection of materials on HECs in 1988, established a National Advisory Council on Ethics Committees, and began publishing a regular "Ethics Committees" feature as part of its journal, the *Hastings Center Report* (67). Now a separate journal, the *HEC Forum*, is being published to explore the ethical and legal issues being taken to HECs throughout the country (68). These issues are also regularly discussed in ethics committee networks that have been established in a number of places, including Michigan, Minnesota, Colorado, the Delaware Val-

ley, Kansas City, and the Minneapolis-St. Paul area.

Perhaps the best indication of the role that HECs can play in measuring and ensuring quality care is a case that brought a torrent of bad publicity to Rush-Presbyterian Hospital in Chicago, a hospital not yet having an ethics committee. The case involved Sammy Linares, a young child in a persistent vegetative state whose father finally resorted to using a handgun to force the medical staff to allow the boy to die apart from mechanical ventilation. Norman Fost, a pediatrician at the University of Wisconsin, later observed that Rush-Presbyterian is "part of a shrinking minority of hospitals in America that does not have an institutional ethics committee to help resolve ethical and legal dilemmas." He observed that an HEC could have helped in the case by reducing the possibility of a negligence action, clarifying the legal situation, and advising the medical staff to "do the right thing" (60).

Ethics Consultation in Hospitals

The use of clinical ethicists (or ethics consultants) is a related effort by some hospitals to address the ethical issues in providing quality care. Not required by the federal government, state governments, or the Joint Commission on the Accreditation of Healthcare Organizations (JCAHO), the expansion of consulting services in some hospitals to include professionals in clinical ethics is a move by these hospitals to encourage physicians, other health professionals, patients, and the surrogates of patients to consider the ethical aspects of clinical cases as an intrinsically important part of good medical practice. The administrators of these hospitals also anticipate that, by having clinical ethicists work with the medical staff and patients on problematic cases, the number of subsequent lawsuits by patients or their families may also be diminished.

Although some ethicists employed by colleges of medicine or university hospitals had begun to do ethics consultations in the early 1980s, the beginnings of a more formalized approach to clinical ethics consultation took place at an NIH-sponsored conference in 1985. This conference, the First National Conference on Ethics Consultation in Health Care, involved approximately 50 professionals invited from a number of universities and hospitals. Illustrating the diversity in the field of clinical ethics, a typical participant at the conference could have had a Ph.D. in philosophy or religious studies, an M.D., an R.N., a J.D., or some combination of these degrees.

By the early 1990s, the interdisciplinary field of clinical ethics has expanded and grown in importance. Most persons in the field belong to the Society for Bioethics Consultation, a multidisciplinary professional organization founded in 1987 and now having its national headquarters in Chicago. The literature on ethics consultations in hospitals has grown dramatically (69–73). Perhaps the best indication of the development of the field is the debate among clinical ethicists themselves regarding the possible need for a licensing or credentialing process, in order to protect hospitals, physicians, and patients from being harmed by uninformed and inadequately trained ethics consultants.

ETHICS OF QUALITY CARE IN INDIVIDUAL CASES

Physicians and other health professionals are motivated and trained to provide quality care that promotes the well-being of their patients. By following the ancient principle of beneficence, physicians and other health professionals adhere to an ethical principle that requires moral agents to advance the important interests of other persons whenever their own proximity, abilities, and efficient alternatives allow them to do so with only minimal risk to themselves.

However, the quality of the care provided in individual cases does not depend solely on the motivation, training, or intentions of the physicians and other health professionals in the case. The patient also has a vitally important role to play, since he or she has the moral and legal right of either consenting to or refusing the medi-

cal treatment recommended by the physician(s) in the case. The ethical principle of respect for autonomy emphasizes the importance of defining and measuring quality care from the perspective of the patient, as well as from the various assessments of quality care by more objective indicators, because, after all, the possibilities of restored health, or at least improved health, or further deterioration of health, or suffering without relief, or the possible end of one's existence are intensely personal matters to the patient.

The ethical principle of justice, which formally calls for the equitable handling of similar (nonmedical) cases, has an important role in helping to define and measure quality care in individual cases. This principle reinforces the principles of beneficence and respect for autonomy by requiring, in most instances, that all autonomous patients be given equal access to the level of available, potentially beneficial medical care they need and desire.

The principle of justice also applies to cases involving nonautonomous patients, regardless of the medical reasons for the lack of autonomy. In these cases the principle of justice supplements the principle of respect for autonomy by requiring that all nonautonomous patients be given equal access (through their surrogates) to similarly beneficial medical care, unless the available treatment is regarded by objective observers as being contrary to an individual patient's best interests. In addition, in cases involving scarce medical resources or requests by patients or surrogates for medically futile treatment, the principle of justice sometimes tempers the principles of beneficence and respect for autonomy by providing the ethical and legal basis for overriding the choices of autonomous patients.

A fourth ethical principle, the principle of nonmaleficence, plays a role in defining and measuring quality care by occasionally placing limits on decisions and actions based on the principle of beneficence. Long associated with the maxim primum non nocere ("above all, do no harm"), the principle of nonmaleficence requires that physicals and other moral agents avoid intentionally or negligently harming other persons. The principle therefore calls on physicians, patients, other health professionals, and the surrogates of nonautonomous patients to assess in individual cases whether the treatment being provided is proving to be beneficial to the patient or whether, on balance, the treatment is producing more burdens than benefits to the patient.

Ethical Analysis of Individual Cases

Questions remain, even with this theoretical analysis of principles, about the ethics of quality care in individual cases. How is it possible to determine the ethically appropriate course of action in a given clinical case? How can the ethics of quality care be compared from one case to another?

Even to raise such questions is problematic, at least for some people. Given the diverse but frequently held notions that moral judgments are relative to individual persons and cultures, that morality and legality are basically the same thing, that ethics is "soft," and that views on matters pertaining to ethics have no more weight than personal opinions, anyone suggesting that individual clinical cases are subject to ethical analysis should be prepared for skepticism.

Let me, therefore, be clear about the claim I am making. I am not claiming that every case has a single "right" way of being handled from the standpoint of clinical ethics, nor am I asserting that the ethics of quality care in individual cases can be discerned only by someone with professional training in ethics. What I am claiming is twofold: (a) all clinical cases have ethical aspects that vary in importance from case to case, and (b) the quality of care in individual cases is improved when the physician(s) and other health professionals are alert to the ethical dimensions of the cases and make informed decisions in relation to these dimensions of the cases.

The use of an "ethics construct" or "ethics work-up" is helpful in analyzing the ethical aspects of cases. One of the first published constructs for analyzing the eth-ical dimensions of cases is, unfortunately, too theoretical to be of much practical use (74). Others are less theoretical, but err in the direction of oversimplifying the complexity of some clinical cases (75, 76).

In my view, the ethical analysis of individual cases is best done with a clinical ethics construct that has seven steps. Step 1 involves identifying the significant medical factors in the case. Examples of medical factors that can be ethically significant include the patient's age, medical history, diagnosis, autonomous status or decision-making capacity, emotional stability, and prognosis with and without treatment.

Step 2 pertains to identifying the significant personal and social factors related to the patient and to the patient's health care. Such factors as the patient's values, religious beliefs, attitudes (e.g., about medical care, physicians, personal responsibility for health care, suffering, health care costs), family situation, and previously expressed preferences (if the patient now lacks autonomy) can be very important in deciding the appropriate course of action in a particular case.

Step 3 focuses on identifying the ethical issue(s) or problem(s) raised by the case. Sometimes ethics consultations in individual cases involve no major problem, but only an individual physician's uncertainty about an ethical aspect (and, not infrequently, a legal or economic aspect) of the case. Other cases involve one or more exceedingly difficult problems that test the analytical skills, knowledge, understanding, and patience of all the parties to the case.

Step 4 consists of identifying the ethical principles involved in the case. The most theoretical aspect of case analysis, this step calls for an explanation of why the principles of beneficence, respect for autonomy, justice, and/or nonmaleficence are relevant to the case. In addition, in some cases step 4 requires an analysis of precisely how some medical interventions can be regarded as beneficial and how others can, on balance, constitute harm to certain patients.

Step 5 involves the identification of alternative courses of action in a case. Depending on the case in question, alternatives might include acting on the basis of an autonomous patient's values and preferences, or according to the medical goal(s) applicable to the case, or on a course determined by an assessment of a nonautonomous patient's best interests. Additional alternatives in many cases would be represented by considerations of the personal values and beliefs of the physicians and other health professionals in the case, the interests of relevant third parties (e.g., family members, hospital administrators, third-party payers), and the law.

Steps 6 and 7 represent the two-part culmination of the case analysis: the identification of the best course of action and an explanation and justification of that decision. Reflective of the medical uncertainty in some clinical cases, the conclusion regarding the appropriate course of action is sometimes difficult to make—with reasonable people occasionally disagreeing about which course of action is preferable.

Nevertheless, this approach to case analysis increases the possibility that ethically appropriate, quality care will characterize individual hospital cases. Moreover, this kind of approach to individual cases allows informed participants to compare the ethics of quality care from one case to another.

The Patient's-Best-Interests Standard

Another approach to individual cases supplements the clinical ethics construct just described and also allows for comparisons to be made about the quality of care in different cases. This approach involves analyzing the variables that constitute the patient's-best-interests (PBI) standard and applying the relevant variables to individual cases, especially cases having patients who lack autonomy because of young age, dementia, brain damage, permanent unconsciousness, or some other reason.

Rather than being merely a slogan common to the practice of medicine, the PBI standard consists of several variables that are helpful in making decisions about treatment options in individual cases. When combined with the clinical ethics construct described above, this standard

for decision making provides important content that helps to define and measure quality care from case to case. The standard is especially helpful in clinical cases involving difficult decisions about initiating, continuing, or abating life-sustaining treatment.

When used in the ethical analysis of cases having adolescent or adult patients with life-threatening conditions, the PBI standard consists of eight variables that can be framed as questions:

1. How severe is the patient's medical condition?
2. What are the chances of correcting or reversing the patient's medical condition with treatment?
3. Can the most important medical goals in the case be achieved?
4. Does the patient have serious neurological impairments that influence decisions about treatments?
5. Does the patient seem to have unrelieved pain?
6. Is the patient experiencing significant physical and/or psychological suffering?
7. Does the patient find life under the present or projected future medical circumstances to be intolerable?
8. What is the proportionality of treatment-related benefits and burdens to the patient? (19)

The last variable pertaining to a determination of a patient's best interests is, in many respects, a summation of the other variables. For the patient, the patient's surrogate (if the patient is nonautonomous), and the patient's physician, a consideration of the benefits of a particular medical intervention to the patient as well as the burdens of that intervention to the patient is the essential point for determining whether administering the treatment or abating the treatment is in the patient's best interests. In making such an assessment, the decision maker(s) arrive at a subjective judgment that includes objective factors, but is not finally reducible to computer printouts, statistical data, or any other quantifiable information.

In the end, a judgment regarding the proportionality of treatment-related benefits and burdens to the patient is a moral judgment. As such, this moral judgment is an important part of an ethical analysis of quality care in individual clinical cases.

References

1. Beecher HK. Ethics and clinical research. N Engl J Med 1966;274:1354–1360.
2. Katz J. Experimentation with human beings. New York: Russell Sage Foundation, 1972.
3. Levine RJ. Ethics and regulation of clinical research. 2d ed. Baltimore and Munich: Urban & Schwarzenberg, 1986:xi–xii.
4. National Commission for the Protection of Human Subjects of Biomedical and Behavioral Research. Research on the fetus: Report and recommendations. Department of Health, Education, and Welfare Publication No. (OS) 76-127, Washington, D.C., 1975.
5. National Commission for the Protection of Human Subjects of Biomedical and Behavioral Research. Research involving prisoners: Report and recommendations. Department of Health, Education, and Welfare Publication No. (OS) 76-131, Washington, D.C., 1976.
6. National Commission for the Protection of Human Subjects of Biomedical and Behavioral Research. Research involving children: Report and recommendations. Department of Health, Education, and Welfare Publication No. (OS) 77-0004, Washington, D.C., 1977.
7. National Commission for the Protection of Human Subjects of Biomedical and Behavioral Research. Institutional review boards: Report and recommendations. Department of Health, Education, and Welfare Publication No. (OS) 78-0008, Washington, D.C., 1978.
8. National Commission for the Protection of Human Subjects of Biomedical and Behavioral Research. Ethical guidelines for the delivery of health services: Report and recommendations. Department of Health, Education, and Welfare Publication No. (OS) 78-0010, Washington, D.C., 1978.
9. National Commission for the Protection of Human Subjects of Biomedical and Behavioral Research. Research involving those institutionalized as mentally infirm: Report and recommendations. Department of Health, Education, and Welfare Publication No. (OS) 78-0006, Washington, D.C., 1978.
10. National Commission for the Protection of Human Subjects of Biomedical and Behavioral Research. The Belmont Report: Ethical principles and guidelines for the protection of human subjects of research. Department of Health, Education, and Welfare Publication No. (OS) 78-0012, Washington, D.C., 1978.
11. Weir RF, ed. Ethical issues in death and dying. 2nd ed. New York: Columbia University Press, 1986:53–58.
12. President's Commission for the Study of Ethical Problems in Medicine and Biomedical and Behavioral Research. Defining death. Washington, D.C.: United States Government Printing Office, 1981.
13. President's Commission for the Study of Ethical Problems in Medicine and Biomedical and Behavioral Research. Securing access to health care. Washington, D.C.: United States Government Printing Office, 1983.
14. President's Commission for the Study of Ethical Problems in Medicine and Biomedical and Behavioral Research. Screening and counseling for genetic conditions. Washington, D.C.: United States Government Printing Office, 1983.
15. President's Commission for the Study of Ethical Problems in Medicine and Biomedical and Behavioral Research. Deciding to forgo life-sustaining treatment. Washington, D.C.: United States Government Printing Office, 1983.
16. Weir RF. Selective nontreatment of handicapped newborns. New York: Oxford University Press, 1984.
17. Federal Register. January 12, 1984:1624–1635.
18. Federal Register. April 15, 1985:14888–14897.
19. Weir RF. Abating treatment with critically ill patients. New York: Oxford University Press, 1989.
20. Application of the President and Directors of Georgetown College, Inc., 331 F.2d 1000 (1964).
21. In re Brooks' Estate, 32 Ill.2d 361, 205 N.E.2d 435 (1965).
22. John F. Kennedy Memorial Hospital v. Heston, 58 N.J. 576, 279 A.2d 670 (1971).
23. In re Osborne, 294 A.2d 372 (D.C. App. 1972).
24. Lane v. Candura, 6 Mass.App.Ct. 377, 376 N.E.2d 1232 (1978).
25. Commissioner of Corrections v. Myers, 399 N.E.2d 452 (Mass. 1979).
26. Satz v. Perlmutter, 362 So.2d 160, aff'd, 379 So.2d 359 (Fla. 1980).
27. Bouvia v. Superior Court, 179 Cal.App.3d 1127, 225 Cal. Rptr. 297 (Cal. App. 2d Dist. 1986).
28. In re Requena, 213 N.J.Super. 475, 517 A.2d 886, aff'd, 517 A.2d 869 (Super. Ct. App. Div. 1986).
29. In re Rodas, No. 86PR139 (Colo. Dist. Ct. Mesa County, January 22, 1987).
30. In re Farrell, 108 N.J. 335, 529 A.2d 404 (1987).
31. In re Quinlan, 137 N.J. Super. 227, 348 A.2d 801, modified and remanded, 70 N.J. 10, 355 A.2d 647 (1976).
32. Superintendent of Belchertown State School v. Saikewicz, 373 Mass. 728, 370 N.E.2d 417 (1977).
33. In re Spring, 380 Mass. 629, 405 N.E.2d 115 (1980).
34. Severns v. Wilmington Medical Center, Inc., 421 A.2d 1334 (Del. 1980).
35. In re Eichner, 102 Misc.2d 184, 423 N.Y.S.2d 580, modified sub nom, Eichner v. Dillon, 73 A.D.2d 431, modified, 420 N.E.2d 64 (1981).
36. In re Colyer, 99 Wash.2d 114, 660 P.2d 738 (1983).
37. Barber v. Superior Court, 147 Cal.App.2d 1006, 195 Cal.Rptr. 484 (1983).
38. Leach v. Akron General Medical Center, 68 Ohio Misc. 1, 426 N.E.2d 809 (1980).
39. In re Hier, 18 Mass. 200, 464 N.E.2d 959 (1984).
40. John F. Kennedy Memorial Hospital, Inc. v. Bludworth, 452 So.2d 921 (Fla. 1984).
41. In re Conroy, 98 N.J. 321, 486 A.2d 1209 (1985).

42. In re Jobes, 108 N.J. 394, 529 A.2d 434 (1987).
43. Corbett v. D'Alessandro, 487 So.2d 368 (Fla. 1986).
44. Brophy v. New England Sinai Hospital, Inc., 398 Mass. 417, 497 N.E.2d 626 (1986).
45. In re Peter 108 N.J. 365, 529 A.2d 419 (1987).
46. In re Gardner, 534 A.2d 947 (Maine 1987).
47. In re Drabick, 200 Cal.App.3d 185, 245 Cal.Rptr. 840 (1988).
48. In re Westchester County Medical Center, 72 N.Y.2d 517, 534 N.Y.S.2d 886, 531 N.E.2d 607 (1988).
49. Cruzan v. Harmon, 760 S.W.2d 408 (Mo. 1988).
50. Cruzan v. Director, Missouri Department of Health, 1990 U.S. LEXIS 3301 (U.S. June 25, 1990).
51. California Natural Death Act, Calif. Health and Safety Code 7185-7195 (1976).
52. Centers for Disease Control. HIV infection reporting—United States. JAMA 1989;262:889–890.
53. Gostin LO, Ziegler A. A review of AIDS-related legislative and regulatory policy in the United States. Law, Medicine and Health Care 1987;15:5–16.
54. Gostin LO, ed. AIDS and the health care system. New Haven: Yale University Press, 1990.
55. Annas GJ. The rights of patients. 2d ed. Carbondale, IL: Southern Illinois University Press, 1989.
56. Teel K. The physician's dilemma—A doctor's view: What the law should be. Baylor Law Review 1975;27:6–9.
57. Youngner SJ, Jackson DL, Coulton C, et al. A national survey of hospital ethics committees. Crit Care Med 1983;11:902–905.
58. Infant Bioethics Task Force and Consultants. Guidelines for infant bioethics committees. Pediatrics 1984;74:306–310.
59. Anonymous. Ethics committees double since 83: Survey. Hospitals 1985;59:60–64.
60. Fost N. Do the right thing: Samuel Linares and defensive law. Law, Medicine and Health Care 1989;17:330–334.
61. Cranford RE, Doudera AE, eds. Institutional ethics committees and health care decision making. Ann Arbor: Health Administration Press, 1984.
62. Ross JW, Bayley C, Michel V, et al. Handbook for hospital ethics committees. Chicago: American Hospital Association, 1986.
63. Cranford RE, Hester FA, Ashley BZ. Institutional ethics committees: Issues of confidentiality and immunity. Law, Medicine and Health Care 1985;13:52–60.
64. Fost N, Cranford RE. Hospital ethics committees: Administrative aspects. JAMA 1985;253:2687–2692.
65. Lo B. Behind closed doors: Promises and pitfalls of ethics committees. N Engl J Med 1987;317:46–50.
66. Weir RF. Pediatric ethics committees: Ethical advisers or legal watchdogs? Law, Medicine and Health Care 1987;15:99–109.
67. Cohen CB. Ethics committees. Hastings Center Report 1988;18:11–14.
68. Spicker SF. Editor's introduction and announcement. Hospital Ethics Committee Forum 1989; 1:233–236.
69. Purtilo R. Ethics consultations in the hospital. N Engl J Med 1984;311:983–986.
70. Self DJ, Skeel JD. Potential roles of the medical ethicist in the clinical setting. Theor Med 1986; 7:33–39.
71. Pellegrino ED. Clinical ethics: Biomedical ethics at the bedside. JAMA 1988;260:837–839.
72. La Puma J, Stocking CB, Silverstein MD, et al. An ethics consultation service in a teaching hospital: Utilization and evaluation. JAMA 1988;260:808–811.
73. Fletcher JC, Quist N, Jonsen AR, eds. Ethics consultation in health care. Ann Arbor: Health Administration Press, 1989.
74. Thomasma D. Training in medical ethics: An ethical work-up. Forum on Medicine 1978;1:33–36.
75. Purtilo RB, Cassell CC. Ethical dimensions in the health professions. Philadelphia: WB Saunders, 1981.
76. Jonsen AR, Siegler M, Winslade WJ. Clinical ethics. 2d ed. New York: Macmillan, 1986.

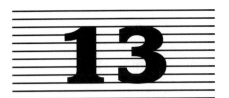

13

Small Area Variations, Practice Style, and Quality of Care

Noralou P. Roos, Ph.D., and Leslie L. Roos, Ph.D.

Traditionally, medicine has been oriented toward care for the individual patient. Using their knowledge base, physicians are seen to intervene to cure or ameliorate the diagnosed illness. Given a choice of treatments, the one most suitable for the patient is selected. This logical model of medical practice implies a tight linkage between needs, interventions, and outcomes, which is radically inconsistent with the results of extensive research on patterns of medical care utilization in Canada, North America, and Western Europe. It suggests a degree of precision in both diagnosis and therapy, a knowledge of patient needs and of effective responses, which is beyond the capabilities of individual practitioners and of the health professions collectively. The blunt reality is that little hard evidence is available to evaluate the effectiveness of many medical acts and procedures, within or outside of the acute care sector, including the commonplace, the high tech, the expensive, and the new.

In the absence of such evidence, opinions within the medical profession differ widely both as to how conditions should be diagnosed and how they should be treated when diagnosed. Patterns of practice vary widely. Amid the resulting diversity, patients of particular physicians or in particular regions might sometimes not receive interventions that would likely do them more good than harm. Patients of other physicians in other regions may receive treatment that would be judged inappropriate or unnecessary if subjected to critical peer review. In short, there can be no basis for a general claim that "more is better," when intervention patterns vary so markedly from region to region, hospital to hospital, physician to physician, and when hard evidence of benefit is so often lacking.

Our description of medical practice, which will be documented by a wide range of evidence, will disconcert many readers. This review is not meant as an exposé. No fingers are pointed nor witch-hunts suggested. Physicians' decision making is influenced by a number of factors, including the psychological dynamics and uncertainty surrounding the short- and long-term consequences of different treatment alternatives.

UNCERTAINTY AND VARIATION
Uncertainty Permeates Medical Practices

Deviations from a logical model of medical practice may be caused by uncertainty

(1). Such a model predicts that, when uncertainty is reduced or eliminated, the forces producing practice variation will greatly diminish. Eddy (1) has described both the uncertainties surrounding how conditions are diagnosed in the first place and how they are treated once diagnosed. For example, in the diagnosis of disease, the line between normal and abnormal findings is often unclear. Many signs and symptoms are common, and knowing which will require treatment is difficult to determine. When two (or three) physicians see the same signs, symptoms, x-rays, or other test results, they are likely to interpret them differently (2, 3).

A similar set of problems surrounds the decision on how to treat diseases once they are diagnosed. For any given patient, a wide variety of procedures "can be ordered in any order and at any time;" the list of procedures that *might* be included in a workup of a patient presenting with chest pain or hypertension could easily take more than a page (1). Even choices between major treatments are by no means obvious. Kassirer and Pauker (4) found that a significant number of clinical problems referred to their division of clinical decision making at Tufts-New England Medical Center for consultation were essentially "tossups." The differences in expected outcomes among the alternative treatments were so small that they were not clinically relevant.

This uncertainty in medical practice revolves around established as well as new and relatively untested areas of medicine. Vayda et al. (5) focused on five common procedures (including cholecystectomy, inguinal herniorrhaphy, hysterectomy, cesarean section, tonsillectomy and adeniodectomy, and colectomy), developing a series of hypothetical cases describing patients. These case histories were mailed to Ontario physicians who were asked to recommend treatment to the patients as described. Recommendations made for every case showed substantial disagreement; for example, 65% of the physicians recommended cesarean section in one case whereas 35% said they would not perform a cesarean on that woman.

Physician consensus panels have also drawn on experts to define the "state of the art" in medical practice. The lack of consensus over appropriate medical treatment in the most common of situations is striking. For example, in a panel examining the appropriateness of various indications for bypass surgery, initial levels of *agreement* among the nine physician panel members ranged from 12.2 to 22.2%, depending upon how stringent the criteria for agreement were. After 2 days of panel discussion, the agreement levels improved somewhat; but, even using the least strict definition of consensus, panel members failed to agree on more than half of the indications for bypass surgery (58.8%) (6).

Not surprisingly, physicians fail to agree on indications for specific procedures because of the substantial uncertainties about the effectiveness of these procedures. Eddy (1) has described a meeting of experts in colorectal cancer detection, all of whom were very familiar with the diagnostic occult fecal blood test and most of whom had participated in two prior meetings on cancer detection. Physicians were asked, "What is the overall reduction in colorectal cancer incidence and mortality that could be expected if men and women over the age of 50 were tested with fecal occult blood tests and 60-cm flexible sigmoidoscopy every year?" The answer to this question is obviously central to estimating the value of fecal occult blood testing. Physician responses as to the value of this test ranged from its being useless to its being capable of wiping out the disease. When these results were communicated to those attending the conference, the physicians "had no idea that they had such differences of opinion" (1).

Uncertainty also permeates medical knowledge about outcomes of even the most common of procedures. When patients are observed over long periods of time after treatment, they typically experience more adverse outcomes than the literature suggests. Thus, although a workshop convened by the National Institutes of Health suggested that following transurethral prostatectomy "the need for further operative treatment is uncommon" (7), the cumulative probability at 8 years of having a second operation was found to be

20.2% (8). When treatments diffuse outside of large hospitals (the site of most evaluations but not where most care is delivered), the outcomes are usually worse (8–10).

Variations and Practice Style

Population-based estimates of health care use (regardless of where the care is received) have been developed to compare usage across countries (11, 12), across states (13, 14), and across smaller hospital service areas (15, 16). These variations occur across all age groups—from children (17), through middle aged (18), to the elderly (13). The implications of these variations have been highlighted in several ways. Using the surgical rates to calculate lifetime probabilities of organ loss, Gittelsohn and Wennberg (19) estimated that in the early 1970s the chances of a Vermont child reaching age 20 with tonsils in place ranged from 40 to 90%, depending on community of residence. If the United States' expenditures on seven common surgical procedures (hysterectomy, tonsillectomy, etc.) were based on the rates of low hospital service areas of Vermont and Maine, the costs were estimated to be $2.4 billion while the bill based on the high-use areas of these two states would be $6.6 billion—in 1975 dollars (20).

Although a number of factors can influence these patterns (21), most of the variation seems explained *not* by underlying health differences in the populations of these different areas but by the practice style of the physicians treating patients (22–26). Some of the most persuasive evidence of the impact of practice style comes from the work on surgical signatures. Wennberg and Gittelsohn (27) have demonstrated marked differences in rates of surgery for five common procedures across several areas in Maine. Rates of hemorrhoidectomy stayed much below the provincial average over each of the 5 years, whereas prostatectomy rates remained high (27). Left undisturbed by feedback and review or by the migration of physicians in and out of the area, the surgical signature of a community remained constant from year to year. Although consistent variation in rates across small areas

points strongly to the influence of physician practice style (since several physicians typically practice in these areas), the evidence is somewhat indirect. However, in Manitoba the surgical workloads of other area physicians remained stable over time when a surgically active physician moved into an area, while population utilization was increased by the new surgeon's activity (17%) (24).

Marked differences in practice patterns among individual physicians seem to underlie the differences in rates. The rate of primary cesarean section across 11 physicians treating low-risk suburban women ranged from 9.6 to 31.8%. Close examination of the data yielded "no obvious explanation for variations in cesarean section rates across physicians" (28). Devitt and Ironside (29) observed several years ago that 85% of one surgeons's patients at the Ottawa Civic Hospital undergoing cholecystectomy had operative cholangiography, whereas none of the patients operated upon by another surgeon had this procedure.

Manitoba patients reporting good or excellent health were found to have very different probabilities of being hospitalized in the 2 years after their interview, depending upon the practice style of their physician. Thirty-three percent of the patients of those physicians scoring high on an index of physician hospital practice style (PHPS) were hospitalized in the 2 years following the interview compared with 20% of the patients of physicians who scored low on the index. Even after controlling for such patient characteristics as age, education, self-reported health status, proximity to death or nursing home entry, and for such system characteristics as supply of hospital beds and occupancy rates, a patient of a physician who scored high on the index was twice as likely to be hospitalized as a patient of a physician scoring low on the index (30).

IS MORE BETTER?
Rates, Innovation, and Outcomes

The North American ethos surrounding the health care system is that "more is better." Expenditures rise every year, and yet headlines constantly decry underexpenditures in the health care system. Does this suggest that high rates identify areas delivering the best quality care? Are areas with the highest hospitalization rates or highest hysterectomy rates delivering the best care to area residents? Examining the hospital records of diabetic cases treated in high-, medium-, and low-rate counties, Connell et al. (31) reported that the patients admitted by physicians in high-rate counties were tested substantially less thoroughly than those admitted in low-rate counties. Intravenous insulin treatment for severe metabolic emergencies was also less appropriately used in high-rate counties.

Some practice patterns are not only costly, but probably have negative implications for health. Both a well-publicized clinical trial in Pittsburgh and extensive Manitoba analyses of administrative data (22, 32) emphasized the desirability of conservative standards for tonsillectomy. Nonetheless, differences across areas remain; children resident in Lethbridge, Alberta are much more likely to have their tonsils removed than are children resident in Edmonton (33).

Assuming that high rates must be better also overlooks the fact that hospitals can be dangerous places. In Steel et al.'s (34) study of patients admitted to a medical service of a university hospital, 36% of the patients were found to have acquired an iatrogenic illness (one caused by treatment); for 9%, the event was considered major (something which was life-threatening or produced considerable disability). Compared with research done over a decade earlier, the risks associated with hospitalization had not been reduced over time, but had, if anything, gotten worse. This has occurred despite the enormous increase in hospital funding over this period, much of which was justified in terms of improving quality of care.

How could this be possible? Orkin (35) has suggested that even relatively innocuous-sounding improvements in care should not be approved without clear demonstrations that the benefits are greater than the risks. His editorial focused on monitoring standards forwarded by the American Society of Anesthesiologists to improve the quality of care for patients undergoing anesthesia. While funding agencies might have had problems generating enthusiasm for these standards (the United States alone has approximately 28,000 operating rooms plus post anesthesia recovery rooms to equip), more monitoring would be expected to benefit the patient. However, since the benefits from the new monitoring equipment are so few (deaths associated with anesthesia are estimated to occur at a rate of less than one per 100,000 anesthetics), the risks need to be carefully considered. The information gained from monitors such as pulse oximetry and capnography, although beneficial in specific situations, does not come without costs and risks.

At the least, these new monitors engender complacency with regard to direct observation of the patient: less attention is directed to the patient and we are lulled into believing that all is well if the monitors do not alarm. However, their alarms sound all too often, spuriously; a recent prospective study in a pediatric hospital noted that alarms (principally pulse oximeters) sounded an average of 10 times per case, every 4.5 minutes. Seventy-five percent of the alarms were false while only 3 percent indicated possible patient risk! (35).

Further questioning of the "more is better" philosophy came from a letter to the *New England Journal of Medicine* in response to the suggestion that anyone over 35 years old planning to take up jogging should be assessed by his or her physician and should consider exercise stress testing. Aside from the $2 billion costs associated with performing 20,000,000 stress tests (a 1980's estimate of the number of joggers in the United States aged 35 years and over), what could be wrong with finding out whether one is fit enough to undertake strenuous physical activity? Unfortunately, the benefits of using a stress test to screen the average person about to commence an exercise program are unknown. Whether the stress test can screen for exertion-induced sudden cardiac death is not clear. However, undergoing a stress test, which in itself carries few risks, is known to result in the identification of certain conditions (sometimes falsely, sometimes correctly), which will lead some physicians to further investigations that carry known risks, and potentially to further treatments, again with certain risks.

Graboys (36) has estimated that the stress testing program described above would result in 2 million individuals undergoing coronary angiography (approximately 10% of asymptomatic persons undergoing stress tests have positive results), and approximately 500,000 people going on to bypass surgery (approximately 25% of such asymptomatic individuals will show some degree of multivessel coronary disease worthy of invasive intervention according to some cardiologists and surgeons). The risks and costs of these subsequent treatments are reasonably clear. A 1% mortality rate has been associated with angiography (2,000,000 procedures would result in 2,000 deaths); bypass surgery carries at least a 2% mortality rate as well as an 8% risk of a perioperative myocardial infarction. At least 10,000 deaths and 40,000 myocardial infarctions might be expected following the 500,000 bypass procedures.

The Case of Bypass Surgery

The growth of coronary artery bypass surgery over the last few years (along with continuing concerns about the population to which this technology is applied) highlights the dangers associated with the "more is better" philosophy. Although Canadian rates are much lower than American rates, they are more than twice British rates; no one knows if this is good or bad (37, 38). Nonetheless, controversies about falling-behind American rates have surfaced repeatedly in Canada over the last several years. Provincial governments have made special allocations to increase the availability of bypass surgery for their residents (38).

Differences within Canada are also large; there is more than a twofold variation in rates of bypass surgery among 12 metropolitan areas (39). For example, the population served by one referral center in Ontario has undergone bypass surgery at a rate almost twice that of a population served by a second referral center (the two areas show rates of bypass surgery of 77.8 versus 42.8 per 100,000 population, respectively (40)). Physicians in one region of Manitoba have referred their ischemic heart disease patients to Winnipeg (the location of tertiary care cardiovascular services) at a much lower rate than those in the other regions (41).

What do the research findings imply for policy makers? Waiting lists are generated by physician behavior, and physician discretion is important in determining who goes first (Morgan CD, Naylor D, Hunter LD, Goldman BS, Baigrie RS, unpublished data). Shortfalls compared to other jurisdictions might be handled, at least in part, by changes in hospital policies. Thus, although Manitoba's rate of coronary artery bypass surgery among the elderly is much less than New England's, Manitoba's rates of cholecystectomy and prostatectomy are somewhat higher (42). Some of the difference in bypass rates could be made up by bringing Manitoba cholecystectomy and prostatectomy rates down and shifting operating room time in the teaching hospitals performing bypass surgery; changes in the need for intensive care would have to be anticipated. Such changes would not necessarily be good (or bad) medicine, but the potential for questioning current usage patterns is clearly there.

As described below, appropriateness studies have shown that, even in areas with relatively low rates of coronary artery bypass surgery, some patients with equivocal or inappropriate indications may well be having surgery. As Canadian cardiovascular surgeons complain about waiting lists and the need to expand surgical programs, some patients with triple-vessel disease (those with quite high probabilities of benefitting) are likely to wait for surgery, while others for whom the benefits of surgery are more doubtful are receiving the operation.

Certain technologies are so important and contentious that population-based programs both to monitor and manage waiting lists and to evaluate outcomes should be instituted. In Canada, such programs for coronary artery bypass surgery have been initiated in Toronto and are planned in Manitoba. By collecting information at several points—from entry onto the waiting list for coronary angiography to coronary artery bypass surgery—the characteristics of patients who do and do not receive these procedures can be studied in a timely manner. Among those who do receive angiography or bypass surgery, patient characteristics can be compared according to their length of time on a waiting list. Although expert panels do disagree among themselves, consensus standards based on expert panels can be applied to the data immediately (43), while information can also be accumulated for outcome studies.

TYPES OF EVIDENCE
Appropriateness and Discretion

Since definitive evidence is lacking, expert opinion has been used to specify what is, and what is not, appropriate care. Analyses based on such expert opinion show high levels of inappropriate and equivocal medical decision making (44). North American studies found only 35% of carotid endarterectomies (45), 14% of tonsillectomies (22), and 80% of pacemaker insertions (46) to be done for appropriate indications. High rates of inappropriate utilization are found in more general reviews of hospital use. Rates of inappropriate admissions ranged from 6 to 19% and rates of inappropriate days of care ranged from 20 to 39% in the studies reviewed by Payne (47).

Some evidence supports the idea that high rates identify discretionary decisions about the delivery of health care and overuse, possibly unnecessary use, of the health care system (48–50). Dyck et al. (15) found a larger proportion (52%) of hysterectomies were inappropriate in the Saskatchewan city with the higher rate than in the city with the lower rate (17%). In a study of 23 adjacent counties in one state, Leape et al. (51) found that 28% of the

variance in rate of coronary angiography was explained by the level of inappropriateness. However, for the other two procedures studied (carotid endarterectomy and upper gastrointestinal tract endoscopy), there was no relationship between surgical rate and rate of appropriately selecting individuals for surgery.

Not only can particular treatments be studied, but hospitalization as a whole can be analyzed in terms of its discretionary or nondiscretionary nature. In Manitoba, the relationship between a physicians's practice style and the type of patient hospitalized was examined to determine if physicians more likely to admit patients to hospitals did so for more discretionary indications and for patients who were less ill. We used the index of PHPS described previously; a physician's score on this index was strongly related to the probability of his or her patient being hospitalized after controlling for factors related to patient health status, access to care, etc. (30, 52).

A 197% difference in hospital admission rates was found between those physicians most and least prone to hospitalize their patients (NP Roos, unpublished data). The range for discretionary use is much less. Physicians scoring highest on this index were 6% more likely to admit patients with a high variation condition and 34% more likely to admit patients with a diagnosis judged to be discretionary. Patients of physicians least prone to hospitalize were also somewhat more likely to show a higher illness level—their patients were 32% more likely to be admitted with a high-risk diagnosis.

Perhaps this lack of correspondence between rates of hospitalization (197% range between categories) and rates of discretionary or inappropriate use (6–34% range between categories) should not be surprising. Wennberg (25) has suggested that: "precisely because so many accepted theories concerning the treatment of common illnesses have not been adequately assessed, the number of potential patients who can be *appropriately* (our emphasis) treated by medical or surgical alternatives is very large indeed." Brook (53) argues persuasively that the bias inherent in our processes of judging appropriateness "may mean that elimination of inappropriate or equivocal uses would improve a population's health, but that increasing appropriate use may only increase health care expenditures."

Cost-Effectiveness and Need

Funding choices about medical treatments need to be made. Government efforts to deal with pressures for new programs force such choices. Decision analysts try to use data of various kinds to answer such critical questions as:

1. Are there treatments providing some benefit to the patient (regardless of cost) that could be expanded?
2. Which treatments are likely to be cost-effective compared with other uses of the funds?

Summarizing information on the comparative cost-effectiveness of a number of programs is difficult. Data from various sources using different methodologies must be forced into a common framework. Table 13.1 summarizes some of Detsky's work (54) on the comparative cost-effectiveness of a number of programs. Choices within groups are extremely difficult to make. Choices between program groups may be suitable. On reexamination, several of the treatments within the moderate and highly expensive groups may well turn out not to bring *any* benefit to the patient.

The calculated cost-effectiveness of some interventions is probably unduly optimistic:

First, the analyses are likely to have been based on efficacy data. Efficacy is concerned with "does a particular treatment work" under ideal conditions, typically on patients selected using a strict protocol in a teaching hospital. Effectiveness studies deal with whether or not a specific treatment works in practice, when the treatment is widely diffused. For example, hospitals where relatively few surgical procedures of a particular type are performed often have poorer outcomes than do those performing larger numbers of the procedure (55). Bypass surgery in particular

shows a very wide range of risk-adjusted mortality among hospitals (10).

Second, most decision analyses are unclear as to the role of comorbidity and age. For example, the selection criteria used in the major randomized clinical trial of bypass surgery (the CASS study) were applicable to a very low percentage (less than 10%) of the patients receiving bypass surgery in CASS participating centers and other hospitals (56, 57). The remainder of the patients were either older or sicker than the CASS group (56). Although the CASS researchers developed a registry to follow individuals who were *not* randomized, most clinical trials do not follow patients with characteristics that may exclude them from randomization (58).

Generally, surgical interventions are less beneficial for older patients and those with more comorbidity. The risks of surgery are greater, whereas the benefits must be reaped over a shorter life span. Decision analysts need to take this into account, as Barry et al. (59) have done for prostatectomy.

Third, the baseline population mortality will vary markedly among areas, even across such large areas as American states (60). Such baseline mortality will affect the judgment as to the benefits and risks of particular interventions (42). Specifically, quality-adjusted life year calculations are likely to be changed when calculated for different populations. The higher the baseline mortality rate in a given area, the lower is likely to be the benefit of interventions that seem expensive in terms of cost/quality-adjusted life-year.

Fourth, the quality of the information used as input into decision analyses is often poor. Although Detsky's summary used some meta-analyses and randomized trials, this is not always the case with published decision analyses. Population-based, nonrandomized research is scarce. Weak research designs tend to be biased toward showing improved outcomes from a new treatment (61–63). Such biases are important because, if the program has a high cost per quality-adjusted life-year, sensitivity testing with small changes in the data may well reveal the new treatment to be of little value.

Table 13.1.
Hypothesized Cost-Effectiveness Ratios[a]

Program	Approximate Cost/QALY Gained[b,c]
Phenylketonuria screening	Money is saved
Coronary artery bypass surgery for left main coronary artery disease	Relatively inexpensive programs (approximately 5–12 thousand U.S. dollars/QALY gained)
Neonatal intensive care, birth weight of 1000–1499 g	
Thyroxine (thyroid) screening	
Treatment of severe hypertension (diastolic blood pressure ≥105 mm Hg)	
Treatment of mild hypertension (diastolic blood pressure 95–104 mm Hg) in men aged 40 years	Moderately expensive programs (approximately 20–70 thousand U.S. dollars/QALY)
New radiocontrast media, provision to 30% of the population at highest risk	
Estrogen therapy for postmenopausal symptoms in women without a prior hysterectomy	
Neonatal intensive care, birth weight of 500–999 g	
Coronary bypass surgery for single-vessel disease with moderately severe angina	
School tuberculin testing program	
Continuous ambulatory peritoneal dialysis	
Hospital hemodialysis	
New radiocontrast media, provision to low-risk patients	Very expensive programs (approximately 200 thousand U.S. dollars/QALY)
Liver transplant	

[a]Adapted from Detsky AS. Are clinical trials a cost-effective investment? JAMA 1989;262:1795–1800.
[b]QALY indicates quality-adjusted life-year.
[c]Reported values were adjusted to United States dollars using the United States Consumer Price Index for medical care for all urban consumers.

Additional uncertainties accompany the cost-effectiveness ratios. Because of the time gap between data collection and publication, proponents of a particular new treatment often claim that the innovation should have a better cost-effectiveness ratio than the literature suggests. Although improvement with experience often does occur (54, 65), Orkin (35) has pointed out that this need not be the case. Given low rates of adverse outcomes, Manitoba data on several common surgical procedures show that increasing expenditures over time do not necessarily translate into significant decreases in postoperative mortality or in the rate of related hospital readmissions (66). Moreover, as an innovation diffuses, new programs typically start up; new physicians and teams have to work up the learning curve.

Outcomes are usually not well-specified for different types of patients. Although

Table 13.1 suggests the very different benefits of coronary artery bypass surgery for two types of patients (those with left main disease and those with single-vessel disease and moderately severe angina), benefits need to be estimated for the other types of patients likely to receive bypass surgery. Often, as has been demonstrated for tonsillectomy, just a small portion of the patients receiving the procedure can be shown to benefit from the surgery (22, 32, 67).

Cost-effectiveness ratios are likely to differ "at the margin" as fewer or more patients receive a procedure. Cross-sectional data (from Manitoba and New England) show no clear relationship between surgical rates and population risk factors (42). As rates increase, a given treatment may bring in older, sicker patients (as appears to have happened with coronary artery bypass surgery) or younger, less ill patients (37). As rates fall, patient risk may increase (cholecystectomy) or decrease (hysterectomy) (66).

Patient Preferences

The shared responsibility "among clinicians, patients and policymakers who act as societal agents" increases the complexity of clinical decision making (68). The expected benefits of any intervention may vary with different patient preferences. Several lines of evidence suggest that patient risk aversion implies lower surgical rates. Specifically, patients seem likely to avoid "a choice that has a high expected utility because it includes a possibility of the worst outcome."

As Wennberg (69) has emphasized, "when offered a choice, patients often choose differently than their physicians." McNeil et al. (70) found that, when confronted by a choice of treatment for lung cancer, subjects preferred radiation therapy, which had higher probabilities of immediate- and 1-year survival, over surgery, which had a higher probability of 5-year survival. Although McNeil et al. (70) further reported that physicians seemed less risk-averse than patients, when physicians are patients they may behave differently. A study of how Canadian oncologists would want to be managed if they had non-small cell lung cancer found that, depending upon details of the conditions, only between 3 and 16% of the lung cancer specialists would wish to be treated with chemotherapy (as recommended in the standard textbooks) (71).

The interactive video-disc technology developed for prostatectomy provides additional evidence (72). After having information on treatment alternatives and outcome probabilities, patients are better able to develop and express their preferences. Preliminary data suggest that, after watching the video, many patients are choosing a "watchful waiting" strategy, postponing prostate surgery as long as the symptoms are tolerable.

PHYSICIAN BEHAVIOR

Increasing information on appropriate treatments or on outcomes associated with different treatments, may, or may not, change physician behavior. Part of the problem may be clinician overconfidence. Baumann et al. (73) noted such overconfidence in two different situations: (a) the treatment of breast cancer by physicians and (b) the management of intensive care patients by nurses. In both situations, clinicians were highly confident that they had made the right decision ("microcertainty") although there was no consensus as to what the optimal treatment would be ("macro-uncertainty").

Although high rates of care are not consistently associated with high rates of inappropriate use, when information on their high-rate practice style is fed back to physicians, rates sometimes fall. When practitioners learned that their rates were substantially above state averages, Wennberg reports a 50% decrease in the rate of hysterectomy; similar changes in practice style following feedback occurred in Maine and Vermont for tonsillectomy and in Norway for lens extractions (18). Physicians in these high-rate areas appear to have recognized that some of their previous operations had been unnecessary.

On the other hand, physicians can be reluctant to change established practice patterns in order to improve quality of care. Research on the behavior of cardiovascular surgeons participating in the CASS study, a major clinical trial that helped develop criteria for coronary artery bypass graft surgery, produced rather discouraging findings (74). Despite their surgeons' cooperation with this high-profile clinical trial, the participating hospitals differed markedly in the extent to which the CASS practice guidelines were followed. Among the 15 hospitals, the number of bypass procedures that took place ranged from 75 to 124% of those expected from CASS guidelines, given the patients' clinical and angiographic characteristics.

Whether physicians left to their own devices reduce only inappropriate and equivocal care is also unclear. Thus, Siu et al. (75) reported from the Rand Health Insurance Experiment that, although cost sharing reduced the rate of admissions to hospitals, it did not reduce the rate of inappropriate admissions. Moreover, the identification of "good practice" and the dissemination of this information is not enough to change practice patterns. For example, a widely disseminated and nationally endorsed cesarean section practice guideline had almost no impact on practice patterns in Ontario, Canada (76), while the National Institute of Health Consensus Conferences have generally failed to stimulate practice style changes in the United States (77). In both of these examples, the guidelines had been communicated; in general, physicians were aware of what they should be doing, but they just were not doing it.

Physicians ideologically resist the monitoring of their practice, particularly if such monitoring can be labeled "cookbook medicine." However, Hampton (78) has argued:

Clinical freedom is dead, and no one need regret its passing. . . . In the days when investigation was nonexistent and treatment as harmless as it was ineffective, the doctor's opinion was all that there was, but now opinion is not good enough.

WHAT HAVE WE LEARNED?

What have we learned from the above review? The research summarized above has demonstrated that:

1. The practice of medicine is very different from one physician to another;
2. A significant amount of care is inappropriate and the rate of inappropriate care is often as high in the low-rate areas as in high-rate areas;
3. The lack of evidence showing clear benefits from procedures, at least as performed on many patients, suggests that existing rates are often too high;
4. Some of the variation is explained by uncertainty;
5. Even when uncertainty is reduced, there is no guarantee that appropriate care will be delivered;
6. Informed patients are likely to prefer more conservative, rather than more

aggressive, treatment (at least where there are risks involved);
7. Both expert panels and cost-effectiveness studies are likely biased such that the benefit of treatments are overestimated. Applying practice guidelines may lower surgical rates in certain areas, but this is not guaranteed.

The politics driving expansion of acute care have been well-documented (38, 79). Continued pressure on health care budgets can certainly be expected. Although the amount of invasive treatment patients wish may be less than that now delivered, informed patients may well value extra information (even if treatment is unlikely to change). Where the risks are very low, and even if efficacy has not been demonstrated to be high, patients and physicians are likely to want better diagnoses. Such interest in extra consultations, laboratory testing, endoscopy, magnetic resonance imaging (MRI), and so on adds to the already existing pressures on the system.

The uncertainties of medical practice and the large variations in the rates of hospitalization for most medical conditions and surgical treatments highlight the interface between population health and the medical care system. Health status (of both individuals and populations) and the effectiveness of medical interventions are related, but "experts" differ greatly in their judgments as to the extent of the relationship and how one affects the other. If the relationship is relatively weak, then funds saved from the health care system can be used for other purposes.

At one extreme, the lack of convincing evidence as to the efficacy and effectiveness of many treatment strategies might suggest that efforts to contain cost can safely focus upon bringing rates of hospitalization for many conditions down toward the lower end of the spectrum of utilization. A more moderate approach would focus on regions whose residents tend to use more resources than others; perhaps utilization in these areas can safely be reduced toward mean levels. This middle-of-the-road strategy may have considerable appeal to government funders in an era of escalating health care costs.

POLICY SUGGESTIONS
Reduce Utilization in High-Rate Areas

The current practice of medicine clearly does not ensure that appropriate care will be delivered to patients. Surprisingly high rates of inappropriate care have been found in both low- and high-rate areas. Even when care has been designated "appropriate," various biases in the system work to overestimate appropriateness and the effectiveness of care. Even RAND's expert panels have been demonstrated to be generous in their assessments of appropriateness. When viewing the same set of research and the same set of patient histories and told to ignore resource constraints, British physicians were much more conservative in their assessment of appropriateness than were United States physicians (80). Thirteen percent of bypass surgery studied was judged inappropriate by United States physicians whereas, viewing the same set of patients, United Kingdom physicians judged 35% of the procedures to be inappropriate.

Iglehart (81) believes that "as provincial plans restrain the use of technology, (Canadian) physicians increasingly face the difficult choice of providing care on the basis of medical need rather than rendering it to all who could benefit." We have argued that the situation is far more complicated. If a portion of the care delivered is inappropriate or of unknown benefit, funds for procedures of proven effectiveness and for increasing the knowledge base should be available from better management and from efforts to restrain areas of high utilization.

What is the basis for thinking that efforts at reducing utilization in high-rate areas will not adversely affect health? First of all, even though socioeconomic factors may affect both rates of utilization and the associated expenses for hospital care (82, 83), in New England (as in Manitoba) the regions with low incomes are not those with the highest hospital utilization rates. Dramatic differences in utilization between Boston and New Haven occur despite demographically similar populations receiving most of their care in university hospitals. Most of the higher utilization in Boston "is devoted to the hospital admission of adults with common acute but often minor illnesses or with chronic diseases. . . . These findings indicate that academic standards of care are compatible with widely varying patterns of practice" (84). Most importantly, regions with high utilization have not been shown to differ systematically from regions with low utilization in terms of access to care, health status, or mortality (23, 26, 41, 48).

Which utilization should be reduced? Targeting *both* areas with high overall utilization and areas that are high in a particular choice of an important surgical or medical treatment identifies a place to start (85). Such changes need to be done with support—both in terms of information and expertise—to maximize the reduction of what is inappropriate and highly discretionary.

New funds for the health care system are difficult to find. Significant funds will be needed to develop practice guidelines, to do outcome assessments, and to monitor practice. Since much more would seem to be gained from improving the quality of care that we are now delivering than from doing more or from doing new things, policy makers and insurers should with good conscience redirect funds from the existing system into the quality assurance and technology assessment activities proposed here. These activities rely on information about providers and patients, so thought must be given to the type and quality of data collected. In many cases, attention to cost-effectiveness in research will suggest "a first cut" at analysis using administrative data. Comparative research may suggest evaluations of particular importance in a given region. For example, comparisons of postsurgical mortality between Manitoba and New England showed relatively poor survival in Manitoba after repair of hip fracture. This procedure has been targeted for special attention. Finally, the "natural experiments" that would take place if rates are reduced would, if organized suitably, provide administrative data for both cost-containment studies and assessment of certain treatments.

Evaluate Treatments

Better information is necessary; Detsky (54) has suggested the (potentially) high cost-effectiveness ratios of clinical trials. Well-designed registry and population-based cohort studies may have similar ratios. New, expensive technologies that *promise* to help at least *some* patients (often without good evidence of benefit) are a particular threat to efforts at cost containment. Their advocates argue that traditional methods of evaluation or technology assessment have been outstripped by the dramatic benefits promised by new technologies. For example, Luepker (86) has summarized care of the coronary heart disease patient as

rapidly evolving, driven by new knowledge and technological innovations. . . . Old methods of clinical trials in epidemiologic surveillance are not rapid or sensitive enough to characterize or justify many of the new treatments. Thus, new methods of testing and surveillance seem essential to better understand and evaluate the population effects of new therapies.

Practice guidelines seem most needed for controversial interventions that have a significant effect on patients or the health care system (87). Procedures showing high variation across service areas suggest professional controversy and the potential for both overuse and inappropriate use. Phelps and Parente (85) have developed an index of expected gain from technology assessment, which combines measures of resource use, the coefficient of variation in rates across regions, and the estimated rate at which the incremental value of a medical intervention changes as its rate of use changes. The index provides a dollar-valued welfare loss for variations that can be used for setting priorities for assessment. The highest index score was generated by coronary artery bypass surgery, but most of the high index interventions were nonsurgical (including hospitalizations for psychosis, cardiac catheterization, chronic obstructive lung disease, and angina pectoris) (85).

The nature and importance of the treatment problem should influence both the methodology and the budget. For example, detailed data on the patient's condition must be collected for thorough assessment of the appropriateness of coronary artery bypass surgery. Higher costs are necessarily incurred in such research, but, if the data are collected concurrently, they can also be used for monitoring purposes and effectiveness studies. On the other hand, administrative data appear suitable for better understanding the differences among Manitoba hospitals in outcomes after hip fracture (88).

Quality of Care Assessment Must Include Judgments of Appropriateness

Recent high-profile efforts to monitor quality of care have focused on comparing mortality rates of patients treated at different hospitals (89). Inhospital reviews often look at deaths, although progress has recently been made in performing target reviews using criteria based on ICD-9-CM diagnostic and procedure codes. Hannan et al. (90) have reported the success of a targeted study (testing 11 explicit criteria) of uniform hospital discharge data when compared with a nontargeted subjective review of the medical record.

Few activities encompassed under quality of care review ask the questions: "Was the admission appropriate in the first place?" "Should the surgery have been done?" "Should the MRI have been performed?" While such questions might be asked as part of utilization review, they are typically not seen as pertinent to reviews of quality of care. Economics aside, modern medical treatments have a significant potential for harm and for producing pain and suffering. Given the enormous variations in physician practice patterns, quality of care assessments must include appropriateness reviews.

Develop Explicit Guidelines Drawing on Nonlocal Sources

If practice guidelines are developed by local practitioners without reference to clinical trial evidence and work done elsewhere, they may well exaggerate local area differences. While the importance of local input to gain acceptance of guidelines should not be underestimated, some education as to the marked variation among well-meaning practitioners must take place.

Leape et al. (87) have reviewed practice guidelines developed in several contexts—by specialty societies, the Clinical Efficacy Assessment Project, the Joint Commission on Accreditation of Healthcare Organizations, etc. These proved to be essentially useless for making assessments as to the appropriateness of a given procedure because such guidelines lack specificity—they are so general as to leave everything up to the judgment of the individual practitioner or review body.

The problem with such guidelines was illustrated in Jessee et al.'s (91) report of nine PSROs' experience with reviewing indications for cesarean section. Using subjective criteria such as "failure to progress in labor" and "fetal distress" led to the identification of 98.9% of the procedures as justified. In contrast, Jennett (92) reports that, after a national group of neurosurgeons developed a set of guidelines for the management of head-injured adults, admission rates fell and mortality was reduced where these guidelines were adopted.

Worthwhile Activities

Pressures for expanding the health care system must not be allowed to drive out funding for other, more worthwhile activities. Three recent studies highlight the various factors at work in trying to both manage health care and ensure good health for all. As seen in Table 13.2, the higher surgical rates found in the United States are associated neither with greater longevity nor with greater public satisfaction with the health care system (42, 93–95). Although, the low levels of American satisfaction with their system are not reflected in general dissatisfaction with their personal health care experiences, compared with the United Kingdom and Canada, "the United States has the smallest proportion of its population who are 'very satisfied' " with these experiences (96).

All countries must look to their health care budgets to find room for outcome assessments, developing practice guidelines, and monitoring the system. Other

Table 13.2.
Admission Rates for Selected Procedures, Mean Life Expectancy, and Satisfaction with Health Care System

Country	Number of Admissions per 100,000 Population[a]					Need to Completely Rebuild System[c]
	Coronary Bypass	Cholecystectomy	Hysterectomy	Operation on Lens	Mean Life Expectancy[b]	
					years	%
Australia	32	145	405	101	76.3	17
Canada	26	219	479	139	76.5	5
Japan	1	2	90	35	79.1	6
Netherlands	5	131	381	68	76.5	5
Sweden		140	145		77.1	6
United Kingdom	6	78	250	98	76.3	17
United States	61	203	557	294	75.0	29

[a]Selected countries for which 1980 data were reported. Data from McPherson K. International differences in medical care practices. Health Care Fin Rev 1989;11:9–20.
[b]Life expectancy was calculated by applying the same methodology to the mortality data for each country. These estimates may differ slightly from the estimates by the countries themselves because of variations in method. Data from 1986 and 1987 were used for all countries. Data from Centers for Disease Control Mortality in developed countries. MMWR 1990;39(13):205–209.
[c]On the survey, the question was worded as follows: "Our health care system has so much wrong with it that we need to completely rebuild it." Data from Blendon RJ, Leitman R, Morrison I, Donelan K. Datawatch: Satisfaction with health systems in ten nations. Health Aff (Millwood) 1990;9(2):185–192.

parts of health care, such as cost-effective health promotion programs that promise to help prevent or postpone major diseases (97) must not be neglected. Perhaps the most important task is to find the political will to manage the health care system in a cost-effective fashion.

References

1. Eddy DM. Variation in physician practice: The role of uncertainty. Health Aff (Millwood) 1984; 3(2):74–89.
2. Koran LM. The reliability of clinical methods, data and judgements (Part 1). N Engl J Med 1975; 293:642–646.
3. Koran LM. The reliability of clinical methods, data and judgements (Part 2). N Engl J Med 1975; 293:695–701.
4. Kassirer JP, Pauker SG. The toss-up. N Engl J Med 1981;305:1467–1469.
5. Vayda E, Mindell WR, Mueller CD, et al. Measuring surgical decision-making with hypothetical cases. Can Med Assoc J 1982;127:287–290.
6. Park RE, Fink A, Brook RH, et al. Physician ratings of appropriate indications for six medical and surgical procedures. Am J Public Health 1986;76:766–772.
7. Grayhack JT, Sadowski RW. Results of surgical treatment of benign prostatic hyperplasia. In: Grayhack, Wilson, Scherbenske, eds. Benign prostatic hyperplasia. Department of Health, Education, and Welfare Publication No. NIH 76-1113, 1975:125–134.
8. Wennberg JE, Roos NP, Sola L, Schori A, Jaffe R. Use of claims data systems to evaluate health care outcomes: Mortality and reoperation following prostatectomy. JAMA 1987;257:933–936.
9. Roos LL, Nicol JP, Cageorge SM. Using administrative data for longitudinal research: Comparisons with primary data collection. J Chron Dis 1987;40:41–49.
10. Steinbrook R. Hospital quality in California. Health Aff (Millwood) 1988;7(3):235–236.
11. Bunker JP. Surgical manpower: A comparison of operations and surgeons in the United States and in England and Wales. N Engl J Med 1970;282:135–144.
12. McPherson K, Wennberg JE, Hovind DB, Clifford P. Small-area variations in the use of common surgical procedures: An international comparison of New England, England, and Norway. N Engl J Med 1982;307:1310–1314.
13. Chassin MR, Brook RH, Park RE, et al. Variations in the use of medical and surgical services by the Medicare population. N Engl J Med 1986;314:285–290.
14. Mindell WE, Vayda E, Cardillo B. Ten-year trends in Canada for selected operations. Can Med Assoc J 1982;127:23–27.
15. Dyck FJ, Murphy FA, Murphy JK, et al. Effect of surveillance on the number of hysterectomies in the province of Saskatchewan. N Engl J Med 1977;296:1326–1328.
16. Knickman JR. Variations in hospital use across cities: A comparison of utilization rates in New York and Los Angeles. In: Rothberg DL, ed. Regional variations in hospital use. Lexington, MA: D.C. Heath and Co., 1982:23–63.
17. Perrin JM, Homer CJ, Berwick DM, Woolf AD, Freeman JL, Wennberg JE. Variations in rates of hospitalization of children in three urban communities. N Engl J Med 1989;320:1183–1187.
18. Wennberg JE. Dealing with medical practice variations: A proposal for action. Health Aff (Millwood) 1984;3:6–31.
19. Gittelsohn AM, Wennberg JE. On the risk of organ loss. J Chron Dis 1976;29:527–535.
20. Wennberg JE, Bunker JP, Barnes B. The need for assessing the outcome of common medical practices. Annu Rev Public Health 1980;1:277–295.
21. McPherson K. Why do variations occur? In: Andersen TF, Mooney G, eds. The challenges of medical practice variations. London: Macmillan, 1990:16–35.
22. Roos NP, Henteleff PD, Roos LL. A new audit procedure applied to an old question: Is the frequency of T & A justified? Med Care 1977;15:1–18.
23. Roos NP, Roos LL. Surgical rate variations: Do they reflect the health or socio-economic characteristics of the population? Med Care 1982;20:945–958.
24. Roos LL. Supply, workload and utilization: A population-based analysis of surgery. Am J Public Health 1983;73:414–421.
25. Wennberg JE. Population illness rates do not explain population hospitalization rates: A comment on Mark Blumberg's thesis that morbidity adjusters are needed to interpret small area variations. Med Care 1987;25:354–359.
26. Wennberg JE, Fowler FJ. A test of consumer contribution to small area variations in health care delivery. J Maine Med Assoc 1977;68:275–279.
27. Wennberg JE, Gittelsohn A. Variations in medical care among small areas. Sci Am 1982;246:120–134.
28. Goyert GL, Bottoms SF, Treadwell MC, Nehra PC. The physician factor in cesarean birth rates. N Engl J Med 1989;329:706–709.
29. Devitt JE, Ironside M. Difficulties in applying patient care audit to surgeons. Bull Am Coll Surg 1975;May:18–21.
30. Roos NP. Predicting hospital utilization by the elderly: The importance of patient, physician, and hospital characteristics. Med Care 1989;27:905–919.
31. Connell FA, Blide LA, Hanken MA. Clinical correlates of small area variations in population-based admission rates for diabetes. Med Care 1984;22:939–949.
32. Paradise JL, Bluestone CD, Bachman RZ, et al. Efficacy of tonsillectomy for recurrent throat infection in severely affected children: Results of parallel randomized and nonrandomized clinical trials. N Engl J Med 1984;310:674–683.
33. Halliday ML, LeRiche WH. Regional variation in surgical rates, Alberta, 1978, and the relationship to characteristics of patients, doctors performing surgery and hospitals where the surgery was

performed. Can J Public Health 1987;78:193–200.

34. Steel K, Gertman PM, Crescenzi C, Anderson J. Iatrogenic illness on a general medical service at a university hospital. N Engl J Med 1981;304:638–642.

35. Orkin FK. Practice standards: The Midas touch or the emperor's new clothes. Anesthesiology 1989;70:567–571.

36. Graboys TB. The economics of screening joggers. N Engl J Med 1979;301:1067.

37. Anderson GM, Newhouse JP, Roos LL. Hospital care for elderly patients with diseases of the circulatory system: A comparison of hospital utilization in the United States and Canada. N Engl J Med 1989;321:1443–1448.

38. Detsky AS, O'Rourke K, Naylor CD, Stacey SR, Kitchens J. Containing Ontario's hospital costs under universal health insurance in the 1980s: What was the record? Can Med Assoc J 1990;142:565–572.

39. Statistics Canada. Coronary artery bypass surgery in Canada. Health Rep 1990;2:9–26.

40. Anderson GM, Lomas J. Regionalization of coronary artery bypass surgery: Effects on access. Med Care 1989;27:288–296.

41. Roos LL, Sharp SM. Innovation, centralization, and growth: Coronary artery bypass surgery in Manitoba. Med Care 1989;27:441–452.

42. Roos LL, Fisher ES, Sharp SM, Newhouse JP, Anderson GM, Bubolz TA. Postsurgical mortality in Manitoba and New England. JAMA 1990;263:2453–2458.

43. Naylor CD, Baigrie RS, Goldman BS, Basinski A. Assessment of priority for coronary revascularisation procedures. Lancet 1990;May 5:1070–1073.

44. Leape LL. Unnecessary surgery. Health Serv Res 1989;23:351–407.

45. Chassin MR, Kosecoff J, Park RE, et al. Does inappropriate use explain geographic variations in the use of health care services. JAMA 1987;258:2533–2537.

46. Greenspan AM, Kay HR, Berger BC, Greenberg RM, et al. Incidence of unwarranted implantation of permanent cardiac pacemakers in a large medical population. N Engl J Med 1988;318:158–163.

47. Payne SMC. Identifying and managing inappropriate hospital utilization. Health Serv Res 1987;22:709–769.

48. Wennberg JE, Freeman JL, Shelton RM, Bubolz TA. Hospital use and mortality among Medicare beneficiaries in Boston and New Haven. N Engl J Med 1989;321:1168–1173.

49. Roos NP, Roos LL, Mossey JM, Havens BJ. Using administrative data to predict important health outcomes: Entry to hosptial, nursing home, and death. Med Care 1988;26:221–239.

50. Paul-Shaheen P, Clark JD, Williams D. Small area analysis: A review and analysis of the North American literature. J Health Politics Policy Law 1987;12:741–809.

51. Leape LL, Park RE, Solomon DH, Chassin MR, Kosecoff J, Brook RH. Does inappropriate use explain small-area variations in the use of health care services? JAMA 1990;263:669–672.

52. Roos NP, Flowerdew G, Wajda A, Tate RB. Variations in physicians' hospitalization practices: A population-based study in Manitoba, Canada. Am J Public Health 1986;76:45–51.

53. Brook RH. Relationship between appropriateness and outcome. In: Hopkins A, Costain D, eds. Measuring the outcomes of medical care. London: King's Fund Centre for Health Services Development, 1990:59–67.

54. Detsky AS. Are clinical trials a cost-effectiveness investment? JAMA 1989;262:1795–1800.

55. Luft HS, Bunker JP, Enthoven AC. Should operations be regionalized? The empirical relation between surgical volume and mortality. N Engl J Med 1979;301:1364–1369.

56. CASS Principal Investigators and Their Associates. The National Heart, Lung, and Blood Institute Coronary Artery Surgery Study (CASS). Circulation 1981;63:(suppl I):I1–I81.

57. Hlatky MA, Califf RM, Harrell FE, Lee KL, Mark DB, Pryor DB. Comparisons of predictions based on observational data with the results of randomized controlled clinical trials of coronary artery bypass surgery. J Am Coll Cardiol 1988;11:237–245.

58. Davis K. Use of data registries to evaluate medical procedures: Coronary Artery Surgery Study and the Balloon Valvuloplasty Registry. Intl J Tech Asses Health Care 1990;6:203–210.

59. Barry MJ, Mulley AG, Fowler FJ, Wennberg JE. Watchful waiting vs. immediate transurethral resection for symptomatic prostatism: The importance of patients' preferences. JAMA 1988;259:3010–3017.

60. U.S. Bureau of Census. Statistical Abstract of the United States: 1990. Washington, D.C.: United States Government Printing Office, 1990.

61. Chalmers TC, Hewett P, Reitman D, Sacks HS. Selection and evaluation of empirical research in technology assessment. Intl J Tech Asses Health Care 1989;5:521–536.

62. Colditz GA, Miller JN, Mosteller F. How study design affects outcomes in comparisons of therapy. I: Medical. Stat Med 1989;8:441–454.

63. Miller JN, Colditz GA, Mosteller F. How study design affects outcomes in comparisons of therapy. II: Surgical. Stat Med 1989;8:455–466.

64. Yeaton WH, Wortman PM. Medical technology assessment: The evaluation of coronary artery bypass graft surgery using data synthesis techniques. Intl J Tech Asses Health Care 1985;1:125–146.

65. Cromwell J, Mitchell JB, Stason WB. Learning by doing in CABG surgery. Med Care 1990;28:6–18.

66. Roos LL, Roos NP, Sharp SM. Monitoring adverse outcomes of surgery using administrative data. Health Care Fin Rev 1987;7(suppl):5–16.

67. Roos LL. Alternative designs to study outcomes: The tonsillectomy case. Med Care 1979;17:1069–1087.

68. Mulley AG. The role of decision analysis in the translation of research findings into clinical practice. In: Gelijns AC, ed. Medical innovation at the crossroads. Vol. I. Modern methods of clinical investigation. Washington, D.C.: National Academy Press, 1990:78–87.

69. Wennberg JE. The paradox of appropriate care. JAMA 1987;258:2568–2569.

70. McNeil BJ, Weichselbaum R, Pauker SG. Fallacy of the five-year survival in lung cancer. N Engl J Med 1978;299:1397–1401.

71. McKillop WJ, O'Sullivan B, Ward GK. Non-small cell lung cancer: How oncologists want to be treated. Int J Radiat Oncol Biol Phys 1987;13:929–934.

72. Wennberg JE. What is outcomes research? In: Gelijns AC, ed. Medical innovation at the crossroads. Vol. I. Modern methods of clinical investigation. Washington, D.C.: National Academy Press, 1990:33–46.

73. Baumann AO, Deber RB, Thompson GG. Overconfidence among physicians and nurses: The "micro-certainty, macro-uncertainty" phenomenon. Soc Sci Med 1991;32:167–174.

74. Maynard C, Fisher L, Alderman EL, et al. Institutional differences in therapeutic decision making in the Coronary Artery Surgery Study (CASS). Med Decis Making 1986;6:127–135.

75. Siu AL, Sonnenberg FA, Manning WG, et al. Inappropriate use of hospitals in a randomized trial of health insurance plans. N Engl J Med 1986;315:1259–1266.

76. Lomas J, Anderson GM, Karin DP, Vayda E, Enkin MW, Hannah WJ. Do practice guidelines guide practice? The effect of a consensus statement on the practice of physicians. N Engl J Med 1989;321:1306–1311.

77. Kosecoff J, Kanouse DE, Rogers WH, McCloskey L, Winslow CM, Brook RH. Effects of the National Institutes of Health concensus development program on physician practice. JAMA 1987;258:2708–2713.

78. Hampton JR. The end of clinical freedom. Br Med J 1983;287:1239–1240.

79. Evans RG, Barer ML. The American predicament. Health Care Fin Rev 1989;Annual Suppl:72–77.

80. Brook RH, Kosecoff JB, Park RE, Chassin MR, Winslow CM, Hampton JR. Diagnosis and treatment of coronary disease: Comparison of doctors' attitudes in the USA and the UK. Lancet 1988; April 2:750–753.

81. Iglehart JK. Canada's health care system faces its problems. N Engl J Med 1990;322:562–568.

82. Mclaughlin CG, Normolle DP, Wolfe RA, McMahon LF, Griffith JR. Small-area inhospital discharge rates: Do socioeconomic variables matter? Med Care 1989;27:507–521.

83. Epstein AM, Stern RS, Weissman JS. Do the poor cost more? A multihospital study of patients' socioeconomic status and use of hospital resources. N Engl J Med 1990;322:1122–1128.

84. Wennberg JE, Freeman JL, Culp WJ. Are hospital services rationed in New Haven or over-utilized in Boston? Lancet 1987;May 23:1185–1189.

85. Phelps CE, Parente ST. Priority setting in medical technology and medical practice assessment. Med Care 1990;28:703–723.

86. Luepker RV. Conclusions. In: Higgins MW, Luepker RV, eds. Trends in coronary heart disease mortality: The influence of medical care. New York: Oxford University Press, 1988:276–278.

87. Leape LL, Park RE, Solomon DH, Chassin MR, Kosecoff J, Brook RH. Relation between surgeons' practice volumes and geographic variation in the rate of carotid endarterectomy. N Engl J Med 1989;321:653–657.

88. Roos LL, Sharp SM, Cohen MM. Comparing clinical information with claims data: Some similarities and differences. J Clin Epidemiol 1991, in press.

89. Brinkley J. U.S. releasing lists of hospitals with abnormal mortality rates. New York Times 1986; March 12:1.

90. Hannan EL, O'Donnell JF, Kilburn H, Bernard HR, Yazici A. Investigation of the relationship between volume and mortality for surgical procedures performed in New York State hospitals. JAMA 1989;262:503–510.

91. Jessee WF, Nickerson CW, Grant WS. Assessing medical practices through PSRO cooperative studies. An evaluation of cesarean birth in nine PSRO areas. Med Care 1982;20:75–84.

92. Jennett B. Variations data from surgeons, for surgeons. In: Ham C, ed. Health care variations: Assessing the evidence. London: King's Fund Institute, 1988:30–31.

93. Centers for Disease Control. Mortality in developed countries. MMWR 1990;39(13):205–209.

94. Blendon RJ, Leitman R, Morrison I, Donelan K. Datawatch: Satisfaction with health systems in ten nations. Health Aff (Millwood) 1990;9(2):185–192.

95. McPherson K. International differences in medical care practices. Health Care Fin Rev 1989;11:9–20.

96. Blendon RJ, Taylor H. Datawatch: Views on health care public opinion in three nations. Health Aff (Millwood) 1989;8(1);149–190.

97. Farquhar JW, Fortmann SP, Flora JA, et al. Effects of community-wide education on cardiovascular disease risk factors: The Stanford five-city project. JAMA 1990;264:359–365.

Section IV

Approaches and Examples for Specific Departments

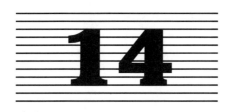

14

Anesthesia

Franklin L. Scamman, M.D.

INTRODUCTION

Quality assurance (QA) in anesthesia is a process that allows for effective identification of potential problems, objective assessment of the cause(s) of these problems, implementation of actions designed to eliminate the problems, and monitoring to assure that the problems have been eliminated. Much has been written and spoken about QA in medical care, yet the true reason for the existence of QA is not clear for many health care providers. Its primary purpose is to assure that patient care, and conceivably outcome associated with that care, be the best possible. It is not to single out individuals to embarrass and harass them, but instead to show that anesthesia is safe, both in terms of outcome and process, and to search for areas of improvement.

The purpose of this chapter is to outline the QA process as formulated by the Joint Commission on Accreditation of Healthcare Organizations (JCAHO) for anesthesia, to give some examples of how other institutions have used this process, and to present our experience with anesthesia QA at the University of Iowa.

The JCAHO

The JCAHO is the primary moving force behind medical QA. JCAHO has clearly defined in the publications that are available for each specialty what the process of QA for medicine is to be. The one for anesthesia, *Monitoring and Evaluation: Anesthesia Services,* was published in 1987 (1). JCAHO supplements this document with standards for quality assurance and surgical and anesthesia services, which are revised yearly (2).

The JCAHO QA Process

The JCAHO has defined a 10-step process, which it requires to be followed when performing QA. These 10 steps are:

1. Assign responsibility for monitoring and evaluating activities;
2. Delineate the scope of care provided by the organization;
3. Identify the most important aspects of care provided by the organization;
4. Identify indicators (and appropriate clinical criteria) for monitoring the important aspects of care;
5. Establish thresholds (levels, patterns, trends) for the indicators that trigger evaluation of the care;
6. Monitor the important aspects of care by collecting and organizing the data for each indicator;
7. Evaluate care when thresholds are reached in order to identify either opportunities to improve care or problems;
8. Take actions to improve care or to correct identified problems;
9. Assess the effectiveness of the actions

and document the improvement in care; and

10. Communicate the results of the monitoring and evaluation process to relevant individuals, departments, or services and to the organizationwide quality assurance program (3).

In addition, JCAHO requires that an anesthesia department perform monitoring and evaluation of the quality and appropriateness of patient care and the clinical performance of all individuals with clinical privileges through monthly meetings of the staff, case review, drug usage evaluation, medical record review, blood usage review, and pharmacy and therapeutics review (4). The entire process of QA must be documented in writing as the policies and procedures of the department/section. This document for the Iowa City Veterans Affairs Medical Center Anesthesiology Service is contained in the Appendix.

These requirements represent a formidable assignment to follow and do take a considerable amount of time and organization. What follows is a discussion of each of the 10 steps.

Expansion on the JCAHO Process

Step 1.   Assign Responsibility

The responsibility for QA efforts belongs with the head or chief of the department/section. He or she is at liberty to delegate this responsibility to competent and qualified individuals, but it is important to remember that evaluation must be at the peer level. Monitoring, however, can be performed by clerks checking for the presence of pre- and post-anesthesia notes in the medical record or by a Certified Registered Nurse Anesthetist (CRNA) abstracting the quality of documentation on an anesthesia record.

Step 2.   Delineate the Scope of Care

For anesthesia, delineation may be as simple as monitoring the activity in the operating suite and post-anesthesia care unit. For our institution, we include the surgical intensive care unit (SICU), obstet-

rics suite, urology suite, ambulatory surgery suite, pain clinic, and other anesthetizing and post-anesthesia care unit (PACU) locations. In other words, any location or function where anesthesia personnel are responsible for patient care falls under the scope of care.

Step 3.   Identify the Important Aspects of Care

For care involving anesthesia for diagnostic or therapeutic procedures, the important aspects are the pre-anesthesia visit, the induction and maintenance of anesthesia, the PACU stay, and the post-anesthesia visit. For the SICU, this might include infection control and details of ventilator and dialysis therapy among others.

Step 4.   Identify Indicators or Monitors

Each aspect of care must have associated with it the ability to measure its quality. For example, the pre-anesthesia note can be evaluated not only by its presence, but by standards that define its optimal content. The anesthetic itself can be monitored by the presence of events that might be associated with less-than-perfect outcome involving the cardiovascular and respiratory systems or regional anesthesia. Fortunately, JCAHO allows each institution to define what and how many the indicators are to be, as long as they give an accurate picture of the scope of clinical practice. Minimal operating room (OR) monitors might include perioperative myocardial infarction and deaths. Our monitors will be described in greater detail in the section on the program at the University of Iowa.

Step 5.   Establish Thresholds

Each indicator or monitor must have associated with it a value or rate (sometimes identified as criteria) that, if exceeded, calls to attention the need for further study and evaluation of the indicator. For example, consider the incidence of patient temperatures in the OR of less than 35°C. Our threshold is 0.9% of the general anesthetics administered. If the rate is higher than this, we might have a problem. Again, the JCAHO allows each QA program to set its own thresholds. For events, it is possible to set a threshold as the mean plus 2 standard deviations above the mean. Additionally, it is possible to set the threshold at the 95% level, such that 95% of the time the rate of the event would be expected to fall below the threshold.

Step 6. Monitor the Indicators by Collecting Data

This process is where many QA programs get bogged down. It is very easy to try to gather too much information of a nonquantifiable nature so that the process of evaluation is impractical. The data in medical records can be of great help. Every patient's chart is coded for diagnoses and procedures on discharge, and medical records should be able to report myocardial infarctions (MIs) associated with procedures. Computerized data bases have been extremely helpful for us (see below) in analyzing data so that thresholds can be linked statistically to the indicator.

Step 7. Evaluate Care When Thresholds Are Reached

A threshold that has been exceeded may indicate a problem. At least, a directed study should be performed to see if there is a problem. At times, this determination cannot be made. For example, the JCAHO recommends that deaths within 48 hours following anesthesia be monitored. The problem here is that most perioperative deaths are a result either of a continuation of the patient's disease or of surgical difficulties. It is very difficult to identify if anesthesia contributed to the patient's demise. Therefore, crude mortality figures do not constitute a very good indicator of how good a particular anesthetist is. On the other hand, if the indicator is that each anesthetist note on the anesthesia record the patient's condition on transport to PACU, that the threshold is 95% compliance, and that an anesthetist undergoing an audit has a compliance of only 65%, then there is definitely a problem in charting.

Step 8. Take Action to Improve Care or Correct Problems

Once a problem has been identified, it is necessary to formulate a plan to correct the problem. It is very important that the action be specific to the problem and that the problem be defined as narrowly as possible to focus the action. For example, if hypothermia is a problem, then educating anesthetists in temperature conservation would be in order. Additionally, warm ORs, heat/moisture exchangers on the airway, and warming blankets might be appropriate.

Step 9. Assess the Effectiveness of the Action

Here is where the QA loop begins to close. If the problem has been identified correctly, and if the action has been appropriate, then the rate of the indicator should drop below the threshold. What was once a problem is no longer a problem, and, hopefully, patients will receive better care.

Step 10. Communicate Results

Oftentimes, problems discovered in anesthesia are not unique to anesthesia but affect other services as well. It is advantageous to share all identified problems with others in the event that their input results in a more-focused solution. In addition, sharing the successes may inspire others in their quest for better patient care.

Future of the JCAHO Process

JCAHO, in 1988, initiated its "Agenda for Change" in which it undertook a rigorous investigation of the indicator-based performance monitoring system. When fully implemented, the system is expected to:

1. Collect continually objective data, which are derived from the application of indicators with respect to performance of key governance, managerial, clinical, and support functions of each accredited health care organization;
2. Aggregate, risk adjust, and analyze the performance data on a national level;
3. Provide comparative performance data to accredited health care organizations for use in their internal quality improvement efforts;
4. Identify trends and patterns in the performance of individual, accredited hospitals that may call for more focused attention at the hospital level;

5. Provide a national performance data base that can serve as a resource for health services research (5).

The anesthesia indicators have been tested in 17 "alpha" hospitals for the past two years and "beta" testing started in 400 hospitals late in 1990. The beta phase is designed to evaluate the following:

1. The ability of hospitals to collect and transmit indicator data to the Joint Commission;
2. The capability of the Joint Commission's information system to receive and analyze such data and provide timely feedback to hospitals;
3. How information related to indicator data may be incorporated into the accreditation process;
4. The reliability and validity of the indicators to assess their potential utility to hospitals and the Joint Commission in the identification of opportunities to improve patient care and services (5).

Part of the beta phase will be to answer the following questions:

1. Does the indicator correctly identify the clinical event that has been targeted for monitoring? This evaluation encompasses the issue of indicator design as well as the potential problems of incorrect or missing data elements.
2. Do the occurrences identified by the indicator merit further review? That is, does the indicator raise substantive questions about performance? (5).

It is anticipated that the beta phase testing will extend through late 1992. The anesthesia care indicators summary list as of September 1990 was as follows:

1. Patients developing a central nervous system (CNS) complication occurring during or within 2 post-procedure days of procedures involving anesthesia administration, subcategorized by ASA-PS class, patient age, and CNS versus non-CNS related procedures. (Author's note: ASA-PS is the abbreviation for American Society of Anesthesiology physical status.)

2. Patients developing a peripheral neurologic deficit during or within 2 post-procedure days of procedures involving anesthesia administration;
3. Patients developing an acute myocardial infarction during or within 2 post-procedure days involving anesthesia administration, subcategorized by ASA-PS class, patient age, and cardiac versus noncardiac procedures;
4. Patients with a cardiac arrest during or within 1 post-procedure day of procedures involving anesthesia administration, excluding patients with required intraoperative cardiac arrest, subcategorized by ASA-PS class, patient age, and cardiac versus noncardiac procedures;
5. Patients with unplanned respiratory arrest during or within 1 post-procedure day of procedures involving anesthesia administration;
6. Death of patients during or within 2 post-procedure days of procedures involving anesthesia administration, subcategorized by ASA-PS class and patient age;
7. Unplanned admission of patients to the hospital within 1 post-procedure day following outpatient procedures involving anesthesia administration;
8. Unplanned admission of patients to an intensive care unit within 1 post-procedure day of procedures involving anesthesia administration and with ICU stay more than 1 day (5).

Although this list might form a core around which a service might want to structure its indicators, it is not sufficient to give an overall picture of the quality of care administered.

For its beta test centers, the JCAHO has prepared a software package to facilitate the collecting and reporting of QA data. The program relies on International Classification of Diseases (ICD-9) discharge codes to detect diagnoses that might indicate that an anesthesia complication occurred. Having identified such a patient, the program then asks for more details, including ICU admissions. For the identified codes, there is opportunity to enter modifiers that explain or mitigate the importance of the complication. Data are sent to the JCAHO via modem or disk monthly so that the national data base may be established. The program allows listings so that the local QA efforts may be enhanced.

QA PROCESS RESULTS FROM THE LITERATURE

The process of QA is inherent to the practice of anesthesia. Each one of us learns from our experience—what we did well and what we did poorly. It is impossible, however, for each of us to manage enough cases to gain sufficient experience and wisdom to avoid all the pitfalls. Therefore, we must learn from the misadventures of others. Our literature is replete with case reports and series of how-to and how-not-to. Anesthesiology, as a medical specialty, was among the first to have undertaken studies in a systematic fashion improving the practice as a whole.

A search of the Medline data base for the union of *anesthesia* and *quality assurance* or *risk management* since 1966 revealed 89 citations. Of these, which were published in a major anesthesia journal or *JAMA,* 26 have appeared since 1988 and only 7 prior to that time. Only two of the 26 directly address QA in a fashion proposed by the JCAHO model (6, 7). What is missing are good prospective studies on the rate of indicators, which include both a denominator as well as a numerator, and a reasonable evaluation of the associated thresholds. In other words, there is very little in the literature to guide one on setting up a "cookbook" QA program.

Review Based on the JCAHO Guidelines

Examining the JCAHO list of beta indicators and recognizing the fact that many of the studies are retrospective, one finds some guidance.

About CNS complications, Hindman (8) estimated the rate of perioperative stroke in vascular and general surgical patients to be 0.37 to 3.5%. The studies he quotes are both from the early 1960s. These rates might be lower now. Skillman (9) states that the rate of permanent neurological

complication following carotid endarterectomy is 5.7%, of thoracic aortic aneurysm is 5.5%, and abdominal aortic aneurysm is less. Dawkins (10) has stated that the rate of permanent paralysis following epidural anesthesia is 0.02%. However, these data offer no help when one is confronted with the need for an estimate of rate for all the cases performed in a surgical suite.

For a peripheral neurologic deficit, the same applies, although nerve damage, according to Cheney (11) is the second most common outcome (15% of the cases) in the ASA Closed Claims Study. Of 1541 cases, 75 involved the ulnar nerve at the elbow, 45 the brachial plexus, and 44 the femoral-sciatic nerves. Nerve block was associated with 25% of the cases and positioning to another 37%. This leaves 38% with no obvious etiology. Again, the denominator is missing.

Concerning myocardial infarction, there is a great deal in the literature about peripheral vascular and coronary artery disease and perioperative myocardial infarction. These studies, however, do not help in trying to determine the overall rate of this event. Our data for the past fiscal year would indicate that there were 22 MIs within 48 hours of surgery from a total of 17,184 cases performed, a rate of 0.12%. Excluded from this rate were any patients who underwent cardiopulmonary bypass.

Data for cardiac and respiratory arrest within the first 24 hours are not available.

Concerning death within 48 hours, it is known that the overall death rate in an operating room from an anesthetic accident now may be as low as none in 244,000 (12). However, this study does not address PACU or SICU events.

Unplanned admissions from most ambulatory surgical centers have been in the 4-5% range. Nausea and vomiting, pain control, and other reasons are about evenly divided as to the cause.

The unplanned admission rate to SICU depends greatly on the definition of "unplanned." At the University of Iowa, unplanned is defined as any admission that is not a craniotomy, a procedure involving cardiopulmonary bypass, or a major otolaryngology, head and neck surgery case.

One of the major difficulties with the

suggested JCAHO indicators is that none of them measure uniquely anesthesia-caused events. An unwanted outcome is related primarily to the patient's age, the severity of illness, the length of the operation, and whether the procedure is an emergency or not. It is a common belief that the practice of anesthesia has become so safe recently that it will be almost impossible to differentiate the anesthesia-related signal from the noise of the insult of surgery and the progression of the patient's disease. It appears to this author that the JCAHO, by using these indicators, will gain a lot of information about the noise and very little about the signal of how to improve the practice of anesthesia.

The Las Vegas Model

Terry Vitez, M.D., when he was in Las Vegas, developed a QA program now called the Las Vegas model (7). This model subsequently has been endorsed by the American Society of Anesthesiologists (14). This model is based on occurrence screening and subscribes to three tenets: determining competence is a human decision; the best indication of competence is outcome; and humans are inherently fallible. Any health care individual, who observes what he or she perceives is an anesthesia management-related event, initiates a review process by submitting an occurrence report to the hospital QA department. Those reports meeting preestablished criteria are investigated by the department collecting the pertinent documents, blinding them as to provider names, and sending them to an anesthesia QA committee member. He or she analyzes the documents and reports to the full committee a judgment on whether the event was related to anesthesia management, on the seriousness of the event, on the class of the errors committed, on the explanation of how the event occurred (with references), and on specific recommendations of how to prevent similar events in the future. The committee, after approving the report, brings it before the full department. Only after the department approves the report does it become part of that practitioner's QA file. Event

profiles are developed for the entire department as a whole and form the basis for the standard of practice. Event profiles of individuals are compared to those of the department and form the basis of judging competence. In order to include those events that are very rare, the department has established minimal levels of competence that every practitioner must meet. The model is considerably more complex than presented here, and the reader may need to review the references personally.

The Las Vegas model has been implemented by many anesthesia departments throughout the United States. However, the only experience reported in the literature is Vitez's (7). During the discussion of the Las Vegas model at the 1989 ASA Annual Meeting, it was pointed out that the model would be very difficult to implement in small departments in which anonymity would be difficult to maintain, or in departments where there are no licensed independent practitioners giving anesthesia. In these cases, the blinded reports could be referred to an outside anesthesia consultant for review and recommendations.

HOW THE UNIVERSITY OF IOWA HOSPITAL'S ANESTHESIA DEPARTMENT DOES QA

In this section, the University of Iowa Hospital's anesthesia QA program will be described. It involves four areas: input, processing output, and evaluation.

Input to the Process

We rely on four major and one minor sources of data: prospective data collection via computer entry sheets from anesthetizing locations and PACUs; clinical chart reviews initiated by data from University of Iowa Hospitals and Clinics (UIHC) Central QA, incident reports, surgery department morbidity and mortality conference, and computer entry sheets; administrative chart reviews for correctness and completeness by personnel from medical records and the anesthesia department; and the post-anesthesia patient question-naires. The minor input is the usual and customary grapevine.

Computer Entry Sheets

In order to implement the JCAHO recommendation that the appropriateness and effectiveness of care be monitored and that this QA monitoring be prospective in design, we have developed a Macintosh™ based data base (13) to follow events in the operating OR and post-anesthesia recovery room (PACU).

Twenty indicators (monitors) were selected to be tracked on every anesthetic. A customized data entry sheet was designed with the help of National Computer Systems (NCS) (Fig. 14.1). The sheet contains an area for demographics (patient, staff, resident ID, and date), for location and type of anesthesia and special considerations, and for the presence of any of the 20 indicators. The bottom half of the entry sheet listed the events (indicators) and the location where the event occurred. The indicators were chosen specifically to be simple and uncomplicated with several opportunities for recording "other events."

The sheet is stamped with the patient's hospital number and handed to the resident in the OR where he or she completes the demographics and OR event areas. When the patient is admitted to the PACU, the resident gives the sheet to the PACU nurse for completion of the PACU data. The data sheets are then scanned by a NCS 3000™ scanner.

The data from the scanner are formatted into a data base on a Macintosh SE running Maxscan™. The data are analyzed and reports are generated by Foxbase™, a d-Base™ software clone for the Macintosh. Data sheets are scanned weekly and reports are generated monthly. The monthly reports stratify the number of events by location and by provider. The aggregate of the monthly data is plotted to obtain secular trends.

Clinical Chart Reviews

There are some indicators that are associated with such severely adverse outcomes that they must be reviewed individually and whenever they occur. Among

these are perioperative myocardial infarction and perioperative death. Because it is customary to make the post-anesthesia visit between 23 and 48 hours after anesthesia, a signal event, such as the above, may be missed. Therefore, we rely upon our central QA service to provide us with data generated from discharge diagnoses. Each month, the hospitalwide program sends us a list of patients, identified by discharge ICD-9 codes, who have had a procedure and who have experienced an MI or who have died. This patient list is entered into a data base that helps track the associated medical record, allows entering the codes for the staff and resident involved, and provides for a synopsis of the case as reviewed by the QA committee. The data base also contains signal cases from the computer entry sheet described above and cases identified as having anesthesia problems from the surgery department morbidity and mortality conference which the QA Committee chairman attends routinely. In addition, the data base contains any patient-related incident reports that reflect anesthesia care.

Administrative Chart Reviews

The anesthesia department has developed standards for charting in the medical record. These standards include the pre-anesthesia visit, the anesthesia record and the post-anesthesia visit. Medical records, in their chart-completion area, identifies the absence of an indicated post-anesthesia note and provides the anesthesia department with the numbers of the patient and the resident. The medical record can then be requested, and the resident can complete his or her note. Additionally, a CRNA spends one-half day per week going to the wards, checking post-anesthesia notes not only for their presence, but also for content. She or he files a report with the chairman of the resident competency committee who counsels wayward residents appropriately. Then the recently retired, former chairman of our QA committee reviews anesthesia records stratified by faculty member so that the QA committee can track how well an individual faculty member supervises his or her residents vis-à-vis charting.

Department of Anesthesia

PT NUMBER	FAC ID	RES ID	DATE MM DD

LOCATION	TYPE OF ANES	SPECIAL	EVENTS
○ MAIN OR	○ GENERAL ET		TOTALLY NORMAL COURSE
○ ASC	○ GENERAL MASK	○ BYPASS	YES
○ L & D	○ SPIN/EPID		○ OR
○ URO	○ REGIONAL	○ CONTROLLED	○ RECOVERY
○ ECT	○ MAC	HYPOTENSION	○ UNPLANNED ADMIT
○ OTHER	○ OTHER		ICU/HOSP

IF ABOVE EVENTFUL, FILL IN BELOW

LOCATION	OR	PACU
CIRCULATION EVENTS		
Cardiac Arrest/Death	○	○
Unplanned Hypotension	○	○
Unplanned Hypertension	○	○
Dysrhythmia/EKG Abnormality	○	○
Other Circulation _____	○	○
AIRWAY/RESPIRATORY EVENTS		
Difficult/Traumatic/Failed Intubation	○	○
Unintended Failure to Extubate/Required Reintubation	○	○
Aspiration	○	○
Desaturation (SaO2 <85 for 2 min or <50 any time)	○	○
Laryngospasm/Airway Obstruction	○	○
Other Respiratory _____	○	○
REGIONAL ANESTHESIA EVENTS		
Unsatisfactory Regional _____	○	○
Technical Difficulties _____	○	○
Wet Tap	○	○
Other Regional _____	○	○
OTHER EVENTS		
Hypothermia (<35)	○	○
Hyperthermia (>39)	○	○
Machine Failure/Equipment Fault _____	○	○
Allergic/Anaphylactoid Reaction _____	○	○
Other _____	○	○

Figure 14.1. The Computer Entry Sheet, used to gather data prospectively on events from the operating room and the PACU. ASC, Ambulatory Surgery Center; L&D, Labor and Delivery Suite; URO, Urology Suite; ECT, Electroconvulsive Therapy Suite; ET, endotrocheal; MAC, monitored anesthesia care.

Post-anesthesia Patient Questionnaires

For several years, our department has been sending out a questionnaire by mail to the majority of patients receiving our services. The questionnaire is reproduced below:

During your recent hospitalization at the University of Iowa Hospitals and Clinics, you required the services of an anesthesiologist.

Would you please take a moment to answer a few questions so that we may attempt to improve our service. Following completion, please place this questionnaire in the self-addressed stamped envelope and mail.

1. Were you seen before your operation by a member of the Anesthesia Department? (Yes, No, Do Not Recall)
2. Were questions asked concerning your physical condition, medical history, and proposed operation? (Yes, No, Do Not Recall)
3. Were the choices of types of anesthesia, and their risks, explained to you? (Yes, No, Do Not Recall)
4. Were your questions concerning your anesthetic answered to your satisfaction? (Yes, No, Do Not Recall)
5. Did you visit with a member of the Anesthesia Department after your operation? (Yes, No, Do Not Recall)
6. Were you satisfied with the anesthesia care that you received? (Yes, No, Do Not Recall)
7. Comments:

These questionnaires are sent out about 6 weeks following the anesthesia. The replies are collated by a CRNA, sorted into the three categories of positive comments, no comments, and negative comments. The CRNA further sorts the negative comments into ones that he or she believes require action by the QA committee and sends them to the QA committee chairman. He or she again sorts them according to action needed or not and enters the ones that require action into a data base to track the course of the action. The action-requiring questionnaires are then copied, and one copy is sent to the faculty member responsible for action. The faculty member performs the necessary action and reports

back to the QA committee chairman. Closed contacts are collated for reporting in the Annual QA Report sent to the central QA program within the hospital.

It is common for a patient, given this opportunity, to express dissatisfaction with some other aspect of hospital or medical care. If another individual, perhaps from a different department, is involved, a copy of the questionnaire is made and sent to the Professional Practice Committee of the College of Medicine. This committee performs an appropriate action and notifies the central QA program within the hospital that that action has been taken. As a check that an action is taken, we inform the central QA program as a risk-control measure that they should expect a response from that committee. This ensures that the potential for follow-up on the complaint is not lost.

Processing the Data

All of the data collected above are reviewed by the anesthesia department QA committee chairman, who relies heavily on the computerized data bases for easy access to information. Each of the data bases can be sorted by event or provider in order to gain information regarding clusters that need further investigation.

Comparing Rates against Thresholds

We now have 12 month's worth of data from the computer entry sheets. The 12 data values for each monitor have been analyzed by mean and standard deviation. The threshold for each monitor has been set at zero for the signal events, or at the mean plus 2 standard deviations for the others. These results will be reported later. Starting with the second year of data collection, if the incidence of a monitor exceeds this value, a directed review will be initiated that will require monitoring all of the medical records containing the event and interviewing the anesthesia personnel involved. That the retrospective review is taking place will be announced at our staff meeting and at the morbidity and mortality conference (M&M), which, in itself, will constitute an educational output and probably reduce the incidence of the event, just because the event will be brought into focus.

Investigating All Signal Events

The chairman of the QA committee reviews the medical records on all signal events. If he or she determines that there might be a quality-of-care issue, the chairman brings the case before the QA committee for discussion, which may include the provider identified. The findings of the committee are recorded in the minutes of the meeting and, if the committee wishes, are included in the provider's credentialing file.

Analyzing Events and Providers for Trends

The data collected from the computerized entry sheets from the ORs and PACUs form the basis for determining the event pattern for the department. Occurrence rates can be determined for each monitor, both for the department as a whole and for individual providers. As is done is the Las Vegas model, the patterns of individual providers can be compared to those of the whole department to identify providers whose practice patterns deviate significantly.

Output of the Process

Memos to and Conferences with Providers

The most common result of an identified error is that the chairman of the QA committee contacts the provider directly. Commonly, these two individuals review the chart together. For minor errors, this is the end of the process. That the conference occurred is noted in the clinical chart review data base. Less frequently, a memo is sent to those involved, asking for a response. Again, this action is noted in the data base. Major errors are discussed before the QA committee and reported to the faculty as discussed above.

Morbidity and Mortality Conference

The clinical chart review data base allows flagging a case for presentation at M&M. Each month, a list of these cases is printed and sent to the M&M coordinator so that he or she may be cognizant of

"good" cases. Because our M&M is a teaching conference that frequently includes didactic material, we do not present all the cases in which the chairman of the QA committee identifies as having anesthesia-related problems. Our M&M frequently contains case presentations in which the providers did a good job and the outcome was favorable.

Faculty Meetings and Resulting Minutes

The faculty meeting is an excellent forum in which to discuss QA matters. Monthly, reports from all of the areas identified in the scope of our anesthesia practice are presented. Problem areas are presented, and the faculty approves plans to reduce the severity of the problem. The problems are tracked on a monthly basis until resolved.

Of great importance is the minutes of these meetings. The JCAHO places great emphasis on being able to verify that problems were found, acted upon, and resolved. Their favorite place to look is faculty minutes. There must be evidence of a detailed and thorough discussion of QA problems on a monthly basis. In addition, there must be evidence that central QA is informed of the above and that they have shared the information with other services involved in the identified problems.

Research Projects

The best mechanism for solving a quality-of-care problem may not be intuitively obvious. For example, nausea and vomiting constitute a major cause of unplanned admission to the hospital following ambulatory surgery, particularly for extraocular muscle surgery. Many techniques have been employed to try to reduce this problem, but it was not until a formal study of the various techniques was undertaken that an effective solution was identified.

Academic Publications

As a result of our QA efforts, our department has several publications. Scamman et al. (13) have reported on the computerized entry sheet. Dull and colleagues (15) have discovered, through the postanesthesia questionnaire, that the majority of anesthesia-related patient complaints are not identified while the patient is still in the hospital. This chapter constitutes a third academic publication.

Privileging and Credentialing

It appears intuitive that anesthesia care providers whose practices are not safe should have their practice restricted. The simplicity of this statement, however, belies the extreme complexity of implementing this process. The QA process is most important in providing data regarding safety and good outcome, and conversely must identify a provider whose practices are unsafe even if his or her outcomes are not health-threatening.

Peer review is extremely important in this process. On the basic level, the "identified individual," to quote the Joint Commission, who is responsible for recommending privileges, may review objective data gathered as part of a prospective process, for evidence of practice problems. There is a great danger here, however. Our computer entry sheets rely on the integrity of the individual to record the problems. It is untenable to use these data in a punitive manner. These data can be used only to identify a problem that the department as a whole is having. Once a problem is identified, then the directed review involving all providers focusing on the problem can be carried out. If an individual provider is identified as an outlier during the directed review, then his or her practice has been compared to that of his or her peers, not based on self-reported information. At this point, evidence of less-than-standard practice can be entered in the provider's credential file.

Other information in the credentialing file that this "individual" may review may include questionnaires with both positive and negative comments, results of QA committee actions, statements relating to the individual's health and evidence of chemical dependency, and letters from other health-care providers.

The process of how an "individual" uses these data to recommend privileges has not been delineated. It has been suspected that in the past an individual, when considering renewal of privileges, has thought that, for example, "Joe is a good old boy and there is

nothing wrong with him. I'll just sign his form." The public and many regulatory agencies now declare that this process is no longer acceptable, that an individual must not be allowed to continue to practice in an unsafe manner, and that objective QA data are the means by which to restrict privileges to safe areas and procedures.

It is difficult to restrict the scope of practice of an individual on a nonvoluntary basis. It is quite probable that this would lead to litigation—an expensive, unpleasant, time-consuming, and lengthy process. In addition, nonvoluntary reductions must be reported to the National Physician Database. However, if the anesthesia community cannot "police" its own, other less knowledgeable, more bureaucratic organizations will do it for us. The solution, as I see it, is to present the *objective* data of unsatisfactory practice to the provider and hope that he or she will voluntarily take steps to correct the deficiencies. The process will have to be monitored very closely, again with *objective* data.

Evaluation of the QA Process

Our QA process is constantly changing in response to the needs of the department. For example, we found that 3 months of prospective data collection in electroconvulsive therapy revealed no problems. Therefore, we collect data there now only on an occurrence basis. The faculty who are interested in regional anesthesia wanted to know not only if a regional anesthetic was not satisfactory, but also if technical problems caused the anesthetic to be unsatisfactory. Therefore, this monitor was added to the computer entry sheet. It was discovered that obstetric patients were being omitted from being contacted via the post-anesthesia questionnaire. They now have been added.

OUR RESULTS

It is very frustrating that we have found little in the way of problems that can be addressed directly and be corrected. That does not mean that we cannot improve our anesthesia care; it means that we need to keep looking.

Computer Entry Sheets

We now have 1 year's worth of data from our computer entry sheets encompassing 12,085 entries. For the past 3 months, the number of sheets processed versus the number of billings yields a submission rate of 80%. This rate is about 10% less than what we would like. We are now comparing, on an individual basis, the submission rate and counseling residents with a rate of less than 75%.

The results from the 20 monitors for the operating rooms are presented in Table 14.1. An event is identified if it is unexpected, unintended, unwanted, and requires treatment. Monitors titled "other" have a blank on the entry sheet where free text may be entered, which is later manually transferred to the data base. Many of these "others" provide input to our morbidity and mortality conference. As noted above, our monitors were selected to be straightforward and simple. Other QA

programs may wish to expand or narrow the range of monitors in this area.

Now that we have criteria or thresholds for our monitors, we expect that in some month in the near future one of our monitors will be above this level, an event that will trigger a directed review. For this review, the patient hospital numbers corresponding to the monitor will be retrieved from the data base and the medical records reviewed by a member of the QA committee who will prepare a report for the committee, which will summarize the findings of the individual cases. The committee, following the QA process, will ascertain if there is a problem. If so, the committee will formulate a solution to the problem and implement the solution. Subsequent tracking of this monitor will determine if the problem has been resolved. The results of this process will be forwarded to central QA.

It is interesting to conjecture at what rate monitors will fall above threshold. If the

Table 14.1.
Results from 1 Year of Prospective Monitoring via Computerized Data Entry Sheets (12,085 Entries)

Monitor	Number	Rate	Criterion (rate + 2 S.D.)
		% total cases	%
Operating room code or death	13	0.11	0.00[a]
Hypotension	103	0.84	1.57
Hypertension	33	0.27	0.73
Dysrhythmia or other ECG abnormality	83	0.69	1.23
Other circulatory events	15	0.12	0.27
Difficult or failed intubation	70	0.72[b]	1.45
Failed extubation	37	0.38[b]	0.96
Aspiration (suspected or proved)	5	0.05[b]	0.17
Desaturation or hypoxia	46	0.38	0.72
Laryngospasm or airway obstruction	63	0.64[b]	1.26
Other respiratory events	51	0.42	0.75
Failed regional anesthetic	63	5.29[c]	8.61
Wet taps on attempted epidural	12	0.89[d]	2.93
Other regional events	22	1.23[c]	3.28
Hypothermia	39	0.39[b]	0.89
Hyperthermia	4	0.04[b]	0.21
Equipment fault	8	0.07	0.22
Allergic or anaphylactoid reaction	6	0.05	0.20
Admitted to hospital or ICU	71	0.59	1.59
Other	187	1.51	6.62

[a]Criterion set at 0.0 by the QA committee.
[b]Based on the number of general anesthetics.
[c]Based on the number of regional anesthetics.
[d]Based on the number of spinals and epidurals. We did not collect data on the number of epidurals.

rate of events for a monitor is normally distributed on a monthly basis implying that the rate would be more than 2 standard deviations above the mean 2.5% of the months (1 of 40), then one could expect 1 of our 40 monitors to be above threshold each month, just on a random basis. If problems were to arise, the number could be greater than this.

As we continue to collect data, we will be interested to see if differences develop among months. For example, would the rate of difficult intubations be higher during the first few months of training, or would the rate of failure of regional anesthesia fall as the new residency class becomes more proficient?

Clinical Chart Reviews

It is in this area where the entire QA process comes together. Last year, QA reviewed 168 medical records that had been identified as being associated with signal events or other problem areas. Each of these records had an entry in a data base that allowed tracking of event, whether anesthesia were responsible for the event, provider(s), resolution of the event, and morbidity and mortality conference status. The data base was sorted by provider to ascertain whether any provider was associated with a greater number of events (none was) or whether there was a pattern of events related to anesthesia cause (none was found). That analysis of this data base yielded little in the way of constructive opportunity to identify and solve problems was disappointing, particularly because medical record review is a slow and tiring process. However, medical record review is vitally important to the QA process and must be considered part of the labor in having an effective QA process.

Post-anesthesia Questionnaire

Our department has been sending out questionnaires to the majority of the patients anesthetized since February 1988. By July 1990, 11,636 questionnaires (representing a 57% return rate) were returned for analysis. Ninety-six percent of the patients were in general satisfied with

their anesthesia care. However, of all the questionnaires returned, 6.8% in the "Comments" item showed some patient dissatisfaction with their experience. Complaints against the provider constituted 23% of these, while 42% were directed against the anesthesia technique. The majority of complaints have been followed up with chart reviews and phone calls. One of our residents was so unpopular with the patients that a series of patient complaints provided some of the documentation used in due process to eject him from our residency program.

These questionnaires have revealed that a significant portion of anesthesia-related complications may not be apparent until the patient has been discharged (15).

FUTURE EFFORTS
Change from Outcome Analysis to Process Analysis

It has become apparent that outcome analysis may not be sensitive enough to detect any but major individual and systematic problems. Part of this lack of sensitivity is because anesthesia-related negative-outcome events are fortunately now quite rare. Even a most-qualified anesthesia provider may have a negative-outcome event without this event indicating the presence of a correctable problem.

Therefore, we have made the assumption that providers who utilize and practice good processes are more skilled and are less likely to have negative outcomes. Unfortunately, it is very difficult to judge anesthesia process except by examining the documentation the provider creates as part of patient care. Our faculty individual who performs the majority of anesthesia record reviews believes that those whom he knows to be the best residents on a clinical basis are also the ones who do the best job of charting. These are also the residents who miss the fewest post-anesthesia notes.

We also think that the computer entry sheet may be an indicator of process, although we have not tested this yet. It is possible that the residents who do the best job of charting also have the highest submission rates. Validation of this easily obtainable process monitor is underway.

Implementation of the JCAHO Beta Test Program

Presently, we are in the process of implementing the JCAHO Beta Test Program at our associated VA Medical Center. We do not know, as of yet, the value of the software package that accompanies this program in terms of discovering areas of anesthesia practice that need improvement. It is apparent that this retrospective system will require a large amount of chart review effort, particularly once a patient has been identified as having a discharge diagnosis, which flags the hospital course for further review. We hope that the data gathered on a national basis will lead to revision and refinement of the monitors that the JCAHO recommends.

Area of Needed Improvement

It is apparent that our QA program needs to improve its image as to purpose and intent among our residents and staff. Many have expressed the feeling that the main purpose of our data collection and analysis efforts is to chastise and humiliate guilty individuals. We suspect that such attitudes are leading to passive-aggressive activities such as noncompliance with charting standards and reluctance to complete computer entry sheets. We understand the difficulty of asking an individual to report events which, in his or her mind, may be used in a punitive manner against that individual. Therefore, we are undertaking an educational program to inform the residents and staff that this is not the case. We hope to engender an attitude that QA is a scientific process of discovering the epidemiology of anesthesia practices that can be improved.

CONCLUSION

Quality Assurance in anesthesia is a process that allows for effective identification of potential problems, objective as-

sessment of the cause(s) of these problems, implementation of actions designed to eliminate the problems, and monitoring to assure that the problems have been eliminated. This chapter has summarized the steps of the process as defined by the JCAHO, adding the mechanisms by which the process is carried out, and outlining a few of the areas where additional progress can be made.

References

1. Joint Commission on Accreditation of Healthcare Organizations. Monitoring and evaluation: Anesthesia services. Chicago: JCAHO, 1987.
2. Joint Commission on Accreditation of Healthcare Organizations. Accreditation manual for hospitals. Chicago: JCAHO, 1990.
3. Joint Commission on Accreditation of Healthcare Organizations. Quality assurance. In: JCAHO. Accreditation manual for hospitals. Chicago: JCAHO, 1990:214
4. Joint Commission on Accreditation of Healthcare Organizations. Quality Assurance. In: JCAHO. Accreditation manual for hospitals. Chicago: JCAHO, 1990:212.
5. From a letter from Dennis S. O'Leary, President, JCAHO to Gary Wilkenson, Medical Center Director, VAMC, Iowa City, IA dated October 11, 1990.
6. Baldock GJ. Quality assurance, standards and accreditation [editorial], Anaesthesia 1990;45:617–618.
7. Vitez TS. A model for quality assurance in anesthesiology. J Clin Anesth 1990;2:280–287.
8. Hindman BJ. Perioperative stroke: The noncardiac surgery patient. Int Anesthesiol Clin 1986;24:101–134.
9. Skillman JJ. Neurological complications of cardiovascular surgery: 1. Procedures involving the carotid arteries and abdominal aorta. Int Anesthesiol Clin 1986;24:135–157.
10. Dawkins CJM. Analysis of the complications of extradural and caudal block. Anaesthesia 1969;24:554.
11. Cheney FW. ASA closed claims study. ASA Newsletter 1989;53:9.
12. Eichhorn JH. Prevention of intraoperative anesthesia accidents and related severe injury through safety monitoring. Anesthesiology 1989;70:572–577.
13. Scamman FL, Todd MM, Jadryev PJ. Computer management of quality assessment monitoring data. Anesthesiology 1990;73:A1039.
14. American Society of Anesthesiologists. Judging clinical competence. Park Ridge: ASA, 1989.
15. Dull DL, Scamman FL, Oltz L, Tinker JH. Long term follow-up for identification of anesthetic complications. Anesth Analg 1990;70:S91.

APPENDIX

**Anesthesiology Service
Veterans Affairs Medical Center
Iowa City, Iowa**

POLICIES OF THE SERVICE
I. The Anesthesiology Service shall be organized, directed, and integrated with other related services or departments of this hospital.
   A. The Chief of the Anesthesiology Service shall be certified by the American Board of Anesthesiology (or its Canadian or UK equivalent) as a specialist in Anesthesiology and must meet the criteria for a staff anesthesiologist. The Chief must hold an academic appointment in the Department of Anesthesia, University of Iowa College of Medicine. The Chief of the Anesthesiology Service shall be clinically competent and possess administrative skills to assure effective leadership of the Service. The Chief of the Anesthesiology Service shall be directly responsible to the Chief of Staff. Duties of the Chief, Anesthesiology Service, or his or her designee include, but are not necessarily limited to:
      1. Recommending appointment and appropriate privileges for staff anesthesiologists and nurse anesthetists. Such appointments shall be processed through the Chief of Staff and the Professional Standards Board.
      2. Maintaining throughout this VAMC a high quality of anesthesia care rendered by staff anesthesiologists, nurse anesthetists, residents, and other trainees assigned to the Anesthesiology Service.
      3. Recommending to the administrative and medical staffs the type and amount of equipment necessary for administering anesthesia and for related resuscitative efforts and ensuring, through an annual review, that such equipment is available.
      4. Developing regulations concerning anesthesia safety.
      5. Ensuring retrospective evaluation of the quality anesthesia care throughout this VAMC, designated the "identified individual." See Section VII.
      6. Maintaining a program of continuing education for staff nurse anesthetists, including in-service training and evaluation of quality-assurance efforts. See Section VII.
      7. Maintaining membership on (or consultant to) the VAMC Cardiopulmonary Resuscitation Committee and Environmental Control (Infections) Committee.
      8. Providing available consultation in the management of acute and chronic respiratory insufficiency, chronic pain, and problems in the care of patients in the Surgical Intensive Care Unit.
      9. Assigning the various anesthesia personnel to cases in a manner which assures that residents and CRNAs are properly supervised by staff anesthesiologists.
   B. When requested, representatives

of the Anesthesiology Service will participate as instructors in the overall hospital program of continuing education and in-service planning.

II. Anesthesia care shall be provided by anesthesiologists, qualified nurse anesthetists, or supervised trainees. A qualified nurse anesthetist or supervised trainee will be available to provide anesthesia care at all times. The administration of anesthesia will be limited to areas where it can be given safely. The same competence of anesthesia personnel shall be available for all procedures requiring anesthesia services, whether elective or emergency. An individual's competence to provide anesthesia care will be reviewed yearly at the time of the performance evaluation, using data gathered from all possible sources, including quality assurance data.

A. Staff anesthesiologists must be certified or eligible for certification by the American Board of Anesthesiologists (or equivalent), must have clinical privileges at this VAMC, must qualify as a licensed independent practitioner, and must be able to perform all of the services usually required in the practice of anesthesiology, including but not limited to being able to:

1. Perform accepted procedures commonly used to render the patient insensible to pain during the performance of surgical, obstetrical, and other pain-producing clinical maneuvers.

2. Support life functions during the period in which anesthesia is administered. This responsibility may include consultation for nurse anesthetists and supervised trainees.

3. Provide appropriate pre- and post-anesthesia management of the patient. This responsibility may include pre-anesthesia consultation with nurse anesthetists and supervised trainees, and reviewing and countersigning their pre-anesthesia evaluations and medication orders.

4. Provide consultation relating to various other forms of patient care, such as respiratory care, cardiopulmonary resuscitation, and special problems in pain relief.

B. Qualified nurse anesthetists must be able to provide general anesthesia under the direction or supervision of the Chief of Anesthesiology or his designee. Nurse anesthetists will not be directed by trainees. Qualified nurse anesthetists shall have competence to:

1. Induce anesthesia.

2. Maintain anesthesia at the required levels.

3. Support life functions during the period in which anesthesia is administered.

4. Recognize and take appropriate corrective action (including requesting of consultation when necessary) for abnormal patient responses to anesthesia or to any adjunctive medication or other form of therapy.

5. Provide professional observation and resuscitative care (including the requesting of consultation when necessary) until the patient has gained control of his or her vital functions.

6. Not undertake procedures for which they have not been certified as being competent.

C. Trainees (residents, medical students, dental students) will provide anesthesia care only under the supervision or direction of the Chief of Anesthesiology or a staff anesthesiologist.

D. When the operating/anesthesia team consists of nonphysicians, there must be a physician immediately available in case of an emergency such as cardiac arrest.

III. Precautions shall be taken to ensure the safe administration of anesthetic agents.

A. Anesthetic apparatus must be inspected and tested by the anesthesia person before use. If a defect is observed, the equipment must not be used until the fault is repaired. See Section VIII for greater detail.

B. Only nonflammable agents shall be used for anesthesia.

C. Because only nonflammable anesthetic agents are used, an isolated power distribution system and its line isolation monitors are not required.

D. The condition of operating room equipment shall be inspected by Engineering on a regular basis and records kept in that department.

E. Anesthesia personnel shall be familiar with air exchange and humidity control mechanisms within the operating rooms.

IV. There shall be written policies relating to the delivery of anesthesia care. These polices shall be approved by the Chief of Staff, reviewed annually, and enforced.

A. There will be a pre-anesthetic evaluation by a staff anesthesiologist, a nurse anesthetist, or a trainee with appropriate documentation in the patient's medical record of the pertinent information relative to the anesthetic and surgical procedure anticipated. When possible, this evaluation will be performed by the anesthesia person who is going to provide the anesthesia care. Except in extreme emergency cases, this evaluation should be recorded prior to the patient's transfer to the anesthetizing area and before any pre-anesthetic medication has been administered. While the choice of agent or technique may be left to the individual administering the anesthetic, the pre-anesthetic note should at least refer to the types of anesthetics (general, spinal, regional, etc.) discussed with and agreed to by the patient. The note should also include a statement that the patient understands the anesthetic and the inherent risks, and that all his or her questions were answered. The patient's ASA physical status, the date, and the time of the note are also required. Patients to be cared for by nurse anesthetists will be evaluated by and have their care prescribed by either a staff anesthesiologist or an anesthesia resident. Pre-anesthesia medication is ordered by either staff or residents. Pre-anesthetic care is monitored by either a direct report or a telephone report between anesthesiology staff and resident trainee or nurse anesthetist. The signature of the responsible staff on the face of the anesthesia record will be documentation that this monitoring has taken place. Compliance with these requirements shall be audited on a quarterly basis. See Section VII.

B. Immediately prior to the induction of anesthesia, the anesthesia person will review the patient's condition. This review will include a review of the medical record with regard to completeness, pertinent laboratory data, and the time of administration and dose of any pre-anesthesia medication. The anesthesia person will appraise any changes in the patient's condition as compared with that noted on previous visits. Evidence of this review will be documented in the patient's medical record.

C. Prior to commencing all anesthetics, the anesthesia person shall check the availability, readiness, cleanliness, sterility (when required), and working condition of all equipment necessary to administer that anesthetic. See Section VIII. Particularly, the ability to institute general anesthesia at any time during a regional anesthetic will be assured. Standard monitoring will consist of ECG, blood pressure, temperature, and pulse oximetry. The anesthesia person may expand the scope of monitoring at his or her discretion.

D. Laryngoscope, airways, breathing bags, masks, endotracheal tubes, and other anesthesia equipment shall be cleaned or disposed of after each use according to policies found in the Infection Control Manual of this facility.

E. Following the procedure for which anesthesia was administered, the anesthesia person or his/her designee shall remain with the patient as long as required by the patient's condition relative to his or her anesthesia status and until responsibility for proper patient care has been assumed by other qualified individuals. Personnel responsible for post-anesthetic care should be advised of specific problems presented by the patient's condition. The same degree of care should be provided when the patient is returned to the nursing floor.

F. Release of patients from the post-anesthetic care unit shall be determined on an individual basis by a member of the anesthesia care team. A progress note shall be entered on the anesthesia record detailing the condition of the patient with reference to mental status, vital signs, time, date, and other pertinent data.

G. A record shall be kept of all pertinent events taking place during the induction of, maintenance of, and emergence from the anesthetic, including the dose and/or duration of all anesthetic agents, other drugs, intravenous fluids, urine output, blood loss

and replacement, vital signs, and quantitative monitors. Compliance with the above requirements shall be audited on a quarterly basis. See Section VII.

H. Post-anesthetic visits shall be made early in the postoperative period and once after complete recovery from anesthesia (24 hrs). At least one note shall be written describing the presence of absence of anesthesia-related complications such as sore throat, dental damage, neurological deficits, or fever, except if the patient is discharged earlier than 24 hours post induction or on a weekend or holiday, and that any questions the patient may have have been answered. Presence of such a note shall be audited on a quarterly basis. See Section VII.

I. Guidelines for the Anesthesiology Service are included in the Infection Control Manual. These guidelines will be reviewed, revised as necessary, and enforced.

J. A quarterly check shall be done of each operating room in which general anesthetics are given to see if the gas scavenging systems are effective. These results shall be recorded in the log book in the anesthesia office and immediate action taken to correct any abnormal reading.

K. The Anesthesiology Service shall comply with all pertinent and applicable sections in NFPA 99.

L. The safe practice of anesthesia shall include:
1. Awareness that general anesthetics are potent cardiovascular and respiratory depressants.
2. Preparation to prevent aspiration of gastric contents, to include, but not be limited to, appropriate application of awake intubation, Sellick maneuver, awake extubation, and cuffed endotracheal tubes.
3. Blood product administration

preceded by check of each product and cross-check with patient identification prior to product administration. If a blood warmer is used, proper temperature will be noted.

4. Attention to patient positioning to avoid nerve damage or other pressure point injury.

5. Careful attention to gas flow meters to include availability of light when the room is darkened for use of operative microscopes, bronchoscopes, or similar devices.

6. Double check of all drugs for certain identification before their administration.

V. The Anesthesiology Service shall hold a staff conference on a monthly basis.

A. The conference will be attended by all staff and CRNAs and the service secretary.

B. The purpose of the meeting will be to discuss affairs of the Anesthesiology Service including but not limited to quality assurance reports, morbidity and mortality case discussions, annual training, announcements, and other Service business.

C. Documentation of the conference shall follow Medical Center Memorandum 88-103.

VI. The Anesthesiology Service Patient-Care Equipment Training Plan.

A. The Anesthesiology Service will conduct orientation of residents on their first day on the service. This orientation will consist of demonstration and check-out on the anesthesia machines and physiological monitors. The purpose of the orientation is to ensure that only qualified individuals operate patient-care equipment. Additionally, the residents will familiarize themselves with the Anesthesia Workroom as to location of drugs, equipment, and manuals. Documentation of this training will be kept by the Service Secretary to include subject, date, and name of resident.

B. The Service will conduct an inservice for permanent staff on a yearly basis to satisfy the requirement of annual continuing education for individuals who use anesthesia equipment. The subjects covered will emphasize safe equipment operation and minimization of clinical and physical risks. This inservice will be documented as a staff meeting with attendance recorded. Additionally, each major item of anesthesia equipment will bear a label indicating who is qualified to use that equipment.

VII. STANDARDS FOR QUALITY ASSURANCE

A. QUARTERLY ANESTHESIOLOGY RECORD AUDIT

1. Surgical patients' medical records will be examined on a quarterly basis for completeness of anesthesia notes and records. Such examination will include:

a. Pre-anesthesia note, which must contain:

1) A review of objective diagnostic data.

2) Evidence of an interview with the patient to discuss the patient's medical, anesthetic, and drug history, the anesthesia plan and its risks and complications including the possibility of transfusion, and the patient's physical status.

b. A review of the anesthesia record, which must contain:

1) Pertinent events such as but not limited to start of anesthesia care, induction, intubation, start of surgery, end of surgery, extubation, and end of anesthesia care.

2) Anesthetic agents and concentrations, and drugs and doses.

3) Intravenous fluid volumes including blood and blood components.

4) Estimates of blood loss and urine output.

c. A review of the post-anesthesia notes, which must contain:

1) A release from the PACU or documentation of a direct admission to the SICU or to the ward from the OR.

2) Evidence that the patient was visited after recovery from anesthesia and that the presence or absence of anesthesia-related complications, such as nausea or vomiting, neurological deficit, hoarseness, or any cardiac or pulmonary complication, is recorded.

2. A record of defects and corrective action will be kept on file and included in the Service's Quarterly Report. Anesthesia team members with significant errors in charting will be notified.

B. ONGOING ANALYSIS OF ANESTHESIOLOGY CLINICAL FUNCTIONS

1. The quality and appropriateness of patient care shall be monitored and evaluated monthly for all anesthesia clinical functions. The scope of these functions includes any anesthesia-related activity conducted within the operating room suite.

a. Information concerning important aspects of care shall be collected routinely. These aspects of care are the preanesthetic evaluation, patient monitoring, equipment monitoring, administration of anesthetics, and post-anesthesia evaluation and care.

b. These data shall be assessed monthly in order to identify important problems in patient care.

c. When a problem is identified, it shall be corrected by appropriate action(s), and the effectiveness of the action(s) evaluated.

2. The results of a, b, and c from above will be documented and reported to the Central QA Coordinator on a quarterly basis through a memo containing the important findings.

3. The Chief of the Anesthesiology Service or his or her designee is responsible for collecting data from the prospective monitors daily, for comparing the data to the criteria monthly, for evaluating variations, for identifying opportunity for improvement, for implementing these opportunities, and for evaluating any improvements.

4. Interesting anesthetics, anesthetics involving morbidity, and anesthetics involving mortality will be presented at the University of Iowa Anesthesia M&M conferences. Minutes of these presentations will be kept on file. The minutes will contain a brief presentation of the anesthetic, a discussion of the management of the anesthetic, and any conclusions relating to the appropriateness of care. The minutes will be reviewed by the Chief of Anesthesiology, and any problem areas will be identified. If a problem is identified, the Chief will formulate a plan of action to minimize the problem, implement the plan, and document, in the quarterly report to the Central QA coordinator, the results of such action.

C. CONTINUING EDUCATION PROGRAM

1. A regular inservice educational program shall be conducted and includes formal and informal presentations by members of the anesthesia care team or others when appropriate.
2. A library shall be maintained for the immediate use of all members of the team. This library shall include texts, current anesthesia journals, technical material on the anesthesia machines, and supplementary material.
3. Members of the team shall be encouraged to attend off-facility continuing education courses as the workload permits. These activities must be sufficient to maintain licensure.

VIII. STANDARDS FOR ANESTHESIA CARE

A. STANDARD FOR ANESTHESIA MACHINES

1. All anesthesia machines are to be equipped with scavenging systems, sphygmomanometers, pin index safety systems, and low pressure guardian systems. Each machine will have an oxygen analyzer. If an anesthesia machine has a ventilator attached, the machine will be equipped with audible alarms to detect low airway pressure and low exhaled volume.
2. Each machine will be inspected on a regular basis for safety and adherence to manufacturer's specifications. Records of these inspections are to be maintained by Bioengineering or the contracted inspector.
3. All anesthesia machines are to be equipped to administer oxygen and nitrous oxide, and are to have at least two vaporizers for volatile anesthetic agents.

B. STANDARD FOR ANESTHESIA MACHINE CHECKOUT

*1. Inspect anesthesia machine for:
   a. machine identification number and record on all anesthesia records.
   b. valid inspection sticker.
   c. undamaged flowmeter, vaporizers, gages, supply hoses.
   d. complete, undamaged breathing system with adequate CO_2 absorbent.
   e. correct mounting of cylinders in yokes.
   f. presence of cylinder wrench.
*2. Inspect and turn on electrical equipment requiring warm-up.
*3. Connect waste gas scavenging system and adjust vacuum as required.
*4. Check that flow control valves are off, that vaporizers are off, that vaporizers are filled, and that filler caps are sealed.
*5. Check O_2 cylinder supplies:
   a. disconnect pipeline supply and return cylinder and pipeline pressure gages to zero with O_2 flush.
   b. open O_2 cylinder; check that there is at least 500 psi pressure.
   c. close valve and observe gage for evidence of high pressure leak.
   d. open cylinder.
*6. Turn on master switch (if present).
*7. Check N_2O and air supplies as above.
*8. Test flowmeters:
   a. check that float is at bottom of tube with flow-control valves closed (or at minimum on O_2).
   b. adjust flow of all gases

through their full range and check for erratic movements of floats.

*9. Test ratio protection/warning system (if present): attempt to create hypoxic and verify correct change in gas flows and/or alarm.

*10. Test O_2 pressure failure system:
  a. set O_2 and other gases to mid-range.
  b. close O_2 cylinder and flush to release O_2 pressure.
  c. verify that all flows fall to zero; open O_2 cylinder.
  d. close all other cylinders and bleed piping pressures.
  e. close O_2 cylinder and bleed piping pressure.
  f. CLOSE ALL FLOWMETER VALVES.

*11. Test central pipeline gas supplies:
  a. inspect supply hoses (should not be cracked or worn).
  b. connect supply hoses, verifying correct color coding.
  c. adjust all flows to mid-range.
  d. verify that supply pressures hold (45–55 psi).
  e. shut off flowmeter valves.

*12. Add any accessory equipment to the breathing system: peep valve, humidifier.

13. Calibrate O_2 monitor:
  a. either calibrate to read 21% in room air or
  b. fill system with 100% O_2 and check that monitor reads near 100%.

14. Sniff inspiratory gas: there should be no odor.

*15. Check unidirectional valves:
  a. inhale and exhale through a surgical mask into the breathing system having disconnected each limb at the "y".
  b. verify unidirectional flow in each limb.
  c. reconnect tubing firmly.

16. Check for leaks in machine and breathing system:
  a. close pop-off valve and occlude system at "y".
  b. fill system via O_2 flush until bag is just full; set O_2 to 5 liters.
  c. slowly decrease O_2 flow until pressure no longer rises above 20 cm H_2O. Flow rate now should be no greater than 200 ml/min.
  d. squeeze bag to pressure of 50 cm H_2O and verify tight system.

17. Exhaust valve and scavenger system:
  a. open pop-off valve and observe release of pressure.
  b. occlude "y" connector and verify that negligible pressure appears with either zero or 5 liters/min flow and that exhaust relief valve opens with flush flow.

18. Test ventilator:
  a. if switching valve is present, test function in both bag and ventilator mode.
  b. close pop-off valve if necessary and occlude system at patient end.
  c. test for leaks and pressure relief by appropriate cycling.
  d. attach reservoir bag at mask fitting, fill system and cycle ventilator; assure filling/emptying of bag.

19. Check suction.

20. Check, connect, and calibrate (if necessary) other electronic monitors.

21. Check final position of all controls.

22. Turn on and set alarms.

Note: Items marked with an * need not

be repeated or may be abbreviated after the initial checkout.

C. STANDARD OF INTRAOPERATIVE MONITORING (From American Society of Anesthesiologists. 1991 directory of members. Park Ridge: ASA, 1991:670–671.)

1. Qualified anesthesia personnel shall be present in the room throughout the conduct of all general anesthetics, regional anesthetics, and monitored anesthetic care.

    OBJECTIVE

    Because of the rapid changes in patient status during anesthesia, qualified anesthesia personnel shall be continuously present to monitor the patient and provide anesthesia care. In the event there is a direct known hazard, e.g., radiation, to the anesthesia personnel which might require intermittent remote observation of the patient, some provisions for monitoring the patient must be made. In the event that an emergency requires the temporary absence of the person primarily responsible for the anesthetic, the best judgment of the anesthesiologist will be exercised in comparing the emergency with the anesthetized patient's condition and in the selection of the person left responsible for the anesthetic during the temporary absence.

2. During all anesthetics, the patient's oxygenation, ventilation, circulation, and temperature shall be continually evaluated.

    a. OXYGENATION

    OBJECTIVE

    To ensure adequate oxygen concentration in the inspired gas and the blood during all anesthetics.

    METHODS

    1) Inspired gas: During every administration of general anesthesia using an anesthesia machine, the concentration of oxygen in the patient breathing system shall be measured by an oxygen analyzer with a low oxygen concentration limit alarm in use.

    2) Blood oxygenation: During all anesthetics, a quantitative method of assessing oxygenation such as pulse oximetry shall be employed. Adequate illumination and exposure of the patient is necessary to assess color.

    b. VENTILATION

    OBJECTIVE

    To ensure adequate ventilation of the patient during all anesthetics.

    METHODS

    1) Every patient receiving general anesthesia shall have the adequacy of ventilation continually evaluated. While qualitative clinical signs such as chest excursion, observation of the reservoir breathing bag and ascultation of breath sounds may be adequate, quantitative monitoring of the CO_2 content and/or volume of expired gas is encouraged.

    2) When an endotracheal tube is inserted, its correct positioning in the trachea must be verified by clinical assessment and by identification of

carbon dioxide in the expired gas. End-tidal CO_2 analysis, in use from the time of endotracheal tube placement, is encouraged.

3) When ventilation is controlled by a mechanical ventilator, there shall be in continuous use a device that is capable of detecting disconnection of components of the breathing system. The device must give an audible signal when its alarm threshold is exceeded.

4) During regional anesthesia and monitored anesthesia care, the adequacy of ventilation shall be evaluated, at least, by continual observation of qualitative clinical signs.

c. CIRCULATION
OBJECTIVE
To ensure the adequacy of the patient's circulatory function during all anesthetics.
METHODS
1) Every patient receiving anesthesia shall have the electrocardiogram continuously displayed from the beginning of anesthesia until preparing to leave the anesthetizing location.

2) Every patient receiving anesthesia shall have arterial blood pressure and heart rate determined and evaluated at least every five minutes.

3) Every patient receiving general anesthesia shall have, in addition to the above, circulatory function continually evalu-

ated by at least one of the following: palpation of a pulse, ascultation of heart sounds, monitoring of a tracing of intraarterial pressure, ultrasound peripheral pulse monitoring, or pulse plethysmography or oximetry.

d. BODY TEMPERATURE
OBJECTIVE
To aid in the maintenance of appropriate body temperature during all anesthetics.
METHODS
1) There shall be readily available a means to continuously measure the patient's temperature. When changes in body temperature are intended, anticipated, or suspected, the temperature shall be measured.

Note: "Continual" is defined as "repeated regularly and frequently in steady rapid succession" whereas "continuous" means "prolonged without any interruption at any time." If any of these requirements cannot be met, they shall be, along with the reasons, noted in the patient's medical record.

D. STANDARD FOR DISPENSING/ SIGNING FOR NARCOTICS— OR
1. Narcotics (DEA Schedule II and III) will be dispensed only after a Controlled Substance Order (VA 10-2321) bearing the patient's name and OR #, name of drug(s), how supplied, quantity of drug(s), and user's signature with date is issued to the OR Charge Nurse. A copy will be retained by the user.

2. After drugs are administered, the user will either sign for the used drug(s) or return the unused drug(s) to the OR

Charge Nurse. The OR Charge Nurse cannot be accountable for drugs left on the cabinet top. User will write on the slip what was used, wasted, or returned. Partial unused ampules must be wasted. Wasting of Schedule II and III drugs must be witnessed with the witness' initials appearing on the VA 10-2321.

3. Drugs should be signed out on the green sheet as soon after use as possible (e.g., after the procedure is completed rather than at the end of the tour of duty).

4. The green sheet must contain the patient's full first and last name, date and time, user's full first and last name, title, and amount used, and balance.

IX. POLICY FOR ENERGY CONSERVATION.
  A. Room temperatures.
    1. When occupied, temperatures in administrative areas shall be set at 21°C for heating and 24°C for cooling. Over weekends, thermostats will be set for energy conservation.
    2. Room temperatures in the operating room shall be set according to patient needs.
  B. Lighting.
    1. Overhead lighting will be turned off when the room is empty.
    2. Use of local lighting (desk lamps) is encouraged.
  C. Windows.
    1. Prime windows and storm windows will be kept closed when the heating and air conditioning systems are in operation.

15

Critical Care Units

John W. Hoyt, M.D., F.C.C.M., F.C.C.P.,
Deborah J. Leisifer, R.N., C.C.R.N.,
and Harry S. Rafkin, M.D.

The history of critical care is barely 35 years old. This history has been replete with technological advances designed to prevent death in the face of life-threatening illness. With all the life support devices and monitoring equipment, "quality care" has seemed synonymous with critical care.

This chapter will examine some of the history of critical care to clarify for the reader the difficulties of performing quality assessment in the intensive care environment. The authors will present examples of quality assurance projects done in the intensive care unit (ICU). Finally, we will take a bottom line approach to analyzing the results of critical care by looking at morbidity, mortality, and length of stay through the lens of the severity of illness classification systems. Only when critical care practitioners have some quantification of severity of illness can they really analyze the result of quality ICU services. It is trivial to tabulate the frequency with which a given protocol is adhered to in the ICU by reviewing records; it is complex to determine if a given protocol reduces morbidity and mortality in a group of critically ill patients with the same diagnosis and similar severity of illness scores.

HISTORY OF CRITICAL CARE

At least three patient care evolutions can be identified that resulted in critical care as we know it today and they were all directed at improving quality of care (1). The first was the opening of recovery rooms in the late 1940s and early 1950s in association with operating rooms and anesthesia departments. Anesthesiologists provided life support and general anesthesia for ever more complicated and prolonged surgical procedures. It became apparent that the job of the anesthesiologist was not complete at the end of a surgical procedure if the patient had not emerged from anesthesia. The surgeon was finished and ready for the next case. There needed to be a monitoring station near the operating room where the anesthesiologist could continue to observe the postoperative patient until the effects of surgery and anesthesia were reversed. As a result, recovery rooms were started, and quality of care improved as adverse reactions during emergence from anesthesia were prevented. Some patients required days to recover from the effects of surgery, and anesthesia and surgical intensive care units evolved from recovery rooms.

A second evolutionary process surrounded the growing understanding of respiratory failure. The polio epidemics of the late 1940s and early 1950s caused many young people to die of respiratory failure when mechanical ventilation was still in its infancy. Initially, negative pressure ventilators and subsequently positive pressure ventilators were used to provide mechanical respiratory support to the dying patient. The etiologies of respiratory failure included neurologic, postoperative, and infectious. Eventually these patients were grouped together in a single area, a respiratory intensive care unit, with skilled nurses and respiratory therapists to improve quality of care and to keep patients alive who would never have survived in the past.

Lastly, continuous electrocardiogram (ECG) monitoring and direct current (DC) defibrillation arrived on the scene of medical care as the understanding of myocardial infarction was evolving. Since ventricular arrhythmias were a common cause of death in myocardial infarction, quality of care improved by grouping patients with acute myocardial infarction in a coronary care unit. ECG monitoring allowed monitor watchers to detect life-threatening arrhythmias early and terminate them with DC defibrillation or prevent them with intravenous lidocaine.

Though not substantiated by well-controlled studies, physicians and hospitals assumed high quality care and patient benefit with intensive care. The 1960s was an era of rapid growth for critical care with the majority of hospitals, particularly large teaching hospitals, establishing one or more intensive care units for monitoring and life support. Champions of intensive care services, "intensivist physicians" specializing in critical care medicine, led the use of a parade of technological advances such as pulmonary artery catheters, portable hemodialysis, parenteral nutrition, intraaortic counterpulsation balloon support, etc.

By the 1980s, two types of patients were presumed to find benefit from the high quality care delivered in the intensive care unit. First, there were patients requiring monitoring to prevent adverse consequences of physiologic changes. For example, patients with a previous myocardial infarction were commonly monitored in the ICU after elective surgery to try and prevent postoperative ischemia and a new myocardial infarction. Second, there were ICU patients requiring active life support

in order to survive an illness. Status asthmaticus with respiratory acidosis refractory to bronchodilator therapy requires mechanical ventilation for survival.

At the present time, United States hospitals have widespread use of intensive care services so that 5–10% of hospital beds are devoted to critical care. If total health care dollars are 11–12% of the gross national product (GNP) (2), then total critical care dollars are 1% of the GNP. Critical care started small with a few patients in the 1950s when death was a natural part of disease. Critical care is now big, one of the biggest hospital expenditures, in an era when death is a less accepted part of any disease or hospitalization.

The meteoric growth in critical care caused a profound change in the delivery of critical care services. When critical care was small, physicians who specialized in life support brought structure and patient care protocols to the delivery of ICU services. Nurses and physicians worked closely in the administration of the ICU and the delivery of patient care. Quality assurance was possible in such an environment because of the limited number of practitioners involved in patient care.

As the presumed benefits of critical care fueled the growth of ICU beds in hospitals across the country, there were never enough intensivists to direct all the new intensive care units. The skills of life support were taught to many physicians in training, and suddenly critical care services were delivered by many physicians in many different intensive care units. Instead of patient care by bedside titration of therapy as occurred with the original champions of critical care, ICU services were delivered by rounding and prescription. The nurse played a central role in this new form of critical care, reporting frequently by phone or via a house officer to the primary attending physician who was providing part-time ICU services. Many variations on life support developed within the same unit, and patient care protocols were difficult to monitor.

In mechanical ventilation for example, some physicians prescribed heavy sedation and muscle relaxants with controlled mechanical ventilation. Other physicians preferred assisted ventilation with a lightly sedated patient. Clinical research failed to demonstrate the value of one technique over another. Quality assurance in that type of ICU is most difficult. Responsibility for care is assigned to many physicians, and the medical director of the unit functions in name only. Step 4 of quality assurance (Table 15.1), identification of indicators, is nearly impossible when a single life support technique is performed in multiple ways.

Three models of intensive care have evolved in the last 35 years of growth in critical care services. The first model is the oldest and is based on the champion of critical care services. These ICU directors have developed into a new specialty of internal medicine, anesthesiology, pediatrics, and surgery called critical care medicine. There is now a prescribed training, an identified body of knowledge, and a mechanism for testing to award certification in critical care. Units operated by trained intensivists are fertile ground for quality assurance activities. The intensivist plays an active role in the policies of the unit and carries the assigned responsibility for patient care as noted in the first step of quality assurance. There is likely to be sameness of delivery of care, which can be monitored and quantified.

A second model is the antithesis of this system. Here there is a medical director in name only or a committee, and responsi-

Tabel 15.1.
The Joint Commission on Accreditation of Healthcare Organizations' 10-Step Process[a]

1. Assign responsibility
2. Delineate scope of care
3. Identify important aspects of care
4. Identify indicators
5. Establish thresholds for evaluation
6. Collect and organize data
7. Evaluate care
8. Take actions to solve problems
9. Assess actions and document improvement
10. Communicate relevant information to the organizationwide quality assurance program

[a]Copyright 1988 by the Joint Commission on Accreditation of Healthcare Organizations, Chicago. Reprinted with permission.

bility is impossible to assign other than to each individual admitting physician or his/her consultants. There is wide variation in patient care protocols, and traditional quality assurance is difficult if not impossible. Later in this chapter we look at the difference in morbidity and mortality in this type of unit versus a more structured unit with full-time critical care physician services.

Between these two models is where most intensive care units reside, particularly those in teaching hospitals with housestaff assigned to the intensive care unit. In that setting, there is usually an assigned medical director or rounding physician who is responsible for the housestaff. The day-to-day care is provided by residents who generally rotate on the ICU service every 2 months. Structured care is more likely with this model than with the second model but not as likely as with the first model since attending physicians likely rotate every week and housestaff every 1–2 months. Quality assurance and monitoring of specific indicators of care are now possible but depend on a strong medical director.

Since the intensivist's approach to structured and administrated critical care services facilitates quality assessment monitoring, the next section of this chapter on critical care will examine the 10-step process of quality assurance as it might be done in a unit with strong nursing and medical directors (Table 15.1). The day-to-day operation of a busy ICU is a marriage between physician and nursing efforts. The final section of this chapter will demonstrate the significant reduction in morbidity and mortality that occurs when this nurse/physician marriage is harmonious.

ICU QUALITY ASSURANCE

The Joint Commission on Accreditation of Healthcare Organizations (JCAHO) has asked that a 10-step process be used to monitor and evaluate the quality and appropriateness of care. The standard from which this is derived is "QA.1. There is an ongoing quality assurance program designed to objectively and systematically monitor and evaluate the quality and appropriateness of patient care, pursue opportunities to improve patient care, and resolve identified problems" (3).

Although the medical literature has little information specific to critical care units, most quality assurance (QA) information from other parts of the hospital can be adapted to critical care.

The technology associated with a special care area poses unique problems. The patients may be at risk simply by their presence in these departments. It is not only important for each unit to verify that quality care is being delivered, but also that a safe environment is being provided. Quality assurance is primarily a means of identifying problems, but is also a means of demonstrating that a high level of care is being delivered to patients. Simply stated, "quality" and "excellence" are synonyms (4); assurance is the "act of making certain" (5).

The most effective way to discuss the specifics of quality assurance in critical care is through examples. Examples from JCAHO literature and from the authors' institution will be used to demonstrate the specifics of QA in critical care.

Unit-based programs of QA are important for two reasons. First, nurses and physicians, working together in the ICU, can effectively monitor the functioning of the unit, while at the same time, provide patient care. Secondly, they are also the best suited to elicit changes necessary to correct problems (6). It should be emphasized that involvement of the nursing staff is important to the success of a QA program in a critical care unit.

Each critical care unit is unique, and the most important aspect of quality assurance is the adaptation of the program to the needs of the particular unit. Various units are staffed differently, physician coverage differs, and technology varies from one critical care unit to another. With that caveat, the 10-step process as it applies to critical care is as follows.

Step 1.   Assign Responsibility

The responsibility for quality assurance in any critical care unit is assigned to the "physician director or chairperson" (8). The physician director is then directed to designate responsibilities for monitoring to other individuals. Despite this statement, the JCAHO fails to review critical care in a manner that might be consistent with that recommendation. First, in the authors' experience with several institutions, a physician reviewer never visits the critical care areas. A physician reviewer visits the operating room and the emergency medicine department, but leaves the critical care units to the nurse reviewer. Second, no effort is made to evaluate physician involvement in critical care quality assurance.

Critical care medicine has evolved as a multidisciplinary specialty with a partnership management of the ICU by a nurse director and a physician director. For that reason, step 1 of the QA process must involve a joint effort from medicine and nursing. QA projects can be developed that look at physician activities as well as at nursing activities, but most projects are likely to look at combined physician and nursing involvement.

Departmental meetings for the ICU should be attended by representatives from all groups on the critical care team. Some members of this committee may have their own quality assurance projects. Physicians, nurses, respiratory therapists, unit secretaries, social workers, technologists, and patient/family coordinators must attend ICU meetings to discuss aspects of care in the department. "As the trend continues toward multi-disciplinary team care for patients, the trend in QA should be toward a multi-disciplinary review of care" (9). Physicians may be asked to do chart reviews; respiratory therapists may be asked to report their findings on quality assurance done routinely by their department. All quality assurance projects should be reported at these meetings. Written reports are sent to the hospital quality assurance committee.

Step 2.   Delineate Scope of Care

Monitoring will depend on the scope of care developed for the department. The scope of care depends on the type of ICU. The following is an example of a scope of care for a 16-bed medical/surgical intensive care unit (M/SICU).

The M/SICU admits patients age 12 years and older. The unit operates on a round-the-clock schedule. The unit is jointly managed by both physicians and nurses with a full-time physician director and his/her associates and a nurse manager and his/her assistants. The physician functions as a critical care attending and automatically sees all ICU admissions. A critical care attending is present in the department 24 hours per day, 7 days a week. The critical care attending supervises the housestaff; and the critical care team provides primary care to ICU admissions, writing all orders and working with the admitting internist or surgeon.

Twenty-four-hour nursing care is provided by an all RN staff. The nurse:patient ratio is 1:1 or 1:2 as determined by patient acuity.

Registered respiratory therapists are present in the department on a 24-hour basis. They are responsible for all ventilator support and therapies. Nurses do not perform any respiratory therapy duties. Ventilator changes and treatments are the exclusive responsibility of the respiratory therapy staff.

The unit monitors ECG, abnormal cardiac rhythms, systemic blood pressure, pulmonary artery pressure, central venous pressure, intracranial pressure, end tidal CO_2, noninvasive blood pressure, electroencephalogram, cardiac output, SvO_2, and SaO_2.

The M/SICU provides life support such as vasoactive and cardiotonic drugs, mechanical ventilation, continuous positive airway pressure, high frequency jet ventilation, thoracostomy tube drainage, pericardial drainage, parenteral and enteral nutrition, plasmaphoresis, transfusion of blood products, endotracheal intubation, continuous arterial venous hemofiltration and hemodialysis, transthoracic pacing, transvenous pacing, fluoroscopy, fluid resuscitation, intraaortic counterpulsation balloon support, gastrointestinal endoscopy, and bronchoscopy.

If a high census and a shortage of ICU beds occur, the medical director has the authority to triage patients for discharge to the floor or to other critical care areas. Patients can be held in the emergency medicine department or recovery room or taken to another hospital.

The M/SICU admits patients with a wide variety of medical and surgical diagnoses and is capable of a broad scope of critical care services.

Step 3.   Identify Important Aspects of Care

Important aspects of care are those provided in the department that are the most important, that are done most often, or carry the highest risk. The JCAHO states that priority should be given to the aspects of care that have one or more of the following characteristics: (*a*) the aspect of care is done frequently or affects a large number of patients; (*b*) the aspect of care is high risk and may have serious consequences if the patient does not receive the care in a correct manner; and (*c*) the aspect of care has previously produced problems within the department (10).

In a medical/surgical intensive care unit there are a number of aspects of care that are done frequently. They include intubation and mechanical ventilation, blood pressure monitoring by use of an arterial catheter, intravenous fluid and medication administration by central venous catheter, and portable hemodialysis by double lumen venous catheter. These life support techniques should be monitored closely because of their high usage rate in any ICU that admits patients with a wide variety of diagnoses.

One aspect of care that has high risk but is used with a lesser frequency than the items listed above is insertion of and monitoring with a balloon-tipped, flow-directed, pulmonary artery (Swan-Ganz) catheter. Frequent thermodilution cardiac output measurements are made with calculation of a hemodynamic profile to better titrate cardiac support. In addition, mixed venous blood oxygen saturation can be intermittently monitored by withdrawing a sample of blood from the pulmonary artery or can be continuously monitored by the use of a fiberoptic pulmonary artery catheter. The process of hemodynamic monitoring is associated with infections, bleeding, damage to the blood vessels of the lung, and other life-endangering complications. All intensive care units that utilize pulmonary artery catheters should consider this an important aspect of care that needs to be regularly monitored to preserve quality care.

Each individual unit should look for aspects of care that have caused problems in the past. For example, if there is a high incidence of hospital-acquired pneumonia, then the infectious disease aspects of respiratory support or mechanical ventilation should be closely and regularly examined.

Step 4.   Identify Indicators

Identifying indicators narrows the monitoring process. "An indicator is a defined, measurable dimension of the quality or appropriateness of an important aspect of care" (11) (Tables 15.2 and 15.3).

Indicators might be equipment malfunction, adverse medication reactions, ICU-incurred trauma, adverse reaction to infections, failure to notify a physician of abnormal lab work within 15 minutes, failure to follow a physician's order, unplanned transfers to ICU, stay in unit over 5 days, ventilator days more than 10 days, reintubations, infection while in the ICU or immediately post transfer, invasive lines in more than 5 days, and development of acute congestive failure and pulmonary edema.

The selection of indicators requires a sound knowledge of the medical literature (12). It is valuable if the nursing and medical staff participate jointly in educational activities such as journal clubs and teaching conferences to be certain that all members of the team are current on standards of care.

No aspect of critical care has changed more in the last few years than the management of myocardial infarction. Most myocardial infarctions seen in the emergency medicine department and finally in the intensive care unit are caused by a

Table 15.2.
Important Aspects of Care[a]

Aspect	Reason
Ventilator management of patients with acute respiratory failure	High risk
Management of hemodynamically unstable patients on vasoactive drugs	High risk, problem prone
Management of patients with septic shock	High risk, problem prone
Management of peritoneal dialysis patients	Problem prone
Management of patients with uncontrolled hypertension	High risk
Management of patients with transfusion reactions	High risk
Transfers to other areas	Problem prone
Use and performance of intraaortic balloon pump	High risk
Insertion of Swan-Ganz catheters and management of such patients	Problem prone

[a]Copyright 1988 by the Joint Commission on Accreditation of Healthcare Organizations, Chicago. Reprinted with permission.

Table 15.3.
Important Aspects of Care with Indicators and Thresholds for Evaluation in the Medical/Surgical Intensive Care Unit at St. Francis Medical Center, Pittsburgh, PA

Aspect	Indicator	Threshold
		%
Insertion of central venous lines via subclavian or jugular route	Chest x-ray taken for proper placement immediately after insertion and before infusion of fluid through line	95
Patient safety	All patients will have proper identification with arm band	95
Documentation	Patients have pain relief documented after administration of medication	85

thrombosis of an epicardial vessel in the heart. This causes myocardial ischemia progressing to necrosis in the muscle distal to the occluded vessel. The patient presents with onset of chest pain and has ECG evidence for new myocardial infarction.

A joint QA project could be developed between emergency medicine and the ICU to look at indicators for myocardial infarction. A very important initial indicator would be the expeditious identification of ECG abnormalities consistent with new myocardial infarction (MI) in patients seen in the emergency medicine department (ED) with new onset chest pain. This identification should occur within 15 minutes of admission to the ED. A second indicator would be the administration of intravenous thrombolytic agents within 15 minutes of making the diagnosis of new MI if the onset of pain is less than 6 hours and the patient has no contraindications to thrombolysis.

A third indicator now moves attention to the ICU to insure transfer and monitoring of the patient within 60 minutes of starting thrombolysis so that reperfusion arrhythmias can be assessed and treated when appropriate. Finally, heparin should be started in the ICU within 15 minutes of completing thrombolysis, particularly if tissue plasminogen activator (tPa) is used since this agent has a short duration of action.

All of these statements are somewhat arbitrary in timing but represent an analysis of the present literature on the treatment of new myocardial infarction. The ICU and ED teams must be aware of changing standards of care for new MI patients and frequently update indicators for monitoring to continuously assure the presence of quality care.

As one may notice, the list of indicators can be very long. It is important to determine which indicators should be monitored and in what order. It is very easy to monitor too many things at once. A schedule can be developed that shows that some indicators may need to be monitored continuously, but some of these indicators can be monitored for short periods of time, especially when no problems are shown to exist. It is important not to be overburdened with monitoring.

Step 5. Establish Thresholds

When establishing thresholds for evaluation, one should be cautioned against setting a threshold of 100%, as it is difficult to live up to a perfect standard. A realistic expectation should be used to determine the percentage of compliance necessary for the indicator.

In most critical care situations where nursing and medical decision making is involved, it is difficult to pick thresholds because of changing standards of care in a high technology aspect of medicine. To refer back to the issue of thrombolysis, one should expect that the threshold for administration of a thrombolysis agent expeditiously after diagnosing new myocardial infarction should be at least 90%. This falls short of 100% and allows for some delays that can be a part of making the diagnosis of new MI when the history and evaluation of the patient are less than clear. Only 3 years ago that was an unrealistic standard. The benefits of thrombolysis were largely understood, but the application of the drug by physicians was still controversial. Three years from now there is likely to be a different standard of care and different thresholds for response.

Step 6. Collect and Organize Data

This chapter contains examples of data collection forms (Figs. 15.1 and 15.2). Possible data sources for monitoring and evaluation are in Table 15.4. A calendar should be developed to illustrate a schedule that should be followed. One needs to determine how often the monitoring will be done.

The process of data collection in critical care can be complicated by the sophistication of monitoring and life support that exists in the ICU. It may be very difficult to have individuals other than ICU nurses or physicians collecting data. Considering the shortage of qualified personnel, particularly of ICU nurses, it becomes very expensive and difficult to employ ICU nurses as data collectors.

With the advance of computer technology, many critical care units are turning to

Form #3

St. Francis Medical Center
Department of Nursing
Data Collection Form

Key * = Met criteria
     - = Did not meet

Dates: Beginning of study _____ End of study _____ Data collector: _____ Sample size: _____

Focus of study: Patient ☐ Staff ☐ System ☐ Objective of monitoring: _____ Census of the day: _____

Aspect of care: _____ High volume ☐ High risk ☐ Problem prone ☐ High cost ☐

Unit numbers

Indicators	Exceptions	Totals	Threshold for Evaluation		Remarks
		*	-	Projected	Actual	
1						
2						

Unit numbers

Indicators	Exceptions	Totals	Threshold for Evaluation		Remarks
		*	-	Projected	Actual	
1						
2						

Original 9/90

Data retrieval method: _____

Figure 15.1. Data collection form. (Courtesy of St. Francis Medical Center Department of Nursing.)

Form #4

Data Collection Form

Dates: Beginning _____

              End of study _____

Data Collector _____

Focus of study   ____ Patient   ____ Staff   ____ System   Objective of monitoring _____

Aspect of care: _____

              ____ High volume   ____ High risk   ____ Problem prone   ____ High cost

Sample size _____

Key   * = Met criteria
        - = Did not meet

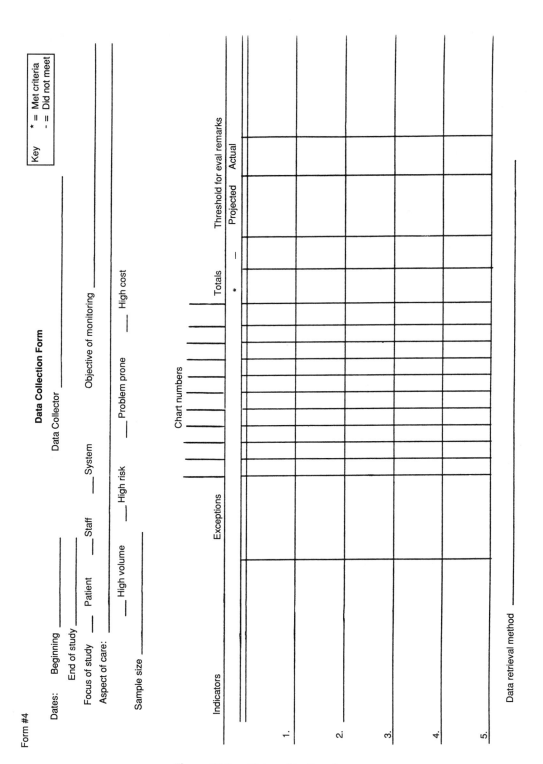

Chart numbers

Indicators

Exceptions

Totals

Threshold for eval remarks

Projected   Actual

* |

1.

2.

3.

4.

5.

Data retrieval method _____

Figure 15.2.   Data collection form.

Table 15.4.
Possible Data Sources for Monitoring and Evaluation[a]

Patient records
Autopsy reports
Laboratory reports
Medication sheets
Incident reports
Department logs
Committee meeting minutes or reports
Infection control reports
Patient satisfaction questionnaires
Direct observation of patients or staff
Utilization review findings
Management meeting minutes
Direct observation
Morbidity/mortality rate review
Personnel performance appraisal
Formal evaluation studies

[a]Copyright 1988 by the Joint Commission on Accreditation of Healthcare Organizations, Chicago. Reprinted with permission.

automatic data collection. Several vendors now offer work station-based, bedside patient data management systems. Many nurse- and physician-patient interactions are done through a bedside terminal that logs events on a time scale for later review. Future quality assurance projects should be developed around such computerized ICU systems to automate as much of the QA data collection and organization as possible.

Step 7.   Evaluate Care

Deficiencies or noncompliance with preestablished criteria noted during evaluation of care can be determined to be a result of deficiency in knowledge, performance, or system. A system deficiency may be an administrative or environmental factor that affects performance (13). Problems can also be caused by equipment deficiencies, documentation deficiencies, and staffing deficiencies.

No step in the 10-step process of QA recommended by the JCAHO for critical care units is more difficult than the evaluation of care. In a previous discussion, three models of critical care delivery were discussed. In the first model with a strong nursing and medical director and primary care of patients, evaluation of care is not a

problem. Policies and procedures are developed by a closed "family," and evaluation of that process is an accounting function.

Since most intensive care units have a more open environment with less control by the nursing and medical director, evaluation of care will depend on the opinion of many admitting physicians. It is here that various techniques of mechanical ventilation or hemodynamic management may lead to situations that are essentially impossible to evaluate. If there is a strong difference of opinion on modes of life support and no clear evidence in the literature to resolve controversy, then evaluation of a given indicator may be impossible. Consider the issue of thrombolysis in myocardial infarction. Beginning heparin administration after thrombolysis is a new and evolving indicator. Some physicians may still prefer to start aspirin administration. Other physicians using longer acting thrombolytic agents may be opposed to heparin. As a result, a 90% compliance of an indicator that heparin must be started expeditiously after completing thrombolysis becomes a matter of opinion among a diverse group of physicians. In a closed unit where a cooperating group of critical care nurses and doctors meet on a regular basis, it is easier to explore a standard in the literature and make a decision about a policy and procedure. Evaluation of that policy and procedure in a unit with good documentation becomes trivial.

Step 8.   Take Action to Solve Problems

When a problem is identified under evaluation of care, action must be taken to solve problems. Problem resolution occurs at two levels within the unit-based QA program, the unit level and the nursing division level (14) (Table 15.5). One may also find that a problem occurred due to a threshold that was set too high. A copy of a form used to document this information can be found in Figure 15.3. This form is also used for reporting through the different committees, the nursing department, and the quality assurance department.

Table 15.5.
Possible Actions to Correct a Problem or Improve Quality of Care[a,b]

Actions if the problem involves deficiencies in systems
Changing communication channels
Using consultant services
Changing organizational structure
Establishing new positions
Changing inventory
Adjusting staffing or redistributing staff
Revising job descriptions
Reallocating resources
Adding or revising policies and procedures
Altering the use of equipment
Purchasing or repairing equipment
Actions if the problem involves deficiencies in staff knowledge
Modifying orientation procedures
Providing focused in-service education
Providing focused continuing education
Circulating written policies and procedures or other informational material
Providing additional reference sources
Actions if the problem involves behavior or performance deficiencies
Revising job descriptions
Informal counseling
Formal counseling
Changing assignments
Disciplinary sanctions (in accordance with staff and professional bylaws)
Placing an individual on probation
Imposing a consultation requirement
Recommending clinical privileges be terminated, modified, or sustained
Reducing staff category or limiting staff prerogatives relating to patient care
Suspending or revoking staff appointments
Transferring to another unit/department

[a]Copyright 1988 by the Joint Commission on Accreditation of Healthcare Organizations, Chicago. Reprinted with permission.
[b]Action is ordinarily implemented through existing channels of department, administration, or medical staff organization. After allowing enough time for the actions to have effect, the effectiveness of action should be assessed, generally using the same monitoring and evaluation procedure that identified the problem originally.

Historically, physicians have clung to a fierce independence in their practice of medicine, which is part art and part science. In many respects, the 10-step quality assurance process attempts to reduce that art and science to something that can be measured, scored, and quantified. There is much resistance to this process of converting the practice of medicine to a series of monitored patient care protocols. In a closed ICU where only a handful of physicians are writing orders, there will be some disagreement on how action should be taken when a "problem" is detected. There should be no difficulty if the problem is a clear deviation from the standard of care. When the problem is a difference of opinion, hard to substantiate in the medical literature, resolution may be more difficult.

In an open-practice, critical care environment with a medical director in name only or a critical care committee with a committee chairman responsible for quality assurance, resolution of problems will be much more difficult. A large portion of life support in critical care cannot be reduced to a series of monitored protocols. Even seemingly simple items such as how long a central venous catheter should be left in place are not simple questions. Variables such as insertion technique, use of bactericidal barriers, dressing changes, and breaks in the line can lead to many different answers to the

ST. FRANCIS MEDICAL CENTER
DEPARTMENT OF NURSING

QUALITY ASSURANCE

DATE: July, 1990   UNIT: N4500 M/SICU   NUMBER OF CASES REVIEWED: 22

DIVISION: Critical Care   ASPECT OF CARE: Documentation

INDICATORS	FINDINGS	DISCUSSION	ACTION/SUGGESTIONS
All patients with central lines will have: (85% threshold) 1. Procedure note written 2. X-ray taken 3. Verification of placement written on chart by MD	20/22 91% 21/22 95% 19/22 86%	Continue to monitor " "	Discuss at dept mtg " "
Patients will have documentation of pain relief after pain med administered 85% threshold	3 pts received 8 doses of med 2 of 8 doses had relief documented 25% compliance	"	Discuss at unit mtg

Figure 15.3. Quality assurance form. (Courtesy of St. Francis Medical Center Department of Nursing.)

question of duration of use of central venous pressure (CVP) catheters.

Step 9. Assess Actions and Document Improvement

During reassessment, it is also helpful to identify patterns that may emerge (15). It is important to attach copies of minutes that reflect department meeting actions that were taken to solve problems. An action that is often listed as a solution is to discuss the results of audits at ICU meetings. If the minutes from the meeting are attached to the audits, there is verification that the action has occurred. Table 15.5 has other suggested actions to correct a problem or improve quality of care. Figure 15.3 gives examples of how steps 7, 8, and 9 may be reported.

Step 10. Communicate Relevant Information to the Organizationwide Quality Assurance Program

An organizational chart is most representative of the reporting mechanism (Fig. 15.4).

Quality assurance can be prospective, concurrent, or retrospective (16, 17). We employ these terms as follows: Prospective studies are developed with a tightly defined protocol to examine a previously identified problem. Concurrent monitoring is done at the same time the patient care delivery is occurring and can be used to show that protocols, unit policy, standards of care, and standing orders are followed. Retrospective monitoring is accomplished via chart review (17). There is no JCAHO standard that determines which method one must use, although it is a good idea to utilize all methods. Other examples of quality assurance are reviews of incident reports and committee meeting minutes. All minutes from meetings should be in the format of topic, discussion, recommendation, and action. Minutes of the ICU meetings should reflect discussion and resolution of problems. This can be accomplished by including this information under old business. The topic of quality assurance should be discussed at all departmental meetings.

Patient complaints are another means of identifying problems. These complaints should be documented and similar complaints can be cause for concern (18).

Incident reports can be logged as a form of quality assurance. The reports can be discussed at ICU meetings listed with discussion, recommendations, and actions. This also allows the ICU staff to look at trends. Documentation of those involved can be done with initials or codes.

ICU patient care statistics should reflect total monthly patients and admissions, number of 24-hour periods of treatment, average daily census, percent occupancy, condition on admission and discharge, use of life support techniques, and invasive procedures. All of this information should be trended on a monthly basis. If a problem develops that can be attributed to staffing, one may wish to look at census

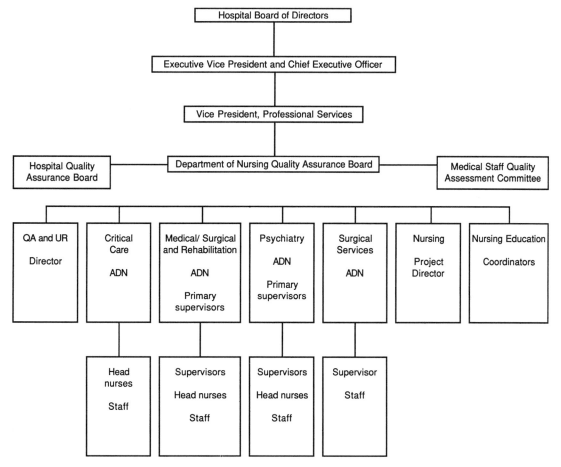

Figure 15.4. Quality assurance organization plan. (Courtesy of St. Francis Medical Center Department of Nursing.)

data to determine if the census changed or the patient acuity increased. Acuity can be determined by the condition on admission and use of various life support techniques.

Charge nurses should be involved in quality management by reporting problems from each shift. These charge nurse reports list cardiac arrests, patient outcome, and incidents such as medication errors and problems with invasive catheters. Access of information during chart review is easier with information from charge nurse reports.

A MACROASSESSMENT OF QUALITY OF CARE IN CRITICAL CARE MEDICINE

Since the inception of ICUs approximately 35 years ago, the concept of the ideal intensive care unit has evolved considerably. Concurrent to our improved understanding of complex pathologic processes seen in critically ill patients has been a growth of equally complex technology. With technological advances, the intensive care environment has become more expensive for society and more stressful for the patient. To justify these financial and psychological investments, early analyses of intensive care attempted to demonstrate a beneficial effect on patient outcome due to hospitalization in an ICU.

Three important questions have evolved with regard to critical care. How does one reliably evaluate quality of care in patients as complex as those cases seen in modern ICUs? Which model of ICU organization increases the potential for the highest quality of care? What is the impact of critical care medicine on improving quality of care?

As is discussed in the previous section, some methods of evaluating quality of care in the ICU have been established. The efficacy of specific therapies and technology must be evaluated. The rate of iatrogenic complications must be monitored. While this type of quality assessment provides useful feedback to ICU personnel and quantifies effectiveness in specific areas, it does not clarify overall benefit rendered by the ICU. Therefore, in addi-

tion to this type of microassessment of the quality of care delivered by the ICU, methods of globally assessing the effectiveness of intensive care units must be established. A macroassessment of this nature involves two steps. First, an evaluation of outcome and ICU utilization must be performed. This encompasses an evaluation of survival rate (outcome), as well as length of stay and inappropriate admissions (utilization). Second, an evaluation of the process through which health care is delivered must occur. The influence of communication among health care personnel on outcome, and the effect of organizational structure of the ICU on outcome, must be elucidated.

With this type of macroassessment, one can now attempt to offer answers to the three questions posed above. The ensuing discussion presents methods for performing a macroassessment of the quality of care in the ICU. Specific methods that evaluate outcome, length of stay, and utilization are presented. The effect of process on ICU outcome is addressed. As part of this latter subject, a review of the principal studies demonstrating the impact of the critical care medicine subspecialty on outcome is presented. Drawing on this discussion, specific recommendations will be made. In particular, those recommendations of the Society of Critical Care Medicine Task Force on Guidelines which are pertinent to this discussion will be mentioned.

Evaluation of ICU Outcome and Utilization

Measurement of outcome refers quite simply to measurement of survival rates. But measurement of outcome is meaningful only when severity of disease is taken into account. Severity of disease scoring systems for critical care patients have been validated, and patient outcome can now be measured in a meaningful manner. Utilization of the ICU is also important. This concept encompasses length of stay in the ICU and appropriateness of admission for monitoring in the ICU. Both are important in this era of cost containment and limited ICU bed availability. Fortunately, these factors can now be assessed by one of the commonly used severity of disease scoring systems. This portion of the discussion will describe reliable and meaningful methods of evaluating ICU outcome and utilization; specific severity of disease scoring systems facilitating these evaluations will be discussed.

Evaluation of Outcome

Evaluation of outcome involves two processes—predicting outcome and measuring outcome. The single most crucial factor in improving medical practice is an accurate prediction of outcome, for only with this information can physicians assess their results. Accurate predictive ability can be done only with the use of a validated severity of disease scoring system. A severity of disease scoring system renders perspective, and therefore meaning, to mortality data. Mortality data can now be used to assess the quality of care within a given ICU and to compare results among several ICUs. Ultimately, accurate prognostication makes it possible to measure the usefulness of intensive care.

Severity of disease scoring systems have been studied by several authors. These analyses have pertained to the medical and surgical ICU population, excluding trauma. The three most effective and commonly used systems will be discussed here and the reader is referred to chapter 7 for details of available systems: the acute physiology and chronic health system (APACHE), the mortality prediction model (MPM), and the therapeutic intervention scoring system (TISS).

APACHE was developed in 1981 by Knaus et al. (19). Although it was validated in subsequent studies, it was found to be cumbersome. In 1985 APACHE II, a more expedient but equally reliable system, was introduced (20). APACHE II is the severity of disease scoring system most useful for quality assurance in that it generates information concerning outcome, length of stay, and potential instability of patients admitted to the ICU for monitoring.

The APACHE program is based on three components: diagnosis (including surgical status), acute physiologic derangement, and chronic health. APACHE II assigns an acute physiology score (APS) and a chronic health evaluation to generate an "APACHE" score. The APS is based on 12 parameters plus age. These parameters were chosen by a panel of experts in critical care medicine. The most abnormal physiologic values collected for each parameter over the first 24 hours of admission are used to compute APS. The greater the physiologic derangement, the higher the APACHE score. Chronic health is measured by the presence or absence of co-morbidities. Components used to generate an APACHE score are shown on Table 7.5.

The APACHE score, diagnosis, surgical status, and chronic health evaluation are then used to predict the risk of mortality for an individual patient through use of a multiple regression logistics equation. This equation and diagnostic categories used by APACHE are shown on Table 15.6. A decision criterion of 0.50 is used. Any patient with an estimated risk of death greater than 0.50 is simply predicted to die. Based on predicted mortality for individual patiets entered into the APACHE system, predicted mortality for the group is generated. APACHE II was initially validated in 5085 patients and has been effectively used in several thousand other patients since then. From this perspective, APACHE is the most reliable, and therefore most utilized, severity of disease scoring system for intensive care patients.

MPM was developed in 1985 by Teres and associates (21) who used statistical analysis (as opposed to a panel of experts) to select variables that correlated best with mortality. Data were collected on 755 consecutive admissions to a single ICU. The authors recorded a total of 137 variables that covered (a) demographics; (b) information on prior ICU admissions; (c) specific organ system failures; (d) measures of functional status; (e) cancer-related variables; (f) arterial blood gases; (g) renal, neurologic, and respiratory variables; and (h) some treatment variables such as concentration of inspired oxygen and units of blood transfused. A multiple linear regression model was then used to determine which variables correlated most highly with mortality.

Table 15.6.
Factors in APACHE System Used to Predict Risk of Mortality in an Individual Patient[a]

Diagnostic Categories

Postoperative admissions
Cardiovascular
  Chronic cardiovascular disease
  Peripheral vascular disease
  Heart valve surgery
  Sepsis (any etiology)
  Hemorrhagic shock
  Post cardiac arrest
Trauma
  Multiple trauma
  Head trauma
Respiratory
  Thoracic surgery for neoplasm
  Post respiratory arrest
  Respiratory insufficiency after surgery
Gastrointestinal
  Gastrointestinal bleeding
  Gastrointestinal surgery for neoplasm
  Gastrointestinal perforation/obstruction
Renal
  Renal surgery for neoplasm
  Renal transplant surgery
Neurologic
  Craniotomy for ICH, SDH, SAH[b]
  Craniotomy for neoplasm
  Laminectomy or spinal surgery

Nonoperative admissions
Respiratory insufficiency
  Asthma, allergy
  Chronic obstructive pulmonary disease
  Pulmonary edema (noncardiac)
  Respiratory infection
  Respiratory neoplasm
  Post respiratory arrest
  Pulmonary embolus
  Aspiration, poisoning, toxic reaction
Cardiovascular insufficiency
  Hypertension
  Congestive heart failure
  Hemorrhagic shock, hypovolemia
  Coronary artery disease
  Sepsis (any etiology)
  Post cardiac arrest
  Dissecting thoracic, abdominal aneurysm
  Rhythm disturbance
Trauma
  Multiple trauma
  Head trauma
Neurologic failure
  Seizure disorder
  ICH, SDH, SAH
Other
  Self drug overdose
  Diabetic ketoacidosis
  Gastrointestinal bleeding

Organ Systems for Classifying Patients
Neurologic
Cardiovascular
Respiratory
Gastrointestinal
Renal
Hematologic
Metabolic

12 Physiologic Variables

Temperature	Oxygenation	Serum creatinine
Mean arterial pressure	Arterial pH	Hematocrit
Heart rate	Serum sodium	White blood cell count
Respiratory rate	Serum potassium	Glasgow Coma Score

Equation to Predict Risk of Mortality
$$\text{Ln} (R/1 - R) = -3.517 + (\text{APACHE II} \times 0.146 + S + D)$$
where
  R = risk of hospital death
  S = additional risk imposed by emergency surgery
  D = risk (+ or −) imposed by specific disease

[a]From Rafkin HS. Assessing the critically ill patient for admission to the intensive care unit. In: Hoyt JW, Tonneson AS, Allen SJ, eds. Critical care practice. Philadelphia: WB Saunders, 1991:19.
[b]*ICH*, Intracranial hemorrhage; *SDH*, subdural hemorrhage; *SAH*, subarachnoid hemorrhage.

MPM establishes a risk of mortality based upon admission data. Therefore, this predictive index is unequivocally independent of therapy. Moreover, MPM provides for reevaluation of the patient's status at 24 and 48 hours. The variables used to score patients at these intervals have also been chosen through statistical analysis and significantly differ in some respects from the variables used at admission. In this way, trends in patient status can be documented, and mortality prediction can be modified according to clinical evolution. Table 15.7 shows the variables used to predict the risk of mortality according to MPM at admission, 24 hours, and 48 hours.

MPM establishes risk of mortality for an individual patient through the use of a multiple linear regression model. The general form of this model is shown on Table 15.7. MPM yields a probability of death that can fall from 0.0 to 1.0. Groups of patients can be categorized into strata defined by estimated probability of death. Within each strata, the number of observed deaths can be compared to the number of predicted deaths.

Although it is less widely used than APACHE, MPM is a validated severity of disease scoring system, and data collection is simpler. MPM accounts for changes in condition that may evolve over the first 48 hours. It can, therefore, be reliably used to assess observed outcome in an ICU. It does not, however, possess the same range of capability as APACHE, as will be discussed.

TISS was established by Cullen and associates in 1974 (22). TISS is composed of 76 monitoring and therapeutic interventions and reflects amount and complexity of therapy required by a patient. TISS is based on the premise that, regardless of the diagnosis, the amount of therapy reflects the degree of physiologic impairment. Table 15.8 shows the components of TISS. Each modality is assigned a weighted score, ranging from 1 to 4, depending on the intensity and complexity of the intervention. Points are totalled, and in this way a TISS score for each 24-hour period can be obtained.

TISS scores are not used to predict outcome per se. However, trends in TISS scores over the first 3 days correlate well with survival (23). While increasing trends in daily TISS scores correlate with increasing severity of disease, decreases in daily TISS scores correlate with decreasing severity of disease and improvement in clinical condition.

At present, APACHE is most often used in conjunction with TISS, and both can be purchased as part of a package. Based on the APACHE score, a predicted TISS score is made available. This serves as a measure to validate whether a patient is being undertreated or overtreated with respect to the severity of illness.

More important, however, is the fact that TISS and APACHE can be used together to clarify the relationship between ICU care and survival. Scheffler and associates (24) looked at 613 admissions in a medical-surgical ICU and performed a two-stage analysis looking at the relationship between amount of therapy and survival. In the first stage, severity of disease was not included; in the second stage, the analysis controlled for severity of disease. APACHE scores were determined during the first 32 hours of admission to the ICU, and probability of survival was determined through use of the APACHE system. TISS scores were recorded during each shift the patient was in the ICU, and all scores were then totaled. The relationship between cumulative TISS points and survival was then studied.

The results are represented by Figure 15.5. When controlling for severity of disease, a U-shaped relationship exists between increments in ICU therapy and probability of survival. As TISS points increase from 0 to 100, the probability of death decreases. As TISS points increase from 100 to 280, the probability of death remains constant. And as TISS points increase from beyond 280 points, the probability of death increases despite implementing aggressive therapy. Crucially, the authors found that without controlling for severity of disease, the relationship between amount of ICU therapy and probability of death appeared to be strictly linear. Increasing therapy did not appear to improve the probability of survival for

Table 15.7.
Factors in Mortality Prediction Model (MPM)[a]

12 Variables and Possible Responses Used to Predict Risk of Mortality in an Individual Patient

Variables	Responses
Presence of coma or deep stupor	Yes or no
Type of admission	Elective or emergency
Cardiopulmonary compression prior to ICU admission	Yes or no
Cancer as part of problem	Yes or no
History of chronic renal failure	Yes or no
Probable infection	Yes or no
Age	
Previous ICU admission within past 6 months	Yes or no
Heart rate at ICU admission	
Surgical service at ICU admission	Yes or no
Systolic blood pressure admission	
Square of systolic blood pressure	

14 Variables used by MPM 24-hour Analysis
Presence of coma or deep stupor
Cancer as part of problem
Emergency admission
Prothrombin time greater than 3 seconds above laboratory standard
Probable shock during first 24 hours
Urine output less than 150 ml in any 8-hour period
Infection confirmed
Pao_2 less than 60 torr mm Hg
Fio_2 greater than 0.50
Creatinine greater than 2 mg/dl
Age
Hours of mechanical ventilation
Number of IV lines
Surgical service

11 Variables used by MPM 48-hour Analysis
Presence of coma or deep stupor
Urine output less than 150 ml in any 8-hour period of day 2
Presence of coma or stupor at admission
Emergency admission
Prothrombin time greater than 3 seconds above laboratory standard
Fio_2 greater than 0.50 during day 2
Cancer as part of problem
Infection confirmed at 48 hours
Age
Total hours of mechanical ventilation in ICU
Total hours of continuous IV vasoactive drug therapy

Form of Multiple Linear Regression Model

$$Pr\,(Y = |1\ X_1, 1\ X_2,...,X_k) = \frac{e\,(B_0 + B_1X_1 + B_2X_2 + ... + B_kX_k)}{1 + e\,(B_0 + B_1X_1 + B_2X_2 + ... + B_kX_k)}$$

where $Pr\,(Y = |1\ X_1, X_2,...,X_k$ denotes the probability that a patient with values of the condition and treatment variables equal to $X_1, X_2,...X_k$ will die (i.e., $Y = 1$).

[a]From Rafkin HS. Assessing the critically ill patient for admission to the intensive care unit. In: Hoyt JW, Tonneson AS, Allen SJ, eds. Critical care practice. Philadelphia, WB Saunders, 1991:21.

Table 15.8.
Description of ICU Active Treatment, ICU Monitoring, and Standard Care Tasks[a]

Active Treatment—ICU

4 Point

Cardiac arrest and/or countershock within past 48 h
Controlled ventilation with or without PEEP[b]
Controlled ventilation with intermittent or continuous muscle relaxants
Balloon tamponade of varices
Continuous arterial infusion
Atrial and/or ventricular pacing
Hemodialysis in unstable patient
Induced hypothermia
Pressure-activated blood infusion
G-suit
IABA (intra-aortic balloon assist)
Emergency operative procedures (within past 24 h)
Lavage of acute GI bleeding
Emergency endoscopy or bronchoscopy
Vasoactive drug infusion (>1 drug)

3 Point

Intermittent mandatory ventilation (IMV) or assisted ventilation
Continuous positive airway pressure (CPAP)
Concentrated K^+ infusion via central catheter
Nasotracheal or orotracheal intubation
Complex metabolic balance (frequent intake and output)
Vasoactive drug infusion (1 drug)
Continuous antiarrhythmia infusions
Cardioversion for arrhythmia (not defibrillation)
Active diuresis for fluid overload or cerebral edema
Active Rx for metabolic alkalosis
Active Rx for metabolic acidosis
Rx of seizures or metabolic encephalopathy (within 48 h of onset)

2 Point

Hemodialysis–stable patient
Fresh tracheostomy (less than 48 h)
Replacement of excess fluid loss

Monitoring—ICU

4 Point

Pulmonary artery catheter
Intracranial pressure monitoring

3 Point

Pacemaker on standby
Arterial line
Measurement of cardiac output by any method

2 Point

ECG monitoring
Hourly neuro vital signs

Standard Care—Floor Care

4 Point

Peritoneal dialysis
Platelet transfusion

3 Point

Central IV hyperalimentation (includes renal, cardiac, hepatic failure fluid)
Chest tubes
Blind intratracheal suctioning
Multiple blood gas, bleeding, and/or STAT studies (>4/shift)
Complex metabolic balance (frequent intake and output)
Frequent infusions of blood products (>5 units/24 h)
Bolus IV medication (nonscheduled)
Hypothermia blanket
Acute digitalization—within 48 h
Emergency thora-, para-, or pericardio-centesis
Active anticoagulation (initial 48 h)
Phlebotomy for volume overload
Coverage with more than two IV antibiotics
Complicated orthopedic traction

2 Point

CVP (central venous pressure)
Two peripheral IV catheters
Spontaneous respiration via endotracheal tube or tracheostomy (T-piece or trach mask)
GI feedings
Parenteral chemotherapy
Multiple dressing changes
Pitressin infusion

1 Point

One peripheral IV catheter
Chronic anticoagulation
Standard intake and output (q 24 h)
STAT blood tests
Intermittent scheduled IV medications
Routine dressing changes
Standard orthopedic traction
Tracheostomy care
Decubitus ulcer
Urinary catheter
Supplemental oxygen (nasal or mask)
IV antibiotics (2 or less)
Chest physiotherapy
Extensive irrigations, packings or debridement of wounds, fistula or colostomy
GI decompression
Peripheral hyperalimentation/Intralipid therapy

[a]From Cullen DJ, Neoneskel AR. Therapeutic intervention scoring systems (TISS). In: Farmer JC, ed. Problems in critical care. Philadelphia: JB Lippincott, 1989:545–562.
[b]PEEP, positive end expiratory pressure.

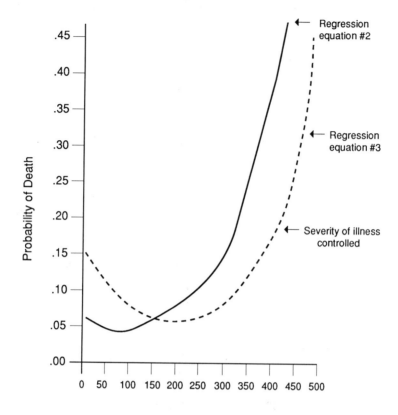

Figure 15.5. Relationship between treatment and survival with and without control for severity of illness. *GWUMC*, George Washington University Medical Center. (From Scheffler RM, Knaus WA, Wagner DP, Zimmerman JE. Severity of illness and the relationship between intensive care and survival. Am J Public Health 1982;72(5)451. © American Public Health Association.)

any of the patients. This message, however, does not represent the truth. On the contrary, by controlling for severity of disease, it is possible to demonstrate a decrease in the probability of survival for a specified group of ICU patients.

This study demonstrates that use of a severity of illness index, such as APACHE, enhances an analysis of the impact of ICU therapy on probability of survival. Had this analysis been performed solely with TISS without controlling for severity of disease, the conclusions would have differed significantly. Instead of implying that increasing total therapy over the course of hospitalization has no positive effect, it suggests to the contrary, that increasing amounts of therapy rendered in the ICU can reduce the risk of mortality for certain patients. The relationship between therapy and outcome are elucidated through use of a severity of disease scoring system.

ICU Utilization

While quality of care may be most classically embodied by the concept of outcome evaluation, an overall assessment of ICU efficiency should include an evaluation of ICU utilization. In this era of limited resources, it is necessary to direct attention to the duration of stay in the ICU. In addition, it is important to direct attention to the nature of patients admitted to the ICU. Particularly germane to this latter issue are patients admitted to the ICU for monitoring. A brief discussion of these issues follows.

Length of Stay

APACHE goes beyond predicting risk of mortality, and also generates the optimal length of stay for the entire group of patients entered into the APACHE program (25). Thus, observed and ideal length of stay can be compared. Although patients should not be discharged before they are satisfactorily stabilized, they should also not remain in the ICU longer than necessary. This would represent poor medical practice and would unnecessarily expose a patient to the potential of iatrogenic complications of the ICU. Moreover, in an era where ICU beds and financial resources are limited, this is an unwise fiscal practice for both the hospital and society in general. Only the APACHE system provides predictions concerning appropriate length of stay.

Identification of Low-Risk Monitor Patients

Finally, APACHE categorizes patients admitted to the ICU for monitoring into those with high risk and those with low risk. Thibault et al. (26) revealed in a series of 2693 admissions to a medical ICU that noninvasive monitoring rather than immediate major intervention was responsible for 77% of admissions. Moreover, only 10% of patients admitted for monitoring required major interventions that justified admission to the ICU. This situation was thought to be representative of many ICUs. Knaus, therefore, developed a system by which APACHE could identify patients admitted to the ICU for monitoring and classify them as either low-risk or high-risk monitor patients (27).

In order to accomplish this, APACHE and TISS are used in a complementary manner. Based on the type and complexity of therapy received during the first 24 hours of ICU care, a patient is classified by APACHE as either an active treatment admission or a monitor admission. APACHE then performs a logistic regression analysis for each monitor admission to predict the risk for receiving subsequent ICU therapy. Predicted risk of receiving subsequent therapy ranges from 0 to 100%. Risk factors used in this regression analysis are APS, surgical status, and major indication for ICU admission. Table 15.9 shows the logistic regression for patient risk factors used in this analysis.

Based on clinical judgment and exami-

Table 15.9.
Logistic Regression of Patient Risk Factors for Receiving Subsequent ICU Therapy When Admitted for Monitoring[a]

Variable	Coefficient	Standard Error	χ^{2b}	p
Intercept	−3.844	0.312	152.09	0.0001
Acute severity of disease[c]	0.113	0.022	26.64	0.0001
Surgical status[d]				
Emergency surgery (Yes = 1)	0.633	0.435	2.11	0.1460
No surgery (Yes = 1)	1.148	0.319	12.93	0.0003
Major indication for ICU admission[e]	−2.340	0.744	9.90	0.0017
Diabetic ketoacidosis, severe electrolyte abnormalities, and drug overdose (Yes = 1)				
Renal failure (Yes = 1)	1.670	0.414	16.28	0.0001

[a]From Wagner DP, Knaus WA, Draper EA. Identification of low risk monitor admissions to medical-surgical ICUs. Chest 1987;92:423–428.
[b]Model χ^2 = 99.05 with 5 D.F.; P = 0.001; N = 778.
[c]APS-12.
[d]Reference group is postelective surgery.
[e]Reference group is neurologic, cardiovascular, respiratory, or gastrointestinal.

nation of individual patient records, the developers of APACHE have chosen a 10% predicted risk as the threshold to distinguish low-risk from high-risk monitor patients. Any patient admitted to the ICU for monitoring, but with less than a 10% chance of receiving immediate active therapy, is considered a low-risk monitor patient. These patients, by inference, do not require ICU therapy.

In conclusion, evaluating the quality of care rendered in the ICU requires an analysis of outcome per se, but also should include a critical evaluation of ICU utilization. Severity of disease scoring systems enable one to perform meaningful and reliable evaluations of these parameters. An analysis of the relationship between therapy and outcome has meaning only when severity of disease is taken into account. In this way, the real impact of medical care in the ICU can be measured. In areas where outcome is suboptimal, the situation can be rectified. Herein lies the best reason to evaluate these parameters through use of severity of disease scoring systems. Quality of care can be improved only with this type of self-critical process.

Influence of Process on ICU Outcome

A macroassessment of quality in the ICU encompasses not only assessment of outcome and utilization, but also an evaluation of the process that produces that outcome. As intensive care units have evolved, varying organizational structures have become rooted in respective hospitals. Moreover, as a consequence of these different structures, the respective roles and relationships between physicians and nurses have tended to vary considerably. Data are now available which suggest that these factors influence outcome. This portion of the discussion will address these issues.

Knaus and associates (28) prospectively assessed the influence of structure and process of intensive care on ICU outcome. These authors evaluated outcome in 13 hospitals with similar technological capabilities but with different organization,

staffing, and commitment to teaching, research, and education. Observed outcome in each of these ICUs was compared to the APACHE-derived predicted outcome. Some hospitals had full-time ICU directors, high nurse:patients ratios, and in-unit teaching and research commitments (level I ICU); some had part-time directors with qualified designates in the hospital at all times, and high to intermediate nurse:patients ratios, (level II ICU); others had part-time directors but relied on coverage by other in-house physicians, and had lower nurse:patient ratios (level III ICU).

The process of health care delivery was found to effect patient outcome significantly (Table 15.10). Specifically, the interaction and coordination of the ICU staff was noted to be the most important factor in determining patient outcome. The best results occurred at hospitals 1 and 4; the worst results occurred at hospitals 3 and 13. Hospitals 1 and 4 were staffed by senior level in-house physicians. They had the most extensive nursing education programs. Educational programs included clinical material for the bedside nurse, as well as managerial material for the charge nurse. Most important of all, continuous and effective communication between physicians and nurses was cultivated and sustained. One structural difference between these two hospitals may have contributed to the difference in ranking. A system of carefully designed clinical protocols created by the senior level in-unit physicians was implemented at hospital 1, but not at hospital 4.

Analysis of the two poorest ranking hospitals reveals noteworthy findings. Hospitals 3 and 13 were both without a full-time ICU director or a part-time unit director. Therefore, there was no senior level physician to influence admission, discharge, or treatment decisions. Furthermore, no clinical protocols were used. Again, organizational differences may explain the slight difference in rankings assigned to these two hospitals. Hospital 3 offered an extensive educational program to the nursing staff. And although this hospital did not have a full-time medical director, the nursing staff met on a daily basis with the private attending during his

Table 15.10.
Structure and Process of Services Given in Intensive Care Units at 13 Hospitals[a]

Hospital Performance	Full-time Unit Director	Controls Decision for		24-Hour In-Unit Physician Coverage	Consistent Senior Charge Nurse	Continuity of Care/ Primary Nursing	Problems with Adequate Nurse Staffing
		Patient Therapy	Admission/ Discharge				
Level I							
1[b]	Yes	Director/staff	Director/staff	Yes	Yes	Yes	None
4	Yes	Director/staff	Director/staff	Yes	Yes	Yes	None
5	Yes	Shared[c]	Director/staff	Yes	Yes	No	None
6	Yes	Director/staff	Shared	Yes	Yes	Yes	Minor[d]
7	Yes	Shared	Shared	Yes	Yes	Yes	None
9	Yes	Shared	Director/staff	Yes	Yes	Yes	Minor
10	Yes	Shared	Director/staff	Yes	Yes	Yes	None
11	Yes	Shared	Director/staff	Yes	Yes	Yes	Minor
12	Yes	Shared	Director/staff	Yes	Yes	Yes	Minor
Level II							
2[e]	Yes	Shared	Attending physician only	Yes	Yes	Yes	Minor
8	No	Shared	Attending physician only	No	Yes	No	Minor
Level III							
3[e]	No	Attending physician only	Attending physician only	No	Yes	Yes	Minor
13[b,e]	No	Attending physician only	Attending physician only	No	No	No	Major

[a]Reproduced with permission from Knaus WA, Draper EA, Wagner DP, Zimmerman JE. An evaluation of outcome from intensive care in major medical centers. Ann Intern Med 1986;104:410–418.
[b]Indicates that standardized mortality rate significantly different ($p < 0.01$) from all others.
[c]Shared indicates that therapy or admission/discharge decisions are shared jointly by attending physician and director/staff.
[d]All hospitals listed as having minor difficulties had organized contingency plans.
[e]Nonteaching hospitals.

rounds with patients. When the attending was not at the hospital, close communications were maintained throughout the day. Hospital 13, the lowest ranked hospital, had no central nursing authority and poor overall nursing organization. There was no formal nursing education program. And crucially, admitting physicians and unit nurses failed to have routine discussions of patient treatment. Communication between nurses and physicians was plagued with disagreement and mutual distrust.

In addition to interaction and coordination of the ICU staff, the administration of the unit was also noted to influence outcome. Eleven of the 13 units had full-time directors; only two of these, hospitals 1 and 4 gave complete control over admission, discharge, and treatment decisions to

the full-time ICU staff. Neither hospital 3 nor 13 gave the unit director authority to influence therapy; instead, all therapeutic decisions were made by the primary attending physician. Optimal outcomes occurred in situations giving the full-time ICU staff either total or shared authority over these issues (Table 15.10). The most common structural system among ICUs evaluated in this study was that where authority for patient care was shared between the ICU and the attending physicians. On the other hand, the poorest outcomes were produced when the ICU director was not involved in these decisions, which were made solely by the attending physician.

This study, the first to evaluate the effect of process of care on outcome in the ICU, sends two important messages regarding quality assurance. Differences in outcome appear to correlate with the effectiveness of interaction and communication between physicians and nurses. In addition, delivering the highest level of health care is facilitated when both physicians and nurses are dedicated on a full-time basis to critical care.

Impact of Critical Care Medicine on ICU Outcome

This specific issue of physician organization in the ICU is paramount. Many retrospective analyses of ICU mortality do not take this factor into account. Early analyses, based essentially on data from the 1970s and early 1980s, aimed to demonstrate a decrease in mortality for specific illness simply due to placement of the patient in an intensive care unit. For example, it was reported that mortality due to myocardial infarction since the development of the coronary care unit (CCU) decreased from 35% in the pre-CCU era to 15% (29). Additionally, other authors pointed out that the intraaortic balloon pump had decreased long-term mortality due to cardiogenic shock to 53%, compared to earlier reports ranging from 62 to 90% (30). And finally, some authors pointed out the decrease in mortality in patients with septic shock due to treatment in the ICU. Although a representative study—prior to intensive care units—revealed a 82% mortality rate in patients with Gram-negative septic shock, later studies performed on ICU patients revealed 63% and 62% mortalities, respectively (31). These results suggest a benefit of intensive care units and make important contributions to our overall appreciation of ICUs. However, during this early stage of ICU development, inadequate attention was directed toward organization and structure of the ICU.

As intensive care medicine has become more complex, the specialty of critical care medicine has developed and evolved. Physicians trained specifically in critical care medicine now administrate many ICUs. Nurturing this development has been the assumption that the presence of on-site physicians dedicated to critical care medicine leads to higher survival rates. Although Knaus' data strongly suggest a benefit derived from on-site physician staffing, this issue still remains controversial in certain circles. Three authors have recently evaluated the impact derived from the presence of physicians formally trained in critical care medicine. Their findings are now presented.

In an early study, Li and associates (32) retrospectively evaluated a community hospital ICU before and after specialized ICU physicians were invited to manage the ICU. Parameters salient to the present discussion that were measured were patient outcome, length of stay, and readmission. Four hundred sixty-three patients admitted to the ICU during the year prior to the change were compared with 491 patients admitted during the year following the change. Severity of illness and other characteristics were controlled by using a stepwise logistic regression analysis, and mortality during the 2 years was compared. When controlling for severity of disease, mortality was significantly reduced during the second year while the ICU was managed by specialized ICU physicians (odds ratio = 0.62, $p = 0.01$, 95% confidence interval, 0.98, 0.45). This difference was most apparent in patients classified as having intermediate risks of mortality, but was, nevertheless, present across all severity of diseases. In addition, improvement in this patient population was most significant among those with cardiac disease or sepsis and was found to result from more frequent and effective use of invasive monitoring such as pulmonary artery catheters. And finally, although the average initial ICU length of stay was not significantly reduced, readmissions to the ICU were reduced from 44 to 29 ($\chi^2 = 4.0$, $p < 0.05$) by the presence of on-site ICU physicians.

More recently, Brown and Sullivan (33) retrospectively evaluated the benefit derived from a full-time ICU specialist in a teaching hospital. Mortality in an ICU over a 2-year period was evaluated. During the first year, patients were treated by their private attending; night coverage was provided by on-call residents in medicine and surgery. During the second year, therapy was shared by a trained ICU physician and the private attending physician; the critical care physician was on call every night and every other weekend. Alternate weekends were covered by an attending anesthesiologist or trauma surgeon. There was no organizational change in nursing or ancillary personnel. Two hundred twenty-three patients were evaluated during the first year, and 216 patients were evaluated during the second year. APACHE II scores were obtained, and both ICU and hospital mortality between the two groups were compared.

The results are depicted in Figures 15.6 and 15.7. The presence of an on-site ICU specialist led to a decrease in ICU mortality from 27.8 to 13.4% ($p < 0.01$). Hospital mortality was also decreased from 35.5 to 24.5% ($p < 0.01$). These decreases in ICU and hospital mortality were apparent in both intermediate and high severity of disease groups. This study suggests that at a university hospital the presence of unsupported in-house resident coverage does not guarantee optimal results. It also confirms and goes beyond the results of Li in that an unequivocal benefit of ICU specialists for severely ill as well as moderately ill patients is demonstrated.

Finally, Reynolds (34) and associates evaluated the impact of critical care physicians on patients with septic shock in a university hospital ICU. Septic shock was chosen because of the high mortality rate seen with this disease. Moreover, during the 20 years prior to this study, mortality rates had not appreciably improved.

In a retrospective study, these investigators recorded mortality due to septic shock in a university hospital medical ICU during two consecutive 12-month periods. During the first interval, the ICU physician staff consisted of faculty from the department of internal medicine and related subspecialties. Medical house officers were assigned to the unit and provided 24-hour in-house coverage of the medical intensive care unit (MICU). Both medical faculty and medical house officers were assigned to the unit on a rotating basis. During the second interval, the MICU was placed under the supervision of specialists formally trained in internal medicine and critical care medicine. In addition to a team of medical residents, two physicians performing post-residency training (fellows) in critical care medicine were incorporated into the ICU team. A formal chain of command from resident to fellow to attending was established. Twenty-four-hour coverage was provided by either a critical care fellow or critical care attending. All patients admitted to the MICU with septic shock during

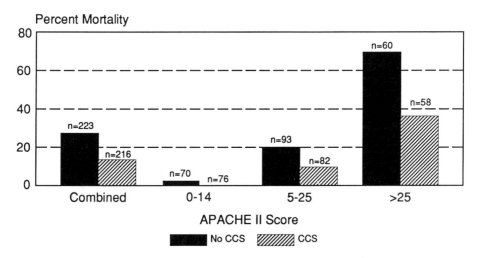

Figure 15.6. Percent ICU mortality versus APACHE II score. (From Brown JJ, Sullivan G. Effect on ICU of a full-time critical care specialist. Chest 1989;96:127–129.)

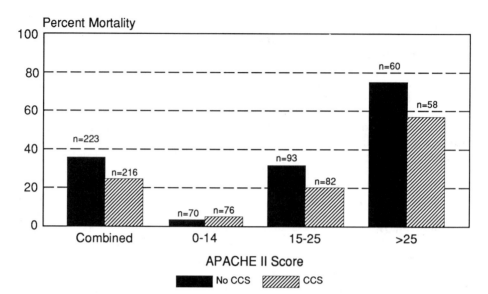

Figure 15.7.   Percent hospital mortality versus APACHE II score. (From Brown JJ, Sullivan G. Effect on ICU of a full-time critical care specialist. Chest 1989;96:127–129.)

these two periods were identified through a chart review.

Mortality among 100 patients with septic shock during the pre-critical care medicine (CCM) interval was compared with mortality among 112 patients with septic shock during the CCM interval. Again, APACHE scores were used to control for severity of disease, and in addition to overall mortality, mortality for each severity of disease subgrouping was compared. The presence of CCM reduced overall mortality from 74 to 57% ($p < 0.01$). This reduction in mortality was seen in all age groups and all levels of severity of disease (Figs. 15.8 and 15.9).

Without any significant advances in medical therapy between these two intervals, the presence of specialists in critical care medicine resulted in a statistically significant and clinically remarkable improvement in survival. Crucially, this improvement occurred with a disease with a mortality rate that has been persistently high for years.

In conclusion, several recent studies demonstrate the importance of process and structure on outcome in the ICU. The presence of a physician trained in critical care medicine and dedicated to the ICU impacts positively on outcome in the ICU. Moreover, effective delivery of health care

in the ICU depends not only on the presence of specialized physicians, but also on nurses specifically trained and educated in the unique complexities of critical care medicine. And most importantly, the benefit derived from the presence of physicians and nurses specialized in critical care medicine is enhanced by a system of synchronized care and effective communication. The process by which health care is delivered in the ICU alters survival.

Specific Recommendations Aimed at Ensuring Quality of Care in the ICU

Several specific recommendations can be made based on the information discussed above. The Society of Critical Care Medicine established a Task Force on Guidelines, and in 1990 published specific recommendations regarding (among other items) the nature of organization and structure of the ICU (35). These recommendations derive in part from data discussed above and are summarized here.

Every ICU should have a director. The director of the ICU should be a physician who on the basis of training can give

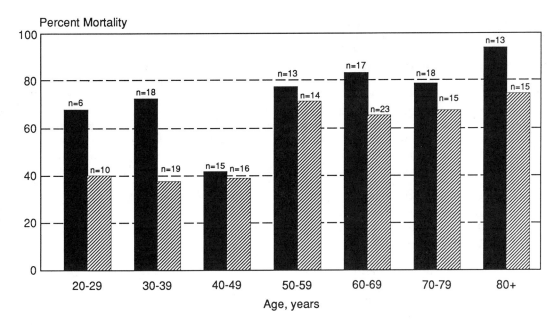

Figure 15.8.   Mortality in patients grouped according to age ($p < 0.01$ for overall significance [χ^2]). *Solid bars* indicate period before critical care medicine; and *slashed bars,* period after critical care medicine. (From Li TCM, Phillips MC, Shaw L, Cook EF, Natanson C, Goldman L. On-site physician staffing in a community hospital intensive care unit. JAMA 1984;252:2023–2027. © 1984, American Medical Association.)

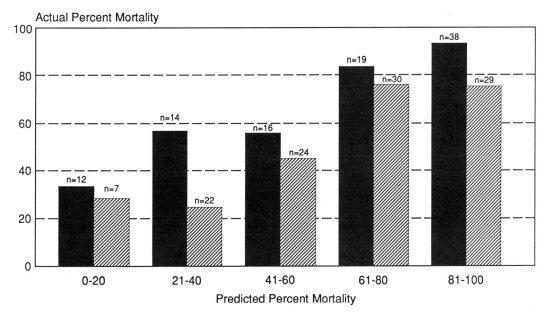

Figure 15.9.   Mortality in patients with Acute Physiology and Chronic Health Evaluation scores corresponding to consecutive mortality intervals ($p < 0.01$ for overall significance [χ^2]). *Solid bars* indicate period before critical care medicine; and *slashed bars,* period after critical care medicine. (From Li TCM, Phillips MC, Shaw L, Cook EF, Natanson C, Goldman L. On-site physician staffing in a community hospital intensive care unit. JAMA 1984;252:2023–2027. © 1984, American Medical Association.)

clinical, administrative, and educational direction to the ICU. Therefore, he/she should be board certified in his/her specialty and, in hospitals that are major teaching institutions or tertiary care facilities, be board certified in critical care medicine. The unit director should also be regularly involved in the care of the patients and at the same time be able to devote adequate time to administrative aspects of unit management. This includes formation and enforcement of unit policies, and education of the staff. In teaching institutions, the unit director must participate in clinical research, participate in continuing education programs in the field of critical care medicine, and participate in the education of physicians and nurses in his/her unit. Finally, the director (or an equally qualified alternate) must be available to the unit 24 hours a day, 7 days a week, for both clinical and administrative matters.

Other physicians must be available to the ICU. Twenty-four-hour in-house coverage is required by a physician who can manage emergencies, such a cardiopulmonary resuscitation, emergency airway management, or shock. In teaching hospitals, physicians dedicated to critical care must be present or immediately available on a 24-hour basis to provide titrated medical care. The need for assistance from other specialties is explicitly recognized, and consultations with other specialists should be available.

A nurse director must be appointed. This individual is responsible for assuring the quality and appropriateness of nursing care. He/she should have a Registered Nurse and a Bachelor of Science degree, as well as Critical Care Registered Nurse certification. In teaching institutions, the nurse director should have previous management experience. Educational activities are equally important, and the Nurse Director must participate in the education of the nursing staff, cooperate with the training of the housestaff, and be prepared to cooperate with clinical research projects.

Finally, the importance of cooperation and harmonious interaction is not overlooked. The guidelines emphasize that "the ICU Director and Nurse Director should collaborate in order to insure the quality, safety, and appropriateness of patient care."

The studies reviewed earlier highlight three critical factors that are required to assure optimal quality of care in the ICU. These are specialization in critical care medicine by both physicians and nurses, close interaction between physicians and nurses, and continuing education for the entire ICU staff. The Society of Critical Care Medicine has incorporated these suggestions explicitly in their formal guidelines.

SUMMARY

As we enter the 1990s, it is becoming increasingly clear that critical care is not synonymous with quality care. There are many problems with health care delivery in the intensive care setting. These problems can be expensive both in dollars and lives. This chapter has reviewed the history of critical care and examined the JCAHO techniques of QA in critical care. Finally, we have looked at the big picture of morbidity, mortality, and length of stay in the ICU. Much work needs to be done to assure quality patient care in the intensive care unit. Much of that work can and will be done as the young specialty of critical care medicine matures into a well-organized and scientifically based part of the health care system.

References

1. Weil MH, Von Planta M, Rackow EC. Critical care medicine: Introduction and historical perspective. In: Shoemaker WC, ed. Textbook of critical care. Philadelphia: WB Saunders, 1989:1–4.
2. Callahan D. Hopes, vain hopes: The pursuit of efficiency. In: Callahan D, ed. What kind of life. New York: Simon & Schuster, 1990:69–102.
3. Joint Commission on Accreditation of Healthcare Organizations. Examples of monitoring and evaluation in special care units. In: Special care unit monitoring and evaluation in perspective. Chicago: Joint Commission on Accreditation of Healthcare Organizations, 1988:11.
4. Brallier M. A quality assurance program to achieve excellence. Nurs Admin Q 1988;18–22.
5. Purgatorio-Howard K. Improving a quality assurance program. Nurs Management 1986;17(4);38–42.
6. Beyerman K. Developing a unit-based nursing

quality assurance program: From concept to practice. J Nurs Qual Assur 1987;2(1);1–11.

7. Finley-Cottone D, Link MK. Quality assurance in critical care. Crit Care Nurse 1985;5(2);46–49.

8. Joint Commission on Accreditation of Healthcare Organizations. Examples of monitoring and evaluation in special care units. In: Synopsis of the ten steps of monitoring and evaluation. Chicago: Joint Commission on Accreditation of Healthcare Organizations, 1988:13.

9. Kanar RJ. The influence of a quality assurance program on patient satisfaction. J Nurs Qual Assur 1988;2(3);36–43.

10. Joint Commission on Accreditation of Healthcare Organizations. Examples of monitoring and evaluation in special care units. In: Step by step through the monitoring and evaluation process. Chicago: Joint Commission on Accreditation of Healthcare Organizations, 1988:15–31.

11. Patterson CH. Perceptions and misconceptions regarding the Joint Commission's view of quality monitoring. Am J Infect Control 1989;17;231–243.

12. Joint Commission on Accreditation of Healthcare Organizations. Examples of monitoring and evaluation in special care units. Chicago: Joint Commission on Accreditation of Healthcare Organizations, 1988.

13. Meisenheimer CG. Incorporating JCAH standards into a quality assurance program. Nurs Admin Q 1983;1–8.

14. Saum MF. Evaluation: A vital component of the quality assurance program. J Nurs Qual Assur 1988;2(4);17–24.

15. Mehnert T. The reassessment process: Key to a meaningful quality assurance program. QRB 1985;127–131.

16. Fein IA, Strosberg MA. Managing the critical care unit. Rockville, MD: Aspen, 1987.

17. Finley-Cottone D, Link MK. Quality assurance in critical care. Crit Care Nurse 1985;5(2);46–49.

18. Bailit HL. Quality assurance and development of criteria and standards. Dent Clin North Am 1985;29(3);457–463.

19. Knaus WA, Zimmerman JE, Wagner DP, et al. APACHE—Acute physiology and chronic health evaluation: A physiologically based classification system. Crit Care Med 1981;9:591–597.

20. Knaus WA, Draper EA, Wagner DP, Zimmerman JE. APACHE II: A severity of disease classification system. Crit Care Med 1985;13:818–829.

21. Teres D, Lemeshow S, Harris D, Klar J. Mortality prediction models (MPM) for ICU patients. In: Farmer JC, ed. Problems in critical care. Philadelphia: JB Lippincott, 1989:585–598.

22. Cullen DJ, Nemeskal AR. Therapeutic intervention scoring systems (TISS). In: Farmer JC, ed. Problems in critical care. Philadelphia: JB Lippincott, 1989:545–562.

23. Girotti MJ, et al. Factors predicting discharge from intensive care: A Canadian experience. Can Anaesth Soc J 1986;33:291.

24. Scheffler RM, Knaus WA, Wagner DP, Zimmerman JE. Severity of illness and the relationship between intensive care and survival. Am J Public Health 1982;72(5):449–454.

25. APACHE II Manual. Acute physiology and chronic health evaluation. Washington, D.C.: APACHE Medical Systems, Inc., 1988.

26. Thibault GE, et al. Medical intensive care: Indications, interventions, and outcomes. N Engl J Med 1980;302(17):939–942.

27. Wagner DP, Knaus WA, Draper EA. Identification of low-risk monitor admissions to medical-surgical ICUs. Chest 1987;92:423–428.

28. Knaus WA, Draper EA, Wagner DP, Zimmerman JE. An evaluation of outcome from intensive care in major medical centers. Ann Intern Med 1986;104:410–418.

29. Mueller HS. Cardiogenic shock. In: Parrillo JE, Ayres SM, eds. Major issues in critical care medicine. Baltimore: Williams & Wilkins, 1984: 87–95.

30. Killip T. Monitoring in the coronary care unit and the role of arrhythmias in myocardial ischemia and infarction. In: Parrillo JE, Ayres SM, eds. Major issues in critical care medicine. Baltimore: Williams & Wilkins, 1984:127–132.

31. Parrillo JE. Septic shock: Clinical manifestations, pathogenesis, hemodynamics, and management in a critical care unit. In: Parrillo JE, Ayres SM, eds. Major issues in critical care medicine. Baltimore; Williams & Wilkins, 1984:111–125.

32. Li TCM, et al. On-site physician staffing in a community hospital intensive care unit. JAMA 1984;252:2023–2027.

33. Brown JJ, Sullivan G. Effect on ICU of a full-time critical care specialist. Chest 1989;96:127–129.

34. Reynolds HN, Haupt MT, Thill-Baharozian MC, Carlson RW. Impact of critical care physician staffing on patients with septic shock in a university hospital intensive care unit. JAMA 1988; 260(23):3446–3450.

35. The Task Force on Guidelines, SCCM. Recommendations for services and personnel for delivery of care in a critical care setting. In: Society of Critical Care Medicine Recommendations, 1990: 28–33.

Suggested Readings

Beyers M. Quality: The banner of the 1980's. Nurs Clin North Am 1988;23(3):617–623.

Bushy A, Roloff D. Interdiscipline implementation of a quality assurance program. Nurs Management 1988;19(7):80I–80P.

Coons M, Donovan C, Kasprow M, et al. Unit or service standards. Nurs Clin North Am 1988; 23(3):639–648.

Coyne C, Killien M. A system for unit-based monitors of quality of nursing care. J Nurs Admin 1987; 17(1):26–32.

Cullen D. Risk modification in the postanesthesia care unit. Int Anes Clin 1989;27(3):184–187.

Deurr BL, Staats K. Quality assurance program evaluation: A view from the unit base. J Nurs Qual Assur 1988;2(4):13–16.

Edmunds L. A computer assisted quality assurance model. J Nurs Admin 1983;13(3):36–43.

Faurer S. A quality assurance program. Am Operating Room Nurses J 1987;45(6):1384–1391.

Finley-Cottone D, Link MK. Quality assurance in critical care. Crit Care Nurse 1985;5(2):46–49.

Fries RC, Heide PW. Establishing a software quality assurance program for microprocessor-based medical equipment. Med Instrumentation 1986;20(3): 156–161.

Harbo JN, Heaney KM. Quality assurance: A reviewer's perspective. Dent Clin North Am 1985; 29(3):589–593.

Harris SH, Kreger SM, Davis MZ. A problem-focused quality assurance program. Nurs Management 1989;20(2):54–60.

Isaac D. Suggestions for organizing a quality assurance program. QRB 1983;68–72.

Jencks SF. Quality assurance. JAMA 1990;263(19): 2679–2680.

Kaluzny A. Quality assurance as a managerial innovation: A research perspective. Health Serv Res 1982;17(3):253–267.

Laessig RH, Ehrmeyer SS, Hassemer DJ. Quality control and quality assurance. Clin Lab Med 1986;6(2):317–327.

Lockwood AH. Percutaneous subclavian vein catheterization: Too much of a good thing? Arch Intern Med 1984;144:1407–1408.

Martin J. From implication to reality through a unit-based quality assurance program. Clin Nurse Specialist 1989;3(4):192–196.

Murphy RA, Williams TW, Ryan CP. Peer review in the 1990's: A look at the Georgia Medical Care Foundation. JMAG 1989;78:549–551.

Pacini CM, Westphal CG. Evaluating the quality of education-practice relationships. Nurs Clin North Am 1988;23(3):671–677.

Patterson CH. Standards of patient care: The Joint Commission focus on nursing quality assurance. Nurs Clin North Am 1988;23(3):625–638.

Pelletier LR, Poster EC. Part 1: An overview of evaluation methodology for nursing quality assurance programs. J Nurs Qual Assur 1988;2(4): 55–62.

Porter AL. Assuring quality through staff nurse performance. Nurs Clin North Am 1988;23(3):649–655.

Poster EC, Pelletier L. Part 2: Quantitative and qualitative approaches to nursing quality assurance program evaluation. J Nurs Qual Assur 1988; 2(4):63–72.

Savorgnani A. Quality assurance activities in healthcare facilities. Milit Med June;154:322–326.

Schroeder P. Directions and dilemmas in nursing quality assurance. Nurs Clin North Am 1988; 23(3):657–664.

Smeltzer C. Evaluating a successful quality assurance program: The process. J Nurs Qual Assur 1988; 2(4):1–10.

Smeltzer CH, Feltman B, Rajki K. Nursing quality assurance: A process, not a tool. J Nurs Admin 1983;5–9.

Summers PM, Nadermann N, Turnis RM, et al. Quality management: Program design. Nurs Clin North Am 1988;23(3):665–670.

Warren JJ. Accountability and nursing diagnosis. J Nurs Admin 1983:34–37.

Wilson C. Designing a quality assurance program evaluation: A process model. J Nurs Qual Assur 1988;2(4):35–44.

Wood J. Bankston K, Bickford B, et al. An effort to identify the optimum method of patient care delivery. Crit Care Nurs Q 1990;12(4):5–9.

16

Emergency Department

Beverly Ringenberg, M.D.

Assessing quality in the emergency department has changed dramatically since the early 1970s when the Joint Commission on Accreditation of Healthcare Organizations (JCAHO) required 12 patient care audits annually and quality assurance (QA) was focused on satisfying these numerical requirements. Several factors have interacted to change all of that: the evolution of the specialty of emergency medicine, the increasing patient demand for high quality, efficient, and compassionate care, and the recognition of the emergency department as a "front door" to the hospital for a significant proportion of hospitalized patients. Now, hospital administrators, liability and health care insurers, and governmental agencies have joined the JCAHO in their efforts to assure high quality and appropriate emergency medical care.

Meeting the demands and expectations of these multiple groups may seem overwhelming in the uncontrolled environment of a busy emergency department (ED). However, a well-planned comprehensive quality assurance program can result in multiple benefits to the emergency department and hospital beyond meeting JCAHO requirements. A program for systematic problem recognition, reporting, and problem solving through quality assurance activities can help emergency department managers address medical and nursing staffing needs, facility renovation and equipment requirements, and liability associated with inadequate documentation (1). The ultimate goal of all quality assurance activities is improved patient outcome and patient satisfaction with care received. Although improvement may be gradual, multifactorial, and difficult to measure, a well-designed quality assurance program with clearly defined feedback loops for action and follow-up will ultimately be rewarding as well as a source of pride for the emergency department staff.

The 1990 JCAHO *Accreditation Manual for Hospitals'* chapter on emergency services includes both quality control (ER.8) and quality assurance (ER.9) standards (2). The quality control standard includes requirements that can be addressed primarily through the establishment of procedures to assure that the emergency department record all tests performed in the emergency department and make them available for follow-up care, that there be a timely method for review of x-ray, electrocardiogram (ECG), and laboratory test results, and that there be a protocol for notifying and recalling patients who require additional or repeat tests. In addition, this standard requires the establishment of a mechanism for review of transfers, blood transfusions, utilization of drugs, and review of medical records.

The quality assurance standard requires that there be a "planned, systematic and on-going process of monitoring, evaluating, and improving the quality and appropriateness of care" that not only identifies trends and opportunities for improvement but also assesses the most important aspects of care (most frequent, highest risk, or those with a tendency to produce problems for patients or staff). In addition, the 1990 standards require the establishment of objective, measurable, and current indicators; regular data collection and evaluation to identify trends or single clinical events needing action; and documentation and reporting of conclusions, recommendations and actions taken. Other JCAHO requirements related to the emergency department quality assurance include medical staff standards on reappointment (MS.5) and pathology and medical laboratory service standards pertaining to decentralized laboratory testing (PA.6.4) (2).

The following section discusses the components of a comprehensive emergency department quality assurance plan to meet these JCAHO requirements with specific examples of chart audit forms, problem reports, presentation of trended data with indicators and thresholds, and examples of how these quality assurance activities can improve care. The following areas are also addressed: epidemiological considerations unique to emergency medicine, some suggestions for how to make a QA program a positive experience for the staff, and specific instructions for implementing or refining a quality assurance program.

SPECIFIC EXAMPLES

The components of a comprehensive quality assurance plan for an emergency department should include the following: (a) an ongoing continuous monitor of quality and appropriateness of patient care, (b) a mechanism for screening all visits for high risk occurrences, (c) a simple and standardized method for incident and problem reporting, (d) a method of assessment of patient satisfaction, (e) a mechanism for short- and long-term problem-specific audits, and (f) equipment checks

and quality control monitoring of laboratory tests performed in the emergency department.

Ongoing Continuous Monitor of Medical Care

Numerous examples of problem-specific or random chart review worksheets have been reported in the literature (3–11). We have considered these examples in designing the chart review checklists used by the physicians and nurses at The University of Iowa Hospitals and Clinics (Figs. 16.1 and 16.2).

A random sample of all emergency department visits on a daily basis can be selected for ongoing review or a focused review of high volume/high risk chief complaints (for example, lacerations, patients discharged with chief complaint of chest pain) or known problem areas may be the focus of several months of investigation (for example, random review has revealed discrepancies among staff in evaluation and treatment of urinary tract infection). To avoid loss of records, it is recommended that charts to be audited be copied prior to the distribution to staff members.

Both nursing and physician aspects of medical care need to be reviewed. Depending upon the volume of the patients seen in the emergency department, the management structure of the emergency department, and the type of charting performed at the institution, medical and nursing audits may be combined or separate. However, efforts should be made to minimize duplication. For example, if both nursing and medical care audits are performed, only one should address documentation of last normal menstrual period. Copies of audited charts should be available for review by the staff being audited. All negative evaluations should require comment by the auditing clinician, and a mechanism for rebuttal should be provided. All discrepancies should be reviewed by the appropriate medical/nursing supervisor or quality assurance committee prior to summation.

Depending on the number of charts audited, monthly or quarterly reports

Criteria	Reviewer Response	Explanation/Comment
1. History complete in view of chief complaint and diagnosis?	☐Satisfactory ☐Unsatisfactory ☐Satisfactory with qualification	
2. Physical complete in view of chief complaint and diagnosis?	☐Satisfactory ☐Unsatisfactory ☐Satisfactory with qualification	
3. Labs complete in view of chief complaint and diagnosis?	Yes No (Explain) No labs done	
4. Were inappropriate blood tests performed?	Yes No (Explain)	
5. Were inappropriate x-rays performed?	Yes No (Explain)	
6. Diagnosis supported?	☐Satisfactory ☐Unsatisfactory ☐Satisfactory with qualification	
7. Treatment appropriate?	☐Satisfactory ☐Unsatisfactory ☐Satisfactory with qualification	
8. Were narcotics ordered?	Yes No	
If yes: a. Justified?	Yes No	
b. Appropriate?	Yes No	
9. Were antibiotics ordered?	Yes No	
If yes: a. Justified?	Yes No	
b. Appropriate?	Yes No	
10. Were other prescription drugs ordered?	Yes No	
If yes: a. Justified?	Yes No	
b. Appropriate?	Yes No	
11. Written instructions: a. Given?	Yes No	
b. Complete?	Yes No	
12. Was patient admitted? a. Yes, indicated b. Yes, not indicated (explain) c. No, not indicated d. No, should have been (explain)		
13. Was consultation obtained? a. Yes, indicated b. Yes, not indicated (explain) c. No, not indicated d. No, should have been (explain)		

Figure 16.1. ED quality assurance physician chart review.

should be compiled. Anonymous reporting by physician with grouped data available for comparison (Fig. 16.3) will provide a tool for self-evaluation for each physician, as well as documentation for annual credentialing of medical staff as required by JCAHO (2). Trended monthly, quarterly, and/or annual data (Fig. 16.4) will help focus on problem areas and demonstrate areas of improved compliance. Although desirable, anonymous individual reporting by each nurse may be complicated by the fact that multiple nurses may care for one patient, numbers may be small for any one nurse, and there may be resistance among the nursing staff toward individual specific reporting.

In addition to meeting JCAHO medical care review requirements and assuring improved documentation of new staff physicians, data from the medical care continuous monitor described above provided

Criteria	Response	Comments
1. Age noted	Yes No	
2. Pediatric weight (if applicable)	Yes No	
3. Initial vitals		
Time recorded?	Yes No	
Complete (R; P; BP; T if possible infectious process; orthostatic BP and P, if possible fluid deficit in adults)?	Yes No	
4. Repeat vitals (if initial abnormal, prolonged stay in ETC, treatment given that effects BP/P)	☐Satisfactory ☐Unsatisfactory ☐Satisfactory with qualification	
5. Mental status recorded	Yes No	
6. Skin perfusion	Yes No	
7. Last tetanus immunization (appropriate with any open wound)	Yes No	
8. LNMP (appropriate with any female of child bearing age)	Yes No	
9. Last meal (if applicable)	Yes No	
10. Allergies (if applicable)	Yes No	
11. Preadmission medications	Yes No	
12. Past medical/surgical history	Yes No	
13. Documentation of treatment prior to arrival	Yes No	
14. Nursing assessment	Yes No	
15. Appropriate nursing intervention based on initial nursing diagnosis	☐Satisfactory ☐Unsatisfactory ☐Satisfactory with qualification	
16. Documentation of procedures/treatment	Yes No	
17. Documentation of patient response	Yes No	
18. Documentation of drugs/IV: (dose/route/time)	Yes No	
19. Complete I & O (if appropriate)	Yes No	
20. Documentation of labs and cultures sent	Yes No	
21. Description and disposition of valuables	Yes No	
22. Nursing note signed	Yes No	

Figure 16.2. Nursing quality assurance chart review.

documentation utilized to support full-time staffing of our emergency department by career-oriented emergency physicians, as "moonlighters" were shown to have higher variation rates. Repeated deficiencies in nursing documentation of temperature have helped support arguments for additional rapid temperature sensing units. Other examples of medical care monitors that have resulted in side benefits to the department have been reported in the literature (12, 13).

Screening for High Risk Occurrences

In contrast to the review of a random sample of selected charts as described

Staff physicians	01	02	03	04	05	Total

Total cases reviewed
Overall variation rate
Criteria
1. History complete
2. Physical complete
3. Labs complete
4. Labs appropriate
5. X-rays appropriate
6. Diagnosis supported
7. Treatment appropriate
8. Narcotics ordered
   a. Order justified
   b. Amount appropriate
9. Antibiotics ordered
   a. Order justified
   b. Amount appropriate
10. Other prescription drugs ordered:
   a. Order justified
   b. Amount appropriate
11. Written instructions
   a. Given
   b. Complete
12. Patient admitted
13. Consult obtained

Figure 16.3. Medical care continuous monitor variation rates by staff physicians.

Overall Variation Rate

	January–March	April–June	July–September	October–December	Total

Total cases reviewed
Overall variation rate
Criteria
1. History Complete
2. Physical complete
3. Labs complete
4. Labs appropriate
5. X-rays appropriate
6. Diagnosis supported
7. Treatment appropriate
8. Narcotics ordered
   a. Order justified
   b. Order appropriate
9. Antibiotics ordered
   a. Order justified
   b. Amount appropriate
10. Other prescription drugs ordered:
   a. Order justified
   b. Amount appropriate
11. Written instructions
   a. Given
   b. Complete
12. Patient admitted
13. Consult obtained

Figure 16.4. Medical care continuous monitor: comparison of overall variation rates per quarter.

above, "generic" screening for certain conditions, situations, or occurrences that may be associated with increased risk is a quality assurance tool that provides incidence data. Errors in clinical judgment or treatment may or may not be present, and, the need for a focused review will depend on perceived risk (for example, a death in emergency department) or deviations from baseline rates. A list of possible generic screens is shown in Figure 16.5. Care should be taken to select relevant screens that meet specific institution and departmental concerns. Moreover, it is reasonable to change the screens periodically as results are evaluated and new high risk occurrences are defined.

Several methods for occurrence screening have been described in the literature. The use of "end of shift" reports has been encouraged by several authors (4, 14, 15) but may not be reliable given the lack of consistent reporting among clinical staff, the underreporting caused by the need to address "real problems" at the time of shift change, and the overreporting if interpersonal conflicts exists. A retrospective re-

view of daily log books by the ED medical director or head nurse may be simple and less time consuming to perform (3). However, these are dependent on consistent record keeping by reliable clerical staff.

A retrospective review of all emergency department charts by clerical personnel (such as a billing clerk) is feasible if screens are well defined and if the emergency department medical record is adapted to highlight these occurrences (3). In this regard computerized data base for demographic and quality assurance screening of all emergency department records has been developed at The University of Iowa Hospitals and Clinics (Fig. 16.6). The chart review and data entry that takes less than 60 seconds per chart are performed by the ED billing clerk. Subsequently, monthly reports with accumulated year-to-date data provide information that can be compared to established thresholds, reviewed by the quality assurance committee, and presented to the emergency department staff.

In addition to providing a format for occurrence screening, this type of com-

---

Patients leaving against medical advice (AMA)
Patients who die in the ED or within 24 hours of admission
Unscheduled returns to the ED
Patients who are transferred
Patients who received blood transfusions in ED
Patients who go to the OR for major procedures more than 3 hours after arrival to ED
Patients who develop wound infections

Figure 16.5.   Generic screens.

Hospital Number: _____   Last Name: _____ First Initial: _____
Date: _____   Birth Date: _____ Sex: _____

Day of Week: _____   Time Discharged: _____   Instructions: _____ (Y/N)
Time Registered: _____   Admitted: _____ (Y/N)   Service: _____
Return Visit: _____ (Y/N)   Deceased: _____ (Y/N)   CPR: _____ (Y/N)

Left AMA: _____ (Y/N)   Wound Repair: _____ (Y/N)
Left Before   Return with Wound Infection: _____ (Y/N)
   Being Seen: _____ (Y/N)   Transferred: _____ (Y/N)

Trauma: _____ (Y/N)   Chest Pain or Arrhythmia: _____ (Y/N)
   Head Injury: _____ (Y/N)   Time of Initial Visit: _____: _____
   Spine Injury: _____ (Y/N)   ED Physician: _____

Figure 16.6.   Demographic/QA data base.

puter data base can provide valuable information relating to treatment times by physician or service, room occupancy rates, and time versus patient volume reports. Furthermore, the data can be used to create lists of important chart numbers for detailed review (for example, transfers, transfusions, cardiac arrest, trauma registry, or patients in research projects).

A year-end report of combined demographic, risk management, and chart monitoring data is shown in Tables 16.1 and 16.2. Data from the computerized demographic/quality assurance data base have been used to improve emergency department medical and nursing staffing and support arguments for triage and the need for additional treatment rooms in our ED. Other authors have described the use of the computer as an adjunct in occurrence monitoring (16, 17). It is likely that as

computerized charting becomes more common place, built-in quality assurance screens may replace retrospective chart review.

Incident and Problem Reporting

A systematic mechanism for documenting, investigating, and summarizing adverse or potentially adverse occurrences (problems, concerns, incidents, etc.) is an essential "on-line" aspect of every ED quality assurance program. In contrast, a haphazard approach of "putting out fires," without systematically documenting and summarizing these incidences makes it more difficult in the long run to address recurrent problems (i.e., repeated equipment failures, doctors who are repeatedly slow to respond to the ED, or a delay in

Table 16.1.
ED Quality Assurance Summary 1989—University of Iowa Hospitals and Clinics

	No. Seen	No. Entered into Data Base	Admits	Unscheduled Return Visits	Patients Leaving against Medical Advice	Patients Leaving before Being Seen	CPR
January	1850	1778	477	51	2	1	4
		96.1%	26.8%	2.9%	0.1%	0.1%	0.2%
February	1612	1542	397	58	3	1	1
		95.7%	5.7%	3.8%	0.2%	0.1%	0.1%
March	1750	1698	461	50	5	3	1
		97.0%	27.1%	2.9%	0.3%	0.2%	0.1%
April	1940	1869	529	49	3	5	3
		96.3%	28.3%	2.6%	0.2%	0.3%	0.2%
May	1861	1776	545	41	4	5	3
		95.4%	30.7%	2.3%	0.2%	0.3%	0.2%
June	1838	1783	559	38	4	3	1
		97.0%	31.4%	2.1%	0.2%	0.2%	0.1%
July	2005	1929	586	58	5	2	8
		96.2%	30.4%	3.0%	0.3%	0.1%	0.4%
August	1973	1915	524	50	7	2	5
		97.1%	27.4%	2.6%	0.4%	0.1%	0.3%
September	2127	2059	610	59	9	2	2
		96.8%	29.6%	2.9%	0.4%	0.1%	0.1%
October	2036	2005	585	52	7	3	1
		98.5%	29.2%	2.6%	0.3%	0.1%	0.0%
November	1843	1775	538	57	1	4	2
		96.3%	30.3%	3.2%	0.1%	0.2%	0.1%
December	1701	1661	496	54	5	6	0
		94.7%	30.8%	3.4%	0.3%	0.4%	0.0%
Total	22,536	21,740	6,307	617	55	37	31

Table 16.2.
ED Charting Summary 1989—University of Iowa Hospitals and Clinics

	No. Seen	Random Chart Audit				
		Chief Complaint Recorded	Discharge Condition Recorded	Disposition Recorded	Mode of Arrival Recorded	Discharge Time Recorded
January	1850	92.0%	70.0%	100.0%	96.0%	86.0%
February	1612	90.9%	81.8%	100.0%	93.2%	93.2%
March	1750	93.7%	91.7%	100.0%	95.8%	95.8%
April	1940	96.3%	90.7%	100.0%	100.0%	94.4%
May	1861	96.1%	82.4%	100.0%	98.0%	90.2%
June	1838	92.3%	90.4%	100.0%	96.2%	90.4%
July	2005	96.4%	94.5%	100.0%	96.4%	90.9%
August	1973	94.5%	87.3%	98.2%	98.2%	96.4%
September	2127	93.2%	84.7%	100.0%	94.9%	91.5%
October	2036	98.2%	93.0%	100.0%	98.2%	96.5%
November	1843	96.0%	92.0%	100.0%	98.0%	96.0%
December	1701	95.7%	87.2%	100.0%	91.5%	89.4%
Total	22,536	94.7%	87.3%	99.8%	96.5%	92.6%

admission because of lack of bed availability).

Although most hospitals have "incident report forms" that are supposed to be used for reporting adverse occurrences, rarely do these lend themselves to adequate reporting of department-specific problems. The fact that these reports are routed outside the department may also prevent reporting of problems that may better be addressed within the department (for example, personnel issues). A department-specific incident report can be developed that makes documentation and categorization of problems easy and efficient (Fig. 16.7) (3, 4, 8). A particular focus for review could be a changed ECG or x-ray reading, unscheduled returns with changed diagnosis, or complications of ED treatment using this tool. Regardless of the format, the forms should be readily available to all staff, and use should be strongly encouraged by the department's medical and nursing directors.

Problems or complaints from outside the department (patient, family, other departments, billing complaints, etc.) should be included in this review process. It may not be necessary to complete a problem report form if the complaint has been received in writing.

The ED medical director or nursing supervisor should promptly address concerns raised by these problem reports. At times, the concern may need extensive review and disciplinary action, at other times the incident may just be filed for future reference in case similar problems occur. Whatever decision is made, the response and follow-up should be documented. All problem reports should be summarized on a monthly or quarterly basis. The data summaries may be stratified by type of complaint (bill complaint, patient complaint, changed ECG readings, etc.) or by physician or department and compared to established thresholds.

Whenever an incident report or problem involves a specific physician or staff member, it is important that the individual be informed and have an opportunity to respond. Annual, physician-specific problems can be summarized as part of the credentialing process (remember to use denominator data—see "Determining the Denominator" below). Recurrent problems relating to issues that often seem "beyond your control" because they involve other departments will be much easier to address if there is a handful of problem reports to bring along when sitting down at the negotiating table. Examples include delays in computed tomography (CT) response, problems with private physicians or specialty residents, or increasing problems with bed availability on a specific nursing unit.

Assessing Patient Satisfaction

One of the primary challenges in emergency medicine is to insure that the high quality medical care that the patient has received is *perceived* as high quality by the patient or family member. The field of emergency medicine is plagued by many factors that may alter that perception: lack of established doctor-patient relationship; need for prioritizing patients; long waits; and a high stress environment for staff and patient. But the fact that good care has been perceived as inadequate causes far more problems than reverse marketing. Patients who feel that their care was inadequate are less likely to accept the physician's diagnosis and treatment plan, take medications as directed, and keep follow-

up appointment (18, 19). Undoubtedly, quality of medical care can be effected. Therefore, it is important to get the patient's "point of view" as part of a total quality assurance program.

Telephone Follow-Up Surveys

In addition to obtaining information concerning how satisfied the patient was with the care that he or she received in the ED, telephone surveys can improve the quality of care by assessing compliance with instructions and response to therapy and by providing further instruction. Most patients appreciate the individualized attention demonstrated by this effort. However, care must be taken to avoid invading privacy or aggravating an already touchy situation (for example, sexually transmitted disease, death in ED, etc.). Obviously, the primary limitation of a telephone survey system is the time-consuming nature of such an endeavor and the need to assure

---

Name:
Hospital Number:
(Stamper plate or sticker may be placed here)

Date of Incident: _____ Time: _____
Date of Report: _____ Time: _____
Reporter: _____

Initial ED Staff: _____
Explain Problem and Action Taken:

Patient-related Problems
☐ Return-Changed Diagnosis
☐ X-Ray/Laboratory/Electrocardiogram Change
☐ Complications of ED Treatment
  ☐ Reaction Medication
  ☐ Wound Infection
  ☐ Other: _____
☐ Patient Complaint
  ☐ Care Given ☐ Bill
  ☐ Other
Service-related Problems
☐ Delay in transfer to floor:
  Floor: _____
  Time Initial Call:
  Time to Floor: _____
☐ Delay in Response to ED
  Doctor/Service: _____
  Time Initial Call: _____
  Time of Arrival in ED: _____
☐ Laboratory Delay (explain):
☐ X-Ray Delay (explain):
☐ Other: _____

Explain Problem: _____

PLEASE PLACE THIS REPORT FORM WITH COPIES OF ED RECORDS (if at all possible) in QA Box. Thanks.

Figure 16.7. Problem report form: emergency department.

appropriate instruction if additional information is given to the patient. However, successful programs have been described even in high volume centers (20, 21).

Patient Satisfaction Questionnaires

Questionnaires are tools commonly used by hospitals, small businesses, and large corporations to assess satisfaction. Whether questionnaires are made available for all patients to pick up as desired, distributed to all patients upon discharge from the emergency department, or mailed to a random sample of patients depends on several factors. The portion of negative responses will probably be somewhat higher if the questionnaires are simply left out for the patients to complete if they choose. The expense of having questionnaires sent out to all patients or making them available to a random sample must be weighed against the benefits of a less representative response group. The marketing value of sending questionnaires to all patients must also be considered.

The questionnaire used at The University of Iowa is shown in Figure 16.8. These are available throughout the department and waiting area, and they are routinely sent to a random 10% sample of all patients seen in the ED. The mailed questionnaires are coded so that random versus nonrandom responses can be separately summarized. The data from the questionnaires are summarized on a quarterly basis, compared to established thresholds, and reviewed with registration, nursing, and physician staff members. Over the years, problems with parking, waiting room, and quality of discharge instructions have

---

Your Opinions	Yes	No
1. Upon presentation to the ED registration desk were you registered:		
Promptly?	☐	☐
Comment: _____		
Courteously?	☐	☐
Comment: _____		
2. After checking in at the desk were you contacted by one of the ED nursing	☐	☐
staff promptly?		
Comment: _____		
3. Were you seen promptly by an ED physician?	☐	☐
Comment: _____		
4. Did you receive courteous and professional care in the ED?	☐	☐
Comment: _____		
5. Were all tests and procedures performed in the ED, including results, explained	☐	☐
to you or your family adequately?		
Comment: _____		
6. If your time in the ED was extended, were you checked on periodically by one	☐	☐
of the ED staff?		
Comment: _____		
7. If you were sent home after your visit to the ED, did you receive written	☐	☐
instructions?		
Did you understand the instructions?	☐	☐
Comment: _____		
8. Were the following features of the ED acceptable?		
Waiting Room	☐	☐
Comment: _____		
Privacy	☐	☐
Comment: _____		
Parking	☐	☐
9. Were you satisfied with the care you received from the ED staff?	☐	☐
Comment: _____		
10. Would you recommend this hospital's ED to your family and friends?	☐	☐
Comment: _____		

Figure 16.8.   Emergency department patient questionnaire.

	1986	1987	1988	1989
Total questionnaires	206	307	385	378
Overall rate:	86%	87%	93%	94%
	(2455/2884)	(3755/4298)	(5039/5390)	(4978/5202)
Item				
1. Registration				
a. Prompt	96%	95%	96%	97%
b. Courteous	94%	89%	99%	99%
2. Contact with nurses				
a. Prompt	93%	96%	94%	93%
3. Contact with physician				
a. Prompt	78%	82%	85%	83%
4. Received courteous/ professional care	92%	95%	95%	94%
5. Adequate explanation of tests/procedures	88%	90%	93%	94%
6. Checked by ED staff periodically	84%	86%	92%	90%
7. Patient instructions				
a. Written	73%	72%	92%	93%
b. Understood	74%	75%	95%	96%
8. Acceptability of				
a. Waiting Room	83%	88%	98%	98%
b. Privacy	90%	95%	97%	97%
c. Parking	74%	79%	92%	95%
9. Satisfaction with care	89%	90%	90%	92%
10. Recommend to family/ friends	89%	93%	92%	96%

Figure 16.9. Emergency department patient questionnaire responses.

shown improvement as each of these problems have been addressed (Fig. 16.9). In addition, the overall satisfaction with emergency department services has gradually improved.

Short- and Long-Term Problem-Specific Outcome Studies

Although the comprehensive program described above can serve as a solid base for a quality assurance program and meet most of JCAHO requirements, a mechanism for performing short- and long-term problem-specific audits can serve as a useful adjunct to problem solving. Problem-specific audits should be designed to address specific areas in a department. The need for such audits may become apparent after a review of data collected from any one of the above methodologies. Several examples of problem-specific audits utilized in our department are described below.

Short-Term Problem-Specific Audits

Temperature Audit. The medical staff noted a persistent problem with documentation of patient temperatures by the nursing staff in our emergency department. It was decided that a detailed review of the medical records for all patients without temperatures charted would better define these deficiencies. Initially, audits were completed of all charts of patients seen over a 2-week period. A list of all diagnoses in which a temperature was not taken was reviewed by the medical staff, and a determination was made on which ones clearly should have had temperatures taken. The data indicated that 9.5% of the patients seen in the ED should have had temperatures measured but in fact did not. After a review of the data at the nursing staff meetings, subsequent follow-up audits at 1 and 3 months showed marked improvement (deficiency rates fell to 5%).

Entrance Utilization Audit. A recognized problem relating to congestion at the ED registration area, thought to be caused by inappropriate utilization of the emergency department entrance, was addressed in another short-term problem-specific audit. Four nursing students, who were required to perform a research project, were scheduled to track who was going in and out of the ED entrance over a 40-hour period. A summary of the data showing that 82% of the people utilizing the ED entrance had nothing to do with the ED was used to document the need to construct a dedicated ED entrance, which has subsequently been approved.

Turnaround Time Audit. Two final examples of problem-specific audits that did not result in dramatic changes were audits of laboratory and x-ray turnaround times. Despite collecting a representative sample of data points, again using nursing students, we found that the average turnaround times were actually not as long as we had often felt, and, despite the fact that they were still longer than we would have liked, there was little change when the results were reviewed with representatives from the other departments. Joint audit efforts between departments may have more potential and might be attempted when departments agree that a problem exists. Several other examples of turnaround time audits have been reported in the literature (12, 22, 23).

Long-Term Problem-Specific Audits

Trauma Care. Depending upon the level of trauma care provided, a detailed audit of trauma care may be an important component of a quality assurance program. The guidelines for review of trauma care and development of a trauma quality assurance program are available through the American College of Surgeons (24). Subsequently, a list of patients appropriate for review can be generated utilizing the computer data base described above. Of interest is the fact that video recording of trauma resuscitation has been reported as a valuable QA and teaching technique (25).

Transfers. A focused review with an audit checklist (Fig. 16.10) can be utilized to ensure that all transfers to other institutions are performed in accordance with established guidelines and Consolidated Omnibus Budget Reconciliation Act (COBRA) legislation. In this high risk area, a review of 100% of charts may be necessary. Again, the list of patients being transferred can be generated using computer-assisted screening of all patients.

Additional topics that may be appropriate for focused short- and long-term problem-specific audits include the following: patients with cardiac arrests, patients requiring physical or chemical restraint, and patients requiring transfusion if this is not part of a hospital wide transfusion quality assurance program. Numerous examples of problem-specific audits have been reported (26–31).

Equipment Checks and Quality Control for the ED Laboratory

Nursing service has traditionally been responsible for performing equipment checks such as crash cart checks, battery checks for defibrillators and other portable equipment, and daily quality control of ED laboratory equipment such as glucometers. However, the medical director should become familiar with these elements of departmental quality assurance and work with the nursing service to establish thresholds and incorporate these and other "environmental" monitors into the departmental quality assurance program.

The pathology and medical laboratory section of the JCAHO Accreditation Manual for Hospitals has clearly defined standards for decentralized laboratory testing (Fig. 16.11). The ED laboratory must have written policies and procedures, maintain records of test performed (accession log) and daily quality control checks, and demonstrate satisfactory levels of competence (proficiency testing). Once again, these requirements seem demanding and undoubtedly will become more strict in the future. Compliance by staff members can be facilitated by creating simple logs that enhance communication within the department and minimize duplication of documentation. Moreover, utilizing commercially available tests that have "built-in" controls, developing procedures that require controls to be run at the same time as the test is run, and contracting with outside agencies to formalize a proficiency testing program will help make the laboratory QA program simple for your staff.

The concept of an "accession log" for recording urinalysis, rapid strep screen, urine pregnancy test, and glucometer results was initially resisted by our staff, as it

---

Date:
Hospital Number:
Name:

(Stamper plate or sticker may be placed here)

Transfer to: _____
Method of transfer: ☐Local ambulance   ☐Law enforcement   ☐Other _____

CHECKLIST

Physician responsibilities
  Documentation of acceptance by receiving   ☐Receiving physician and title documented
    facility   ☐Date and time of acceptance documented
  Documentation of stabilization prior to transfer   ☐Diagnosis documented
                                        ☐Emergency care provided to assure patient stable for transport documented
                                        ☐Condition at time of transfer documented
  Documentation of patient/family   ☐Patient informed and agrees to transfer
                                        ☐Family informed and agrees if patient is not competent

Nursing responsibilities
  Documentation of records sent   ☐Copy of ED records
                                        ☐Results of laboratory/electrocardiogram/x-ray
  Nursing documentation   ☐Handling of valuables
                                        ☐Report called to receiving facility

COMPLETED CHECKLIST SHOULD BE ATTACHED AND FILED WITH ED CHART COPIES

(This is not to be sent with the patient and is not part of the medical record)

Figure 16.10. Transfer documentation.

PA.6.4.1 If diagnostic clinical laboratory testing for the organization's patients is done within the organization, outside a central laboratory
  PA.6.4.1.1 Personnel responsible for test performance and those responsible for direction/supervision of the testing activity are identified;
  PA.6.4.1.2 Personnel performing tests have adequate, specific training and orientation to perform the tests, and demonstrate satisfactory levels of competence.
  PA.6.4.1.3 Current written policies and procedures are readily available and address
    PA.6.4.1.3.1 specimen collection;
    PA.6.4.1.3.2 specimen preservation;
    PA.6.4.1.3.3 instrument calibration;
    PA.6.4.1.3.4 quality control remedial action;
    PA.6.4.1.3.5 equipment performance evaluation; and
    PA.6.4.1.3.6 test performance;
  PA.6.4.1.4 Quality control checks are conducted on each procedure each day the procedure is performed, and identified problems are resolved; and
  PA.6.4.1.5 Appropriate quality control and test records are maintained.

Figure 16.11. Decentralized laboratory testing.

appeared to create duplication of effort. However, within several weeks of posting the log beside the laboratory desk, it became clear that the log actually reduced duplication of tests because results were documented immediately, and the need for verbal communication of results was eliminated. In addition to record keeping of daily controls and documentation of actions taken if problems are encountered, utilizing test procedures that had built-in controls can improve efficiency, (for example, rapid strep screens or urine pregnancy test).

Performing controls on tests like Gram stain and pulmonary function tests devices may be more time consuming and problematic, especially when they require the cooperation of the physician staff. One of the simplest ways to assure that controls are being checked by all physicians performing the test is to have the controls done at the same time that the test is performed (have control Gram stain slides with both Gram-positive and Gram-negative organisms on a slide available in the laboratory at the same time the patient's Gram stain is performed). There should be a readily available log for the physicians to record control and patient results. The idea of performing Gram stain controls was initially resisted at our institution, but now the physician staff agree that being able to check the control slide to verify correct staining has increased confidence in the Gram stain readings.

Finally, proficiency testing (performance of a given test on an unknown sample) can be arranged with independent laboratories on a contract basis. The results should be kept in a notebook for easy reference at the time of laboratory review.

EPIDEMIOLOGICAL CONSIDERATIONS

There are several epidemiological features that should be considered when developing or refining a quality assurance plan.

Selection of a Representative Sample

Care should be taken to make sure that the quality assurance program covers all major aspects of medical care in your ED. The quality assurance program should be customized to the hospital's population and primary problem areas. For example, an ED that serves as a regional trauma center should ensure that the care of the major trauma patients is monitored utilizing a specifically developed continuous monitor of medical and nursing care in the ED and develop risk occurrence screening methodologies specific for trauma patients such as patients who die in the ED or x-ray suite. In contrast, an ED that sees a large number of elderly patients with acute cardiac conditions may want to develop a continuous monitoring review process for patients with a chief complaint of chest pain, such as a monitor of promptness of initiation of thrombolytic therapy, and set up occurrence screening methodology that pick up complications related to thrombolytic therapy or adherence to do-not-resuscitate (DNR) documentation protocols.

In addition to making sure that the quality assurance plan addresses a representative sample of the patient population, efforts should be directed to monitoring a representative sample of the medical staff. For example, an ED in a teaching institution with residents working in the ED should provide information feedback to the residents as well as the staff concerning chart monitoring, occurrence screening when appropriate, and adverse outcomes involving a resident. Another quality assurance challenge occurs in emergency departments where a large number of patients are seen only by private physicians or only by specialty services (teaching hospitals without ED residency programs). The ED medical director might consider working with these other physicians to establish mutually agreeable parameters to follow (for example, time of arrival of private physician or consultant) and develop a method for review of a random sample of charts.

Finally, the actual number of charts reviewed should be enough to give a good overall picture, but not be overburdening to the staff or quality assurance committee. For a randomly selected review, a 5% sample is probably adequate. In contrast, a diagnosis-specific sample may include all patients with a given condition or a maximum that totals no greater than 5% of the overall population (for example, all lacerations for a given month, not to exceed 5% of the ED volume for that month). When the number of physicians or nurses involved is high and the overall patient volume is low, summarizing data on a quarterly basis will give a better picture of individual staff performance.

Determining the Denominator

When reporting the results of QA monitors, one needs to remember that there are numerous epidemiological factors that may influence the absolute number of adverse outcomes, problem reports, or charting errors. For example, some physicians prefer to work more nights (a time when there may be more patients leaving against medical advice), others may work fewer weekends because of seniority (and therefore may be less likely to have problems with people complaining about waiting times), and some people work fewer hours (less chance for all adverse occurrences). Although not perfect, the good method to report occurrences or deficiencies is to be sure that the appropriate denominator is being used (i.e., number of charts audited for a given physician or the number of patients seen by a given physician). The methodology does not reflect variations due to unequal distribution of "high risk" shifts. However, these factors must be considered when results are reported for annual credentialing or staff counseling.

INTERACTION WITH STAFF

Fortunately most ED managers no longer have to convince their reluctant staff that quality assurance is necessary. Even the most reluctant accept it as a necessary evil (32). Currently, the challenge is to develop a quality assurance program that can be enthusiastically supported by the staff because tangible results can be seen from their efforts. Certainly, the key elements in making this possible include keeping it simple, choosing relevant issues, involving all staff, using anonymous reporting, and providing feedback.

Keeping It Simple

It is important that clerical functions, such as the selection of charts to be copied, the distribution and collection of audited charts, and the summarization of results, be performed by support personnel rather than medical or nursing staff if at all possible. Some departments have a dedicated quality assurance coordinator who may perform these tasks as part of his or her overall duties and responsibilities. However, when this is not the case, these functions can be assigned to unit clerks during slow hours or departmental secretaries.

When performing the nursing or medical audit, the clinical staff should be able to use a checklist format requiring a written comment only if a negative response is checked. Written comments should be educational and brief. Importantly, care should be taken to make sure that the clinical staff are not auditing items that could be more easily monitored by clerical staff at the time of occurrence screening (times, condition on discharge, disposition, etc.).

As trivial as it may sound, the courtesy of having the charts to be audited delivered to the staff and having a conveniently located central collection area for completed audits undoubtedly improves compliance. Additionally, general reminders of when audits are due may be necessary to encourage staff. If noncompliance becomes a problem, it may be necessary to track how many records are being distributed to each staff member and how many are returned.

Choosing Relevant Issues

One of the most important aspects of a good quality assurance program is to try to make it relevant, rather than be just a "paperwork exercise" (7). Unfortunately, there is not always agreement on what is relevant and there are some relevant issues that may be more difficult to change, such as abuse of the ED by certain patient populations. Thus, deciding what is relevant should follow group discussion but be guided by leadership that directs activities to meet requirements of the various groups (JCAHO, hospital quality assurance committee, etc.). The focus should have the potential for facilitating needed change.

Relevant issues may be high risk/high volume areas, such as chest pain or lacerations, or departmental issues like difficulties in admitting patients, or inadequate documentation of patient vital signs. Quality assurance activities may also seem more relevant if they are educational. For example, it may be educational to audit the medical care of all female patients who were discharged with the diagnosis of nonspecific abdominal pain and find out what proportion of them had unsuspected chlamydial infections.

Involving All Staff

Establishing a quality assurance committee is probably the best way to assure representative input from all staff and is clearly recommended by most experts (33, 34). However, many of us find ourselves wanting when looking for volunteers for the quality assurance committee. This may be especially true in EDs that are small or are experiencing shortages because of high volume or understaffing. Many times the ED medical director or nursing supervisor may carry out most of the quality assurance responsibilities.

Whether there is an active quality assurance committee or not, the entire staff should be involved in the quality assurance process. The review of quality assurance activities should be a routine part of all medical and nursing staff meetings. Ideally all staff would perform auditing functions, either on a rotating basis by month or a daily basis with charts routinely distributed to all staff members. In general, sharing the load creates more of a peer review environment than a boss-

employee review process, and it is generally better accepted. Certainly, objective criteria should be defined to provide standard assessment by multiple observers (35).

Anonymous Reporting

Care should be taken to insure that the staff do not feel singled out for punitive purposes by departmental quality assurance efforts. Although reports can be individualized by staff member (as shown in Figure 16.3), all names should be deleted from distributed reports. Staff members should be able to compare themselves to peers whose activities are included in an overall report in order to make a self-assessment. As emphasized above, the denominator data are essential. Appropriate ED managers should be aware of individual results in order to provide guidance and assure thorough evaluation of the employee.

Information Feedback

The importance of feedback cannot be overemphasized (6, 10, 15). The staff must be informed of the results of the ongoing medical and nursing monitors as described above. They ought to be informed when there are complaints or problems attributable to their care. Importantly, they ought to be aware of how quality assurance activities have resulted in desired changes in the department.

A copy of the ED record and audit form should be made available for review and comment by the audited physician/nurse. Some room for comment or "rebuttal" should be allowed, and discrepancies should be resolved by the appropriate medical/nursing supervisor or QA committee. The results of monthly and quarterly reports should be reviewed at staff meetings, and trended data should be reviewed quarterly.

Providing feedback when there are complaints or problems can be more sensitive. Nevertheless, staff members should be aware of concerns raised and allowed to respond. Sometimes a copy of the "problem report" form with a copy of the chart attached can simply be sent to the staff member marked "for your information" or "for your review and comment." At other times, the physician or nurse must be contacted by phone or in person to discuss the issues involved. Specific positive and negative comments made about the medical or nursing care on the patient satisfaction questionnaire should be shared with the involved staff members as well. Some indication of appreciation for a job well done should be included when a strong positive comment is received such as "the nurse that took care of me was so thoughtful and caring." A copy of the ED record should be attached when negative comments are made so that the staff member can review the circumstances surrounding the complaint.

Finally, it is important to take the time to let the staff know that their quality assurance efforts are appreciated and are being used to improve quality of care. This may be as straightforward as telling them how good the department did during a recent JCAHO review or, more importantly, reviewing for them how quality assurance data have been used to support staffing changes, the need for new equipment, or the need for a new facility.

SPECIFIC INSTRUCTIONS FOR IMPLEMENTING AN EMERGENCY DEPARTMENT QUALITY ASSURANCE PROGRAM

Whether just beginning to establish an overall quality assurance plan or refining an existing departmental plan, the 10-step process recognized by JCAHO (Fig. 16.12) is a simple format to utilize (2).

The first step is to establish who is responsible for quality assurance within the department. A quality assurance committee with physician and nursing representation is encouraged to establish a departmental teamwork approach to quality assurance and avoid duplication of effort. Representatives from registration, security, laboratory, radiology, etc., can also be included depending on the size of the department and management structure. A definite timetable for completion of the departmental quality assurance plan needs to be established and regular meetings scheduled.

The quality assurance committee should first attempt to define the "scope of care" provided in the ED and then identify the most important aspects of the care provided. Obviously, the scope of care in emergency medicine is very broad and therefore difficult to define. However, the most important aspects of care may be more straightforward such as the identification and stabilization of significant illness or injury.

Once the most important aspects of care at a given institution are defined, identifiable and quantifiable indicators for monitoring these aspects of care should be defined. When refining a quality assurance program, indicators that have been determined to be helpful, retrievable, and reproducible in the past may be chosen. Thresholds, or action levels, that establish a minimum level of compliance beyond

---

1. Assign responsibility for monitoring and evaluation activities;
2. Delineate the scope of care provided by the organization;
3. Identify the most important aspects of care provided by the organization;
4. Identify indicators (and appropriate clinical criteria) for monitoring the important aspects of care;
5. Establish thresholds (levels, patterns, trends) for the indicators that trigger evaluation of the care;
6. Monitor the important aspects of care by collecting and organizing the data for each indicator;
7. Evaluate care when thresholds are reached in order to identify either opportunities to improve care or problems;
8. Take actions to improve care or to correct identified problems;
9. Assess the effectiveness of the actions and document the improvement in care; and
10. Communicate the results of the monitoring and evaluation process to relevant individuals, departments, or services and to the organizationwide quality assurance program.

Figure 16.12. 10-Step monitoring and evaluation process.

Table 16.3.
Overall ED Quality Assurance Plan

Standards/Indicators	Threshold	Data Collection Mechanism (Analysis Frequency)
Provide high quality medical care to all ED patients		
a. Rapid triage of patients presenting with a chief complaint of chest pain or irregular heart beat:		
1. Nursing vital signs within 5 minutes of registration	>95%	ED data base (monthly/yearly)
2. Thrombolytic therapy, if appropriate within 1 hour of presentation to ED	>95%	ED data base and chart audit (monthly/yearly)
b. Trauma patients requiring head, chest, or abdominal surgery to OR within 3 hours of presentation to ED	>90%	ED data base (monthly/yearly)
c. Nursing and medical care consistent with current standards of care		Nursing and medical care chart audit. Diagnoses to be audited selected based on common or high risk presentation. Changed biannually (quarterly/yearly)
d. All new patients discharged from the ED to receive written discharge instructions	>95%	ED data base (monthly/yearly)
e. Wound infection rate for wound repaired in ED by ED resident/staff	>97.5%	ED data base (monthly/yearly)
f. O negative and type specific blood transfusions justified	>97.5%	Notified by blood bank, reviewed by ED medical director (annually)
g. Problem reports—Any problem noted or reported relating to medical care should have problem report completed and forwarded to medical director as soon as possible.	>1% of all patients seen in ED/month	Monthly summary of problem reports relating to medical care (monthly/yearly)
Patients/families satisfied with care given		
a. Patient satisfaction survey		
1. Registration prompt and courteous	>95%	Survey (quarterly/yearly)
2. Contact with nurse prompt	>90%	Survey (quarterly/yearly)
3. Contact with MD prompt	>90%	Survey (quarterly/yearly)
4. Courteous and professional care	>90%	Survey (quarterly/yearly)
5. Explanation of tests	>90%	Survey (quarterly/yearly)

which intervention will be taken should be defined. Care should be taken to establish thresholds that are reasonable and reflect the relative importance of the indicator. For example, establishing a threshold of >90% for successful cardiac resuscitation in patients who arrest in the ED would be wonderful but is unobtainable. In contrast, a threshold of >98% successful intubations in the ED would be appropriate. For new indicators, it may be difficult to define an appropriate threshold. In this case, the quality assurance committee should agree upon an acceptable minimum and be flexible to change that may be necessary in the future.

Methods for monitoring have been described earlier in this chapter. Whether

Table 16.3—*continued*

Standards/Indicators	Threshold	Data Collection Mechanism (Analysis Frequency)
6. Checked on periodically by staff	>90%	Survey (quarterly/yearly)
7. Instruction received and understood	>95%	Survey (quarterly/yearly)
8. Acceptability of waiting room, privacy, parking	>95%	Survey (quarterly/yearly)
9. Overall satisfaction with care	>90%	Survey (quarterly/yearly)
10. Recommend to family and friends	>90%	Survey (quarterly/yearly)
b. Monitor high risk behaviors		
1. Left against medical advice	>1%	ED data base (monthly/yearly)
2. Left before being seen	>1%	ED data base (monthly/yearly)
3. Unscheduled return	>1%	ED data base (monthly/yearly)
c. Problem reports—Any patient complaints about care received, bills, etc. should be forwarded to medical director as soon as possible	>1%	Monthly summary of problems relating to patient satisfaction (monthly/yearly)
Maintain high safety standards		
a. Minimize risk to staff for needle sticks		
1. Incident reports	>0.1%	Incident report (monthly/yearly)
2. Other injury incident reports	>0.1%	Incident report (monthly/yearly)
b. Minimize risk to patients— Mislabeled laboratory tests	>0.1%	Incident report (monthly/yearly)
c. Problem reports—Incident reports and/or problems related to safety of patients or staff members should be reported to head nurse as soon as possible	>0.1%	Incident report (monthly/yearly)
Services provided and care given are well documented		
a. Nursing and medical care well documented		Nursing and medical care continuous monitor (quarterly/annually)
b. Required JCAHO information completed		
Chief complaint, mode of arrival, conditions, disposition, time of discharge	>95%	ED data base (monthly/annually)

obtained from random chart audits, occurrence screening, problem/incidence reports, patient satisfaction questionnaires, problem-specific audits, or departmental quality control checklists, data can be collected and organized for each defined indicator. On a monthly or quarterly basis, data should be evaluated and compared to established thresholds. When thresholds are exceeded, the results should be shared with the staff and methods to improve care

identified. An example of an overall ED quality assurance plan with defined standards, indicators, thresholds, methods of data retrieval, and schedule for data collection and analysis is shown in Table 16.3.

Continual reassessment through monthly and quarterly monitoring will determine the effectiveness of actions taken and provide documentation. If follow-up studies do not show improvement, the quality assurance committee and staff must reevaluate the threshold and decide whether expectations are too high or additional changes can be made to try to improve compliance. Finally, results, actions taken, and effectiveness of interventions should be regularly communicated to the overall hospital quality assurance program. This external feedback loop, outside the ED proper, demonstrates the commitment of the ED to excellence in the delivery of emergency care and can improve the image of the ED throughout the institution.

CONCLUSION

There is no one "right" way to assure high quality emergency medical care. Without a doubt, ED quality assurance begins with a qualified and dedicated emergency department medical and nursing staff. These individuals are the best ones to define standards, indicators, and thresholds, and, undoubtedly are the most qualified to determine interventions that will improve the quality of the ED care. However, the ED is often overcrowded, understaffed, and underappreciated, making quality assurance often seem like a time-consuming and bureaucratic exercise. Understanding these facts can help ED directors and hospital quality assurance coordinators work with the ED staff to develop a comprehensive quality assurance plan that meets JCAHO requirements and addresses concerns of the ED staff, while attempting to minimize daily time commitment of professional staff. Utilizing checklists for medical care audits, using convenient department-specific incident/problem report forms, and streamlining quality control in the departmental laboratory, while developing clerical support for computerized occurrence screening, data summary, and problem-specific audits can improve emergency department quality assurance.

Staff involvement in the development or refining process, as well as regular feedback to all involved staff is essential. Directly linking quality assurance activities and interventions to improved patient outcome may be difficult. However, if the ED staff come to appreciate the connection

between departmental quality assurance activities and changes that are implemented within the department that further help them deliver high quality emergency medical care, the patient will undoubtedly benefit as well.

References

1. Holbrook J, Aghababian R. A computerized audit of 15,009 emergency department records. Ann Em Med 1990;19(2):139–144.
2. Joint Commission on Accreditation of Healthcare Organizations Emergency Services (ER). *Accreditation Manual for Hospitals*. Chicago: JCAHO, 1990.
3. Schneiderman N, Wiseman M, eds. Quality assurance manual for emergency medicine. Dallas: American College of Emergency Physicians, 1987.
4. Whitcomb JE, Stueven H, Tonsfeldt D, Kastenson G. Quality assurance in the emergency department. Ann Emerg Med 1985;14(12):1199–1204.
5. Sniff D. The evolution of a quality assurance program. QRB 1980;6(1):26–29.
6. Overton DT. A computer-assisted emergency department chart audit. Ann Emerg Med 1987; 16(1):68–72.
7. Greene CS, Walter JJ. The problem-oriented review in the emergency department. Top Health Rec Manage 1984;5(2):39–45.
8. Edwards C. Quality assessment in the emergency room of a small rural hospital. QRB 1984;10(4): 119–123.
9. Cohen AG, Tucker E. Department of nursing implementation of JCAH standards: A quality assurance program applied. Hosp Top 1980; 58(2):38–40.
10. Harchelroad FP Jr, Martin ML, Kremen RM, Murray KW. Emergency department daily record review: A quality assurance system. QRB 1988; 14(2):45–49.
11. Waskerwitz S, Unfer SM. Quality assurance in emergency pediatrics. Pediatr Emerg Care 1987; 3(2):121–126.
12. Smeltzer CH, Curtis L. Analyzing patient time in the emergency department. QRB 1986;12(11): 380–382.
13. Wagner PL, Stapleton JA, Stein R, Wadina C. Care of the child with fever: A quality assurance study. QRB 1984;10(10):325–330.
14. Sollars GM. Emergency department quality assurance: Perspectives from the teaching hospital. Top Health Rec Manage 1984;5(2):47–53.
15. Stair TO. Quality Assurance. Emerg Med Clin North Am 1987;5(1):41–50.
16. Kuypers ME. A computerized log and integrated quality assessment program for the small emergency department. QRB 1989;15(5):144–150.
17. Cantrill SV. Use of computers in emergency department practice. Emerg Med Clin North Am 1987;5(1):155–165.
18. Yeh C. Effective patient relations. Emergency Organization and Management Series. Dallas:

American College of Emergency Physicians, 1986.

19. Comstock LM, Hooper EM, Goodwin JM, et al. Physician behaviors that correlate with patient satisfaction. J Med Law 1982;57:105–111.

20. Jones J, Clark W, Bradford J, Dougherty J. Efficacy of a telephone follow-up system in the emergency department. J Emerg Med 1988;6(3): 249–254.

21. Varian DW. Patient telephone callback [Correspondence]. Ann Emerg Med 1986;15(3):383.

22. Wilbert CC. Timeliness of care in the emergency department. QRB 1984;10(4):99-108.

23. Noland TM, Oberlaid F, Boldt D. Radiological services in a hospital emergency department— An evaluation of service delivery and radiograph interpretation. Aust Paediatr J 1984;20:109–112.

24. American College of Surgeons Committee on Trauma. Quality assurance and education in the emergency department. Bull Am Coll Surg 1980;65(2):34–35.

25. Hoyt DB, Shackford SR, Fridland PH, et al. Video recording trauma resuscitation: An effective teaching technique. J Trauma 1988;28(4):435–440.

26. Kresky B, Mangano L. Study of drug overdose patients in an emergency department. QRB 1980;6(7):15–18.

27. Moran MT, Hewitt ME, Michocki RJ, Antos M.

28. Keith KD, Bocka JJ, Kobernick MS, Krome RL, Ross MA. Emergency department revisits. Ann Emerg Med 1989;18(9):964–968.

29. Edlich RF, Widler BJ, Silloway KA, Nichter LS, Bryant CA. Quality assessment of tetanus prophylaxis in the wounded patient. Am Surg 1986;52(10):544–547.

30. Ciulla MR, Salisbury SR, McSherry E. Quality assurance in DNR (do not resuscitate) decisions— The role of chaplaincy: A case report and a 92 patient group study. J Health Care Chaplain 1988;2(1):57–80.

31. Schade J. An evaluation framework for code 99. QRB 1983;9(10):306–309.

32. Carlson R. Debunking the myths and horrors of quality assurance. Emerg Med News 1990 (April) 17, 35.

33. Flint LS, Hammett WH, Martens K. Quality assurance in the emergency department. Ann Emerg Med 1985;14(2):134–138.

34. Kresky B, Cohen A. Considerations for evaluation of patient care in emergency departments. QRB 1980;6(12):8–15.

35. Council on Medical Service. Quality care. JAMA 1986;256(8):1032–1034.

Housestaff management of pharyngitis in a university emergency department. Am J Emerg Med 1987;5(6):550–553.

17

Hospital Dentistry

James J. Crall, D.D.S., M.S., S.M., and Raymond P. White, Jr., D.D.S., Ph.D.

Dentistry is predominantly an ambulatory diagnostic and treatment service. Although the types of services can be similar, hospital dentistry differs from dental care provided outside the hospital setting in several ways that have important implications for quality assurance. For example, while general dentists retain a prominent role in most hospital dental departments, dental specialists provide a greater proportion of services within the hospital compared to community-based care. Those specialists most active in hospital dental departments include oral and maxillofacial surgeons, pediatric dentists, maxillofacial prosthodontists, and periodontists. Increased specialty care generally implies a higher percentage of limited-care patients (i.e., patients who seek care for specific, often acute conditions and who do not return for periodic diagnostic and preventive services as is the more general model for community-based dental care). The case mix of hospital dental departments also consists of a higher proportion of medically compromised patients and in some areas medically indigent patients, factors which must be considered in evaluating appropriateness and outcomes of care. Lastly, in addition to providing primary care services in outpatient clinics, hospital dental departments provide an expanded scope of services including treatment in emergency room and operating room settings.

Formal quality assessment and quality assurance activities are not pervasive in dentistry, in part because of the nature of the dental care delivery system. More than 95% of all dental services are provided in private practices, over 85% of which are operated as solo or two-person offices (1). With relatively few exceptions, private dental offices are not evaluated routinely by any regulatory or accrediting body. Moreover, since less than 3% of dental services are financed through public expenditures (2), dental care providers have had limited interaction with intermediaries responsible for overseeing care provided through public programs (e.g., Professional Review Organizations). Formal dental quality assurance programs generally are found in accredited group practices and institutional settings (3); however, those entities comprise only a small proportion of all dental care facilities. Another factor contributing to the relative underdevelopment of quality assurance programs within hospital dental departments has been the limited review that dental departments historically have received during hospital accreditation site visits. In light of the above, it is not surprising that quality assurance in dentistry is at a stage of development that is more on par with initiatives in other ambulatory care fields, and accordingly less developed than systems that are operational for inpatient care (4). However, as is true throughout most ambulatory care sectors, considerable attention has been directed toward the development of effective quality assurance programs of late.

A major focus of quality assurance programs in hospitals and throughout health care has been the development of indicators and standards of care. Although the formulation of indicators and standards is at a relatively early stage throughout much of dentistry, "important elements of quality care" have been defined for medical care (5) and should serve as a useful framework for further development of indicators and standards in dentistry. These important elements that reflect on processes of care, but at the same time have significant relationships to outcomes, emphasize that quality care: (*a*) is concerned with optimal improvement in the patient's level of physical and social functioning and comfort, in addition to physiological status; (*b*) emphasizes health promotion, disease prevention, and early detection of conditions; (*c*) is provided in a timely manner, without undue delay in initiation of care, inappropriate curtailment or discontinuity, or unnecessary prolongation of care; (*d*) seeks to achieve informed cooperation and participation by patients in the care process and decisions concerning care; (*e*) is based on accepted scientific principles and proficient use of appropriate technological and professional resources; (*f*) is provided with sensitivity to the stress and anxiety that illness and disability can generate and with concern for the patient's overall welfare; (*g*) makes efficient use of technology and other health system resources; and (*h*) is sufficiently documented in the patient's record to enable continuity of care and peer evaluation.

Quality assurance has become a major focus within hospital dental departments during the latter half of the 1980s for a variety of reasons. Many of the agents responsible for that change are external in origin, stemming from organizations and entities outside the hospital. However, in addition to satisfying increased accreditation and regulatory requirements, there is evidence that benefits can accrue to hospitals through the implementation of effec-

tive quality assurance programs. For example, hospitals and medical/dental staffs that have combined to self-insure against malpractice claims have seen the cost of their malpractice programs reduced following the implementation of comprehensive quality assurance/risk management programs (6). While many affected individuals continue to view quality assurance activities as burdensome and ineffective, proposed modifications in the approaches used to evaluate and improve quality (i.e., the JCAHO's Agenda for Change (7)) and advancements in data collection methods are expected to increase the effectiveness and acceptance of systems designed for those purposes. Consistent with the implementation of those new approaches is an increased emphasis on monitoring and improving outcomes of care.

MAJOR INFLUENCES ON HOSPITAL DENTISTRY QUALITY ASSURANCE

Major influences on hospital dental quality assurance have come from accrediting bodies such as the Joint Commission on Accreditation of Healthcare Organizations (JCAHO), from organizations representing professional constituencies (e.g., the American Dental Association (ADA), American Association of Oral and Maxillofacial Surgeons (AAOMS), and American Academy of Pediatric Dentistry (AAPD)), and more recently from regulatory agencies (e.g., the Health Care Financing Administration (HCFA) and Professional Review Organizations (PROs)).

JCAHO Standards

Over time, the JCAHO has stressed different dimensions of quality in its hospital accreditation process. In recent years, the predominant focus has shifted from structural aspects to processes and outcomes of care (7). The following examples of standards and requirements from the most recent JCAHO *Accreditation Manual for Hospitals* (*AMH*) (8) are cited to highlight evaluation criteria felt to be of particular relevance to hospital dental departments. References to specific sections are indicated within brackets ("[ ]"). Although extensive, the referenced sections should not be viewed as an exhaustive specification of all criteria relevant to the evaluation of hospital dental care.

The Quality Assurance (QA) chapter comprises only a small portion of the *AMH*. Through the QA chapter, the JCAHO has outlined significant organizational linkages involving the QA program and requirements related to the 10-step monitoring and evaluation process that is intended to assist in the identification of high priority quality-of-care issues. In essence, the QA chapter outlines a mechanism for conducting a quality assurance program, but the substance of what needs to be monitored is contained in various other chapters of the *AMH*.

In most hospitals, dentists with clinical privileges function together in a department of dentistry and are members of the medical staff. In hospitals participating in professional graduate education, care also may be provided by house staff under the supervision of members of the medical staff. Rules and regulations regarding the supervision and privileges of house staff must be delineated [MS.2.9]. The JCAHO Medical Staff (MS) and Quality Assurance (QA) Standards both mandate that each department have a quality assurance program in place that includes quality assessment and risk management functions [MS.6, QA.3]. The departmental chairperson is responsible for implementing a quality assurance program to monitor and evaluate the quality and appropriateness of care rendered by individual clinicians in each department. JCAHO standards specify that the chairman of the department is responsible for recommending clinical privileges for each member of the department [MS.3.9] and that continued membership on the medical staff requires a performance review at least biennially [MS.3.5]. This focus on activity of individual dentists represents a shift in emphasis by the JCAHO, but is consistent with approaches adopted by regulatory agencies (e.g., the HCFA and National Practitioner Data Bank (9)).

Diagnostic and treatment procedures provided in emergency room, operating room, and hospital clinic settings must be monitored and evaluated. Care provided in both emergency rooms and operating rooms, regardless of whether services are provided on an outpatient or inpatient basis, must conform to specific JCAHO quality standards that apply to all medical staff activity in those areas (e.g., Emergency Room Standards (ER)). In addition, because of the extensive scope of diagnostic and treatment services typically provided in the course of rendering comprehensive oral health care, standards from numerous other chapters of the JCAHO *AMH* apply to most activities of most hospital dental departments.

Because dental clinics in most institutions serve ambulatory patients, Standards for Hospital-Sponsored Ambulatory Care Services (HO) apply. For example, the scope of dental services planned and provided must be included in the overall hospital mission and plan [HO.1.1]. Dentists who provide care only in dental clinics must have appropriate clinical privileges [HO.1.4], and dentists and dental auxiliaries must participate in relevant continuing education programs, including cardiopulmonary resuscitation training [HO.2.1]. Policy manuals developed for dental clinics must reflect general hospital ambulatory care policies as well as specific policies related to the provision of dental care [HO.3]. Policies must be in place to ensure that patients have a voice in decisions affecting their care and understand their responsibility in planned treatment [HO.3.4]. Policies and procedures that address the provision of surgical and anesthesia services in dental clinics are mandated [HO.3.5] (dental procedures are considered surgical services). Appropriate visual and auditory privacy is required, a situation often difficult to obtain in many crowded hospital clinics [HO.4.2]. Adequate equipment, drugs, and supplies must be available for medical emergencies [HO.4.5]. Documentation of care in the medical record must meet specific guidelines [HO.5], which may require the recording of information not commonly documented in most dental records. Standards also specify that the quality and appropriateness of care rendered in the clinic must be included as part of the hospital's quality assurance program [HO.7], and that steps be taken to facilitate improvement in the quality of patient services [HO.6].

Virtually all dental clinics provide diagnostic radiology services, which commonly are not available through radiology departments. Standards for Diagnostic Radiology Services (DR) require that dentists have delineated clinical privileges for all radiology services they provide [DR.1.1]. The hospital's director of diagnostic radiology services must be a physician certified by the American Board of Radiology [DR.1.2]; however, responsibilities for providing consultations and establishing policies and procedures for radiology services, including the implementation of a quality assurance program, may be delegated to qualified personnel within dental departments [DR.1.3]. Policies and procedures must be in place to assure that radiology services provided in dental clinics are provided in an effective and safe manner [DR.2]. Guidelines for protecting personnel and patients from radiation must be adhered to [DR.2], a requirement that can be problematic in some dental clinics designed to support a wide range of care (e.g., diagnostic, restorative, surgical services) for numerous patients at the same time.

In many hospitals, dentists provide a variety of surgical and anesthesia services in outpatient clinics, and this care is expected to meet the same quality and appropriateness standards that apply to inpatient care [HO.1.5]. Responsibilities for recommending outpatient surgical privileges and for monitoring and evaluating surgical activity in outpatient clinics remain with the chairman of the department of dentistry [SA.1.3]. In nearly all hospitals, patients may be given oral, inhalation, or parenteral sedative or anesthesia agents in addition to local anesthesia for dental treatment; accordingly, Standards for Surgical and Anesthesia Services (SA) apply. The responsibility for anesthesia services provided in dental clinics lies with the director of anesthesia services [SA.1.4],

but may be delegated to qualified individuals (e.g., the chairman of the department of dentistry or his or her designate). In all cases, specific clinical privileges must be delineated for each individual who provides outpatient anesthesia services [SA.1.2]. Policies and procedures for preanesthesia evaluation, drug administration, monitoring of patients during treatment, and appropriate discharge procedures must be specified and adhered to [SA.1.5]. The quality of anesthesia services provided in dental clinics must conform to hospitalwide standards [SA.2] and must be monitored and evaluated as part of departmental quality assurance mechanisms [SA.4].

As noted earlier, the sections from the *AMH* cited above do not represent every instance in which standards apply to hospital dental departments. For example, no mention was made of specific Infection Control (IC) Standards even though infection control is obviously an extremely important aspect of delivering quality dental care in hospitals. Likewise, Standards for Plant Technology and Safety Management (PL) apply throughout the hospital. In fact, very few JCAHO standards for hospital accreditation specifically refer to dentists or dental care *per se*. However, as formal organizational components and members of the medical staff, dental departments and staff dentists are expected to comply with the numerous JCAHO standards that apply to the delivery of care in hospital settings.

Professional Organizations

The American Dental Association through its Office of Quality Assurance, the American Fund for Dental Health, and the W. K. Kellogg Foundation have sought to further the development and dissemination of quality assessment and quality assurance approaches for dentistry (e.g., computer applications, consumer involvement, oral health status measures, and quality assessment instruments) (10). Through its membership on the JCAHO board, the ADA also has endorsed the JCAHO's "Agenda for Change." The

AAOMS recently published criteria for treatment and standards of care in nine areas of oral and maxillofacial surgery that should serve as a useful guide for evaluation of hospital surgical practices (11). Similarly, the American Academy of Pediatric Dentistry has begun a process of developing and adopting guidelines that should aid in the evaluation of pediatric dental care (12).

Regulatory Agencies

Regulatory agencies (e.g., HCFA and associated PROs) acting on behalf of federal programs historically have had limited influence on dental care since very few inpatient dental services are covered under Medicare, traditionally the primary focus of HCFA/PRO review. However, HCFA, acting through the PROs, recently has expanded its activities using a method known as generic screening to review ambulatory care procedures provided for patients covered by the Medicare and Civilian Health and Medical Program of the Uniformed Services (CHAMPUS) programs (13). The program works as follows. A sample of patient charts is requested by the PRO, whereupon a review specialist (usually a nurse) compares the documentation provided for a particular episode of treatment with explicit screening criteria. Records that do not pass the initial screen then undergo implicit review by a physician who may request additional information from the hospital and involved dental staff. Experience thus far in hospital dental departments indicates that problems identified through this process commonly are related to deficiencies in documentation. For example, blood pressure may be recorded appropriately during a procedure via an automated monitor, but not documented adequately in the patient's records. Deficiencies such as these are easily remedied through attention to the quality screen criteria. In addition to actions that can impact directly on a provider's or institution's capacity to provide certain types of care, adverse review by the PRO can affect reimbursement for services provided to Medicare or CHAMPUS recipients.

SCOPE AND ORGANIZATION OF QA ACTIVITIES FOR HOSPITAL DENTAL CARE

The overall hospital quality assurance plan must include an ongoing review and evaluation of all clinical activities, regardless of whether they occur in operating rooms, ambulatory care areas, or emergency rooms. The plan also must include provisions for risk management [QA.1.4]. The responsibility for developing the quality assurance plan for all clinical activities lies with the medical staff [MS.1, QA.1]. Often the medical staff has a quality assurance committee or medical care evaluation committee that provides oversight for all departmental plans and communicates the findings and recommendations of quality assurance activities to the executive committee, which in turn is responsible for communicating information and recommendations directly to the governing body of the hospital [MS.3.5, QA.1.2].

The chairman of each department is responsible for all professional and administrative activities of staff members with clinical privileges in that department [MS.3.9, MS.6]. Accordingly, the chairman of the department of dentistry is responsible for the department having a written plan for monitoring and evaluating clinical activities. The plan should describe the departmental quality assurance program's objectives, organization, scope, and mechanisms for overseeing the effectiveness of monitoring, evaluation, and problem-solving activities [QA.1.3]. The departmental plan must be coordinated with those of other departments, reviewed annually, and revised as necessary. The department of dentistry must hold monthly meetings to consider findings that accrue from implementation of its quality assurance plan [MS.3.7]. Reports of findings from monitoring and evaluation activities and any actions taken to improve care should be communicated through appropriate established channels [QA.3, QA.4].

Organization of Quality Assurance Activities

The QA plan for the department of dentistry can be organized according to five major areas: (*a*) risk management and loss prevention, (*b*) provider credentialing and granting of privileges, (*c*) intradepartmental peer review, (*d*) administrative monitors, and (*e*) monitoring of dental laboratory services (14). Examples of specific activities within each of these areas are listed in Figure 17.1. Findings from monitoring activities related to these areas can serve as the focus for evaluations and discussions at mandatory monthly departmental quality assurance meetings and should form the basis for decisions regarding the need for further reviews, policy changes, and assessments of actions taken to remedy previously identified problems.

Risk Management and Loss Prevention

Major objectives of the risk management and loss prevention program include reductions in the frequency of preventable adverse occurrences that lead to liability claims, decreased risk for patient injury associated with clinical care, reductions in the number of claims filed, and cost control for claims that do emerge (6). Activities at the departmental level related to those objectives include the submission of incident reports and monitoring and evaluating adverse occurrences. In this context, an incident is any perceived or actual negative impact, outcome, or reaction related to patient care, or other medical or administrative occurrence that deviates from what might be considered the normal course of patient treatment. Incident reports usually involve a written description of an injury, adverse outcome, or mishap filed by members of the hospital staff. Occurrence screening was developed to overcome certain deficiencies inherent in incident reporting and record audit procedures and involves adapting generic screening criteria to provide for timely evaluation of the contribution of provider error to adverse events along with risk control (15).

Provider Credentialing and Granting of Privileges

JCAHO standards specify that the chairman of each department is responsible for recommending clinical privileges for each

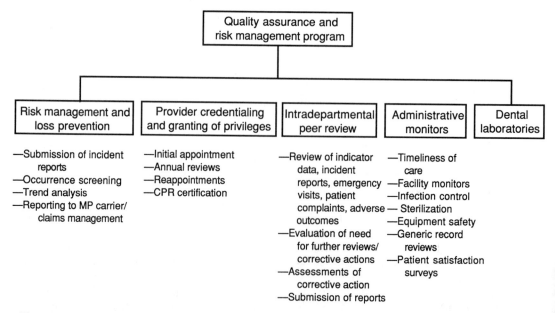

Figure 17.1. **Proposed scope and organization of a quality assurance and risk management program for departments of hospital dentistry.**

member of the medical staff and for continuing surveillance of the professional performance of all individuals who have delineated clinical privileges in the department. Initial appointments generally are based upon a review of provider credentials (e.g., training, experience, licensure, board certification status), past performance as a health care provider, and current competence. Once appointed, each staff member must be reviewed at least once every 2 years prior to reappointment. Relevant findings from quality assurance activities are to be used as part of the reappointment process. Although no specific expectations, other than cardiopulmonary resuscitation training, are included in JCAHO standards, each individual applying for reappointment is expected to have completed continuing education activity pertinent to their clinical privileges. As is the case for all clinical departments, the recommendation from the chairman of the department of dentistry is forwarded through the hospital committee process to the credentials committee for their review and subsequently to the executive committee and governing board of the hospital.

Intradepartmental Peer Review

Through its Agenda for Change (7), the JCAHO has begun to place increasing emphasis on the monitoring and evaluation of data that reflect on quality of care. The JCAHO has stated that by the early 1990s it will expect accredited organizations to go beyond simply demonstrating their potential to improve care (via descriptions of peer review and other quality assurance processes) and actually demonstrate quality improvement over time as evidenced by periodically collected data on clinical indicators (7). Thus, intradepartmental monitoring and evaluation of indicator data will constitute an increasingly important element of departmental quality assurance activities. The JCAHO has become quite specific with regards to what it expects in the way of monitoring and evaluation. The prescribed process outlined in the QA chapter of the most recent *AMH* (8) consists of 10 steps and can be summarized as follows: identification of

the most important aspects of care (i.e., procedures or treatments that are considered to be high risk, high volume, or problem-prone); use of measurable indicators to systematically monitor those aspects in an ongoing manner; evaluation of care when thresholds are reached in order to identify opportunities for improvement or problems related to appropriateness and quality of care; taking actions to improve care or solve problems and evaluation of the effectiveness of those actions.

In the view of the JCAHO, clinical indicators are objective measures of quantifiable aspects of patient care that can be used as guides to monitor and evaluate quality and appropriateness of care (16). Indicators do not serve as direct measures of quality, but rather act as screens or flags to direct attention to specific performance issues that should be the subject of more intense peer or administrative review (16). A potential use of clinical indicators is to signal significant variations in treatment outcomes among providers of similar services (i.e., variance analysis). Staff members whose patients are experiencing more problems than expected or whose practice patterns differ significantly from accepted norms (derived from analyses of aggregate data collected over time) might be considered for additional review. As noted previously, widely accepted indicators have not been developed for many aspects of dentistry. However, professional organizations representing prominent specialties involved in hospital dental care are actively involved in developing and evaluating clinical indicators as part of the process of creating guidelines, quality assurance criteria, and standards of care (11, 12). Individual hospital dental departments also have entered into the process of indicator development for general dentistry (17, 18). Although the use of data-based monitoring and evaluation processes is a relatively new concept within clinical departments, expectations are that this approach will become more commonplace and will be facilitated by advances in electronic records and clinical information systems.

Hospitals are usually willing to provide assistance in gathering data for departmental review provided that the process is not onerous. Working together, staff members within a department can identify and select indicators to monitor care. Selection of a limited number of valid and reliable indicators is more likely to increase acceptance and effectiveness. Extensive lists of indicators are difficult to monitor on a protracted ongoing basis. Establishment of indicator thresholds that trigger further evaluation currently is left to individual departments until large-scale field testing can be accomplished. Obviously certain occurrences (e.g., death during or after elective surgery) should be treated as sentinel events with each case being reviewed. Other indicators (e.g., postsurgical wound infection in trauma patients) might represent clinical circumstances that occur with some expected frequency, leading to the establishment of thresholds based on relative rates (e.g., greater than 10% in the case of postsurgical infection in trauma cases).

It bears reemphasizing that indicators are not meant to be used as the sole basis for judgments about clinical performance, but rather are designed to signal areas or individuals that warrant further review. It is anticipated that in many instances, review of indicator data will result in suggestions for improving clinical practice that will benefit all patients treated within the department or service. As an example, transfusion of homologous blood might be chosen as an indicator for orthognathic surgical care. Given the status of autologous blood programs, additional transfusion of homologous blood would be unusual. Review of indicator data could lead to changes in practice policies that would lessen the likelihood of homologous blood transfusion (e.g., collection of more than one unit of predonated autologous blood for certain patients). Other examples of potential uses of indicator data to improve overall performance include monitoring of radiograph retake rates to recognize types of patients for whom additional attention is warranted, alter practice patterns, or identify providers in need of additional training. Responses of this nature are consistent with the intent of JCAHO standards for quality assurance programs and recognized methods of quality improvement.

Within any given clinical discipline, indi-vidual practitioners often have different ideas about appropriate patient care practices. It is likely that the departmental chairperson's evaluation tasks will be made easier, but not eliminated, by the acceptance of guidelines, criteria, and standards of care. Decisions regarding acceptable levels of clinical performance will continue to be based on peer review and, to some extent, personal judgment. However, indicator data should provide objective information over time with respect to practices and providers.

Administrative Monitors

Administrative monitors generally consist of reports based on data routinely collected by nondepartmental personnel from various support services. Examples include visit data, which can be used to monitor timeliness of care, and results of periodic assessments of compliance with infection control, radiation hygiene, and safety programs. Results of record reviews conducted by hospital administrative personnel and hospitalwide patient satisfaction surveys represent additional sources of information that can be used to monitor various aspects of care.

Monitoring of Dental Laboratory Services

Dental laboratories constitute another support area whose services are more directly linked to the technical quality of many dental treatments. Quality assurance regarding dental laboratory services generally takes the form of quality control monitoring (e.g., inspection of fabricated restorations and prostheses at various steps prior to delivery to patients). Lately, an additional focus of considerable attention concerns infection control practices during the transfer of potentially infective materials between patients and laboratory personnel (e.g., impression materials that have been in contact with blood and/or saliva).

Additional Quality Assurance Responsibility

In addition to monitoring patient care within the dental department, the chairperson is responsible for reviewing hospitalwide quality assurance reports for items that might impact the department. For example, the activity of the pharmacy and therapeutics committee should be monitored for issues that might impact on care provided within the dental department (e.g., recommendations for antibiotic usage). The department of dentistry is affected by activity of the medical records committee. The transfusion review committee monitors blood product usage. Hospital risk management activity that follows an incident report also should be incorporated into the chairman's review.

Conversely, the executive committee acts on behalf of the medical staff to develop institutional policy. In most instances, the chairman of the department of dentistry serves on the executive committee and in this role has the opportunity to influence actions that will positively impact care across the institution as well as in the dental department.

QUALITY ASSURANCE ACTIVITIES WITHIN HOSPITAL DENTAL DEPARTMENTS

Hospital dental departments vary considerably in terms of organization, numbers of staff, and scope of services provided. In cases where the dental staff is large and the department of dentistry divided into divisions, the chairman of the department may seek help from division chiefs in accomplishing quality assurance tasks. This delegation can be particularly helpful because in many instances the chairman may be trained in one dental specialty, whereas the clinicians being evaluated provide a different type of specialty care or practice as general dentists. The following sections describe quality assurance activities according to major categories of services commonly provided in hospital dental departments.

Oral and Maxillofacial Surgery

Most oral and maxillofacial surgeons are eligible by training to take the certifying examination offered by the American Board of Oral and Maxillofacial Surgeons. Most surgeons satisfactorily complete the examination and become board-certified within a few years after finishing their training programs. Board certification is viewed as a criterion for evaluating competency by the JCAHO and most hospitals; however, individuals applying for medical staff membership and delineated clinical privileges also must be evaluated according to additional criteria (e.g., relevant training, clinical experience, and current competency). Some hospitals require a separate review process for surgeons who desire privileges to perform certain procedures involving higher risk or newer technologies (e.g., laser surgery). As the use of those technologies becomes more commonplace, privileges to perform the same procedures may be granted to board-certified applicants without special review based upon the level of training and competency expected of individuals who have passed the board examination.

Oral and maxillofacial surgery treatments with the greatest potential to produce serious adverse consequences if performed inappropriately generally involve procedures carried out in the operating room (e.g., dentoalveolar surgery, orthognathic surgery, surgery involving the temporomandibular joint, treatment of traumatic injuries, reconstructive surgery, and reconstructive implantology). The JCAHO-mandated surgical case review is one mechanism for monitoring and evaluating those relatively high risk services. In addition, JCAHO standards mandate that each clinical department have written indications for surgical procedures and that the indications for surgery for each surgical case be discussed, preferably in advance of the procedure. Discussing cases in advance of surgery remains a logistical problem in most institutions. Anesthesia services constitute another category of relatively high risk services performed by oral and maxillofacial surgeons in outpatient areas.

A comprehensive listing of indicators for treatment and outcome indicators for the above areas is beyond the scope of this chapter; however, the AAOMS has developed an extensive document detailing parameters for nine designated areas that cover the spectrum of care provided by oral and maxillofacial surgeons (11). The AAOMS parameters consist of sections detailing indications for care, therapeutic goals, factors affecting risk, standards of care, and indicators of desirable and undesirable outcomes. Examples of indicators of adverse outcomes for surgical procedures include the following: death or respiratory and/or cardiac arrest during hospitalization; iatrogenic injury during surgery; unplanned exploratory procedures associated with surgery; unplanned admission to intensive care, temperature greater than 101° at 72 hours postsurgery or failure to ambulate within 48 hours following elective surgery; reintubation, tracheostomy, or unplanned intubation for longer than 12 hours following surgery; unplanned transfusions during or following surgery and repeat surgery or readmission within prescribed times following surgery.

With respect to high volume procedures, dentoalveolar surgery is generally the most common oral and maxillofacial surgical procedure conducted in outpatient areas. Indicators identifying postsurgical problems include return to the emergency room for bleeding and additional treatment for wound infection. While all postsurgical bleeding problems might be reviewed, the threshold for review of wound infections following removal of infected teeth might be based on a preselected rate founded on prior experience or reports in the literature (e.g., review of all cases if infection rate is greater than 10%). Indicators appropriate for other conditions commonly treated by oral and maxillofacial surgeons include nonunion of jaw fracture (obvious when patients return for a second corrective surgery), wound dehiscence following preprosthetic or reconstructive surgery, blood transfusion in patients having temporomandibular joint surgery, discrepancy between presurgical and postsurgical diagnosis for pathology cases and altered sensory perception following dentoalveolar surgery.

Outpatient oral surgery procedures often involve conscious sedation, deep sedation, or general anesthesia. Specific JCAHO standards exist regarding the lev-

els of evaluation and monitoring required for sedated or anesthetized patients. Indicators requiring further evaluation might include patients identified as having periods of apnea when only conscious sedation was intended and unanticipated endotracheal intubation with the use of general anesthesia. The task of reviewing anesthetic records using indicators to identify cases for further evaluation is required by JCAHO standards. Indicators that target the length of time before discharge are becoming more commonplace. Compliance with specific criteria for discharge following anesthesia (e.g., physiological status, level of functioning, and identification of the person responsible for care following discharge) has received additional attention in recent JCAHO standards.

Oral and maxillofacial surgery staff activities for emergency patients provided in clinics or the emergency rooms also must be monitored and reviewed. Both diagnostic and surgical procedures must be included. Review of diagnostic radiology processes applies to all dental staff members; however, oral and maxillofacial surgeons are expected to see that diagnostic radiology services are adequate for trauma patients receiving oral and maxillofacial surgical care.

Pediatric Dentistry

The scope of pediatric dentistry encompasses a variety of preventive, diagnostic, surgical, and rehabilitative treatment approaches that share a common basis with other areas of dentistry, but are modified based on consideration of the mental, psychological, and physical development and oral health care needs of children. In addition, pediatric dentists traditionally have contributed significantly to providing preventive and rehabilitative dental services for individuals with special needs (e.g., developmental disabilities), regardless of age. Pediatric dentists frequently provide services in hospital outpatient clinics, operating rooms, and emergency rooms.

Pediatric dentists can become board-eligible by successfully completing an accredited program of training and making application to the American Board of Pediatric Dentistry. Once eligible, candidates have 8 years in which to complete a certifying examination process that consists of four sections: written examination, oral examination, case documentation, and site-visit/clinical simulation. Successful completion usually requires a minimum of 5 years. Approximately 25% of the 3000 members of the AAPD were board certified as of 1989 (19). The JCAHO specifies that board certification is one criteria to be considered in evaluating applicants to hospital medical staffs. Departmental chairpersons also may choose to use board status as a guide in delineating clinical privileges.

Aspects of pediatric dental care that might be considered to be relatively high risk (and in some hospitals, high volume) generally involve oral rehabilitative treatments provided in the operating room and services rendered on an outpatient basis in conjunction with the administration of conscious or deep sedation. Within the hospital, JCAHO standards for surgical case review and anesthesia services obviously apply. In addition, the AAPD has developed guidelines for the elective use of sedation and general anesthesia in pediatric dental patients that specify goals of treatment and responsibilities for case selection, informed consent, documentation, monitoring, and recovery (20). More recently, the AAPD has adopted quality assurance criteria for care provided under sedation and general anesthesia (20) (as well as for a broad spectrum of pediatric dental services (12)), which contain indications for treatment and outcome indicators. Previously cited surgery and anesthesia indicators that might be selected to signal further review include patients experiencing apnea when only conscious sedation was intended, unanticipated intubation, prolonged recovery and/or unanticipated admission following sedation or general anesthesia provided on a same-day surgery basis. Treatment of patients who have significant medical complications constitutes another potential high risk area in pediatric dentistry. Compliance with requirements for documentation of medical alerts and evidence of compliance with recommended prophylactic antibiotic coverage when indicated are examples of criteria that can be applied for the evaluation of care provided to medically compromised patients. Pediatric dentists also frequently treat trauma patients; however, major trauma cases usually are referred to or treated in conjunction with oral and maxillofacial surgeons.

High volume pediatric dental services generally consist of diagnostic, preventive, and restorative procedures performed on an outpatient basis, along with pulpal therapy and management of developing occlusions. Candidates for relevant indicators include rates of radiograph retakes, compliance with recommended guidelines for radiograph usage, replacement rates for restoration, and need for retreatment or extraction following pulp therapy. Pediatric dentists frequently function as primary care providers for some patients and as referral-based specialists for others. Continuity of care is an obvious criterion for evaluating dental care provided for pediatric patients, regardless of whether the pediatric dentist serves as a primary care provider or provides care on a referral basis.

General Dentistry

General dentists within the hospital dental department typically provide a broad scope of diagnostic, rehabilitative, and surgical services. What distinguishes general dentistry in the hospital from general dental care provided outside the hospital is not so much the nature of the services, but rather the characteristics of the patients treated in hospital settings. Patients treated in hospital dental clinics often have significant associated medical conditions or developmental disabilities (21). Accordingly, generalists in hospital dental departments can actually receive referrals from community-based dentists as well as from physicians. Studies have shown that patients seeking hospital-sponsored ambulatory dental services are more likely to come from underserved areas (21) and are more likely to seek care on an emergent or episodic basis (22). Increasingly, general dentists who provide care in hospital settings have acquired formal postgraduate training via general practice residencies. Although hospital-based general dentists are not eligible for board certification, additional credentialing for generalists is provided by various organizations including the Academy of General Dentistry.

In addition to treatment of medically compromised patients, services considered to be relatively high risk for general dentists include procedures performed while patients are under sedation or general anesthesia and treatment of trauma patients admitted through the emergency room. JCAHO standards and indicators outlined above apply. Additional evaluation criteria and indicators have been developed specifically for hospital-based general dentistry quality assurance programs (17, 18, 23). Most programs currently rely extensively on some form of record audit procedure. Additional review criteria for structure and process-related aspects of general dental practice, regardless of the type of clinical setting, have been proposed as *Guidelines for Criteria and Standards of Acceptable Quality General Dental Practice* (24).

THE FUTURE OF QUALITY ASSURANCE IN HOSPITAL DENTAL DEPARTMENTS

The leadership of professional organizations, regulatory agencies, the hospital industry, third-party payers, and patient advocacy groups anticipate that quality assurance will become an accepted management tool and an essential part of health care delivery. The challenge for developing effective programs for evaluating and improving the quality of care provided in hospitals, as well as in other health care settings, is to create systems and approaches that serve all parties who have a stake in the delivery of care. To the extent that those objectives can be accomplished, quality assurance programs will contribute to better care being provided to patients.

Through its Agenda for Change, the JCAHO will continue its quest to improve the process of quality assurance. The development of clinical indicators is expected to become increasingly pervasive across clinical disciplines and institutions. Evaluations of centrally collected aggregate data on indicators of treatment processes and outcomes from numerous institutions will allow hospitals and clinicians to adopt a broader, more objective view of patient care. A key factor related to the continued success of programs designed to assure and improve quality is the balance between the burden or costs imposed by the programs' operations and the benefits that accrue (or are perceived to accrue) to various parties. In that regard, more efficient methods for collecting, storing, and transmitting information electronically will undoubtedly become increasingly important (25).

Several dental specialty groups, notably those traditionally prominent in providing hospital-based care, have begun the process of developing, testing, and revising practice guidelines, quality assurance criteria, and standards of care. On a broader front, the American Dental Association has embarked on a process of developing practice parameters that will aid in the definition of appropriateness for a wide range of dental services (26). Beyond that, guidelines for predoctoral and advanced dental education programs and standards for accreditation are being modified to stimulate the development of comprehensive quality assurance programs within institutions that provide dental training and to prepare future professionals to carry out quality assurance activities (27). Future accreditation guidelines for all advanced education programs are expected to include specific quality assurance activities, the format of which will undoubtedly follow the process established by the respective specialty groups and the JCAHO.

References

1. ADA Bureau of Economic and Behavioral Research. The 1988 survey of dental practice. Chicago: American Dental Association, 1988.
2. Health Insurance Association of America. Source book of health insurance data, 1989. Washington, D.C.: Health Insurance Association of America, 1989:51.

3. Burakoff RP, Demby NA. Quality assurance: Historical perspective and critical issues. Dent Clin North Am 1985;29:427–436.
4. Palmer RH. The challenges and prospects for quality assessment and assurance in ambulatory care. Inquiry 1988;25:119–131.
5. American Medical Association Council on Medical Service. Quality of care. JAMA 1986;256:1032–1034.
6. Morlock L, Lindgren OH, Mills DH. Malpractice, clinical risk management and quality assessment. In: Goldfield N, Nash DB, eds. Providing quality care: The challenge to clinicians. Philadelphia: American College of Physicians, 1989:225–257.
7. O'Leary DS. The Joint Commission's Agenda for Change. Chicago: Joint Commission for Accreditation of Healthcare Organizations 1987:1–10.
8. Joint Commission on Accreditation of Healthcare Organizations. 1991 Accreditation manual for hospitals. Chicago: Joint Commission on Accreditation of Healthcare Organizations, 1990.
9. Federal Register, October 17, 1989;54:42722–42734.
10. Klyop J. The dental professions's commitment to quality assurance. Dent Clin North Am 1985;29:523–530.
11. American Association of Oral and Maxillofacial Surgeons. 1991 Parameters of care for oral and maxillofacial surgery: A guide for practice, monitoring and evaluation (AAOMS parameters-91). Chicago: American Association of Oral and Maxillofacial Surgeons, 1991.
12. AAPD Policy and Procedures Committee. Guidelines and quality assurance criteria for pediatric dentistry. Chicago: American Academy of Pediatric Dentistry, 1991.
13. Institute of Medicine Division of Health Care Services. Medicare: A strategy for quality assurance, Vol. I. Lohr KN, ed. Washington, D.C.: National Academy Press, 1990:281–283.
14. M Cleveland, Director of Patient Services, School of Dentistry, University of North Carolina at Chapel Hill, NC, personal communication.
15. Mills DH. California Medical Association and California Hospital Association. Report on the medical insurance feasibility study. San Francisco: Sutter Publications, 1977.
16. Joint Commission on Accreditation of Healthcare

Organizations. Characteristics of clinical indicators. QRB 1989;15:330–339.
17. Presentation by Dr. Thomas Griffin at 131st Annual Session of the American Dental Association, Boston, October 14, 1990.
18. The Bowman Gray School of Medicine Department of Dentistry. Quality assurance plan for the Dental Service of North Carolina Baptist Hospital. Winston-Salem, NC: Wake Forest University, 1990.
19. American Board of Pediatric Dentistry. American Board of Pediatric Dentistry Report—1990. In: 1989–90 AAPD annual reports. Chicago: American Academy of Pediatric Dentistry, 1990:323
20. American Academy of Pediatric Dentistry. Guidelines for elective use of conscious sedation, deep sedation, and general anesthesia in pediatric patients. In: AAPD oral health policies: 1990–91. Chicago: American Academy of Pediatric Dentistry, 1990:108–111.
21. Koch AL, Schoen MH, Marcus M. The hospital-sponsored ambulatory dental services program. Part I: An evaluation of patient access. Spec Care Dentistry 1987;7:246–252.
22. Schoen MH, Marcus M, Koch AL. The hospital-sponsored ambulatory dental services program. Part II: An evaluation of dental services. Spec Care Dentistry 1988;8:6–12.
23. Bailit HL, Gotowka T, eds. Guidelines for the development of a quality assurance audit system for hospital dental programs. Chicago: American Dental Association, 1983.
24. Schoen MH, Freed J, Gershen JA, Marcus M. Guidelines for criteria and standards of acceptable quality general dental practice (special emphasis on group practice). J Dent Educ 1989;53(11):662–669.
25. Barnett GO, Winickoff RN. Quality assurance and computer-based patient records. Am J Public Health 1990;80:257–258.
26. American Dental Association News. House gives parameters a green light. Chicago: American Dental Association, November 5, 1990:6, 16.
27. ADA Commission on Dental Accreditation. Accreditation standards for dental education programs. Chicago: American Dental Association, 1988.

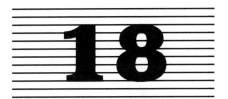

Obstetrics and Gynecology

Willie A. Andersen, M.D.

"That's the way I always do it and it seems to work out okay."
Anonymous

Although this general statement of quality assurance has been prevalent, the Joint Commission on Accreditation of Health Care Organizations (JCAHO) requires far more in its "Agenda for Change." The JCAHO program emphasizes the assessment of actual patient outcomes rather than the capacity of each health care facility to deliver good quality of care (1). While the quality assurance buzz phrase bounces around with many interpretations and definitions, in this chapter something that is very personal to each practicing gynecologist will be discussed. Quality assurance as a process is an opportunity to maximize the care of each patient we encounter, and it is a way to improve the care of our patients continuously over time. It is a system utilizing appropriate standards that allows physicians in gynecology to monitor the care of each patient and to assure ourselves that it is the best care that we can deliver. Quality assurance also is a system that provides appropriate intervention measures to correct significant deviations from standards when necessary (2).

It is important to emphasize that quality assurance is *not* utilization control—a system that assures that there is a demonstrated need for the use of care and services. Nor is quality assurance a utilization review—the evaluation of services provided in relation to their necessity and appropri-

ateness. True quality assurance is also *not* risk management—a system to minimize risk of financial lost to health care providers or to minimize risk to patient's safety (2).

Although quality assurance is *not* a process for credentialing, reappointment, privileging, or recertification of practitioners, it can be interfaced for such purposes. Participation in quality assurance programs strongly reinforces the physicians' commitment to lifelong learning and is therefore an objective criteria for such things as privileging or credentialing (2).

In obstetrics and gynecology, scientific discoveries and technologic innovations have led the public, in many instances, to expect more of the practitioner than can be delivered (3). There is a significant dollar cost to application of these "miraculous" developments and those who are bearing the brunt of financing health care, are now asking about the quality of care they are receiving for their health care dollars (3). These two additional reasons demand that the gynecologist be supremely interested in developing standards and participating in quality assurance programs.

In the implementation of any effective quality assurance program there are a number of barriers to overcome. These include the following: (*a*) the natural reluctance of physicians to having one's professional performance exposed and reviewed, and (*b*) the lack of hospital administrative support (3). Many physicians feel that they, through participation in educational programs, interdepartmental conferences, and self-education, provide their own quality assessment. Paramedical support to the effectively run quality assurance programs costs dollars that must come from existing tight hospital administrative budgets. However, in the context of a commitment to excellence in patient care, every practicing gynecologist must decide that quality assurance is an individual, moral obligation. The "conscience of the specialty" does not allow us to carry on when "hearing, seeing and doing nothing" (3).

HISTORICAL REVIEW

Jason Purcell would claim that Sir James Young Simpson, the Scot obstetrician, "fathered" quality assurance because of his mid-19th century practice of systematically recording and analyzing surgical results in hospitals (2). In 1913, the American College of Surgeons was formed and set standards relevant to medical staff, patient records, and diagnostic and therapeutic equipment. JCAHO assumed the responsibility for hospital quality of care in 1951 and in 1953 initiated specific kinds of medical staff monitoring such as transfusion, pharmacy and therapeutics, and surgical care reviews (2). The American College of Obstetricians and Gynecologists began the development of its own quality assurance interest with the 1972 publication, *Indices for Use in Peer Review of Obstetrics/Gynecologic Practice* followed by *Indices for Outcome Audits* in 1977. A more workable and comprehensive monograph followed in 1981—*Quality Assurance in Obstetrics and Gynecology*, which was followed by *Standards for Obstetric/Gynecologic Services*, initiated in 1989 (1).

In 1986, the American College of Obstetrics and Gynecology (ACOG) formed from the Task Force on Quality Assurance, which first determined what issues should be addressed in an ACOG quality assurance program. This gave rise to *Quality Assurance in Obstetrics and Gynecology*, which, in essence, defines quality assurance in gynecology. Under the leadership of Dr. Irving Meeker the task force developed "clinical indicators" and "criteria sets," which represent the standard base levels of acceptable care, below which no gynecologist or hospital should fall. The manual is specifically designed to apply to all hospital departments of obstetrics and gynecology, no matter what the size, location, or level of service. It is notable that many procedures and diagnoses were not included either because the technology was still evolving or because professional judgment regarding efficacy was too diverse (1). Internal reviews by pertinent ACOG committees were used to assure that the task force recommendations were consistent with other college advisories. The task force report was meant only to be a beginning, and it was stressed that ongoing review and update of recommendations and positions were an absolute necessity.

THE AMERICAN COLLEGE OF OBSTETRICS AND GYNECOLOGY PROGRAM

Quality Assurance in Obstetrics and Gynecology presents in great detail the ACOG's effort and methodology (1). At its heart, to identify problem areas is a generic screening process that is organized in such a way that nonphysician personnel can accomplish the majority of the work. Nonphysician participation is critical if any program like this is to be truly functional.

The ACOG program is based on evaluating clinical care on the basis of clinical indicators and clinical criteria sets. The areas chosen by the ACOG were to represent events that cover a broad range of activities. Although not all-inclusive, it was the assumption that, if selected activities had been carried out well, similar activities were likely to be handled appropriately as well. The chosen indicators and criteria could be *and* were made to be altered specifically by any given institution as it seemed appropriate.

Clinical Indicators

The Task Force on Quality Assurance developed a series of clinical indicators (Table 18.1). These are to be used by ab-

Table 18.1.
Gynecologic Clinical Indicators[a]

1. Unplanned readmission within 14 days
2. Admission after a return visit to the emergency room for the same problem
3. Cardiopulmonary arrest
4. Occurrence of an infection not present on admission
5. Unplanned admission to special (intensive) care unit
6. Unplanned return to operating room for surgery during the same admission
7. Ambulatory surgery patient admitted or retained for complication of surgery or anesthesia
8. Gynecologic surgery, except radical hysterectomy or exenteration, using 2 or more units of blood or postoperative hematocrit of less than 24 vol% or hemoglobin of less than 8 g
9. Unplanned removal, injury, or repair of organ during operative procedure
10. Initiation of antibiotics more than 24 hours after surgery
11. Discrepancy between preoperative diagnosis and postoperative tissue report
12. Removal of uterus weighing less than 280 g for leiomyomata
13. Removal of simple cyst or corpus luteum of ovary
14. Hysterectomy performed on woman younger than 30 except for malignancy
15. Gynecologic death

[a]From Quality assurance in obstetrics and gynecology. Washington, D.C.: The American College of Obstetrics and Gynecology, 1989. Reprinted by permission.

stractors, who would review all gynecologic discharges and flag patients' records when they contained material indicating the need for further physician review or evaluation. The clinical indicators were designated to describe a threshold of provider activity below which most physicians would consider the care to be substandard (1). All records flagged by the paramedical screeners would then be reviewed by the local quality assurance panel, which would include physicians, before the care provided is judged to be substandard. Education should be the initial technique to deal with most deviations from standard care, and this could be on an individual physician basis or on a group basis, for instance, specific topics to be addressed during educational programs when a problem

involves several departmental staff members. The ACOG has developed sample data collection forms for use in review of all gynecologic discharges (Table 18.2 and Figure 18.1).

The review of clinical indicators can subsequently be used to develop trending for either an individual or a department. This aspect of quality assurance does become complicated by medicolegal nuances. However, for quality assurance to have any impact, deviation from normal trends by a particular physician *must* be investigated and discussed, and the deviation rectified.

Clinical Criteria Sets

Criteria sets represent the second part of the quality assurance system of the American College of Obstetricians and Gynecologists. To measure or evaluate any activity, it is necessary to compare it to some acceptable standard (1). Again, while the ACOG provides guidelines for the gynecologic procedures, it has chosen to indicate that considerable local variation is possible. The criteria sets, again, describe a threshold of provider activity below which most physicians would agree was substandard care. Criteria sets were developed in consultation with appropriate ACOG committees and commissions, and all relevant ACOG publications have been used in this development. Criteria sets, of course, will continue to evolve.

Criteria sets allow evaluation of the appropriateness of surgery performed by practitioners within any given department. Clinical criteria sets can be used to review the entire department's experience with a given procedure on an intermittent basis, for example, to review on a yearly basis the appropriateness of hysterectomy, etc. Use of the criteria sets could be ongoing or on-line, but the specific application of the criteria sets is made within the context of local institutional abilities. The nine criteria sets developed are found in the Appendix.

The administrative organization of quality assurance in gynecology should be centered on the Department of Obstetrics and Gynecology in each local institution.

Table 18.2.
Sample Data Collection Form: Gynecologic Clinical Indicators[a]

Patient _____ Hosp. # _____ Disch Date _____

Date of Surgery _____ MD Code # _____

Adm Hct _____ Hb _____ Lowest Hct _____ Hb _____

1. Unplanned readmission within 14 days	Y	N
2. Admission after a return visit to the emergency room for the same problem	Y	N
3. Cardiopulmonary arrest	Y	N
4. Occurrence of an infection not present on admission	Y	N
5. Unplanned admission to special (intensive) care unit	Y	N
6. Unplanned return to operating room for surgery during the same admission	Y	N
7. Ambulatory surgery patient admitted or retained for complication of surgery or anesthesia	Y	N
8. Gynecologic surgery, except radical hysterectomy or exenteration, using two or more units of blood or postoperative hematocrit of less than 24 vol% or hemoglobin of less than 8 g	Y	N
9. Unplanned removal, injury, or repair of organ during operative procedure	Y	N
10. Initiation of antibiotics more than 24 hours after surgery	Y	N
11. Discrepancy between preoperative diagnosis and postoperative tissue report	Y	N
12. Removal of uterus weighing less than 280 g for leiomyomata	Y	N
13. Removal of simple cyst or corpus luteum of ovary	Y	N
14. Hysterectomy performed on woman younger than 30 except for malignancy	Y	N
15. Gynecologic death	Y	N

[a]From Quality assurance in obstetrics and gynecology. Washington, D.C.: The American College of Obstetrics and Gynecology, 1989. Reprinted by permission.

The appropriate size and scope of each committee should depend on the department itself. There will need to be a quality assurance committee chairman—usually the department chairman—as well as a representative from hospital administration and nursing. The quality assurance committee in gynecology should meet regularly, although, again, the exact timing is proscribed by institutional size. The gynecologic quality assurance groups also must regularly and formally interact with other hospital committees including: (a) the tissue committee, (b) the pharmacy committee, (c) infectious control, and (d) credentialing. Again, whereas these interactions may be as often as monthly or as infrequently as semiannually, the report guidelines must be defined from the onset.

All those involved in quality assurance activities are protected under the Health Care Quality Improvement Act of 1986. All records used in quality assurance activities should enjoy absolute confidentiality. This confidentiality must extend to the patients involved in review as well as to the physicians providing care. The ACOG recommends that material summarized by abstractors and prepared for quality assurance committee review be "coded" with individual practitioners' quality assurance numbers instead of names. If necessary, such codes can be broken by the department heads.

ASSESSMENT OF ACOG GUIDELINES

Although the ACOG Task Force invested considerable time and effort into developing both the gynecologic clinical indicators as well as the criteria sets, are the specific recommendations valid and logical for general application? There are limited data to answer this question. One way to assess the guidelines is to see if, indeed, they do represent frequently occurring events, events that have significant effect on patient health, or events that can be of a preventative or health maintenance nature.

In the United States, the most common hospital discharge diagnoses (1988) in women of reproductive age were: (a) pregnancy with delivery, (b) pregnancy with an abortive outcome, and (c) infections or inflammations of the female pelvic organs.

Provide numbers of procedures done within this hospital during the most recently completed quarter and year.

Procedure*	Quarter 1 2 3 4 (Circle one)	Year 19____
Gynecologic mortalities		
Inpatient surgical procedures		
Outpatient surgical procedures		
D&Cs, not related to pregnancy (69.09) Inpatient		
Ambulatory		
Conizations (67.2)		
Laparoscopies Sterilization (66.2)		
Other (54.21)		
Laser procedures Lower genital tract		
Other		
Hysterectomies Abdominal (68.4)		
Vaginal (68.5)		
Exploratory laparotomies (54.11)		
Operations for urinary stress incontinence Abdominal (59.4–59.6)		
Vaginal (59.3, 59.7 all)		

*Numbers in parentheses are ICD-9-CM codes, which may be applicable for some, but not all, procedures.

Figure 18.1 Sample Department Gynecologic Data Summary. (From Quality assurance in obstetrics and gynecology. Washington, D.C.: The American College of Obstetrics and Gynecology, 1989. Reprinted by permission.)

The sixth most common discharge diagnosis was disorders of menstruation. Likewise, in the reproductive age groups, the most common nonobstetrical operation was hysterectomy with 655,000 cases in 1988. This was followed by salpingo-oophorectomy, either unilateral or bilateral (552,000), and then by operations for tubal occlusion (406,000) and diagnostic dilation and curettage (D&C) (143,000) (4).

Based on this pattern of indications for both admission and operative procedure, it would seem that both clinical indicators and gynecologic criteria sets reflect the pattern of gynecologic problems and procedures generally encountered. This is further amplified if one looks at the age group of 45–64 years in women where hysterectomy is the most common operation followed by salpingo-oophorectomy, either bilateral or unilateral (4). The criteria sets, however, could emphasize further assessment guidelines for patients with venereally acquired inflammatory disease and endometriosis.

Cancer in women represents the second leading cause of death overall and the most common cause of death in women age 45–64 (4). Cancer prevention/early detection should be a major concern for all gynecologists. The criteria sets address the issue of cervical and endometrial cancer— the two gynecologic malignancies that have the best chance for screening and detection/treatment at an early stage. The ACOG guidelines, however, do not address the issue of either breast cancer screening or colon/rectal cancer screening. While it is primarily an outpatient concern, all patients admitted to the gynecology service should have plans made for breast and colorectal screening as outlined by the American Cancer Society. Stool guaiac would seen almost mandatory for any woman in the postmenopausal age group who is to undergo pelvic surgery.

Finally, the ACOG guidelines do not address the issue of the most common cause of death in females—atherosclerotic cardiovascular diseases. Although this is, again, primarily an outpatient evaluation/treatment issue, cholesterol assessment for inpatients of the appropriate age group would seem a most cost-efficient consideration.

It is difficult to document, but the application of quality assurance processes compatible with the ACOG guidelines can make a difference. Gambone et al. (5) showed a decrease in the overall frequency of hysterectomy and an increase in the histologic verification rate based on preoperative diagnoses in their study of 657 hysterectomies in a large teaching hospital. Although long-term outcomes in patients who have had a hysterectomy need to be compared with the outcomes of alternative forms of therapy, both surgical and nonsurgical, with respect to efficacy, safety, and cost, the consistent application of a quality assurance process appears to facilitate greatly the comparison of effectiveness and appropriateness of various therapies for each indication (5).

Although problems exist with any arbitrary set of standards, if the quality assurance process is to proceed, some initial decisions must be made. The guidelines of the ACOG *must* be adopted and interpreted at a local level and *must* be flexible enough to undergo continuous change. It is the communication and introspection facilitated by the program that allows adaptation and improvements that will keep up with the advances in science and technology.

SUMMARY

The opportunity to apply quality assurance concepts in the care of gynecologic patients is an opportunity to improve health care delivery to women. Quality assurance measures have implications that spill over into peer review, utilization review, privileging, and credentialing, but all clinicians must *first* concentrate on advantages to improve patient care. Although at its heart is education, quality assurance must possess the power of corrective action.

Quality assurance is not an option; it is a moral imperative, and it is required by the JCAHO. The American College of Obstetricians and Gynecologists has provided a very flexible outline for the application of a reasonable quality assurance program that can be adapted to any clinical practice and institutional character (1). Its conceptual design is anchored by a flexible list of clinical indicators, easily identified by paramedical personnel, and can be tracked in an "on-line" fashion from hospital discharges. In addition to these indicators, there are clinical criteria sets that allow, again in a most flexible manner, the establishment of standards of decision making and care, which can then be applied to clinical gynecologic practice. The standards are not based on the most sophisticated technology or concepts, which would not be expected to be present at all institutions.

The application process is straightforward.

1. *Meet and communicate.*   Through the local gynecologic department, set up meetings with the local hospital admin-

istration to establish a quality assurance committee in gynecology. The first task is to design and adopt the local standards that are unanimously agreed upon by the gynecologic practitioners. Next, select local guidelines for the frequency and type of screening, and then detail, in advance, the frequency of local quality assurance meetings.

2. *Demand help.* The local hospital administration should provide paramedical personnel for on-line tracking of clinical indicators through either medical records or admission/discharge personnel. Ideally a hospital nurse epidemiologist should be in charge of this screening process.

3. *Initiate a prospective screening process with clinical indicators.*

4. *Conduct intermittent retrospective analysis via criteria sets.* Criteria sets can be utilized for review in a retrospective intermittent manner depending on the volume of local practice. One could agree to check one of the criteria sets every 6 months or perhaps every 3 months and in this way include all nine indicators in the course of a few years.

5. *Review.* The quality assurance committee in the department should report semiannually or annually on the status of review, and problem areas should be identified for general discussion within the entire department. This will result in both education and analysis and modification of criteria sets on a local level.

The ultimate application of what is a most detailed and comprehensive manual for quality assurance, however, depends on the determination of an individual institutional administrator (with adequate personnel/financial support), coupled with the dedication of concerned clinicians. With the attitude of "the patient first" it would seem that all caring physicians are compelled to provide unrestrained support and enthusiasm.

References

1. Quality assurance in obstetrics and gynecology. Washington, D.C.: The American College of Obstetrics and Gynecology, 1989.
2. Purcell G Jr. Quality assurance/utilization management and risk management: Deterence to professional liability. Clin Obstet Gynecol 1988;31:162–168.
3. Malkasian GD Jr. The conscience of the specialty. Obstet Gynecol 75:1–4, 1990.
4. Statistical Abstract of the United States 1990. 110th ed. Washington, D.C.: United States Bureau of the Census, 1990.
5. Gambone JC, Reiter RC, Lench JB, Moore JG. The impact of a quality assurance process on the frequency and confirmation rate of hysterectomy. Am J Obstet Gynecol 1990;163:545–550.

APPENDIX

Gynecologic Criteria Sets[a]

Unless otherwise stated, **each** numbered and lettered item (except contraindications) **must** be present.

Procedure: Dilation and curettage (D&C 69.09)

Indication: Abnormal uterine bleeding in women of reproductive age (626 all, except 626.0, 626.1, 626.5, 626.7)

Confirmation of Indication:
History of abnormal uterine bleeding persisting for two cycles or more*

Actions Prior to Procedure:
1. Obtain endometrial sample in office†
2. Determine that attempted hormone treatment (estrogen/progestogen) was not successful
3. Consider metabolic disturbances
4. Consider bleeding diathesis
5. Consider pregnancy

Contraindication:
Acute pelvic inflammatory disease

---

*Except for profuse bleeding requiring treatment.
†Except when unable to perform sampling in office.

Procedure: Hysterectomy, abdominal (68.4) or vaginal (68.5)

Indication: Leiomyomata (218.0–281.9)

Confirmation of Indication:
Presence of 1 or 2 or 3 or 4
1. Asymptomatic myomata associated with a uterine size equal to or larger than that after 12 weeks of gestation,* determined by physical examination or ultrasound examination
2. Excessive uterine bleeding evidenced by *either* a or b:

a. Bleeding for more than 8 days during more than a single cycle and profuse bleeding† requiring additional protection
b. Anemia due to acute or chronic blood loss

3. Pelvic discomfort caused by myomata associated with a uterine size equal to or larger than that after 12 weeks of gestation
a. Acute and severe
b. Chronic lower abdominal or low back pressure
c. Bladder pressure with urinary frequency not due to urinary tract infection

4. Rapid growth in size of uterus/myomata, to a point equal to or larger than uterine size after 12 weeks of gestation

Actions Prior to Procedure:
1. Confirm by cytologic study the absence of cervical malignancy
2. Obtain endometrial sample or perform D&C (when abnormal bleeding is present)
3. Correct anemia
4. Consider patient's medical and psychologic risks concerning hysterectomy

Contraindication:
Desire to maintain fertility, in which case myomectomy may be considered

---

*Transverse measurement of at least 8 cm or weight of 280 g or more.
†For example, large clots, gushes; limitations on activity.

---

[a]From Quality assurance in obstetrics and gynecology. Washington, D.C.: The American College of Obstetrics and Gynecology, 1989. Reprinted by permission.

Procedure: Hysterectomy, abdominal (68.4) or vaginal (68.5)*

Indication: Abnormal uterine bleeding in women of reproductive age (626 all, except 626.0, 626.1, 626.3, 626.5, 626.7)†

Confirmation of Indication:
1. History
   a. Excessive uterine bleeding
      1. Bleeding for more than 8 days during more than a single cycle
      2. Profuse bleeding requiring additional protection‡
   b. No history of a bleeding diathesis or use of medications that may cause bleeding
   c. Negative effect on patient's quality of life
2. Failure to find on physical examination uterine or cervical pathology that would cause abnormal bleeding
3. Laboratory data
   a. No finding of endometrial neoplasia
   b. No malignancy found in cytologic studies of cervix
4. No finding of endometrial polyps (by D&C, hysterectomy, or hysterogram)

Actions Prior to Procedure:
1. Consider patient's medical and psychologic risks concerning hysterectomy
2. Determine that attempted hormone treatment (estrogen-progestogen) was not successful

Contraindication:
Desire to maintain fertility

---

*Evaluation of the quality of care provided with this procedure, when performed for the indication listed, will be possible through "trending."
†Other diagnoses that should also be evaluated according to these criteria include menorrhagia (626.2, 627.0), hypermenorrhea (626.2), dysfunctional uterine bleeding, menometrorrhagia (626.2), and polymenorrhea (626.2).
‡For example, large clots, gushes, limitations on activity.

Procedure: Diagnostic laparoscopy (54.21)*

Indication: Chronic pelvic pain (625.9)

Confirmation of Indication:
Pelvic pain for more than 3 months without demonstrated cause

Actions Prior to Procedure:
1. Obtain meticulous history concerning pain
2. Evaluate the following systems as possible sources of pelvic pain:
   a. Gastrointestinal
   b. Lower urinary
   c. Musculoskeletal

Contraindication:
Severe cardiorespiratory disease

---

*Evaluation of the quality of care provided with this procedure, when performed for the indication listed, will be possible through "trending."

Procedure: Cone biopsy of cervix, diagnostic (67.2)

Indication: Cervical intraepithelial neoplasia (233.1, 622.1)

Confirmation of Indication:
Presence of 1 or 2 or 3 or 4 or 5
1. Microinvasive carcinoma of cervix found on colposcopically directed biopsy
2. Cervical intraepithelial neoplasia found on endocervical curettage
3. Cervical cytology report suggesting disease more severe than that found by colposcopically directed biopsy
4. In situ adenocarcinoma of cervix
5. Inability to perform a satisfactory colposcopy

Actions Prior to Procedure:
1. Perform colposcopy with multiple directed biopsies of the cervix
2. Perform vaginal inspection with biopsy if indicated

Contraindication:
1. Known invasive carcinoma of cervix beyond micro invasion
2. Acute pelvic inflammatory disease or cervical culture positive for gonorrhea or chlamydia

---

Procedure: Cone biopsy of cervix, therapeutic (67.2)

Indication: Cervical intraepithelial neoplasia (233.1, 622.1)

Confirmation of Indication:
Demonstration (by exocervical or endocervical biopsies) of cervical intraepithelial neoplasia without invasion
Actions Prior to Procedure:
1. Perform colposcopy with multiple directed biopsies of the cervix
2. Perform vaginal inspection and biopsy if indicated
Contraindications:
1. Invasive carcinoma of cervix
2. Acute pelvic inflammatory disease or cervical culture positive for gonorrhea or chlamydia

---

Procedure: Hysterectomy, abdominal (68.4) or vaginal (68.5)*
Indication: Chronic pelvic pain in the absence of significant pathology (625.9)†
Confirmation of Indication:
1. No significant pathology found on laparoscopic examination
2. Presence of pain for more than 6 months with negative effect on patient's quality of life
Actions Prior to Procedure:
1. Document failure of a therapeutic trial with, for example, one or more of the following:
    a. Oral contraceptives
    b. Diuretics
    c. Nonsteroidal antiinflammatory drugs
    d. Induced amenorrhea
2. Evaluate the following systems as possible sources of pelvic pain:
    a. Urinary
    b. Gastrointestinal
    c. Musculoskeletal
3. Evaluate patient's psychologic and psychosexual status and counsel
4. Confirm by cytologic study the absence of cervical malignancy
Contraindication:
Desire to maintain fertility

---

*Evaluation of the quality of care provided with this procedure, when performed for the indication listed, will be possible through "trending."

†Other diagnoses that should be evaluated according to these criteria include pelvic congestion (625.5); pelvic varices (456.5); uterine retroversion (621.6); congenital anomalies (752.3); mild endometriosis (617–617.9); minimal pelvic adhesions (614.6); broad ligament window (620.6); first-degree uterine prolapse (618–618.9); and mild adenomyosis (617.0).

Procedure: Surgery for stress urinary incontinence, including
1. Retropubic procedures (59.5)
2. Needle suspensions (59.6)
3. Urethral plication (59.3, 59.7 all)
4. Sling procedures (59.4)
Indication: Stress urinary incontinence (625.6)
Confirmation of Indications:
1. History of involuntary loss of urine with increased intraabdominal pressure in the absence of bladder contractions
2. Some evidence of urethral descent (eg, Q-tip, visual) on physical examination, with observation of other factors often associated with stress incontinence (e.g., cystocele, rectocele, hypoestrogenism)
3. Demonstration of involuntary loss of urine
Actions Prior to Procedure*:
1. Obtain cystometrogram
2. Obtain urinalysis and culture
Contraindications:
1. Urinary tract infection
2. Neurologic cause of incontinence
3. Fistulas

---

*Additional procedures that may be helpful in making the diagnosis include cystourethroscopy, diary of urinary pattern, and urethral pressure profile.

Procedure: Oophorectomy, unilateral (65.3), or ovarian cystectomy (65.29)*
Indication: Asymptomatic ovarian cyst in women of reproductive age (220, 620 all)
Confirmation of Indication:
Presence of 1 or 2 or 3
1. Pelvic examination finding of cyst mass that is 8 cm or larger

2. Persistence of a 6–8-cm mass for two cycles
3. Presence of cystic mass that is multilocular or has solid components, as confirmed by ultrasound examination

Actions Prior to Procedure:

Perform vaginal examination no more than 24 hours before procedure to confirm persistence of mass

---

*Evaluation of the quality of care provided with this procedure, when performed for the indication listed, will be possible through "trending."

19

Ophthalmology

Ronald V. Keech, M.D., and
Thomas A. Weingeist, M.D., Ph.D.

Quality assessment plays an increasingly important role in the practice of ophthalmology. The Joint Commission for Accreditation of Healthcare Organizations (JCAHO) has developed progressively complex standards regarding the assessment of quality that must be satisfied in order to attain certification (1). Carefully monitored and clearly documented prospective evaluations of quality have replaced retrospective audits (2). Additionally, quality of care must also be considered in determining the privileges and reappointments of physicians (3).

The expanding burden of medical expenses has prompted an interest by the government and private insurers in the quality of care as a method to monitor the utilization of medical services and control costs (4, 5). Ophthalmology has experienced a greater share of this intrusion than many other specialties. This is primarily due to the financial strain on third party payers caused by the more than one million cataract surgeries performed each year (6). At the prompting of government and private insurers, peer review organizations (PROs) and second opinion programs have been created to assess the quality of cataract surgery and other ophthalmic procedures (7). The "Alternative Cataract Surgery Payment Demonstration Project" currently proposed by the Health Care Financing Administration (HCFA) is likely to have an even greater impact on ophthalmology than all other "quality" control measures (8).

The quality of medical care can be defined and measured in a variety of ways. From the physician's perspective, quality is usually based on technical aspects of care. The highest quality is measured by the best diagnostic workup or tests, or the most effective treatment with the lowest rate of complications. Quality of care can also be defined from the patient's point of view, which may be very much different from the physician's. Patient's concerns often focus on the interpersonal aspects of providing care. The physician's willingness and ability to communicate play a significant role in this perception of quality (9). Still another view of the quality of medical care is from a broader, community perspective. The economics and distribution of health care are included under this definition.

In this chapter, we focus on aspects of quality that pertain to the development of a quality assurance program in ophthalmology. The clinician's perception of quality and its assessment are primarily emphasized, although patient concerns are also considered. Many issues of quality assessment that lack adequate information or are highly controversial will not be addressed. Among these are the accessibility, economics, and legal issues of the quality of medical care.

The chapter is divided into four sections. The first section reviews the standards suggested by the JCAHO for establishing a quality assurance program. Next, the results of a national survey of quality assessment and assurance techniques used in ophthalmology are presented. These include the organization of departmental quality assurance programs, data collection techniques, and methods for analysis. Third, we note some of the possible problems associated with quality assessment and assurance that are especially applicable to ophthalmology. Finally, specific instructions are given for implementing a basic quality assurance program in ophthalmology.

JCAHO STANDARDS AND OPHTHALMOLOGY

The standards set by the JCAHO are often the introduction to the assessment of medical quality for physicians. Hospitals and other health organizations that seek accreditation from this agency must meet standards for the practice of medicine which help to assure quality. The JCAHO suggests using high priority issues to monitor and evaluate the quality of care effectively at both a hospital and departmental level. The Commission's recommendations include identifying important aspects of care, developing appropriate monitors for these aspects of care with threshold levels, and establishing an approach to solving quality of care problems. The JCAHO has outlined a 10-step process to aid in achieving these recommendations (1).

Applying the JCAHO standards and recommendations to a departmental quality assurance program requires considerable planning in order to be effective. The most difficult task is determining the important aspects, or targets, of care that are to be monitored and developing appropriate indicators of the quality for these. As defined by the JCAHO, important aspects of care include those activities that occur in large numbers, are associated with high risk, or have a tendency to produce prob-

lems. Areas of care that fall into one or, preferably, more of these categories should be considered for more in-depth quality assessment. For example, although all ophthalmic surgical procedures usually undergo at least a cursory evaluation of quality, a more detailed review of the preoperative indications, complications, and results may be indicated for the most frequent operations. In most ophthalmology departments, these include cataract, retinal detachment, strabismus, and glaucoma surgeries. Less common procedures with exceptionally high risks such as ocular and orbital cancer surgeries may also warrant more emphasis.

Common office or clinic-based activities may call for an assessment of quality. All laser surgeries and other "minor" surgical procedures are reasonable areas to evaluate. They are performed frequently and have well-defined risks. Less risky clinical activities that might also be evaluated for quality are fluorescein angiography (10) and pupillary dilation of young children with cycloplegic drugs (11). Still other procedures are performed so frequently that they may be assessed for quality even though traditionally they have resulted in few problems. Refraction and applanation tonometry are two of the most common activities performed by ophthalmologists. The incidence of abrasions following applanation tonometry and the lack of a documented refraction have been used as indicators of quality in an outpatient setting (12).

Some medical care activities have a very low risk for serious adverse occurrences and are not considered important by many physicians. Nevertheless, they may deserve an assessment for quality because they create problems for the patient. From the patient's perspective, a long waiting time for an appointment, a long wait during the appointment, and the inability to complete the necessary evaluation in a single visit constitute significant quality of care concerns. Scheduling problems with patient clinic visits and ancillary tests and procedures such as photography, perimetry, or echography are aspects of care that may prompt an assessment of quality. In our clinic temporal artery biopsies receive more intensive assessment of quality than other more frequently performed or risky procedures because they incur difficulties with scheduling and staffing.

QUALITY ASSURANCE SURVEY

We surveyed ophthalmology departments or services throughout the nation for information on how they managed quality assurance. A questionnaire was mailed to 110 ophthalmology department chairmen listed in the most recent directory of the Association of University Professors of Ophthalmology. Based on a previ-

ous study of pediatric departments (13), we asked questions about the organization of the quality assurance program, the methods for gathering and analyzing data, and how this information was used to improve quality (Table 19.1). Seventy-seven questionnaires were returned, with six physicians stating they did not have an organized ophthalmology department or service. The results of this survey are based on the 71 complete or partial responses to the questionnaire by the department chairman or an assigned physician.

Fifty-six physicians reported that their department had an organized quality assurance program with a written plan. The number of full- or part-time staff physi-

Table 19.1.
Quality Assurance Questionnaire

1. Do you have a written departmental quality assurance (QA) plan?
2. Approximately how many physicians are reviewed under your departmental QA program?
3. Who performs the majority of the departmental QA functions?
4. If you have a departmental QA committee, what individuals make up the committee?
5. How often does your QA committee meet?
6. In what manner do you share the QA findings with the department?
7. What support personnel do you actively use to collect/interpret data?
8. Note (from the list below) what items are *routinely* reviewed in your hospital. Check the appropriate column for the committee which is involved in the review (may be more than one):

	Hospital QA committee	Department QA committee	Other
Infection rates	_____	_____	_____
Drug usage	_____	_____	_____
Utilization review items	_____	_____	_____
Unplanned readmissions	_____	_____	_____
Operative complications	_____	_____	_____
Morbidity/mortality	_____	_____	_____
Indications for surgery	_____	_____	_____
Medical records review (i.e., IOP, VA, H&P)[a]	_____	_____	_____

9. How is the issue of "morbidity and mortality" handled?
10. Check any of the QA areas below in which you have specific criteria or an established protocol for evaluating:
    _____ Surgical case reviews
    _____ Pre/post operative discrepancies
    _____ Operative complications
    _____ Preoperative indications
    _____ Medical outcomes
11. Are the QA findings used for physician accreditation or reappointment?
12. Do you use a computer in your QA activities? If so how?
13. Do you perform any QA related to ambulatory care?
14. Describe any other QA activities that your department performs that were not addressed in this questionnaire?

[a]IOP, intraocular pressure; VA, visual acuity; H&P, history and physical.

cians evaluated within the quality assurance plans ranged from 3 to 75. The median number of physicians was 13 with a mean of 25. The head of the department is responsible for the quality of care within his or her organization. Only 14%, however, handled this activity personally. A staff member was assigned the responsibility in 59% of the departments, whereas 21% handled the activity primarily as a committee. The four remaining quality assurance programs were managed exclusively by hospital personnel or by a hospital-based quality assurance service.

The size and makeup of the departmental quality assurance committee was also considered. Twenty percent of the questionnaires gave no response. Six physicians stated specifically that all quality assurance within their department was handled by a single staff member with occasional help from the department administrator. The remaining 51 physicians reported that their department or service has an ophthalmology quality assurance committee. Of these 51 committees, the makeup of members varied considerably. Forty-one (80%) programs included ophthalmologists as committee members. Less than half of the committees included administrators (37%) or nurses (33%). Only 8% of the quality assurance committees have other physicians (i.e., anesthesiologists) as members who are not ophthalmologists, and 16% of the committees include a variety of personnel such as administrators from outside the department, medical record technicians, social workers, and pharmacists. Two programs (4%) also have at least one resident on their quality assurance committee.

In response to questions regarding the frequency of meetings and the distribution of information, the departmental quality assurance committees were fairly consistent. Fifty-eight (82%) of the 71 physicians who returned questionnaires indicated that their quality assurance committees meet monthly, eight meet quarterly, and four only as needed. It is not entirely clear from the survey how many of these responses referred to departmental or hospital quality assurance committees. Of the 51 programs, however, that have an organized departmental quality assurance committee, 39 (76%) have monthly meetings, 11 (22%) have quarterly meetings, and one (2%) committee has a meeting "only when necessary." Of these 51 programs, 33 (65%) noted that they share their findings with the department by reporting at a monthly faculty meeting. Thirteen (25%) committees report to their departmental members at a faculty meeting in addition to written correspondence. One (2%) program conveys information to other department members by letters or memos only, two (4%) programs have no procedure, and two (4%) use unspecified means to convey information to other department members.

Ninety-three percent of the physicians responding to the survey stated that their department or service uses other personnel in addition to committee members to collect and analyze data. Thirty-seven (52%) programs use registered nurses as all or part of this support group. Eight (11%) programs rely entirely on medical record technicians and an additional 18 (25%) include them as a part of their support group. Other personnel are used to collect or analyze data in 35 (49%) programs. The latter included ophthalmic technicians, computer personnel, residents, physicians, secretaries, operating room supervisors, and hospital quality assurance technicians.

We asked about issues that are commonly addressed in hospital or departmental quality assurance programs. These include infection rates, drug usage, utilization review items, unplanned admissions, operative complications, morbidities and mortalities, indications for surgery, and medical records review. The majority of ophthalmology departments or services represented in the questionnaires rely upon either their hospital or departmental quality assurance committee to evaluate these issues. Whereas more than one committee or group is often involved with each issue, it was clear from our survey that hospital quality assurance committees are more than twice as likely (75%) as departmental quality assurance committees (31%) to collect and analyze data on infection rates, drug usage, and utilization review items.

Unplanned readmissions, operative complications, morbidities and mortalities, and preoperative indications are slightly more likely to be reviewed routinely by the departmental quality assurance committee (75%) than by a hospital committee (58%). Thirteen percent of the responders noted that their hospital or departmental quality assurance committees did not routinely review one or more of these issues. Additional areas that are reviewed on a regular basis by some departmental quality assurance committees include photography, unplanned admissions, and surgical outcomes for selected procedures.

The management of morbidities and mortalities was also considered in this questionnaire. Of the 70 responses to this question, four (6%) noted that a hospital committee routinely reviewed all morbidities and mortalities. The remaining 66 physicians who responded to the question stated that their departments had some method for evaluating morbidities and mortalities. Twenty-six programs (37%) manage it exclusively by a periodic, usually monthly, conference, and 13 (19%) rely upon written reports to the quality assurance committee from the physician involved. Sixteen (23%) additional programs use both a periodic conference and a written report to document morbidities and mortalities. The 11 (16%) other responses indicated that the department includes morbidities and mortalities in their regular (daily or weekly) rounds with five of these also submitting written documentation to the department quality assurance committee.

An important area of concern in quality assurance is the development of criteria for judging the quality of care. Regarding this, we asked if the ophthalmology departments have specific criteria for evaluating surgical case reviews, preoperative and postoperative discrepancies, operative complications, preoperative indications, and medical outcomes. Eight percent of the programs have no specific criteria for any of these areas. Seventy-six percent of the programs have criteria for the evaluation of surgical case reviews, 70% for operative complications, and 66% for preoperative indications. Forty-six percent

have criteria for medical outcomes and 48% have criteria for preoperative and postoperative discrepancies. Seven (10%) physicians also commented that their programs have criteria for other areas of care such as medical records review, postoperative infections, and blood transfusions.

A common function of quality assessment is to provide information for determining clinical privileges and reappointing medical staff. Of the 71 returned questionnaires, 31% noted that their departments do not use quality assurance information for assessing the qualifications of the medical staff or for determining their reappointment. Several of these negative responses also added, however, that they were "considering" or "should" use this information for that purpose. The remaining 69% physicians who responded to the questionnaire stated that quality assurance information is reviewed as part of the process for establishing the credentials of their medical staff, for reappointing the medical staff, or for both.

Since the collection and analysis of data can be extremely time consuming, we determined the number of programs that used computers within the department to aid in their quality assurance activities. Of the 71 responses, 45% stated that their quality assurance program depends on one or more computers to retrieve, track, or analyze quality assurance data. Eighteen programs (25%) use a computer for one or two of these activities, and 14 programs (20%) use a computer for all three. Three additional programs (4%) use information collected from computers within the hospital-based quality assurance service.

The move toward ambulatory care in ophthalmology has made the quality assurance process more complex. In light of this, we asked the physicians to describe any departmental quality assurance activity related to ambulatory care. Seventy-two percent of physicians commented that their department performs some type of ambulatory quality assurance activity. Eighteen percent stated that their department does not perform any quality assurance activity related to ambulatory care, and 10% of physicians gave no response. The most common quality assurance ambulatory care activity described was a periodic review of outpatient records. Additional activities that were mentioned included the evaluation of laser treatment indications, a review of outpatient complications for retrobulbar anesthesia, the assessment of oculinum injections, the monitoring of contact lens complications, and the evaluation of fluorescein angiography for adverse occurrences.

To complete our survey, we asked if any of the ophthalmology departments performed additional quality assurance activities not addressed in our questionnaire. Twenty percent of the physician respondents described additional departmental quality assurance activities including a morbidity review of fluorescein angiography, a review of all invasive procedures, follow-up and documentation of abnormal laboratory values, a review of resident performances, and a survey of patient satisfaction.

CONSIDERATIONS IN QUALITY ASSESSMENT

There are a number of potential problems associated with the assessment of the quality of medical care that have implications for ophthalmology. Some of these problems are related to the size of the department, the need for obtaining the support of physicians and determining patient care responsibilities, and the special focus on outpatient care.

The small size of most ophthalmology departments can cause problems in the quality assessment process. A quality assurance program will require extra work from a small staff who are already burdened by numerous administrative responsibilities. Due to the limited number of staff members, ophthalmologists may have to review their own cases for quality assurance. In some situations, it may even be necessary for physicians other than ophthalmologists to assess the quality of ophthalmic care. The small size of the department may also hamper the development of quality assessment criteria; it has been suggested that these criteria are best determined by a panel of at least five to as

many as 13 experts (14, 15). This approach, however, is difficult for ophthalmology departments, which often have only one physician with expertise within a particular subspecialty. In this situation, professional or personal bias may distort the quality assurance process. A better alternative would be to have criteria for major issues of care drafted by a regional or national committee of ophthalmologists recognized within their field. This approach is being used by the American Academy of Ophthalmology with the development of guidelines on "preferred practice patterns" for a number of ophthalmic disorders (16). Although it has received criticism for being too restrictive (17), this type of program may provide more comprehensive and less biased quality assessment criteria than other methods.

Active and enthusiastic involvement of physicians is crucial in order to develop an effective quality assurance program (18). There are a number of reasons, however, why it is difficult to obtain physician support. The additional work of monitoring and evaluating medical care is generally a significant burden for physicians who already have busy schedules of patient care, teaching, and research. Physicians are also wary because of the misuse and distortion of quality assessment information. The propriety of public disclosure of hospital mortality rates has encouraged tremendous public debate (19) with little evidence that it measures quality (20). Information on medical quality is often used more as a means for controlling costs rather than for improving quality (21, 22). In ophthalmology, there is growing evidence that preauthorization and second opinion programs have little effect on the quality of cataract surgery (23). Finally, increasing competition among existing health care systems has prompted the use of quality assessment information as a technique for marketing medical care. In the near future, hospitals as well as individual practitioners will no doubt be advertising their "results" with little attention given to the multitude of confounding factors affecting medical outcomes.

Although there are a number of reasons why physicians may be discouraged, it is imperative that they actively participate in the development and application of quality assessment information. Medical practitioners can provide the most accurate picture of the important areas of care and the appropriate elements that should be used to judge quality. Physician involvement can be promoted in a number of ways. It is essential that quality assessment and assurance be established as a priority by the hospital administration, by the medical staff, and especially by the head of the department or service. Moreover, the hospital should actively aid the clinical department in developing a quality assurance program and supporting its collection and analysis of data. Sufficient support personnel should be made available within the department. Another helpful approach is to use quality assurance programs to assist physicians in utilization review and cost control matters. Intervening with payers, interpreting new practice guidelines or requirements, soliciting for changes in inappropriate requirements, and educating physicians in regard to the need for proper documentation are activities that can be performed by departmental or hospital quality assessment personnel to support physicians and to encourage a more positive attitude toward quality assurance (24).

Perhaps the most important approach to overcoming physician mistrust is to emphasize an educational rather than a punitive approach (25). The departmental quality assurance program should be developed and viewed as an organization to support physicians in attaining and maintaining the best possible medical care. Physicians with less than optimal skills can be identified and aided in improving their level of care. This should be encouraged in a supportive educational manner as much as possible. Punitive approaches that publicize findings and threaten to restrict or suspend privileges should be used only as a last resort when the practitioner is resistant to other recommendations. The evidence from industrial quality assessment studies suggests that a punitive approach lowers morale and does not result in long-term improvements (26).

Many ophthalmology departments are associated with large teaching hospitals,

which may have unique quality assurance problems due to their size and complexity. When a number of different physician specialists are participating in the management of a patient, the responsibility for the quality of care becomes complex and the peer review process may be unfair (13). For example, at our institution a diabetic patient who underwent retinal detachment surgery was subsequently considered to have received suboptimal care. At our hospital, all appropriate consultations were obtained for a foot ulcer related to the diabetes, all recommendations were followed, and the patient was discharged from the hospital with the retina attached. Following the discharge, however, the patient was examined by another physician who recommended rehospitalization for the foot ulcer. The peer review organization found fault with the original care and penalized the ophthalmologist. Neither the consultants nor the physician who recommended rehospitalization were subject to any review of *their* quality of care. Another example applicable to all institutions involves the hospitalization of children for postoperative nausea and vomiting, or prolonged drowsiness following strabismus surgery. If the rate of postoperative hospitalization is higher than the accepted standards, it may indicate poor quality of care. However, there is often no clear distinction made as to whether the ophthalmologist, anesthesiologist, or both physicians are responsible for the quality of care in this situation.

The rapid turnover of house staff in training institutions also poses problems regarding the timeliness and effectiveness of quality assurance methods. Criteria for assessing quality are commonly used as a method for screening cases that require further review. Nevertheless, whereas trends in the care provided by residents can be followed, a particular physician's problem in surgery may not be fully recognized until his or her cases are compared with normative data. For example, a resident may have a vitreous loss rate twice that of other residents or staff. This may not be apparent until the total number of cases are compared. By that time, the physician may have completed the specific surgical rotation or even the residency, thus allowing little opportunity to improve quality.

The movement toward outpatient care in ophthalmology raises additional quality assurance concerns. It may be difficult to obtain appropriate medical information from office records, especially if they are kept in separate facilities. For example, a record of laser procedures will usually note any initial discomfort or adverse reactions during the procedure. A delayed rise in intraocular pressure or inflammation, however, may not be detected until the patient is seen in the physician's office where the data are documented on a separate record. There is currently no accurate and economical method to obtain medical information under these circumstances (27–29).

DEVELOPMENT OF AN OPHTHALMOLOGY DEPARTMENT QUALITY ASSURANCE PROGRAM

This section provides information for developing and implementing a basic quality assurance program within an ophthalmology department or service. Almost all of the suggestions mentioned have been or are in the process of being implemented in the Department of Ophthalmology at the University of Iowa Hospitals and Clinics. We have attempted to make the instructions specific, although they are not intended to be restrictive.

It is apparent from our survey that there is no standard approach to the development of an ophthalmology department quality assurance program. Quality assurance methods are modified based on a number of factors including the size and makeup of the hospital or department and the presence of a hospital-based quality assurance support service. In a small department, for example, the chairman may elect to manage quality assurance with little or no input from other staff members. Ten of the 71 physicians who completed questionnaires in our survey noted that quality assurance was handled exclusively by the chairman. For larger ophthalmology programs, the department chairman is more likely to assign the responsibility to a staff physician who chairs a quality assurance committee (30).

A departmental quality assurance committee will ideally be made up of several ophthalmologists, usually representing a spectrum of ophthalmic subspecialties. If the department has an ophthalmic pathologist, he or she should also be included in order to provide timely reports on clinical and pathological discrepancies. Although an optimum number of committee members has not been determined, we recommend a committee consisting of at least three physicians.

Other committee members may include administrators, nurses, quality assurance technicians, or physicians from other departments. A committee with a broad representation is more likely to provide better recognition and understanding of quality assurance problems. In our experience, a department administrator and a nurse familiar with quality assurance have helped to identify concerns, collect necessary data, and offer solutions to quality assurance problems (31). One or more coordinators from the hospital quality assurance support service may also be included in department quality assurance meetings, especially when the program is in its formative stages. Concern about confidentiality does not appear to be a significant reason for excluding nonphysicians from quality assurance committees (24).

Physicians who are not ophthalmologists may also be included as members of the ophthalmology department quality assurance committee, although according to our survey this is an uncommon practice. Neurologists, anesthesiologists, or other physicians who have similar patient care concerns may provide insight regarding quality assurance problems in ophthalmology. Most of these physicians who are on ophthalmology quality assurance committees, but are not ophthalmologists, have full- or part-time appointments within the department of ophthalmology. In our department, we call on physicians who are not ophthalmologists for help when indicated for specific quality assurance problems but do not include them as regular members of the quality assurance committee.

It is vital that the quality assurance department committee have support personnel to collect and screen data. Preferably, this includes one or more individuals familiar with medical terminology and trained in quality assurance techniques. Medical records technicians or nurses often fulfill this position. Smaller hospitals may use the same quality assurance support person for all the clinical departments. Eye departments with large clinical and surgical volumes, however, will usually employ someone within the department on a full- or part-time basis to perform this task.

Once the structure of the department's quality assurance program has been established, the initial task of the quality assurance committee is to identify the important aspects of care that should be targeted for quality assessment. These are most often diagnoses, conditions, or procedures that are part of the departmental care process (Table 19.2). They may be derived from a number of different sources. The most valuable source for determining areas of care that are important in ophthalmology is the department staff. After reviewing the literature and evaluating all past quality assurance data, each quality assurance committee member should be asked to develop a list of important aspects of care. If additional input is desired, other staff members may be interviewed or surveyed. This approach has the advantage of making the faculty aware of the importance of quality assurance.

Another valuable source for quality of care issues are the nurses, technicians, and other ancillary personnel who work with patients. Their perception of quality care is often different from the physician's. Finally, the patient provides still another perspective regarding quality of care. All patient complaints should be directed to the quality assurance committee. Additional information can be obtained from patient surveys or interviews. Questions regarding convenience, understanding, confidence, improvement, and satisfaction are helpful in identifying areas of importance in which quality can be improved.

Still another source might be the guidelines or requirements for important areas of medical care established by organizations outside of the health care facility, which must be met in order for hospitals to receive accreditation, reimbursement, or to obtain other desired benefits. We have previously discussed the recommendations suggested by the Joint Commission for Accreditation of Healthcare Organizations. They offer guidelines for specific hospital and department quality assurance activities including surgical case review, morbidity and mortality monitoring, and infection control. Other private and government-sponsored peer review organizations have guidelines for hospital utilization and surgery indications. All of these guidelines should be carefully reviewed and, when appropriate, incorporated into a departmental quality assurance program.

Finally, the hospital quality assurance program may be a source for important areas of care that should be assessed. For a number of years, most hospitals have had programs for the collection and analysis data on hospitalwide areas of care. These often include areas such as drug usage, employee and patient safety, infection control, laboratory and pathological usage and accuracy, blood usage, and surgical morbidity and mortality. The ophthalmology quality assurance committee should monitor all of the information from the hospital's quality assurance program that applies to their department.

The quality assurance committee should develop a priority list from the important areas of care that are targeted for quality assessment. The frequency of occurrence of these elements and their associated risks will aid in determining which should receive the highest priority. For example, a small improvement in the quality of care for cataract patients is likely to benefit a large number of patients. In comparison, an equal improvement in the quality of care for an epikeratophakia procedure would be less important since it is rarely performed and has an impact on only a few patients. The severity of the risk is another factor that may affect the importance of the area of care. Procedures with very high risks such as optic nerve sheath fenestra-

Table 19.2.
Important Areas of Care and General Criteria

Important Areas of Care	General Criteria
I. Surgery	
A. Surgical procedures	1. Avoidable cancellations
	2. Surgical delays
	3. Operative reports not dictated within 24 hours
B. Specific surgical procedure (i.e., see Table 19.3)	1. Preoperative indications
	2. Medical record documentation
	3. Indication for admission
	4. Operative complications
	5. Pathologic diagnosis
	6. Postoperative course
	7. Functional outcome
II. Outpatient clinics	
A. Nonsurgical trauma cases	1. Medical record documentation (i.e., visual acuity, retinal examination)
	2. Diagnostic evaluation
	3. Treatment protocol
B. Temporal arteritis	1. Medical record documentation
	2. Biopsy (i.e., timeliness, adverse occurrences)
	3. Pathologic confirmation
	4. Treatment
C. Pediatric dilation	1. Adverse reactions
D. Chloral hydrate sedation	1. Indications
	2. Adverse reactions
	3. Home contact
E. Others (i.e., fluorescein angiography, minor surgical procedures, laser procedures)	1. Adverse reactions
III. Miscellaneous	
A. Incident reports, patient complaints, physician complaints	1. Number reviewed and a written response sent
B. Patient surveys	1. Waiting time
	2. Satisfaction
IV. Areas addressed by hospital QA service	
A. Infection rates	1. Incidence per inpatient hospital days
B. Drug utilization	1. Indication for antibiotic usage
	2. Narcotic usage
C. Mortalities	1. All cases reviewed for appropriateness of care
D. Blood usage	1. Indications

tion may benefit from the assessment of quality even though they are rarely performed. Ocular and orbital cancer procedures are also uncommon, but carry severe consequences if the management is less than optimal. They should be among the initial elements of care for which quality is assessed.

Other factors may influence the choice of the important areas of care that deserve quality assessment. Those areas that re-

quire extra record keeping and analysis would be less desirable topics for an initial departmental quality assessment. Information on the patient's opinion of the quality of care, for example, is usually not included in a standard medical record and would require an independent survey (32). Additionally, areas of care that are already being evaluated by other hospital quality assurance programs usually do not need to be duplicated. For instance, most hospitals have established programs for evaluating and controlling infections. It is unlikely that a separate analysis of infection rates by a departmental quality assurance committee would be productive unless a problem was first detected by the hospital program.

For each important area of care, the quality assurance committee will need to develop suitable criteria or indicators of quality. Medical criteria are "predetermined elements against which aspects of the quality of medical service may be compared" (33). Although development process can be extremely complex (34, 35), the quality assurance committee should be able to draft useful criteria for assessing the care provided within the department based on the scientific evidence in the literature, previously published criteria, and the experience of the staff members.

Whenever possible, the criteria for assessing the quality of care should be derived from the scientific basis of clinical practice. Many aspects of medical care, however, do not have definitive scientific evidence of efficacy (36, 37). Moreover, with few exceptions (38), the majority of the medical information is not directly applicable to the quality assessment process. Additional sources of information on the development of criteria for assessing quality may include the guidelines or standards available from other organizations. For example, the American Academy of Ophthalmology (AAO) has published minimum criteria for cataract surgery (39). The Academy is also developing a series of pamphlets on preferred practice standards that offer "accumulated clinical knowledge" on diagnostic and therapeutic modalities for cataract, diabetic retinopathy, open angle glaucoma, and other ocular conditions (16). Local peer review organizations are another source for guidelines regarding surgical indications and utilization.

Finally, the most valuable source for developing quality assessment criteria will be the clinical staff. With guidance from the quality assurance committee, the staff members should be able to provide useful criteria that closely reflect the clinical situation. For example, each member may be asked to list the indications, operative complications, and the desired outcome for each surgical procedure he or she performs. The staff may also note the essential information they expect to be documented in the medical record, the diagnostic tests indicated, and the appropriate treatment options for a specific medical diagnosis. Table 19.3 illustrates the criteria developed at the University of Iowa for assessing the quality of cataract surgery.

The criteria for assessing the quality of care may require considerable review and modification during the initial stages of development. In our department, the quality assurance committee developed a general format of preoperative indications and operative complications for ophthalmic surgery. All of the services were asked to follow this format and prepare a list of criteria of quality for the important aspects of care within their subspecialty. These criteria were, in turn, revised by the quality assurance committee. For example, the retina specialists determined that intraocular (vitreous, retinal, subretinal, and choroidal) hemorrhage should be included as an operative complication for a vitrectomy. However, since these procedures often have hemorrhage, this criterion proved to be too general resulting in excessive "complications" that had little to do with the quality of care. In order to provide a more useful measure of quality, the committee modified the criterion to include any intraocular hemorrhage that resulted in premature termination of the procedure or in an additional medical or surgical intervention.

Once suitable criteria have been developed for the important aspects of care, it is necessary to establish thresholds or standards for these criteria. "Standards are professionally developed expressions of the range of acceptable variation from a norm or criterion" (33). The methods for deriving these vary. Data may be obtained from the literature, although they should be applied with caution due to variations in procedures and case mix. Data from hospital records or previous audits can also help to set thresholds. If no data are available, then thresholds may have to be determined by a prospective analysis.

Table 19.3.
Criteria for Cataract Surgery

A. Preoperative indications
   1. Lens opacification on slit lamp examination
   2. Best corrected distance visual acuity 20/50 or less
   3. Reasonable explanation that decreased visual acuity is secondary to the cataract
   4. Cataract causing amblyopia
   5. Cataract causing glaucoma or iritis
   6. Cataract obscuring observation or treatment of posterior pole lesion
B. Medical record documentation
   1. Visual acuity
   2. Description of cataract
   3. Status of other eye
   4. Intraocular pressure
   5. Retinal or echographic examination
   6. Pupil reaction
   7. Type and level of functional impairment
   8. Explanation if:
      a. visual acuity of eye to be operated is best corrected to 20/40 or better
      b. previously operated eye has not obtained 20/50 or better visual acuity
C. Indications for admission
   1. Level and severity of coexisting disorders
   2. Consultations
D. Operative complications
   1. Retrobulbar hemorrhage
   2. Posterior capsule tear
   3. Vitreous loss
   4. Expulsive hemorrhage
   5. Iridodialysis
   6. Posterior lens dislocation
   7. Pseudophakic malposition
E. Postoperative course
   1. Readmission
   2. Outpatient surgical or medical intervention
      a. Repair of wound leak
      b. Anterior chamber/vitreous tap for suspected endophthalmitis
      c. Pseudophakic repositioning or replacement
      d. Treatment of postoperative ocular hypertension
   3. Number of postoperative visits
   4. Time to final refraction
F. Functional outcome
   1. Percent of patients with visual acuities $\geq$ 20/40 (subdivided according to known or suspected preexisting macular disorder)
   2. Patient satisfaction

The level at which the threshold is set will be dependent upon the information desired. When it is necessary to identify every noncompliant case, the threshold level should be set at 100%. This is particularly important for quality of care problems that are clearly defined, easily correctable, and may result in severe adverse outcomes. For example, within our department, we identify and screen 100% of the cases resulting in mortality, endoph- thalmitis, or incomplete removal of a malignancy. All cataract cases with a preoperative visual acuity of 20/40 or greater are also reviewed. If the threshold is intended to identify a trend for a specific diagnosis, condition, or procedure, it should be set between zero and 100%. A review of the quality of care is triggered only when the established threshold level is exceeded. Examples of criteria for which this approach may apply include vitreous loss during cataract surgery, postoperative visual acuity following cataract surgery, and wound leaks following penetrating keratoplasties.

At the University of Iowa, the hospital quality assurance support service provides threshold information for a number of adverse occurrences including those associated with the administration of medication, injuries, and selected surgical procedures. The thresholds are determined from the data collected from the preceding year and compared with the results for the current month. In the department of ophthalmology, threshold information has been established or is in the process of being established for selected surgical complications and outcomes. These include vitreous loss during cataract surgery, visual outcome following cataract surgery, retinal reattachment rates, and alignment following strabismus surgery. Although we rely upon threshold information for comparing trends, it is used cautiously and selectively. The variations in severity of given conditions and the presence of other medical conditions are difficult to quantitate, yet they can have a major influence on data used to determine thresholds.

The sources of the quality assurance data will vary depending upon the personnel available and the areas of care selected for review. Usually some data are provided to department committees from a hospital quality assurance program. This may include items such as hospital and departmental infection rates, mortalities, drug usage, operating room utilization, and chart documentation. Very small ophthalmology departments or services may depend entirely upon the hospital programs for all their quality assurance information. In larger departments, however, most information on the quality of care is collected and screened by members of a departmental quality assurance committee or their support staff.

At our institution, we use a technician trained in quality assurance to screen medical records for preoperative indications, appropriate chart documentation, operative complications, and other selected topics. Most of these cases are reviewed further by a physician before being reviewed at the quality assurance committee meeting. Additional data are collected by other assigned personnel. All cases regarding clinical and pathological discrepancies are reviewed and reported to the committee by the ophthalmic pathologist. A log of minor surgical procedures and related activities is maintained and reported on by ophthalmology nurses. Morbidity and mortality data are provided from a number of different sources including written reports from each ophthalmic service, presentations at department rounds, and hospital autopsy reports.

Most departmental quality assurance programs collect and analyze large volumes of information. Computer systems have been developed to aid in this process (35, 40); however, they are not extensively used in ophthalmology. In our survey, 45% of the respondents stated that their departments used computers for retrieving, tracking, or analyzing quality assurance data. At our institution, we use computers to provide hospital-based information and pathology data. In addition, we are developing computer programs for collecting and analyzing data on preoperative indications, record documentation, and operative complications.

Even with the aid of computers, however, the collection and analysis of quality assurance data are time consuming. Random sampling techniques, when properly performed, can reduce the time and effort and still provide adequate information on quality. A review of all the cases of cataract surgery for a specified period of time, for example, may reveal an extremely low rate of complications. Based on these data, it may be justified to review a small percentage of randomly chosen cataract operations on a continual basis. A more thorough review may be indicated if the sampled cases demonstrate a variation from the previously established threshold. In our department, every record that contains the diagnosis, condition, or procedure that we have previously targeted for the assessment of quality is evaluated by a physician, nurse, or quality assurance technician. After all of the records have been assessed for at least 6 months and the noncompliance rate is found to be below the designated threshold, the quality assessment review is reduced to a 10% random sample of cases.

In addition to developing methods for data collection and analysis, the quality assurance committee must establish procedures for the management of this information. The quality assurance committee should meet at least monthly and clearly document the activities of each meeting. The mechanisms for evaluating, correcting, and reassessing quality of care problems need to be clarified. Finally, methods should be instituted for conveying the appropriate quality assurance information to the department staff and the necessary hospital committees. A written plan for outlining the departmental quality assurance program will help formalize this process and provide continuity. The plan should include a description of the quality assurance organization, as well as its scope, objectives, and methods for evaluating and monitoring quality assurance. The JCAHO has made recommendations for the development and content of a written quality assurance plan (1).

In our department, quality assurance committee meetings are held on a monthly basis to discuss all appropriate data and to make recommendations. The committee provides a summary of the meeting minutes to the department head who, in turn, approves it for submission to the hospital executive committee. All recommendations are sent to the department head who may take action or call upon the committee for additional information. The minutes of the quality assurance committee are also summarized at a monthly meeting of the department faculty.

SUMMARY

Quality assessment is an increasingly important topic in medicine. The field of medical quality assessment has expanded in the past few years primarily as a result of the urging of government and private insurers. This has resulted in an excessive emphasis on cost and utilization controls and less concern about issues that are directly relevant to the quality of care.

Ophthalmology has experienced a significant impact from cost and utilization control measures in the name of quality assessment.

Rather than allow others to guide the development of quality assessment, clinicians need to take an active role in formulating quality of care issues important to ophthalmology and establish standards based on the best scientific information. Our survey illustrates the increasing interest in quality assessment among ophthalmology departments nationwide. It also demonstrates, however, that there is considerable room for improvement in many programs. Twenty-one percent of the respondents do not have a written quality assurance plan, and 28% do not have a departmental quality assurance committee. There is enough information on quality assessment currently available to provide a foundation for the development of a quality assurance program. We offer one approach for developing a departmental quality assurance program that we think can have a positive effect on the quality of care within opthalmology.

References

1. Joint Commission on Accreditation of Health Care Organizations: Accreditation manual for hospitals. Chicago: Joint Commission on Accreditation of Health Care Organizations, 1990.
2. Lerhmann RD. Joint commission sets agenda for change. QRB 1987;13:148–150.
3. Murchland JB. Quality assurance and recertification. Aust N Z J Ophthalmol 1988;16:255–257.
4. Jensen AD. Cataract PPOs. Arch Ophthalmol 1990;108:501–502.
5. Ruther M, Black C. Medicare use and cost of short-stay hospital services by enrollees with cataract. Health Care Financ Rev 1987;9:91–99.
6. Stark WJ et al. Trends in intraocular lens implantation in the US. Arch Ophthalmol 1986;104:1769–1770.
7. Dans PF, Weiner JP, Otter SF. Peer review organizations: Promises and pitfalls. N Engl J Med 1985;313:1131–1137.
8. Jenson AD. Cataract PPOs. Arch Ophthalmol 1990;108:501–502.
9. Vuori H. Patient satisfaction—an attribute or indicator of the quality of care. QRB 1987;13:106–108.
10. Halperin LS, Olk RJ, Soubrane G, Coscas G. Safety of fluorescein angiography during pregnancy. Am J Ophthalmol 1990;109:563–566.

11. Apt L, Gaffney WL. Toxic effects of topical eye medication in infants and children. In: Tasman W, Jaeger EA, eds. Biomedical foundations of ophthalmology. Philadelphia: JB Lippincott, 1989;3:3–7.

12. Oswald EM, Winer IK. A simple approach to quality assurance in a complex ambulatory care setting. QRB 1987;13(2):56–60.

13. Weichsel ME Jr, Greenberg SA. Structuring a departmental quality assurance program: A survey of academic pediatric departments. QRB 1989; 15(5):153–155.

14. Donabedian A. Explorations in quality assessment and monitoring. Vol. II. The criteria and standards of quality. Ann Arbor: Health Administration Press, 1982:180–182.

15. Williamson JW. Formulating priorities for quality assurance activity: Description of a method and its application. JAMA 1978;239(7):631–637.

16. Sommer A, Weiner JP, Gamble L. Developing specialtywide standards of practice: The experience of ophthalmology. QRB 1990;16(2):65–70.

17. Winograd LA. When will they ever learn? Ophthalmol Management June 1990:4.

18. Miller ST, Flanagen E. Growth and development of physicians in quality assurance: An ontogeny for quality assurance managers. Quality Review Bulletin 1988;14(12):358–362.

19. Medicare hospital mortality information 1986. Washington, D.C.: Health Care Financing Administration, 1987.

20. Green J, Wintfeld N, Sharkey P, Passman LJ. The importance of severity of illness in assessing hospital mortality JAMA 1990;263(2):241–246.

21. Berwick DM: Measuring health care quality. Pediatr Rev 1988;10(1):11–16.

22. Gary BH, Field MJ, eds. Committee on utilization managment: Controlling costs and changing patient care? The role of utilization management by third parties. Washington, D.C.: Institute of Medicine National Academy Press, 1989.

23. Vibbert S, ed. PRO cataract preprocedure review: Huge waste of money [Editorial]. Utilization Rev 1990;18(17):1.

24. Falk D, Seifert GR, Kahane AJ, Harm RC. Motivating medical staff participation in quality assurance: Views from a surveyor and a provider. QRB 1989;15(10):298–301.

25. Council of Medical Service. Guidelines for quality assurance. JAMA 1988;259(17):2572–2573.

26. Berwick DM. Continuous improvement as an ideal in health care. N Engl J Med 1989;320(1):53–54.

27. Norman LA. Evolving principles of office quality assurance. West J Med 1988;149(2):230–233.

28. Edwards C. Development of a surgical case review system. QRB 1988;14(11):332–335.

29. Benson DS, Gartner C, Anderson J, Schweer H, Kirchgessner R. The ambulatory care parameter: A structured approach to quality assurance in the ambulatory care setting. QRB 1987;13(2):51–55.

30. Schachat AP, Lee PP, Wu W C-S. A quality assurance program for an inpatient department of ophthalmology. Arch Ophthalmol 1989;107:1293–1296.

31. Clanton C, Means ME. Quality and appropriateness of care. Ophthal Nursing Tech 1988;7(4):130–133.

32. Steffen GE. Quality medical care. JAMA 1988; 260(1):56–61.

33. Task Force on Guidelines of Care. American Medical Association Advisory Committee on PSRO: PSROs and norms of care. JAMA 1974; 229:166–171.

34. Dubois RW, Brook RH: Assessing clinical decision: Is the ideal system feasible? Inquiry Spring 1988;(25):59–64.

35. Fifer WR: Quality assurance in the computer era. QRB 1987;13(8):266–270.

36. Roper WL, Winkenwerden W, Hackbarth GM, Krakauer H: Effectiveness in health care: An initiative to evaluate and improve medical practice. N Engl J Med 1988;319(18):1197–1202.

37. United States Preventive Services Task Force. Guide to clinical preventive services: An assessment of the effectiveness of 169 interventions. Baltimore: Williams & Wilkins, 1989:ii.

38. Williamson JW. Improving medical practice and health care: A bibliographic guide to information managment in quality assurance and continuing education. Cambridge, MA: Ballinger, 1977.

39. American Academy of Ophthalmology. Minimum criteria for cataract surgery (Minimum criteria for ophthalmic care). San Francisco: American Academy of Ophthalmology, 1987.

40. Shanahan M. Confronting the software dilemma: Specifications for a QA/RM information management system. QRB 1988;14(11);345–347.

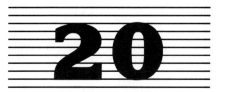

Otolaryngology, Head and Neck Surgery

Sidney T. Dana, M.D., and Martha J. Ryan, R.N., M.H.A.

In 1987 the American Academy of Otolaryngology-Head & Neck Surgery (AAO-HNS) gave the following directive to the quality assurance (QA) committee: present guidelines and criteria for maintaining quality medical and surgical care but emphasize professional judgment as the primary component. The QA committee was created as a subcommittee of the cost containment committee by the AAO-HNS, because economic considerations were considered important when defining surgical guidelines. If that were not the case, it could have been subordinate to another committee such as medical ethics or professional liability. The economic benefit of indications for surgical procedures obviously favors those who pay rather than those who provide services because defined indications tend to limit surgical opportunities. Therefore, the medical profession is encouraged to develop guidelines before standards are imposed by government and industry. If "quality care" is a cost containment issue, then it may be in conflict with the concern that "professional judgement be the primary component of quality medical care." Recognizing this conflict, the QA committee became independent of the cost containment committee. In addition, the QA committee also decided to produce two documents: one to satisfy immediate Joint Commission on Accreditation of Healthcare Organizations

(JCAHO) requirements and a second to address the more comprehensive development of specific practice parameters.

The AAO-HNS is a democratic organization composed of about 9000 medical specialists represented by an elected board of directors. Policies need to be flexible and broad in order to be accepted by the membership. Clinical indicators developed by the QA committee in 1988 provided a starting point for the AAO-HNS to focus its attention on practice guidelines. It deliberately chose to identify quality-related elements, which could survive criticism and win approval by the membership for surgical management of the 20 most frequently performed procedures. To that extent the document was successful. Nevertheless, the indicators were not specifically designed to satisfy hospital requirements. In 1988 the guidelines were based on the concept of *justifying the surgery* by matching an appropriate diagnosis based on minimal criteria. The next stage of indicator development scheduled for release in 1991 will emphasize a logical and more complete documentation to *justify the diagnosis* for each procedure. Professional judgment will certainly be encouraged, and procedure-specific postoperative observations, risks, and outcome studies will also be initiated.

The JCAHO, unlike the AAO-HNS and the American Medical Association (AMA)

is not a democratic or political organization. It establishes policies and expects compliance from its hospital constituency. Noncompliance results in nonaccreditation, which eventually has a harmful economic consequence. Primarily motivated by concern for patient safety in the delivery of health care, the JCAHO requires institutional self-evaluation for the purpose of continual improvement. One of the most important sources of information used to monitor quality according to specific criteria is the patient record. The review and analysis process of this record is easiest when there is compliance with an objective list of criteria. This is a characteristic of the "generic review" and may be performed by any member of the hospital staff. It provides lists of numbers that facilitate comparison. Another way to examine records is to use logical arguments such as: "How was the diagnosis made?" "How was it solved?" "What was the benefit to the patient?" This is one of the formats for the "focused review," best performed by a physician rather than non-professional staff. The focused review is difficult and time consuming, but it has the potential for providing the most useful information about quality patient care and practitioner standards of practice.

Clinical medicine (patient care) is the combined application of art and science. To the extent that science is based on logic, it can be objectively studied, evaluated, monitored, measured, and required to conform with the rules of logic. However, the practice of medicine is incomplete if it is examined only as a science; the art of medicine is a vital and necessary component. Whereas the science of medicine may be evaluated by all, the individuality or art of a physician is more easily judged by peers.

A quality assurance plan is biased toward the scientific part of medicine because science is more amenable to criteria development and thus easier to implement. The art of medicine seems to thrive on the exceptions to the norm, while the science seeks to establish universal standards. It may be impossible to identify by documentation a physician who is honest, performs surgery competently, or has skill in physical diagnosis. The best we can do

in our attempt to insure quality care is to limit the definition and concentrate on what is most easily improved upon; specifically one should ask what can be learned and accomplished by a reasonable person.

There are concerns with the current trends nationally, for example, one may ask whether the JCAHO, which seems to reflect societal expectations, is leading us toward the concept of the generic physician and the generic hospital. It is an issue raised by those who predict that the new regulations will force physicians to practice "cookbook medicine." This probably depends on how quality assurance leaders and regulators interpret their roles. We think that future changes will emphasize the highest individual achievable goals and not comparisons or national averages.

JCAHO STANDARDS

In the 1991 edition of the *Accreditation Manual for Hospitals*, an outline for quality assurance, which became effective in 1985, is presented. Its design at first appears deceptively simple; each of four standards is followed by several required characteristics. The first standard (QA.1) defines the program as "an ongoing quality assurance program designed to objectively and systematically monitor and evaluate the quality and appropriateness of patient care, pursue opportunities to improve patient care, and resolve identified problems." Required characteristics describe a formal written plan sensitive to effective patient care, problem solving and risk management. There should be a hospitalwide program actively supported by, and representative of, clinical and administrative staffs.

Years ago a writer once said on public radio, "If the Russian contribution to literature is the novel, then the American contribution must be the technical bulletin." The first quality assurance standard (QA.1) is probably the perfect example of concise and informative writing. Each word is important and meaningful. There are two words, "quality" and "appropriateness," that deserve some consideration. To define "appropriateness" as suitable or fitting, one must consider outcome (result). This subject was discussed by Dr. R. Heather Palmer at a continuing medical education and quality assessment conference sponsored by the American Medical Association in Chicago on May 11, 1990. She made a distinction between the prescription (procedure) and the patient. Is it appropriate to recommend a costly, complicated, heroic treatment for a dying patient? She defined appropriate care as, "the probability of benefit to the patient exceeding the probability of disbenefit" and stated that an important outcome consideration is "a change in the health status of the patient attributable to care."

An example of inappropriate expense and testing is demonstrated in the treatment of a simple nasal fracture. When a patient with an acutely deformed nose goes to an emergency facility, a plain view x-ray of the face is often routinely ordered. The emergency room physician believes it is good medical management and helpful to the consultant. However, the nose is supported by bones so accessible to physical examination that specialists rarely find an x-ray necessary. Another example is routine ordering of tympanometry for evaluation of the middle ear. An unusual example occurred when tympanometry was reported as "flat and possibly indicating serous otitis media" in a patient with congenital atresia (absence) of the ear canal! The purpose of these examples is to point out that clinical knowledge and experience may be required to recognize when a "good" test or procedure is a "bad" choice, a decision not always obvious to a nonphysician, who initially reviews hospital records based on criteria.

The word "quality" is defined on the basis of experience, ethic, culture, etc. In order to apply it to a system of measurement, however, the definition used by Philip B. Crosby in his book, *Quality is Free,* may be the most useful. He states, "quality is conformance to requirements." At first this appears to be mechanical and insensitive. Yet, the more one thinks about monitors, indicators, evaluations, standards, parameters, and guidelines, the more one will realize that the common denominator is "requirement." If that is how we are to

evaluate quality, then it must be viewed in terms of conformance. Nevertheless, this definition of quality will certainly be debated by physicians during the next few years.

The second standard (QA.2) defines the broad scope of a quality assurance program. The required characteristics include monitoring and evaluation of patient care by all individuals with clinical privileges through monthly meetings, surgical case review, drug and other pharmaceutical use evaluation, medical record review, and blood usage review. There is a specific requirement that activities of surgical services (QA.2.2.15) be included. Relevant findings from these reviews are considered part of the basis for medical staff appraisal and reappointment, privilege renewal, and determination of competence to practice.

It is safe to assume that by now every otolaryngology department leader in the country has been made aware of the increased responsibility of hospitals to document compliance with the new quality assurance standards. Much more comprehensive and detailed organizational activity is demanded. This may be especially burdensome to the smaller institutions and departments because they have limited staff resources and lack of available time from volunteer staff. Technical assistance for departments throughout the United States has become an important activity of the AAO-HNS since 1988. Requests for information are handled every week by the chairman of the QA committee and the director of socio-economic affairs. Because the inventory of otolaryngologic procedures is so large and the procedure for development of specific guidelines somewhat cumbersome, responding to every request is impossible at this time. The *American Medical News* (June 8, 1990) reported what Egon Jonsson, Ph.D., director of the Swedish Council on Technology Assessment in Health Care, said about guidelines in Sweden: "Often it took two years for specialists to come to a consensus on a treatment guideline; by the time it was put into practice, it was outdated."

A few years ago after endoscopic sinus surgery evolved as a new method, lectures and continuing medical education (CME) credit courses began to proliferate. In the spring of 1990, the AAO-HNS QA committee began to respond to many calls from otolaryngology chairpersons and hospitals around the country asking for guidelines and advice about credentialing physicians whose only training had been a 2-day course. Our response was that there are proposed guidelines not yet approved by the Academy, and the department chairperson still had ultimate responsibility for recommending staff privileges to the hospital administration. It is becoming increasingly apparent that the development of a method to measure and improve quality of patient care will be a major medical activity and contribution during the decade of the 1990s. Thus, we believe it will assume historic importance as we enter the 21st century.

The third standard (QA.3) deals with, but poorly describes, the monitoring and evaluation process focused on high priority quality care issues. It is the most important and controversial of the four standards and is better defined under Required Characteristics, focusing on high priority quality care issues. Indicators to monitor activities are used to identify trends or patterns of care but may also be used to assess important single events. An attempt is made to identify situations most likely to provide the opportunity to improve care or correct deficiencies in care. The most comprehensive description and guide to application is found in Chapter 4 of the *Guide to Quality Assurance* published by the JCAHO in 1988. This chapter is devoted to the 10-step monitoring and evaluation process. Because of its importance in the hospital setting, we will describe it as completely as possible and present numerous examples relevant to the otolaryngology department.

10-STEP MONITORING AND EVALUATION PROCESS

Step 1.   Assign Responsibility

a. Department chairperson
  1. Reports to medical executive committee
  2. Reports to medical QA committee
  3. Appoints departmental QA officer

b. Department QA officer
  1. Develops departmental QA plan
  2. Oversees plan
  3. Recommends and defines focused reviews
  4. Presents monthly report to department

c. Department members
  1. Assigned to focused review, verify fairness and accuracy
  2. Share presentation of findings with QA officer
  3. Discuss QA issues at monthly department meeting
  4. Approve criteria and standards of practice

Above is the department organizational plan for assignment of responsibility. Every member is expected to participate. In some departments it may be traditional to choose a chairperson who is the most senior or best clinician, but a department is better advised to choose a chairperson and QA officer on the basis of leadership skills, ability to motivate, and enthusiasm for the task. The complaining, critical, negative personality will never achieve success because a QA plan requires cooperation from members and commitment to goals. "What you accept, you teach" is the best advice we can offer. If poorly documented illegible charts are approved, they will be the model for the future in that department. The hospital administration also has a responsibility to educate and support department leaders. Successful implementation of a QA plan is too large a task for one person. The AAO-HNS has begun to recognize this fact and is preparing to become an active resource for the many department chairpersons and QA officers throughout the country.

Step 2.   Delineate Scope of Care

a. Inventory of clinical activities
  1. Surgical and medical procedures
  2. Type of patients served
  3. Type of practitioners providing care
  4. Sites and times when care is provided

Although this inventory appears to be bookkeeping busy work, it is intended to aid subsequent steps of monitoring and evaluation. If the department does not list a certain procedure such as liposuction for removal of excessive submental fat, then no department members are expected to have credentials to perform that procedure, and it will not be included in focused reviews. If audiologic services and a licensed audiologist are not available in the institution, then an out-of-hospital referral system needs to be identified for inpatients requiring those diagnostic procedures. Finally, if there is insufficient coverage for consultative services to the emergency department during nights and weekends, then those patients will have to be referred to another institution where proper services are available. In other words, the hospital needs to define the services that it is expected to provide and how to make an appropriate referral for services not available—a more common problem in smaller communities served by a single otolaryngologist.

Step 3. Identify Important Aspects of Care

a. Prioritize the procedure and diagnosis inventory
   1. Most commonly performed procedures
   2. Highest risk procedures
   3. Most serious diagnoses

A year-end survey of medical records sorted by code number will give a clear picture of volume for each procedure and diagnosis. High volume, high risk, or problem-prone aspects of care should have the highest priority for monitoring and evaluation. In most departments, adenotonsillectomy is a high volume, low risk procedure, but is associated with sufficient complications to qualify. Tympanostomy tube insertion is high volume, low risk, and has very few complications, although the frequency of infections due to postoperative contamination probably qualifies it for outcome review. Mastoidectomy for cholesteatoma may be low volume but is associated with the high risk of facial nerve injury, and for this reason deserves review. Outpatient removal of small sebaceous cysts is low to medium volume, and

neither risky nor associated with significant complications. Therefore, it would be relegated to generic, rather than focused, review. This kind of information will eventually be collected by enough departments so that national statistics can be developed and used for comparative analysis. How will they be used? Will teaching hospitals often having the greatest volume of complicated high risk problems request their own list for comparison? Will hospitals with only a few stapedectomies annually be compared with those where a single surgeon may perform 100 or more each year? Will patients and physicians have access to information that identifies the high volume hospitals for a specific problem and seek these out for care in the expectation that they will be treated by the most experienced physicians? These are the kind of issues that may be raised when data are developed and access to it is obtained.

Step 4. Identify Indicators

Indicators and the monitoring process examine the following:

a. Identify opportunities to improve patient care
b. Identify and correct important problems
c. Identify patterns or trends warranting evaluation
d. Identify single hospital events or outcome events that warrant evaluation
e. Determine presence or absence of opportunity to improve patient care
f. Determine how to improve care or correct problem

Indicators are also required to consider issues that:

a. Occur frequently
b. Place patients at risk
c. Create risk when care is incorrect
d. Create risk when care is not provided
e. Create risk when care is not indicated
f. Cause problems for patients and staff

Indicators include clinical criteria (sometimes referred to as standards, guidelines, or practice parameters). They are objective, measurable, and based on current knowledge and clinical experience. These indicators include procedures and outcomes. Data collected are related to frequency and importance of single events, patterns of care, and outcomes.

Indicators of Structure. Structures are the elements that facilitate care such as therapy and testing resources, equipment, adequacy of staff for delivery of a specific treatment, etc. For example, an in-hospital audiology unit is a testing resource. Laryngectomy speech training or cochlear implant patient training provide highly specialized therapy. Specialized equipment is needed for complex facial fracture repair and endoscopic sinus surgery.

Indicators of Process. Process of care includes justification for surgical procedures based on clinical experience of the staff as well as authoritative sources in the literature. These indicators depend more on objective rather than subjective data in order to facilitate the development of monitoring criteria. For instance, a tonsillectomy is advocated because of documented failure of medical management for recurrent infection during a specific period of time. In this case the patient has a shared responsibility to seek treatment from a primary care physician before a surgical option is recommended.

Indicators of Outcome. These include complications as well as short- and long-term results both beneficial and detrimental to health. An example is information obtained by a 1-day surgery center from discharged patients who have been asked to respond to specific questions such as, "Was there any evidence of bleeding requiring treatment during the week after surgery?"

Our first experience with "indicators" occurred at the beginning of 1987 when the department of otolaryngology was directed by the hospital administration to "develop indicators for the most commonly performed procedures." We assumed that "indicators" meant indications, and we proceeded to design a document that listed the reasons (indications) for those procedures found to be most frequently performed in our institution. The JCAHO describes these procedure justifications as "indicators of process." Being among the first in the country written by and for otolaryngologists, they were shared with about 40 hospitals during the year before the AAO-HNS 1988 clinical indicators were published.

Because we thought that quality begins at home (in the office), both the physician and office nurse were trained to identify indications developed for the 20 most frequently performed procedures. Each indication was given a code number, and department members were asked to indicate that code on the hospital record in order to motivate use of specific language and to make it easier for the reviewer to determine compliance. This was especially helpful when reviewing records that were difficult to read. It also discourages "doctor rhetoric" and forces the writer to review accepted indications. No attempt was made to reeducate after the familiarization period was passed. In retrospect this was a minor mistake. The code compliance increased from 50 to about 80% in the initial phase and dropped back to 25%, because we exerted no pressure on the physician to stay with the coding system. Nevertheless, working with coded indications did result in sufficient familiarization so that we could document that 95% of the charts had satisfactory indications for surgery during the next 2 years. This was a vast improvement in reviews of patient histories with minimal documentation such as "frequent tonsillitis," "deviated septum 3+" and "dull ears." Actually, those chart notations were made by very competent clinicians whom we believed practiced quality medicine. You just would not be able to document it from their charts.

How do these justifications help identify problems or potentials for improvement? First, they do so in a negative way. If a procedure was performed without approved indications, then the reviewer could challenge the assumption that such a procedure was truly warranted. The departmental meeting is the most desirable place to address this issue because the controversy is then debated openly by professional peers.

At our institution, Community-General Hospital of Syracuse, we discovered that local anesthesia cases caused problems for patients and staff and created risk when care was not provided. The standard care for all patients in the operating room was to have the electrocardiogram (ECG) and vital signs continuously monitored during each procedure. When a local anesthetic was administered by the surgeon, as in the case of nasal septal surgery, the circulating nurse had the monitoring responsibility. Each time this nurse was preoccupied with other duties, the monitoring was temporarily discontinued. Furthermore, the nurse was not trained to evaluate ECG changes, so the task created safety problems and some risk to the patient. Our solution was to require a member of the anesthesia department to be present during all procedures even though that person was not responsible for administering the local anesthetic. Although this decision increased the cost of the procedure for the patient or insurance company, it was considered justified because the potential risk was diminished. Thus, we had a situation where cost containment was of secondary importance to quality (safe) care.

The above example was a patient safety concern originating in the nursing service, which had become sensitive to quality care issues. In the future, we expect that many of the quality indicators will evolve from this kind of experience and reasoning. Surely, we are not in a position to anticipate all of these problems. That is why a QA plan should be written as a blueprint, which not only forms a basis for implementation and action, but also allows for growth as experience is gained in the QA environment. It is a process of gradual evolution requiring the experiences of health care providers to recognize specific needs.

Justifications serve quality in a positive way, which is even more desirable. They force the physician to self-evaluate each case before making the decision to recommend that procedure for care in an institution that operates under a quality assurance program. In other words, *quality begins in the office.* Since the patient encounter starts in the doctor's office, that is the logical starting place for the quality-sensitive document to originate. The attending physician has the choice of either accepting those justifications agreed upon by his/her peers or defending reasons for recommending an exceptional procedure. Reasonable and logical defense should be easily accepted, but it does place a new kind of responsibility on the physician who, until now, took the position that a license to practice medicine was sufficient justification for any medical decision.

Indicators of outcome are a unique problem. The majority of otolaryngic procedures are performed on outpatients who go home within a few hours after surgery, and recovery is deemed satisfactory. The reason for the surgery, i.e., improvement of breathing (nasal septum surgery), restoration of hearing (stapedectomy), or decreased infection (tonsillectomy), is not known for some weeks or months afterward. In these examples, the outcome data in the patient's chart contain more information pertinent to nursing and anesthesia departments than to otolaryngology. This does not imply there are not some important data such as bleeding control, return to the operating room, severe dizziness requiring hospitalization, etc. Nevertheless, none of these issues answers the question, "Did the treatment help the patient?"

Intermediate and long-term outcome data for 1-day patient surgery remain an unresolved challenge. At Community-General Hospital, an outcome study to assess postoperative complications was completed with the assistance of the nursing department. It is customary in our 1-day surgery unit for a nurse to call each patient on the day after surgery. He or she routinely asks if recovery is satisfactory and if there are any problems regarding hospital and home care. Our modification was to have the nurse make a second call a week later and inquire whether there was any subsequent evidence of bleeding or infection requiring the doctor to prescribe treatment or the patient to go to an emergency room. Some of the members of the department were critical of this study because they considered it beyond the authority of the hospital to make inquiries after 7 days even though they had no objection to the same questions asked within 24 hours of surgery. Their reaction surprised us because in this study not only were complications minimal but also the outcome demonstrated excellent patient care.

Subsequently, we asked the staff to approve a long-term nasal surgery study in which we proposed to ask questions about improvement in breathing 6 months after surgery. Here the resistance was stronger. One member of the staff refused both approval and participation. He stated that he did not want to expose himself to criticism because it might reflect poorly on his ability even though he was convinced that his results are probably as good as others. When asked what he routinely tells his patients about the probability of risk or benefit, his response was that he used statistics learned as a resident in addition to his impression of outcomes in private practice even though there are no organized data to support that contention. Another department member said that the hospital has no right to review outcomes once the patient has been discharged because, in his opinion, such information is privileged.

These two examples illustrate the challenge we face in developing meaningful outcome statistics. As long as participation is voluntary, it appears that complete and accurate information is not possible. One solution is for the hospital to establish a policy mandating participation as a requirement for staff membership. A single hospital in a community cannot set such a policy without alienating members of the medical staff and thereby encouraging them to take their work elsewhere. This would obviously be a poor economic decision on the part of the private hospital. We do not yet know whether or not the JCAHO has the interest or the authority to make this a requirement for all hospitals.

Whereas the future for outcome studies is uncertain in the private sector, it is less of a problem for government-financed hospitals and clinics. In those institutions where all physicians are paid employees, the administration has greater freedom to establish policies without fear of veto from the staff. Unfortunately, the skill and experience of much of the staff at those institu-

tions may be at a different level than the best private hospitals. The outcome from surgery performed by residents is not comparable to their teachers or other experienced physicians. Much has been written about this subject in recent years in articles discussing the results of stapedectomies in training programs.

Step 5. Establish Thresholds for Evaluation

After indicator data have been collected and sorted, a certain percentage of cases may "fall out," i.e., fail to meet approved criteria. A reasonable percentage or threshold is predetermined. When that number has been exceeded, more intensive evaluation is required. An example is postoperative parotidectomy accumulation of serous fluid beneath the flap. This is not an unusual finding, but if the number of occurrences for the staff or a particular staff member exceeded normal expectations, then the department would be obliged to determine if there is sufficient reason to recommend a change in technique. Other examples are adenotonsillectomy bleeding rate, which might be 2.5%, or a tympanostomy tube infection rate of 5%. The threshold for facial nerve paralysis might be 0% for mastoidectomy but 100% for parotid carcinoma surgery. Thresholds for evaluation are an interesting problem for clinicians to study and develop. They should provide many opportunities for discussion and publication of articles in the coming years. Monitoring thresholds for outpatient procedures presents additional difficulty because there is so little information to review during the few hours required to recover from anesthesia. The only solution may be for every institution to develop its own outcome studies.

Step 6. Collect and Organize Data

The purpose of step 6 is to determine from the indicators where the appropriate data will be located, retrieved, and assembled in order to be evaluated. Indicators pertaining to surgical justification are located in the history and physical portion of the patient record. Indicators for the use of medications are found in medication sheets, physicians' orders, and nursing notes. Outcome indicators are located in patient records and post discharge patient questionnaires. Although the location of information is usually obvious, it may be helpful when defining indicators to include a source reference.

Data collection need not be exclusively assigned to a member of the administrative staff. Physician participation is also a valuable adjunct to his/her understanding of the validity and fairness of the process.

Step 7. Evaluate Care

Qualified staff members (especially physicians) analyze the collected data to determine if there is compliance with criteria. They also look for problems, opportunities to improve care and undesirable patterns. When indicated, a more intensive evaluation by peer review is required for a specific problem or individual. A convenient and democratic opportunity for peer review is the monthly department meeting, which for this purpose functions like a quality assurance test tube, a place where ideas and criticism combine to create better methods and cooperation. Whenever the review is performed, it is followed by recommendations for action or information.

Step 8. Take Actions to Improve Care and/or Correct Problems

Based on evaluation recommendations, the department must decide what corrective action is to be taken. The need for correction is based on evidence supporting the decision that a problem was caused by insufficient knowledge, system defects, or deficient behavior. A corrective plan identifies, "*who or what* is expected to change; *who* is responsible for implementing action; *what* action is appropriate; and *when* change is expected to occur." In-service education, policy change, and counseling are common forms of corrective action.

A parotidectomy review revealed a high number of postoperative hematomata and serum collections requiring patients to return to the operating room for drainage. Initially the blame was placed on a new wound suction device, but a more careful

evaluation based on interviews of personnel revealed that some recovery room nurses were simply unfamiliar with its proper use. All department members and hospital staff were given in-service education. The following year there were no suction incidents even though more parotidectomies were performed. In this example taken from real experience, education was the corrective action, resulting in improved patient care.

Step 9. Assess Actions and Document Improvement

This is an opportunity for the department to meet, evaluate the effectiveness of the corrective action documented by subsequent reviews, and determine if the problem is resolved or continuing. It may be necessary to take a different approach for unresolved problems. If the only solution requires higher authority, then appropriate medical staff/hospital channels are used.

Step 10. Communicate Relevant Information to the Organizationwide Quality Assurance Program

The frequency and route of formal reports are determined by the hospital QA plan and medical staff bylaws. The board of directors is ultimately responsible. A recommended format for documentation of review in the departmental meeting includes the following: conclusions, recommendations, actions taken, and evaluation (CRAE). This information may affect patient care by other hospital departments. QA activity is also utilized in the reappointment process for medical staff.

Finally, the last standard (QA.4) states that the hospital plan assures compliance with previous standards. The status of problems is tracked, and the plan is reevaluated annually.

IMPLEMENTATION

The ideal quality assurance program *motivates* the physician to provide and document the highest level of contemporary care, *facilitates* review and evaluation of that care by both professional and nonprofessional staff, and *encourages* public confidence in the institution and physicians providing health care. The program should be "user friendly" so that it is understood by all physicians and perceived as a helpful adjunct rather than as an impediment.

The following quotations by P. B. Crosby offer sound advice: "Being part of a team is not a natural human function; it is learned." "Cooperation does not mean that you have to abandon any personal standards." "But most of all, do not be *uncooperative*. That guarantees you will be ignored." Because it is the nature of physicians to have that master-of-the-ship, I-know-what-is-best attitude, real cooperation, not the illusion of cooperation, was one of the greatest challenges we encountered.

We did not assume that physicians would ask the quality manager to develop a program and support that choice with enthusiasm. Nor did we fall into the trap of asking a quality manager to provide the department with a "canned" or commercially available generic format, one that the physicians would either reject or fail to support. Neither approach works. One by one, physicians must be exposed to and convinced of the benefits of quality monitoring and individual involvement. Of course, the process can be accelerated by hospital policy, but that does not guarantee automatic acceptance and cooperation. Before a program can be effectively presented, the leader must be trained. If necessary, a different leader must be recruited. The hospital has a responsibility for education and motivation before setting that person afloat in a hostile sea.

A FINAL THOUGHT

We have described the otolaryngologic approach to quality assurance and its relationship to recent JCAHO standards. This chapter is difficult to end because each experience has led to changes and new beginnings. A quality assurance plan is a statement of good intentions, not a promise that the job will be well done, or insurance against loss or harm. It is an act of faith to think that total quality assurance can be attained, and it is this belief that motivates us toward excellence.

Suggested Readings

1988 Clinical indicators for otolaryngic-head & neck surgery. Arlington, VA: American Academy of Otolaryngology-Head & Neck Surgery, 1988.

Crosby PB. Quality is free. New York: McGraw-Hill/Mentor, 1980.

Guide to quality assurance. Chicago: Joint Commission on Accreditation of Healthcare Organizations, 1988.

1991 Accreditation manual for hospitals. Chicago: Joint Commission on Accreditation of Healthcare Organizations, 1990.

Medical staff monitoring and evaluation—Departmental review. Chicago: Joint Commission on Accreditation of Healthcare Organizations, 1988.

Morgan-Williams G, Jesse WF. The first step in quality assurance. Mich Hosp May 1987; 22–29.

The quality letter for healthcare leaders. Rockville, MD: Bader & Associates, 1991.

Ziegenfuss JT. Toward a definition of roles for physicians in quality assurance. Quality Assurance and Utilization Review. May 1987;36–41.

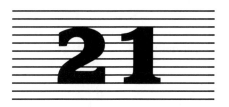

Pediatrics

Timothy R. Townsend, M.D.

INTERPRETATION OF CURRENT JOINT COMMISSION ON ACCREDITATION OF HEALTHCARE ORGANIZATIONS (JCAHO) STANDARDS

The JCAHO standards applicable to a pediatric department in a hospital are found in the 1989 edition of the *Accreditation Manual for Hospitals* published by the JCAHO (1). Which standards apply to a particular pediatric department will depend on how a department is organized to deliver its services to infants and children. If a department consists only of acute inpatient facilities with no hospital-sponsored outpatient facilities (either ambulatory care or pediatric emergency), no intensive care units for either newborns or older infants and children, no pediatric surgical specialties, and no rehabilitation or special care units such as a renal unit, then only certain standards will apply. If, however, a department is organized such that many and diverse services are provided, then standards for each of those services will apply. A tertiary care, freestanding, children's hospital would be an example of a pediatric department upon which virtually all JCAHO standards would apply ranging from standards for diagnostic radiology services and dietetic services to surgical and anesthesia services and utilization review. Many of the standards relating to these varied services are covered in other chapters, and since most pediatric departments are organized not to provide a complete diversity of services, these standards will not be discussed here. The reader is encouraged to examine the organization of his or her department to identify the components of service for which the department is responsible and refer to the *Accreditation Manual for Hospitals* and other chapters in this book for guidance concerning applicable standards.

There are seven JCAHO standards that apply to all pediatric departments regardless of their organizational structure. Those seven are referred to as the Medical Staff Standards.

Responsibility for compliance with each of the standards will rest solely or partially on members of the pediatric department depending on the hospital's organizational structure. In the case of a freestanding children's hospital, all seven will be the sole responsibility of the department. In those hospitals where pediatrics is one of several departments, the responsibility for meeting Medical Staff Standards will be shared in a medical staff organizational structure. Appointed or elected representatives from the department to the hospital's medical staff committees will need to contribute to those specific aspects of the standards that are relevant to pediatrics.

For example, in Standard 4, delineation of clinical privileges, the pediatrics department would determine if American Board of Pediatrics certification is required for staff privileges or, in delineating privileges for certain invasive procedures, whether a certain number of supervised procedures need be performed before privileges for that procedure are granted. In addition, pediatrics as well as other departments are to comply with Standard 3, which requires that each department and its chairman are specifically delegated the responsibility for being accountable for all professional and administrative activities in the department, for continued surveillance of professional performance, for defining the criteria for clinical privileges, for identifying for each member of the department their clinical privileges, and for assuring the monitoring and evaluation of the appropriateness and quality of care in the department. In hospitals not organized into departments, those physicians caring for infants and children will need to comply with the Medical Staff Standards based on their scope of services in an integrated fashion with other physicians on the medical staff.

Standard 6 is the standard that places the responsibility on the department for systematically monitoring and evaluating the quality and appropriateness of care and treatment of its patients. To assist departments in implementing a process to comply with Standard 6, the JCAHO has published two booklets: scoring guidelines, which it uses to evaluate compliance with Medical Staff Standards during an accreditation survey, and a "how to" for setting up a departmental monitoring and evaluation process (2, 3). This process is referred to as the 10-step process and a description of each step follows.

Step 1. Assign Responsibility

The chairperson of the department has ultimate responsibility for monitoring and evaluating the quality and appropriateness of care delivered to patients. He or she may assign specific activities to one or more physicians in the department and

they in turn may assign portions of the task to ancillary or other support personnel as appropriate. A written plan delineating the specific tasks, activities, and responsibilities is helpful.

Step 2. Delineate Scope of Care

This is simply a rather exhaustive inventory of the activities and services provided by the department. These services and activities might be broadly categorized into types of patients receiving services (e.g., by diagnosis for each age group served) and by types of diagnostic or therapeutic activities (e.g., tests such as echocardiogram or throat cultures, drugs such as ampicillin or aminophylline, blood products such as packed cells and Rh immune globulin, surgical or invasive procedures such as cardiac surgery or hyperalimentation). When making the inventory, estimate, as accurately as possible, the numbers of episodes of each service or activity. This will help in step 3.

Step 3. Identify Important Aspects of Care

Since it would be inefficient to monitor and evaluate all aspects of care provided in the department, efforts should be focused on the most important. To help determine which are the most important, three criteria for selection are suggested: high volume, high risk, and problem prone. High volume can be determined from step 2, which identified those services or activities with large numbers of episodes of care. High risk might be defined as "if the care given is not exactly correct or if care when it should have been given was not, then serious consequences will be suffered by the patient." Problem-prone services or activities are those that might have caused the department or a specific group of patients problems in the past. This latter criteria often will be highly individual for each department. For example, if the chest x-rays of young infants taken during the night shift are often of poor readability, this could be a problem-prone activity worthy of focus.

Step 4.   Identify Indicators

An indicator is a variable that measures an aspect of the structure, process, or outcome of patient care. Structure may be thought of as the environment in which care is delivered such as types and availability of equipment, qualifications of personnel, or timeliness of delivery of a particular service. Process is the care that is or is not delivered such as diagnostic or therapeutic maneuvers or ancillary services rendered. Outcome is the result of the care that is or is not delivered such as the success or failure of a particular operation measured in terms of short- or long-term return of patient function. Indicators may be thought of as events that occur, or fail to occur, depending on the point of view or judgment of those defining the indicator. Since the quality of care is determined by many factors, many of which require judgments that may be difficult to define, an indicator by itself cannot be a measure of quality (4). Indicators or events relating to medical care then become screens to identify the aspect of structure, process, or outcome that needs to be further evaluated, often in a judgmental sense, to determine if the quality of care was good, bad, or unaffected. The judgment of quality can be made during the identification of indicators by selecting those indicators that reflect cause-and-effect relationships between specific aspects of structure, process, or outcome (see "Epidemiological Considerations" for a discussion of this concept).

As screens, indicators can be evaluated for their epidemiologic characteristics such as validity, reliability, sensitivity, specificity, and predictive value (5). As with any screen, an indicator must have a precise "case definition" in order to determine if the event being measured occurred or not. As a practical matter, an indicator should measure an event that can be assessed with reasonable ease. For example, to use as an outcome indicator the event "IQ above 100 at 5 years of age" to assess the quality of head sonography among premature infants in a particular hospital's new-born intensive care unit would be impractical. Indicators may be single-event indicators (sentinel events) where each time the event occurs there is a further evaluation to determine if the quality of care was good, bad, or unaffected. Usually rare events are those measured by this type, and they measure a serious aspect of the structure (e.g., all the ventilators are in use when an asthmatic in respiratory failure is admitted), process (e.g., the heart wall is perforated during cardiac catheterization), or outcome (e.g., fatal aplastic anemia following chloramphenicol therapy) of care. Indicators may be used to develop rates when the event contributes to the numerator of a rate, and the denominator is the population at risk for the event. Rates should be used when the event being measured has an expected frequency of occurring irrespective of the quality of care provided. However, when rates are compared over time or between populations, the issue of confounding (e.g., case-mix, secular trends, etc.) makes interpretation problematic. As long as rates are kept in the perspective that they are simply screens to give guidance to address the question of why a particular rate is occurring, they can be useful tools.

Step 5.   Establish Thresholds for Evaluation

For each indicator, as noted above, there should be a definition as to when the indicator's screening function should trigger an in-depth evaluation to determine if the quality of care is good, bad, or unaffected. Some indicators will have a threshold of 0 or 100%. Zero percent indicators would be sentinel event indicators where each event would be evaluated. One hundred percent indicators would be those where the event must always occur (e.g., a signed informed consent prior to surgery) and the failure to occur triggers an evaluation. Thresholds other than 0 or 100% are rates and the expected frequency of occurrence, as determined by the scientific literature, judgment, or prior experience, irrespective of the quality of care, which will determine where the threshold is set.

Step 6. Collect and Organize Data

This step is important to consider in completing steps 3, 4 and 5 in that if the data are too difficult to collect in a meaningful fashion then the particular important aspect of care as identified by an indicator may not be able to be evaluated. In this case, either a different indicator must be chosen or the aspect of care must await the development of different data systems to be evaluated. It is important to know when to stop collecting information about an important aspect of care. If over a reasonable period of time, such as a year, no quality problems are noted for a particular aspect of care, it is appropriate to document the fact that no problem was found and focus effort on some other important aspect of care. Persons in the health care setting particularly skilled at helping with step 6 are those familiar with data sources, data collection, and data management (e.g., infection control, quality assurance, medical records, and computer systems). Those with research experience may be particularly sophisticated and helpful.

Step 7. Evaluate Care

The purpose for using a screening technique (indicators) to evaluate the appropriateness and quality of care is so that those who must evaluate the care can do so efficiently. If the indicators identify too many events where the care was appropriate and of high quality, the process is inefficient. Equally inefficient but often more difficult to quantitate is when an indicator fails to identify poor quality. Those individuals given the responsibility of evaluating the quality and appropriateness of care should have two fundamental characteristics. First, they should be knowledgeable enough about the care given to determine its quality and appropriateness, and second, they should be in a position to help effect change if any deficiencies in care are found. The peer review process is important in this respect in that in screening many aspects of care a particular member of a department may

need to have the quality or appropriateness of his or her care evaluated, and only other members of the department with similar backgrounds and experiences would be knowledgeable enough about the care and be in a position to help correct any deficiencies found.

Step 8. Take Actions to Solve Identified Problems

Most problems are caused by defects in knowledge, organization, or performance. Once a problem has been identified in step 7, the defect may be obvious or additional evaluation may be needed to find the cause of the problem. Once the cause has been identified, it is often useful to develop a written plan of corrective action. This will delineate what the problem is, what needs to be done by whom in what time frame, and what the expected outcome of the corrective action might be.

Step 9. Assess Actions and Document Improvement

Continuing the screening process through the use of indicators, provided they are sensitive and specific enough to detect difference in care, should be adequate for this assessment. If the plan of corrective action is completed as outlined in step 8 and the indicator performance improves, then there is a reasonable assumption of cause and effect between the problem and the quality or appropriateness of care. If, however, there is no improvement or worsening of the indicator performance, then the indicator should be examined for its performance characteristics and the cause-and-effect relationship between the problem and the care should be questioned.

Step 10. Communicate Relevant Information to the Organizationwide Quality Assurance Program

The documentation of the monitoring and evaluation activities themselves, the actions and results of those activities, and the communication to the organizational structure are important for several reasons. First, the governing body of the organization is both legally and ethically responsible for the care provided by the organization. Second, in recent years those receiving health care services, and those who pay for it, seek assurance that quality and appropriate care are provided. Finally, it would seem natural that any professional would want to document the quality of his or her professional activities. Professionals set themselves apart from others by having special knowledge and skills. Within groups of professionals, special knowledge and skills separate one group from another such as pediatricians and nonpediatricians who care for infants and children. This special knowledge and skill is based on the assumption that those with the special knowledge or skill can give "better" care (e.g., a pediatrician can give better care for infants and children). Those with the skill and knowledge usually are anxious to document what sets them apart such as board certification or subspecialty status, so documentation of quality should be an expected physician trait.

In Standard 6 there are several additional elements that are required of departments such as surgical case review, drug usage evaluation, medical record review for clinical pertinence, blood usage review, pharmacy and therapeutics function, risk management activities, and other review functions. The 10-step approach noted above can be used to address each of these elements. Although the JCAHO suggests that all operations and invasive procedures be reviewed, it seems more efficient to use the high volume, high risk, problem-prone approach to select those on which to focus.

SPECIFIC EXAMPLES

Two examples of the quality and appropriateness of care monitoring and evaluation that can be done in a pediatric department follow. The 10-step process will be shown for each, except for steps 1 and 2 in which the department chairperson has assigned the responsibility to the quality assurance physician advisor for the depart-

ment who shares or delegates parts of the tasks to the quality assurance coordinators assigned by the quality assurance department of the hospital to work with pediatrics.

Example 1.   Suspected Bacterial Meningitis

An important aspect of care for the department is treatment of infants and children with suspected bacterial meningitis (step 3). This was determined by examining the lists of diagnoses for the preceding year and finding that 23 infants and children older than 1 month of age were admitted with meningitis, and the risk of death or long-term disability was high if proper and timely therapy was not undertaken. Antimicrobial treatment regimens for suspected bacterial meningitis designed to treat the three most common pathogens had been ceftriaxone for the past year, and no problems had been identified with its use and no child had failed to receive it. Recent evidence suggested that administering a corticosteroid, dexamethasone, before or at the same time as the first dose of antibiotics, improved patient outcomes and the side effects, such as gastrointestinal bleeding, were rare and treatable (6). The use of dexamethasone for suspected bacterial meningitis was chosen as a high risk, relative high volume aspect of care for monitoring and evaluation.

Two indicators were developed to screen the care given to infants and children with suspected bacterial meningitis (step 4):

Indicator 1. Dexamethasone, 0.5 mg/kg every 6 hours for 4 days.
Indicator 2. First dose of dexamethasone must be administered before or within 15 minutes after the first dose of ceftriaxone.

The thresholds for both were set at 99% (step 5). Possible exceptions for both indicators might be moribund patients in whom life support attempts precluded an orderly usage and timing of the drug.

Since all patients with suspected bacterial meningitis are admitted, the medical record, which also included the emergency room record, would be the source document for collecting and organizing data (step 6). The quality assurance coordinators concurrently review all charts of all inpatients and would collect these indicators on all patients with an admitting diagnosis of suspected bacterial meningitis. The medication administration record and the emergency room sheet were searched to determine the timing of the administration of the drugs. During the first 3 months, five patients with suspected bacterial meningitis were admitted, one (20%) was not treated with dexamethasone, and two (40%) received their first dose more than 15 minutes after ceftriaxone.

The records of the three patients were reviewed (step 7). In all three cases, there was no obvious reason for not using dexamethasone (case 1) or for the delay in its administration (cases 2 and 3).

After discussion with the three different physicians whose patients were case 1, 2, and 3, it was apparent that a lack of knowledge of the use of the drug and the timing of its first dose was the problem. A brief letter from the quality assurance physician advisor to the department chairperson outlined the problem and proposed an action plan of a one-page educational letter to the staff outlining the studies on which dexamethasone use was based. The educational letter was sent.

Over the 9 months following the letter, continued monitoring of the medical records of all patients admitted with suspected bacterial meningitis revealed no case in which dexamethasone was not used and only one case in which the time interval was 18 minutes. Since this did not seem to be a deviation sufficient to affect the quality of care nor did it seem sufficient to revise indicator 2, no further action was taken.

Results of the experience with these two indicators was presented to the departmental quality assurance committee meeting (step 10). The report was attached to the committee minutes, which were sent to the hospital quality assurance committee and included in that committee's report to the board of trustees.

Example 2. Diphtheria, Pertussis, Tetanus (DPT) Immunization of Preterm Infants

The department has a 30-bed newborn intensive care unit (NICU) that serves as a tertiary referral center and admits about 600 sick, often preterm, newborns. About one-third of patients admitted spend at least 2 months in the NICU, many with pulmonary disease due to their prematurity. Even mild respiratory infections can have severe consequences in these patients. Thus, an important aspect of care in this high volume of patients is to prevent pertussis (step 3). In addition, there had been debate within the department for many years as to when preterm infants should start their DPT immunizations. Some argued that the infant should be 48 weeks postconception, and some argued that the infant should weigh at least 5 pounds. The result was that many infants were not immunized during their highest risk period, the first 6 months of life. A recent study indicated that the immune response and side effects of DPT were the same in preterm infants and full-term infants when the first dose is given at 2 months of age regardless of birth weight or gestational age (7). Administering DPT immunization to preterm infants in the NICU at 2 months of age was chosen as a high risk, high volume, problem-prone aspect of care.

One indicator was developed to screen the care given to patients in the NICU who were 2 months of age (step 4):

Indicator. All infants in the NICU at 65 days of age are to have received a DPT immunization between 60 and 65 days of life.

The threshold for this indicator was set at 95% (step 5). Possible exceptions for this indicator may be a contraindication to immunization (e.g., evolving neurological disorder).

The source document for collecting and organizing data would be the medical record of infants in the NICU (step 6). The order sheet and medication administration record were reviewed when an infant in the NICU became 65 days of age. To facilitate review, the quality assurance coordinator who reviewed NICU records kept a card with the list of names of all infants who were 50 days of age and would be expected to become 65 days of age in the next 2 weeks. This card was updated weekly. During the first month, 20 infants became 65 days of age, and none had received DPT immunization.

Since it was unlikely that all 20 infants had a contraindication to immunization and the neonatologists had been consulted during the indicator development suggesting that knowledge deficiency was not the problem, it was assumed that an organizational problem existed (step 7).

Discussion with all of the neonatologists confirmed that knowledge was not a problem. They indicated that, in a busy NICU with many critically ill patients, remembering to order a DPT immunization for infants who often were "feeding and growing" and not critically ill was difficult. The quality assurance coordinator suggested that, since she generated a list of infants each week who would become 65 days old that week, she might be able to help remind the neonatologists. At the next neonatology division meeting, it was agreed that the coordinator would give a copy of her list to the head nurse in the NICU, and she would put a sticker "Evaluate for first DPT" on the order sheet of each infant approaching 65 days of age. The neonatologists would evaluate the patient for contraindications, document their results, and, if there were no contraindications, write the order for DPT vaccine. This approach was briefly outlined in a letter from the quality assurance physician advisor to the department chairperson, with copies to all neonatologists and nursing staff (step 8).

Over the next 5 months following the institution of the "sticker" reminder, 93 infants reached 65 days of age and 91 (99%) received DPT (step 9). Since this was above the threshold of 95%, no action was taken.

Results of the experience were presented to the division of neonatology by the coordinator, who also noted how good the documentation in the medical records was for the two infants who did not receive DPT vaccine because they had evolving neurological disorders. The results were reported to the departmental quality assurance committee, then to the hospital's quality assurance committee and to the Board of Trustees (step 10).

EPIDEMIOLOGICAL CONSIDERATIONS

Quality of medical care is a complex concept. The definition of quality of health care will depend on the context of the assessment (8). Donabedian proposed three approaches to the assessment of quality: structure, process, and outcome. A judgment of the quality of care could be made (*a*) directly by examining the processes of care or (*b*) indirectly by examining the settings in which care is provided (structure) or by examining the effects of care on the health of individuals or populations (outcomes) (8). However, to assess care using this approach, one assumes a cause-and-effect relationship between particular elements of structure and process (or between process and outcome or between structure and outcome). For example, if drugs A and B are effective in treating asthma, then choosing between them cannot be used to assess the quality of care of asthma. However, if drug A is more effective than drug C, then a judgment about the care of asthmatics can be made concerning physicians who choose drug C rather than drug A. Epidemiologists are well trained in assessing the strengths of casual associations. Such skills are helpful in selecting elements of structure, process, and outcome for assessing quality. In example 2 in the preceding section, the strong causal association between the process, administering DPT vaccine, and the outcome (prevention of pertussis) made for an ideal approach to judge the quality of care of those who did or did not administer the vaccine.

In addition to using an epidemiologic

approach in evaluating causation to determine what is important to assess, the
concept of case definition can add efficiency to the process. If, for example, an
indicator "stroke following cardiac surgery" were to be developed, many cases of
"watershed strokes" (analogous to changing a hot water heater in a home and the
water is brown for a while after the new
heater is installed due to "shaking up the
system"), which occur with predictable
frequency and are nonpreventable, would
be included. If the "case definition" was
changed to "non-watershed stroke defined
by computed tomography following cardiac surgery" then only those patients in
whom anticoagulation or bypass pump
problems or other process of care difficulties might have occurred are reviewed,
making the assessment process more efficient. Keeping track of indicator performance in terms of a simple "true-positive"
"false-positive" tabulation, compared to a
judgment of deficient quality or no deficiency in quality, will often highlight indicators that may need better "case definitions."

Many epidemiologic skills are helpful in
the day-to-day management of the quality
assurance process. Data quality is important, particularly reproducibility. Periodically, having two persons reviewing the
same medical record independently to
identify indicators helps assure the medical staff that the data are of high quality.
Paying attention to the basic epidemiologic
principle—that when rates are developed
the denominator selected must reflect the
population at risk for being included in the
numerator—is important. In example 1 in
the previous section, the denominator was
patients with suspected bacterial meningitis because they are the ones at risk for
failing to receive dexamethasone appropriately. Patients with suspected viral meningitis, chemical meningitis, or leukemic
meningitis would not be included.

INTERACTING WITH
THE STAFF

An old Native American saying captures
the essence of much of human interactions: "To know a man you must walk a
mile in his moccasins." If we attempt to see
an issue as we imagine that another person
might, trying to identify their bias, attitude, or mindset, we can have a clearer
understanding of why they view a particular issue as they do and we can better
identify common ground to resolve the
issue. What follows are three examples of
different staff persons with differing but
fairly typical biases, attitudes, or mindsets
and some of the approaches that can be
used to find a common ground to resolve
issues.

Physician A has been in private practice
for 16 years. His longevity on the hospital's
staff has forced him, reluctantly, to serve
on several committees, but he has not
taken a leadership role in hospital affairs.
His rapport with the infants and children
in his practice is excellent but less good
(not bad but mostly just cordial) with their
parents. He has now been assigned to the
departmental quality assurance committee
and immediately becomes hostile to the
quality assurance staff on nearly every
issue raised. He thinks quality assurance is
a waste of time, he accuses the quality
assurance staff of being spies for the hospital, and he says that he practices high
quality pediatrics as do his colleagues, and
therefore, quality assurance is unnecessary.

Put yourself in physician A's position.
He is in private practice as he is probably
fiercely independent and not used to dealing with regulatory or external controls.
His reluctant involvement with the hospital as an organization fits with this independent mindset. Being in private practice
means he deals with patients one at a time
and he does not think epidemiologically or
feel comfortable with rates, screening
methods, populations, or data bases. He
simply may be more comfortable around
children than adults, so adults may have to
work harder to relate to him. How can
common ground be reached on the issues
he raised? He says that he practices high
quality medicine. He does, and that must
be recognized. He must be educated that
for years medicine in general did not pay
much attention to documenting the quality
of care provided; it took an attitude of

"trust me, I know what is best," and now patients and payers are asking for proof. His assistance is needed to show how good his and his colleagues care is; and if any areas for improvement can be found, he and his colleagues are in the best position to find them and fix them. Having been in private practice and having avoided involvement in the hospital organization probably has insulated him from local and national changes in the medical care system. He probably lacks knowledge of how the hospital's quality assurance structure fits in with regulatory, accrediting, and payer requirements. His only contact with this part of the outside world is the "business" part of his practice, probably 90% of which is handled by his office staff. A thorough explanation of the big picture, defining, as best as possible, the rationale for each part of the picture, may help him understand the role of quality assurance. Finally, he thinks quality assurance is a waste of time. To him, productive time is taking care of infants and children. That is what he was trained to do, and that is what he has devoted his life to. He is absolutely right, and that must be appreciated. However, if it can be pointed out to him that most all pediatricians on the staff are in the same situation and that if no pediatrician steps forward, then, by default, someone else will come in and set the rules. At this juncture, a negotiated settlement can be offered. His time will be respected by having a quality assurance structure as efficient as possible so that only those issues that must be decided by a pediatrician are brought to his attention. In exchange, he will buy into the process and cooperate in a mutually respectful working relationship.

Physician B is the chairperson of the pediatrics department. She is a busy person who spends little time seeing patients and a great deal of time with budgets, administrators, and endless meetings. She has been told by the hospital's chief executive officer that pediatrics must develop a quality assurance program, and she delegates the task to one of the younger physicians in the department. Her mindset is that this is a low priority, and she is too busy.

Put yourself in physician B's position. The idea of a quality assurance program is not hers; she was told to do it. The hospital's management often tells departments that it wants certain things done, and this was given neither high nor low priority. There was no crisis that brought this request from management. How can a common ground be reached such that the departmental leadership can give quality assurance higher priority (and the rest of the department's members will sense that priority) yet not intrude on the time and focus of a busy leader? Both communication and negotiation skills are helpful. Simply getting one-half hour of her time for an initial meeting may be difficult. However, one might stimulate her interest by indicating the need to explain briefly the importance of quality assurance and outline the structure of the program that the chief executive officer recently sent to her. In the meeting, give a brief outline of the program and focus on the major goal—visible leadership. Propose a plan that is respectful of her time. Ask her to give a 5-minute progress report and an appeal for cooperation in this necessary task every 3 months at the departmental staff meeting. In exchange for that commitment one could meet with her for no more than 15 minutes before that quarterly staff meeting and give her a prepared text that she can use for the progress report.

Physician C finished his training last year and is the newest member of the department. He is energetic and trained at a place that had a very active quality assurance program. He has been delegated the task by the department chairman to develop the departmental quality assurance program. He has not built up his practice yet, this is his first departmental responsibility, and he has plenty of time on his hands. His mindset is that he is going to take on this task with great gusto, he is going to develop 50 indicators using the JCAHO 10-step model, and this will be the best program in the region.

Put yourself in physician C's position. He just came from a hotshot training program, he knows the latest treatments and diagnostic techniques, and he can bring the other pediatricians up to the high standards of the academic mecca he came from by using the quality assurance program. How do you find a common ground that will not alienate his colleagues yet preserve his enthusiasm, energy, and prior experience with quality assurance? Simple, honest communication is useful. Let him know that you understand his mindset and offer to be an honest sounding board for his ideas before he approaches his colleagues. Let him know that you will try to understand his point of view because you heard an old Native American saying that captures the essence of much human interaction: "To know a man you must walk a mile in his moccasins."

SPECIFIC INSTRUCTIONS FOR IMPLEMENTING A QUALITY ASSURANCE PROGRAM

Very little published data exist that describe the structure and activities of quality assurance programs in pediatric departments (9, 10). Most of the meager, published literature specific to pediatrics focuses on appropriateness of use of medical services (11–14) or outcomes of care (15, 16).

Werchsel and Greenberg surveyed 37 academic pediatric departments (19 university or public hospitals, 6 children's hospitals, and 12 others), and 25 (68%) responded to the survey. All respondents had a quality assurance program, and three-fourths reported that a committee guided the quality assurance activities. Three-fourths reported that nondepartmental personnel, such as full-time hospital quality assurance nurses, participated in their quality assurance activities. Eighty-four percent reported that medical care evaluation studies were regularly performed as part of their activities, and more than one-half of the programs evaluated either death and autopsy data, nosocomial infection data, unplanned transfers to intensive care units, unplanned readmissions, serious complications or drug usage. Over three-fourths of all programs review individual cases and have a morbidity and mortality conference as part of their activi-

ties even though it was noted that these were more educationally oriented than being quality of care reviews. Less than one-half of the programs use quality assurance data for physician credentialing or privilege delineation. Although the authors did not include questions in their survey concerning the reasons why particular program structures or activities were chosen, the structure and activities appear to be strongly influenced by JCAHO standards.

The JCAHO has published guidelines for structuring and implementing quality assurance programs (17). Several different models for both hospitalwide and department-specific (although somewhat generic) programs are suggested in the above referenced JCAHO publication. These can be helpful to hospitals that have little experience with a program or to departments that are just beginning to develop a program within an already existing hospitalwide program. The 10-step model, particularly steps 2 and 3 delineating the scope of care and identifying important aspects of care, is particularly helpful in organizing an approach to developing a program. A common temptation for those implementing a program, once they have defined what the department does and what is most important, is to try to take on too much. Not everything on the list of "most important" must be tackled immediately. Resources are limited and a priority list, written into a departmentwide plan, should give both direction to the program and methodical thoroughness to the approach.

Two other very important selection criteria should be applied to the lists of what the department does and what is most important so as to focus resources for quality assurance activities and to put the activities on a sound, rational footing. The purpose of a quality assurance program is to evaluate the quality and appropriateness of care. Quality, as was noted earlier, can be judged only when there is a cause-and-effect relationship between a structure and a process of care, a structure and an outcome of care, or a process and an outcome of care. Appropriateness of care, which can be thought of as "was the right thing done for this patient," is more difficult to determine. Considerable research is currently underway to evaluate "what is the right thing for this type of patient." Up until now, however, the general approach to appropriateness has been expert consensus panels that develop criteria for patients who should receive a particular treatment or procedure. A department can utilize these concepts of quality and appropriateness as selection criteria for evaluating the lists of what a department does and what is most important. The medical literature should be the guide for deciding what structures, processes, or outcomes are causally related as demonstrated by well-designed studies. Both the medical literature and a departmental consensus panel can be used for developing appropriateness of care criteria. A word of caution: the development of appropriateness criteria can be difficult and frustrating, and techniques such as decision theory and branching analysis, concepts newly introduced into medicine, are appearing in this field of research. To the average clinician, appropriateness criteria look like "cookbook" medicine and a substitute for clinical judgment. Despite its frustrations and difficulties, setting up appropriateness criteria often brings to light issues or choices that had not been part of the traditional clinical judgment such as patient preference, cost of different treatment options, and access to care.

Finally, there is a temptation simply to adopt a canned program from another department or another hospital. Doing so bypasses the intellectual exercises of understanding why any one aspect of the program exists. For example, if another hospital's pediatrics department has as an indicator "unplanned admission to the intensive care unit" and it is adopted without examining what your department does and what is important (it may be that unplanned admissions rarely happen and when they do there is no cause-and-effect relationship between the patient's prior care and what prompted the admission) the program will look like make-work with no benefit. This is not to say that some aspects of the program may need to exist for regulatory, accrediting, or payer purposes, but they should be identified as such and those that evaluate quality and appropriateness of care should be thoroughly conceived and defensible to intellectual scrutiny.

SUMMARY

The goal of a quality assurance program in a department of pediatrics is to assess the quality of care provided. Quality of care is defined by the context of the assessment, and three approaches have been suggested: structure, process, and outcome. A judgment concerning quality can be made only when there is a cause-and-effect relationship between any two elements of structure, process, or outcome. The JCAHO provides a model to fashion a quality assurance program; but the elements of structure, process, and outcome that will be evaluated are left to the individual pediatric department. The tools of epidemiology—from critical examination of the medical literature to determine cause-and-effect relationships between elements of structure, process, and outcome to the functional activities of surveillance and data quality, manipulation, and interpretation—are important in developing a credible program for assessing quality of care.

References

1. Accreditation Manual for Hospitals, 1989. Chicago: Joint Commission on Accreditation of Healthcare Organizations, 1988.
2. Hospital Accreditation Program: Scoring Guidelines. Chicago: Joint Commission on Accreditation of Healthcare Organizations, 1988.
3. Medical Staff Monitoring and Evaluation: Departmental Review. Chicago: Joint Commission on Accreditation of Healthcare Organizations, 1988.
4. Anonymous. Characteristics of clinical indicators. QRB 1989;15:330–339.
5. Crede WB, Hierholzer WJ. Surveillance for quality assessment: III. The critical assessment of quality indicators. Infect Control Hosp Epidemiol 1990;11:197–201.
6. Tauber MG, Sande MA. Dexamethasone in bacterial meningitis: Increasing evidence for a beneficial effect. Pediatr Infect Dis J 1989;8:842–844.
7. Koblin BH, Townsend TR, Munoz A, Onarato I, Wilson M, Polk BF. Response of preterm infants to diphtheria-tetanus-pertussis vaccine. Pediatr Infect Dis J 1988;7:704–711.

8. Donabedian A. Quality assessment and assurance: Unity of purpose, diversity of means. Inquiry 1988;25:173–192.

9. Werchsel ME, Greenberg SA. Structuring a departmental quality assurance program: A survey of academic pediatric departments. QRB 1989; 15:153–155.

10. Nakayama DK, Sartz EW, Gardner MJ, Kompare E, Guzik E, Rowe MI. Quality assessment in the pediatric trauma care system. J Pediatr Surg 1989;24:159–162.

11. Kemper KJ. Medically inappropriate hospital use in a pediatric population. N Engl J Med 1988; 318:1033–1037.

12. Kemper KJ, Fink HD, McCarthy PL. The reliability and validity of the pediatric appropriateness evaluation protocol. QRB 1989;15:77–80.

13. Perrin JM, Homer CJ, Berwick DM, Woolf AD, Freeman JL, Wennberg JE. Variations in rates of hospitalization of children in three urban communities. N Engl J Med 1989;320:1183–1187.

14. Wise PH, Eisenberg L. What do regional variations in the rates of hospitalization of children really mean? N Engl J Med 1989;320:1209–1211.

15. Braveman P, Oliva G, Miller MG, Reiter R, Egerter S. Adverse outcomes and lack of health insurance among newborns in an eight-county area of California, 1982 to 1986. N Engl J Med 1989;321:508–5112.

16. Pollack MM, Ruttimann UE, Getson PR. Accurate prediction of the outcome of pediatric intensive care: A new quantitative method. N Engl J Med 1987;316:134–139.

17. The Joint Commission Guide to Quality Assurance. Chicago: Joint Commission on Accreditation of Healthcare Organizations, 1988.

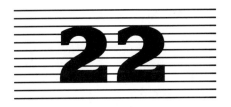

Psychiatry

Michael A. Fauman, Ph.D., M.D.

In 1715 the Dutch physician Herman Boerhaave, who many considered the greatest clinician of his day, proposed the following criteria for the diagnosis of "madness" in his *Aphorisms: Concerning the Knowledge and Cure of Diseases* (1).

If melancholy increases so far, that from the great motion of the liquid of the brain the patient be thrown into a wild fury, it is call'd madness. (Aphorism 1118)

He followed this with specific treatment criteria.

The greatest remedy for it is to throw the patient unwarily into the sea, and to keep him under water as long as he can possibly bear without being quite stifled. (Aphorism 1123)

There has been significant progress in the quality of psychiatric services since that time. Some of the elements of this progress will be discussed in this chapter. However, it is well to remember that even the scientific clinical criteria of today may appear stale in the light of history!

Unlike internal medicine, the pathophysiological bases of most major psychiatric diseases are unknown. There are, as yet, no blood tests for depression, mania, schizophrenia, or anxiety. Unlike surgery, psychiatry cannot definitively remove the diseased parts of the personality leaving behind a functioning system free of illness. However, psychiatrists generally do not despair about the state of their field.

On the contrary, modern discoveries in psychopharmacology, the neurosciences, and the behavioral sciences have given modern psychiatry the capacity to treat many previously untreatable illnesses. These include major depression, manic-depressive illness, obsessive-compulsive disorders, and the broad spectrum of anxiety-related illnesses such as phobias and panic disorders. If the schizophrenias and severe personality disorders still elude a definitive treatment, we are comforted by the similar struggles of our colleagues in other areas of medicine who fight to cure cancer and the degenerative diseases. If the process and outcome of psychotherapeutic treatment cannot be easily measured we know that much of the internist's and surgeon's art, which often determines the difference between a good and bad outcome, is similarly based on judgments that are not easily measured.

What is true about the specialty of psychiatry is also true of its quality assurance (QA). Modern psychiatry is a broad medical specialty that encompasses many diverse treatment approaches. Some of these are simple to monitor whereas others present special assessment problems. This chapter will describe psychiatric quality assurance and highlight the similarities and differences between it and the quality assurance of other medical specialties. First, a brief outline of the specialty of psychiatry will help place the unique problems associated with psychiatric quality assurance in perspective and identify significant differences between psychiatry and other medical specialties. Second, the history of psychiatric quality assurance will be described to highlight the areas in which it differs from the QA of other medical specialties. Third, psychiatric quality assurance will be discussed in the context of the specific requirements of the Joint Commission on Accreditation of Healthcare Organizations (JCAHO) as presented in the *Accreditation Manual for Hospitals* (*AMH*) (2). Finally, the steps necessary to set up a psychiatric QA system will be outlined.

BRIEF OUTLINE OF THE SPECIALTY OF PSYCHIATRY

The diagnostic process in psychiatry depends on data gathered from observations of the patient's behavior, mood, thought processes, and thought content. Mood and thought content usually cannot be verified independent of the patient's report. However, many psychiatric illnesses have distinctive behaviors that occur coincidentally with specific disorders of mood and thought content. Their presence helps to validate the patient's reports of internal feelings and thoughts. For example, depressed patients often exhibit psychomotor retardation, a combination of depressed affect, reduced motoric activity, and slowed thinking. Patients suffering from disturbed thought processes often demonstrate this problem through a disrupted ability to communicate. The data for psychiatric diagnosis is primarily elicited from the clinical interview and the mental status examination. The expanded mental status examination administered by a psychiatrist serves a role analogous to the neurological examination administered by a neurologist. It should include information derived from the patient's report of his or her own thought content and mood (e.g., auditory hallucinations, depression, anxiety), as well as the examiner's observations of the patient's thought processes (e.g., loose associations, paranoid ideation, confusion) and behavior (e.g., psychomotor retardation, pacing, hand wringing, verbal

or physical threats). In the process of diagnosis, psychiatry struggles with many of the same conceptual questions as other fields of medicine. Most notable is the difficulty in determining normalcy or delineating the boundary between normal and abnormal conditions. For example, is an individual who occasionally talks to himself or who feels chronically disillusioned with life suffering from a psychiatric disorder? This problem is analogous to the determination of the boundary between normal and abnormal physiological parameters such as the blood pressure or blood glucose level.

Psychiatrists commonly use sets of explicit criteria in the diagnostic process (Table 22.1). The American Psychiatric Association's *Diagnostic and Statistical Manual* (3rd edition, revised) (*DSM*-IIIR) contains one set of diagnostic criteria that has been accepted as a standard by many clinicians (3). However, psychiatrists also use other criteria sets that may be better suited for diagnosis in specific areas. Since there are no pathognomonic signs for psychiatric illness, diagnosis consists of comparing the patient's signs and symptoms to the criteria for a specific psychiatric syndrome. Like the diagnosis of angina or congestive heart failure, the degree of fit between the symptoms and the criteria will vary. The cluster of criteria in each *DSM*-IIIR diagnostic category describes a quasi-prototype of a psychiatric syndrome and includes options to allow for the normal variation in the clinical presentation of different patients suffering from the same disease process. Even so, it is not unusual to find patients who cannot be fit into any single category because one or more of the necessary criteria for that category are not fulfilled or because the patient fulfills the criteria for more than one category. This latter area of comorbidity is a subject of active research in psychiatry.

The initial challenge in all psychiatric diagnoses is the distinction between organic and so-called functional disease processes. An organic mental disorder is a disorder of thought, mood, anxiety, or behavior that has a clearly discernible physical or biochemical cause. Psychiatrists are always alert to the possibility that the psychiatric disorders they are treating

Table 22.1.
Examples of Criteria for the Diagnosis and Treatment of Depression

Diagnosis of depression
1. The patient reports either a depressed mood or decreased capability to experience pleasure from activities (anhedonia).
2. The patient has experienced four of the following symptoms
   a. Loss or gain of a significant amount of weight
   b. Persistent thoughts of death, thoughts of suicide or a suicide attempt
   c. Persistent fatigue or loss of energy
   d. Persistent difficulty sleeping (insomnia) or excessive sleeping (hypersomnia)
   e. Feelings of excessive or inappropriate guilt or a feeling of worthlessness
   f. Difficulty concentrating or making decisions
   g. Generalized agitation or slowing in thought, movement, and behavior

Treatment of depression with a tricyclic antidepressant medication
1. None of the following contraindications are present
   a. Cardiac conduction delay
   b. Intolerance to antidepressant side effects
   c. Previous nonresponse to a similar antidepressant medication
2. Pretreatment workup includes electrocardiogram (ECG) and complete blood count (CBC)
3. One of the following medications is prescribed at a level not exceeding the maximum dosage shown below. (Reduce the maximum dosage by one-half for patients over the age of 65)

imipramine	(300 mg max dose)
amitriptyline	(300 mg max dose)
desipramine	(300 mg max dose)
doxepin	(300 mg max dose)
amoxapine	(300 mg max dose)
nortriptyline	(150 mg max dose)
protriptyline	(60 mg max dose)

4. If the medication is prescribed at less than the maximum dosage, one of the following reasons is documented.
   a. There is a sufficient therapeutic response at a lower dose
   b. The patient is intolerant of the medication's side affects at the maximum dose.

Response of depression to treatment
1. Patients who receive a diagnosis of depression will be rated on the Hamilton Depression Rating Scale (HDRS) before treatment
2. The initial HDRS score will be above 20
3. Patients will be rated on the HDRS five (5) weeks after the initial diagnosis or at discharge
4. The second HDRS score will be 50% or 10 points below the initial score

---

mask or presage an underlying physical illness. Examples of organic mental disorders include: psychosis associated with adrenal disease; confusion, irritable behavior, or personality changes caused by brain injury or infection; and psychotic behavior secondary to the abuse of illicit drugs such as phencyclidine and amphetamines. However, the presence of an organic disease does not always mean that it is the etiological basis for a concomitant psychiatric illness. A distinction must be made between psychiatric syndromes that are caused by an underlying physical illness and those that are a psychological reaction to a physical illness. Depression in response to chronic illness is an example of the latter.

A functional disease process is a psychiatric illness that has no discernible physical etiology. This does not mean that there is no physical etiology for the illness. The functional grouping merely reflects the present state of knowledge about the pathophysiology of the disease process. Clearly, psychiatric illnesses that respond to medication must have some physical etiology. Examples of functional illnesses include: dysthymic disorders, adjustment reactions, schizophrenia, bipolar disease, and phobias. Most psychiatric care involves the diagnosis and treatment of functional disorders. However, the term functional is controversial and its use is declining.

There are three broad groups of psychiatric treatment: psychotherapy, behavior therapy, and biological therapy (i.e., electroconvulsive therapy (ECT) and psychopharmacology). Psychotherapy is the oldest and probably the most prevalent mode of psychiatric treatment. The techniques used in the various psychotherapies are based on specific theories of the structure of personality, the cognitive organization of the mind, and the nature of human social interaction. Contemporary psychotherapies include: psychoanalysis, cognitive therapy, group therapy, family therapy, and client-centered therapy. The best known psychotherapy is Freudian psychoanalysis. It is based on the concept of dynamic conflict between unconscious thoughts and feelings. Psychoanalysis and its derivative therapies are called "dynamic" psychotherapies. The theory postulates that symptoms are a reflection of the patient's unconscious attempt to reach a compromise between discordant thoughts and feelings and thus resolve the conflict. Psychoanalysts treat patients by asking them to "free associate" or say whatever comes to their mind without censoring their thoughts. The analyst then interprets the unconscious or "latent" meaning of the associations. Complete treatment usually require four to five therapy sessions a week for several years. Only a small number of psychiatrists choose to be trained as psychoanalysts. However, the theory has had an impact far beyond the actual practice of psychoanalysis because it forms the core paradigm of many briefer "dynamic" therapies and is the most prevalent theory taught in psychiatric training programs.

Patients who cannot benefit from or afford psychoanalysis are treated in less intensive psychotherapy for one or two therapy sessions a week over a period of several months or years. Like psychoanalysis, these therapies try to help the patient examine and make changes in multiple aspects of his or her life. Intensive psycho-therapies may be based on the same dynamic theories as psychoanalysis or on other theories of the structure of the mind and personality. Psychotherapies that attempt to make significant changes in many areas of a patient's life require a substantial investment of time and money. However, as fiscal resources become more limited, the emphasis has switched from intensive psychotherapy to the brief psychotherapies that focus on helping the patient deal with one specific, distressing event in his or her life such as a divorce or the diagnosis of a serious medical illness. The entire course of brief therapy may last for only 10–20 sessions. Other therapies, such as group therapy, are also increasingly used because they are cost efficient, treating several patients at one time. They also may be effective for patients with personality disorders who have difficulty understanding how their behavior provokes negative responses from other people. All of the psychotherapies are similar. They depend on a patient reporting internal thoughts and feelings to a therapist who responds by trying to help the patient understand how the feelings produce his or her discomfort. There is no way to validate the information reported by the patient other than by tracking the internal consistency of the reports from session to session and observing the patient's behavior. When successful, the psychotherapies can produce dramatic as well as multiple, subtle changes in the patient's thought processes, mood, and personality. However, the complexity and variability of acceptable treatment approaches make it difficult to monitor the process of psychotherapy, and the subtlety of changes in the patient makes it is difficult to find a few easily measurable parameters that can be used to assess the outcome of therapy. Psychiatrists and psychologists are aware of these problems and are actively conducting research on the question of outcome in psychotherapy.

The behavior modification therapies differ from the dynamic psychotherapies in two ways. First, they depend on the identification of a specific measurable behavior that becomes the target of therapy. Second, there is no attempt to explain the

behavior's etiology by postulating unconscious mental processes. The goal of behavioral therapy is the increase or decrease
in the selected behavior. For example, the
target might be a hand washing ritual
associated with an obsessive-compulsive
disorder. The goal of therapy would be to
decrease the number of times the patient
washes his or her hands each day. Behavior therapies are effective in the treatment
of anxiety disorders, such as phobias,
obsessive-compulsive disorders, and habits, such as smoking. They also may be
applicable whenever a specific problem
behavior can be identified and measured.
Biofeedback therapy is similar to behavior
therapy. It attempts to help the patient
modify an abnormal physiological parameter such as elevated blood pressure or
deficient peripheral circulation that cannot
normally be observed without specialized
monitoring equipment. The monitoring
instrument converts the physiological parameter into a visual, auditory, or tactile
signal that varies in direct relation to the
intensity of the physiological parameter.
The patient learns various techniques to
modify the physiological process in the
desired direction. Since behavior modification depends on the designation of a
specific behavior or physiological parameter to be altered, it is well suited for
outcome monitoring in quality assurance.

Proponents argue that each school of
psychotherapy or behavior therapy is pure
in the sense that treatment within the
paradigm follows specific rules based on
the theoretical basis of the field. However,
this is often not the case. In many situations, the actual treatment approaches of
the various schools overlap. For example,
psychoanalysts commonly identify and
point out their patient's cognitive errors in
thinking, and client-centered therapists
talk about empathy in a manner similar to
that in psychoanalysis. Furthermore, modern behavior therapy depends upon the
establishment of a warm therapeutic relationship between the therapist and patient
that does not preclude identifying the
specific behaviors that need modification.
This relationship is similar to the "therapeutic alliance" described by practitioners
of the dynamic therapies.

The most dramatic advances in psychiatric treatment during the last 40 years have
been in the field of biological psychiatry,
specifically psychopharmacology (4). The
first widely used psychiatric drugs were
the antipsychotic medications (i.e., neuroleptics, major tranquilizers). Developed
in the early 1950s to treat schizophrenia,
they are effective in decreasing the thought
disorder and agitation that are common
symptoms of the illness. Neuroleptics are
also effective for psychotic agitation associated with organic brain disorders and
affective disorders such as major depression or bipolar disorders. However, they
do not cure psychosis; they ameliorate the
symptoms of the disorder. On the other
hand, the antidepressant medications can
cure depression. Unlike the neuroleptics
that have a therapeutic effect immediately,
antidepressants may take 2–3 weeks to
show any appreciable clinical effect. Several classes of antidepressant medication
have been developed. Patients who do not
respond to one class may respond to
another. Lithium was discovered to be an
effective treatment for manic disorders in
the 1940s, but was not officially approved
for use in the United States until the early
1970s. It is the treatment of choice for
manic episodes associated with bipolar
disorders. However, patients must stay on
lithium indefinitely to prevent a relapse.
Significant advances have also been made
in the development of powerful antianxi-
ety medications (i.e., anxiolytics, minor
tranquilizers). The most common minor
tranquilizers belong to a class of medications known as the benzodiazepines. They
are most effective for the short-term treatment of anxiety. Most psychiatrists use
medication and psychotherapy or behavior
therapy in the treatment of depression,
anxiety, and even schizophrenia. The combination of the two modes of treatment
produces a better therapeutic effect than
either one alone.

Based on this brief discussion, the essential elements of psychiatric practice can be
summarized as follows. (*a*) The pathophysiological etiology of most major psychiatric diseases is unknown. (*b*) Most
psychiatric clinical data consist of reports
by patients of their internal thoughts and

mood that are difficult to verify independently. The subjective and complex nature of psychiatric information often requires the development and use of multiparameter rating scales. (*c*) Psychiatric illnesses are generally not associated with significant physiological parameters that can be monitored during treatment. (*d*) Psychiatrists use very few physical procedures in the diagnosis and treatment of patients. (*e*) Several different types of psychotherapy may be effective in treating the same condition. (*f*) Successful treatment with psychotherapy often produces multiple subtle changes in the patient's personality that are difficult to measure objectively. (*g*) Most psychopharmacological agents have their major effect on the patient's thoughts and mood and produce few, if any, physical changes, other than side effects, which can be objectively monitored.

USE OF CRITERIA IN PSYCHIATRY

Criteria are statements that define appropriate clinical care. Professionals define criteria based on their clinical experience and the current scientific literature. Criteria can be classified as *implicit* or *explicit*. Implicit criteria depend on the assessment of the quality of care by expert professionals based on their clinical experience without the use of a set of detailed predetermined rules. The evaluation, by a group of peer review physicians, of the treatment of an individual patient for depression is an example of the use of implicit criteria. Clinical supervision is another example of the application of implicit criteria. Explicit criteria are sets of rules or guidelines that are clearly specified before an assessment is made. Many quality assurance standards contain explicit criteria that stipulate the elements of care for a specific clinical process. Explicit criteria usually relate to the structure (i.e., resources), process (i.e., provision), or outcome (i.e., results) of care (5, 6). There are criteria for many areas of psychiatric care including: diagnosis, pharmacologic therapy, ECT, behavioral therapy, and various types of psychotherapy. Table 22.1 in-

cludes examples of criteria for the diagnosis of major depression, treatment with an antidepressant medication, and outcome of treatment. The American Psychiatric Association is developing an extensive series of "practice parameters" that will include criteria defining acceptable treatment for many psychiatric disorders. Like all standards, the practice parameters will only guide psychiatrists treating patients. Each clinician must use his or her clinical judgment to determine when they should be followed or modified. When a clinician deviates from the standards he or she must document the reasons for the deviation.

USE OF CLINICAL INDICATORS IN PSYCHIATRY

Indicators are well-defined measurable clinical variables that can be used to monitor the provision and outcome of diagnosis and treatment or events that affect the provision of these services (7–11). Medical staff often find the idea of an indicator confusing because they think of it as a monolithic concept. In reality, a clinical indicator is a complex parameter that has several characteristics (Table 22.2). For example, an indicator can include a specific set of explicit criteria, a physiological parameter, or a behavioral event. The concept of a clinical indicator is not new. In 1981, Chambers et al. (12) defined an indicator condition as a frequently occurring treatable clinical situation that often included several criteria. Lane and Kelman (13) developed indicators for pregnancy, and Kessner et al. (14) described the use of tracers or "identifiable health problems" to monitor care. However, none of these systems described quantifiable elements of care that could be measured. A contemporary indicator might best be thought of as a quantifiable answer to a question about the quality of care. For example, "how many patients with schizophrenia were treated according to explicit criteria for the use of neuroleptic medications" or "how many patients on tricyclic antidepressant medication experienced significant electrocardiogram (ECG) changes?" Table 22.3 pre-

Table 22.2.
Characteristics of Psychiatric Indicators

1. Subject of indicator
   What is the main clinical subject of the indicator? (e.g., patient diagnosis, psychotherapy, pharmacotherapy, patient behavior, accidents, etc.)
2. Component of care addressed
   What element of care does the indicator address? (e.g., structure (resources), process (provision of care), outcome (results of care))
3. Specificity of indicator
   Is the indicator specific to one service or treatment modality or is it a general screening indicator that applies to widespread aspect of care, crossing several medical services and disciplines? (e.g., discharge against medical advice (AMA), patient falls)
4. Clinical parameter measured
   a. Criteria of care
      Is the indicator a measure of compliance with an explicit criteria of care? (e.g., criteria for the diagnosis of depression, criteria for the treatment of bipolar disorder with lithium)
   b. Adverse events
      Is the indicator a measure of a specific event associated with patient or staff behavior? (e.g., patient falls, patient assaults, inappropriate patient sexual activity, administration of an incorrect medication, suicide attempt)
   c. Physiological parameter
      Is the indicator a measure of a physiological parameter associated with treatment? (e.g., nosocomial infection, blood pressure following antihypertensive treatment, tardive dyskinesia)

sents a list of possible psychiatric indicators classified by clinical topic. The Joint Commission's use of indicators will be discussed later in this chapter.

HISTORY OF QUALITY ASSURANCE IN PSYCHIATRY

The unique elements of psychiatric diagnosis and treatment discussed previously militated against the early development of meaningful quality assurance programs. As a result, psychiatry lagged behind the other medical specialties in the organization and implementation of these activities for many years. The Community Mental Health Centers (CMHC) Act of 1963 contained general requirements for quality assurance activities. This law induced the National Institute of Mental Health (NIMH) to begin addressing the problems associated with quality assessment of psychiatric services. The first major NIMH supported venture to study this problem was the Psychiatric Utilization Review and Evaluation (PURE) Project, a joint undertaking of the Connecticut Mental Health Center and Yale University (15). The PURE approach depended on the development

of specific treatment criteria, which were used in evaluating the quality of care (16). Additional pressure for quality assurance arose with the creation of the Medicare and Medicaid programs (Public Law 89-94, 1965), which included a requirement for retrospective utilization reviews in all facilities seeking reimbursement under the Medicare and Medicaid systems. Despite these programs, quality assurance in psychiatry during the 1960s was generally rudimentary. Requirements were vague and few people knew how to set up an effective quality assurance system. During the 1970s, several factors helped the development of psychiatric quality assurance programs including: the activities of the American Psychiatric Association (APA) and the NIMH; new federal health care legislation; an increased emphasis on quality assurance by the JCAHO; and protests by third party payers over the rising cost of medical care (7, 17–25). Some of these factors were applicable to all medicine but many were specific to psychiatry. It is difficult to single out any one of these organizations or events as more important than another because they mutually influenced each other. In one sense, they were individual expressions of a general sense

Table 22.3.
Examples of Psychiatric Quality Assurance Indicators

General screening indicators
  Unexpected death
  Suicide
  Discharge against medical advice
  Fall leading to injury
  Severe drug reaction
  Incorrect medication administered to a patient

Diagnostic indicators
  Documentation in medical chart of criteria for *DSM*-IIIR diagnosis
  Failure to diagnose an organic brain disorder

General treatment indicators
  Written integrated treatment plan within 3 days of patient's admission
  Progress note written for each identified problem at least 3 times/week
  Use of physical restraints
  Use of patient seclusion

Pharmacologic indicators
  More than two different medications of same class prescribed in 5 days
  Antiparkinsonian medication prescribed without documented side effects
  Antidepressant medication prescribed according to explicit guidelines
  Lithium prescribed according to explicit guidelines
  Patient on neuroleptic develops tardive dyskinesia
  Patient on neuroleptic develops neuroleptic malignant syndrome
  Physician and patient discussion of medication side effects documented
  Patient signs informed consent for use of neuroleptic medication

Electroconvulsive therapy indicators
  Patient evaluated for increased intracranial pressure before ECT
  Patient achieves a generalized seizure during ECT treatment
  Physiological injury due to ECT or anesthesia
  Significant memory loss after ECT treatment

Substance abuse indicators
  Substance abuse problems are identified and treatment initiated
  Drug withdrawal is recognized and treated without medical complications

Medical records indicators
  Physical examination and history are recorded within 12 hours of patient's admission
  Documentation that abnormal laboratory results have been noted by physician
  Documentation of patient's response or lack of response to medications

Behavior indicators
  Suicide attempt
  Goal-directed violence against another person
  Agitation (functional psychotic or organic based) leading to injury

Admission, discharge, transfer indicators
  Delay in discharge due to difficulty in placement
  Transfer to a medical or surgical service
  Transfer to another psychiatric facility
  Readmission within 1 month after discharge

that quality assurance was a concept whose time had come even if it was not then and is still not entirely clear how it should be achieved.

Federal Legislation and Psychiatric Quality Assurance

The quality assurance program included in the original Medicare and Medicaid programs (Public Law 89-94, 1965) was ineffective. This led to the 1972 amendment of the Social Security Act (Public Law 92-603) that established the Professional Standard Review Organizations (PSROs) (7, 22, 23, 26). The PSROs reviewed the clinical services in each institution reimbursed under the Medicare, Medicaid, and Title V programs (Maternal and Child Health Program and Crippled Children's Services). Each PSRO developed explicit clinical criteria based on "model criteria sets" that were being developed by various national medical specialty groups under the coordination of the American Medical Association (AMA). The American Psychiatric Association responded by developing its Model Criteria Sets in 1974 (27). The PSRO quality assurance requirements did not apply to those programs funded through the Community Mental Health Centers Act of 1963. Therefore, in 1975 Congress passed the Community Mental Health Centers Amendments (Public Law 94-63). It contained three new quality assurance requirements: (a) the development of a set of national standards for all CMHCs; (b) the development of quality assurance programs in each CMHC; and (c) the use of quality assurance data in the evaluation of CMHC programs. The National Institute of Mental Health took the lead in the development of QA standards for the CMHCs. Two sets of standards were developed, one by the NIMH directly and a second by the Joint Commission under contract from the NIMH. The former draft standard was submitted to Congress in 1977 in compliance with the first QA requirement of the new law. The latter resulted in the publication of a JCAHO accreditation manual for CMHCs. Although similar, there were significant dif-

ferences between the two standards (18, 28). The new act also incorporated several features intended to make sure that the quality assurance programs that were to be developed in each CMHC could interface with the PSRO quality assurance requirements (18). However, the draft standards were never enacted and the Community Mental Health Amendments of 1975 were subsequently repealed.

In 1982 Congress passed the Tax Equity and Fiscal Responsibility Act (TEFRA) (Public Law 97-248, 1982) that created the Peer Review Organizations (PROs) (29). The general review provision of the PROs included psychiatry. In 1983, amendments to the Social Security Act (Public Law 98-21) created the Medicare Prospective Pricing System (PPS) that introduced the Diagnosis-Related Group (DRG). The DRG system was an attempt to categorize medical diagnoses so they could be compared, from institution to institution, on parameters such as the length of stay. Most psychiatric services have been excluded from the DRG system because psychiatric diagnosis categories do not readily correlate with parameters such as the length of stay. However, there have been recent attempts to apply DRGs to psychiatric patients who fall under the Medicaid and Medicare systems.

American Psychiatric Association and Quality Assurance

The American Psychiatric Association began to be active in quality assurance in the 1960s when it encouraged the Joint Commission to develop separate standards for psychiatric facilities (23). In 1973, the APA created an Ad Hoc Committee on PSROs to respond to the review requirements of the PSRO legislation (Public Law 92-60, 1972). The committee was responsible for developing the APA's model criteria sets for use in the review of clinical diagnosis (30, 31). The Ad Hoc Committee on PSROs was dissolved in 1974 and replaced by a new Task Force on Peer Review that began preparing a set of broad peer review guidelines for the practice of psychiatry.

The Task Force developed the current quality assurance guidelines of the APA contained in the 3rd edition of the *Manual of Psychiatric Peer Review* (4). The manual defines psychiatric peer review as, "a review process by psychiatrists concerned with utilization review, quality review, continuing education, advocacy for improved care with intermediaries, and cost control" (32, p. 3). In essence, psychiatric peer review, so defined, corresponds to quality assurance as defined by other specialties. During the 1970s most district branches of the APA set up independent peer review committees to oversee the quality of care provided by individual psychiatrists.

The APA also recognized the need for the creation of clear and consistent criteria for psychiatric diagnosis. The 2nd edition of the association's *Diagnostic and Statistical Manual* (*DSM*-II, 1968) included a general description of the major psychiatric disorders with few specific necessary and sufficient criteria for the diagnosis. Clinicians had a great deal of leeway in the diagnosis. As a result, the validity and reliability of the diagnostic process was difficult to determine. In response to these problems, the APA developed the 3rd edition of the *Diagnostic and Statistical Manual* (*DSM*-III, 1981) that contained specific inclusion and exclusion criteria for the diagnosis of psychiatric disorders. The current version of the manual is a revision of the 3rd edition (*DSM*-III-R) (3). Work is progressing on the 4th edition (*DSM*-IV) that will be accompanied by research support material substantiating the diagnostic categories and criteria.

Third Party Payer and Psychiatric Quality Assurance

Third party payers have exerted substantial pressure for the development of quality assurance and utilization review programs in psychiatry. The American Psychiatric Association became involved in the peer review process in 1974 when the Department of Defense's Civilian Health and Medical Program for the Uniformed Services (CHAMPUS) and insurance carriers in the Federal Employees Health Benefit Program (FEHBP) announced that they

were cutting mental health benefits. The cuts were motivated by cost-containment concerns and questions about the efficacy of some of the treatment modalities they had been reimbursing (17). The third party payers agreed to rescind their cutbacks when the APA pledged to work with them to develop a review process for inpatient and outpatient care. In 1977, CHAMPUS contracted with the American Psychiatric Association to develop a quality assurance review system for psychiatric inpatient and outpatient services and the American Psychological Association to create a quality assurance peer review system for outpatient psychological services (33–36). Private insurance groups followed the lead of CHAMPUS in contracting with the professional groups for peer review of patients covered under their programs (37, 38).

The American Psychiatric Association's program used psychiatrists in each district branch as peer reviewers (36). The therapist submitted detailed treatment about each reviewed case. The reviewers used explicit and implicit criteria to determine whether care was being provided in an appropriate manner. The CHAMPUS program's strengths included its use of senior expert reviewers, establishment of uniform treatment report formats, and use of empirical data to develop explicit criteria. Its weaknesses came from the exclusive reliance on potentially inaccurate data submitted by providers and the reliance on reports of the process of care rather than its outcome (34, 38). Furthermore, there was little information concerning the cost-effectiveness of the program when compared to other methods of quality assurance. Finally, there was some evidence suggesting that the theoretical orientation of the senior peer reviewers had an effect on their judgment of the appropriateness of care (39–42).

JCAHO and Psychiatric Quality Assurance

The Joint Commission has played a role second only to the federal government in the development of standards for mental health facilities. The Joint Commission publishes the *Accreditation Manual for Hos-*

pitals (*AMH*), which contains its general quality assurance standards (2). In 1970, the JCAHO established the Council on Accreditation of Psychiatric Facilities in response to encouragement from the American Psychiatric Association (23). This was followed by the development of separate sets of standards for adult psychiatric services, child and adolescent psychiatric services, community mental health centers, and alcohol and drug abuse programs. The Joint Commission subsequently combined these standards in the *Consolidated Standards Manual* (*CSM*). The *CSM* is used to survey freestanding and chronic care psychiatric programs not eligible for survey under the *AMH* (25). The *AMH* is currently used to evaluate psychiatric services in general medical hospitals.

In 1975, JCAHO developed an audit system of retrospective review of medical care called the Performance Evaluation Procedure for Auditing and Improving Patient Care (20, 43). These audits were not effective in psychiatry because they focused on a very narrow element of care (e.g., the treatment of bipolar disorder with lithium), required a large amount of resources to complete and were rarely used to modify treatment policies. In the 1980 edition of the *AMH*, the Joint Commission broadened the number and scope of required quality assurance activities to focus on problem identification, assessment, and resolution (44). Many medical staff members continued to have difficulty with the problem identification process. In the 1985 revision of the *AMH*, the Joint Commission responded by introducing a 10-step process to guide monitoring activities (9). This was followed in 1986 by a new program called the "Agenda for Change" that stressed the outcome of clinical care rather than the process of providing care (10, 11, 45–47). To assess clinical outcome, JCAHO began to develop a series of indicators or screening devices for monitoring high volume, high risk, or problem-prone areas of clinical practice (46). Currently, there are no JCAHO indicators for psychiatry. Therefore, it is the responsibility of each psychiatry department to develop its own indicators.

APPLICATION OF CURRENT JCAHO QA REQUIREMENTS TO PSYCHIATRY

There is no separate section on the specialty of psychiatry in the AMH or the CSM. Therefore, psychiatric QA follows the general JCAHO QA requirements in each manual. Since the requirements in the two manuals are similar, this chapter will discuss only the QA standards contained in the AMH. The effective application of the Joint Commission's quality assurance standards to the field of psychiatry depends upon their reconciliation with the unique aspects of psychiatric diagnosis and treatment discussed earlier. The first three standards (QA.1–QA.3) in the quality assurance section of the Joint Commission's 1991 *Accreditation Manual for Hospitals* contain the required characteristics for the development, scope, and activities of a QA program (2). These standards will be examined in terms of their implementation in psychiatric practice that differs in some ways from their application to other medical specialties. The fourth standard (QA.4) refers to the administration and coordination of the hospital's overall quality assurance program. This process is no different in psychiatry than the other medical specialties and will not be discussed further.

Establishment of a Quality Assurance Program (QA.1)

The initial standard (QA.1) contains the general quality assurance requirements for the health care organization and stipulates that it must do the following: establish a quality assurance program (QA.1.1); monitor the quality and appropriateness of patient care (QA.1.2); develop a written quality assurance plan (QA.1.3); and integrate risk management and quality assurance functions (QA.1.4,QA.1.5) (2). These general organizational requirements are as applicable to psychiatry as to any other medical specialty. In psychiatry, the process usually begins with the appointment of a director of quality assurance and a QA committee who are responsible for creating a written QA plan and developing a

QA program. The plan must include provisions for the establishment of ongoing clinical monitoring of patient care. The QA section of the *AMH* contains guidelines for identifying important aspects of care to monitor. Functional links must be established between the psychiatry QA committee, the health care organization QA committee and the risk management department. The association between psychiatry and risk management must be a two-way relationship. Psychiatry must trust the risk management department with confidential information about patient care that could prove embarrassing to individual clinicians. Conversely, risk management must supply psychiatry with information about events that could, or do, adversely affect patients and might lead to litigation. This information should be used to identify and correct possible clinical problems.

Scope of the Quality Assurance Program (QA.2)

The second standard (QA.2) stipulates the scope of the quality assurance program by describing the type of activities it must include. There are several required characteristics in this standard that apply to psychiatry.

Monthly Departmental QA Meeting (QA.2.1.1.1)

The psychiatry department must hold monthly meetings to discuss the results of the ongoing monitoring program. Effective monitoring activities usually provide a significant amount of information to be discussed in the meetings. However, quality assurance meetings must do more than discuss monitoring data to be successful. The major goal of the meeting should be to identify and solve problems related to the provision of appropriate clinical care. Participants should be reassured that the proceedings of the meeting are confidential. The tone of the meeting should be nonaccusatory, starting with the premise that the participants are competent and doing their best to provide quality care. Each participant will find that his or her decisions are the subject of inquiry at some point during the meetings. If individual clinicians feel under attack, they will become defensive and secretive about their clinical decisions and will find ways to avoid participating in the meetings. Eventually they will start to obstruct the quality assurance process. In this sense, it is important for the director of quality assurance to be associated with a clinical service so that he or she will not be considered to be immune from scrutiny in the QA process. Perhaps most important is the establishment of an atmosphere of inquiry in which clinicians feel they can openly discuss problems that arise in the care of their patients. The emphasis on a scholarly problem-solving approach does not mean that clinicians can abrogate responsibility for their decisions. Those practitioners who consistently display poor clinical judgment can be managed through the credentialing process or confronted about their performance in private conferences with the department chairman or discipline chief.

Drug Usage Evaluation (QA.2.1.1.3)

The prescription of psychotrophic medication by physicians has been studied many times (48–51). Generally, concern has focused on the discovery of the following prescribing patterns: (a) prescription of medication at dosages that are above the maximum recommended level; (b) polypharmacy; (c) prolonged prescription of medications without documentation of sufficient indications for continued treatment; and (d) the prescription of psychotrophic medications for psychiatric illnesses in which they are not indicated. However, some investigators have noted that many of these studies do not take into account the variability of patient presentation nor the appropriateness of the drug standards that were used (52). Other studies show that nonpsychiatrists prescribe a significant amount of psychotrophic medication in a manner that is not consistent with accepted guidelines (49, 53). Therefore, psychotrophic drug usage monitoring probably should extend beyond the field of psychiatry. The prescription of psychotrophic drugs is one area in psychiatry where quantitative treatment standards are clearly established. There are effective medications for the treatment of psychosis, affective disorders, obsessive-compulsive disorders, anxiety disorders, and other psychiatric problems. Each of these classes of medications has appropriate indications and recommended dosage ranges. As a result, this area of practice has become a prime focus for quality assurance monitoring in psychiatry.

Several general guidelines for the use of psychotrophic medication can be discussed. The initial consideration in the monitoring of drug usage is whether the physician has made an appropriate decision to use or not use a specific medication for a particular illness. This can be a difficult clinical decision because there are psychiatric disorders, such as depression, where antidepressant medications are indicated in some circumstances and psychotherapy in others. These judgments require a significant amount of experience. When a medication is prescribed, its use should be consistent with the generally acceptable practice of the profession. For example, antidepressant medication should not be prescribed for patients who are acutely psychotic because it may exacerbate the patient's psychosis. Neuroleptic or antipsychotic medication is generally the treatment of choice for acute psychosis. For patients who are suffering from a major depression, antidepressant medication should be administered in amounts that ensure that the medication reaches an adequate blood level for successful treatment. Some drugs require specific pretreatment laboratory tests before they are given to the patient. For example, treatment with lithium requires prior evaluation of thyroid and kidney function. The accepted practice in the treatment of patients with psychotropic medication is to avoid polypharmacy. Generally, it is not appropriate to prescribe more than one medication of the same class at the same time. These psychopharmacologic guidelines can be found in the *Peer Review Manual* of the American Psychiatric Association and in several textbooks on the subject. However, guidelines represent an expression of the *average* standard of care that may not fit individual outlier cases.

There must be a mechanism that allows the clinician to deviate from the standard in cases that do not seem to respond to accepted practice. Currently there are few specific rules to cover these situations. In fact, this is a very complex problem that raises significant questions about the nature of psychiatric diagnosis and treatment that cannot be discussed in depth in this chapter. Some clinicians suggest that this is when the art of medicine is most important. Others suggest that this is when the clinician's biases in judgment are most apparent. Nevertheless, it seems reasonable under these circumstances to allow the physician a moderately free hand to treat as he or she sees fit as long as the reasons for the decision are documented in the patient's medical chart. This documentation should include some objective assessment of the patient's condition before and during the course of treatment.

Medical Record Review (QA.2.1.1.4)

Successful clinical management theoretically depends on accurate records of a patient's diagnosis, treatment, and response to treatment. The Joint Commission has stipulated that the medical staff must routinely collect information about the quality of the medical records. This review should assess the completeness, clarity, accuracy, timeliness, and clinical pertinence of the record. The Joint Commission requires the following elements in a complete medical record: medical history, comprehensive physical assessment, diagnostic and therapeutic orders, reports from consultants, reports of diagnostic tests and all procedures, progress notes, a statement of the conclusions drawn from the history and physical examination, and a treatment plan (46). Psychiatric records are more complex than medical or surgical records because they must include an account of the patient's psychiatric and physical problems. In addition, they must document any interactions between the physical and psychiatric illness in the form of organic brain disorders or psychiatric reactions to physical illness. However, not all psychiatric records are identical in terms of the type of medical information they should contain. The psychiatrist's responsibility for the patient's medical problems differs depending upon whether the patient is treated in an inpatient or outpatient setting.

The psychiatrist has the total responsibility for the physical as well as the psychological care of hospitalized patients because they are not free to act on their own to seek help for physical problems. However, it would be inappropriate to expect a psychiatrist to treat all of the patient's physical problems without the help of other medical specialists. The inpatient medical chart should ideally include the following information about the patient's physical care: (*a*) a complete physical and medical history; (*b*) a list of identified physical problems; (*c*) requests for consultations from the appropriate specialists for the identified problems; (*d*) documentation that the consultation responses have been read and considered, and appropriate action has been taken to implement the recommendations for the care of the patient; (*e*) documentation that arrangements have been made for the consultant to see the patient in follow-up or officially take over the management of the patient's physical problems; (*f*) documentation of any presumed relationship between the patient's physical and psychiatric problems; and (*g*) ongoing notes documenting the progress in treatment of the identified physical problems.

In the outpatient setting, the psychiatrist has less responsibility for the patient's medical problems. If he or she identifies or suspects that the patient has a physical problem, the psychiatrist should urge the patient to seek medical attention for the problem from the appropriate specialist. The psychiatrist is not a primary care physician and therefore is not responsible for the patient's total medical care. The patient's chart should contain documentation of the psychiatrist's observations and recommendations to the patient as well as some assessment of the possible relationship between any physical problem and the patient's psychiatric problem. As long as the patient can act independently, it is his or her responsibility to seek the appropriate medical care.

The content of the psychiatric portion of the patient's medical record again reflects those aspects of care the psychiatrist is responsible for providing. Although many nonpsychiatric mental health professionals play an important role in the treatment of the patient, the psychiatrist remains ultimately responsible for the patient's care. Each nonpsychiatric mental health profession has its own requirements for quality assurance that will not be discussed here. In some ways, the required documentation of psychiatric problems is simpler than medical problems because the psychiatrist is solely responsible for this aspect of the patient's care. Furthermore, there are fewer differences between the responsibilities for inpatient and outpatient psychiatric care. The patient's record should contain the following information within the first 24–48 hours of the patient's admission to an inpatient service: (*a*) a psychiatric and social history; (*b*) a list of past and present psychiatric medications; (*c*) a complete mental status examination; (*d*) assessment of suicidal or homicidal ideation or intent; (*e*) a formulation or synthesis of the patient's psychiatric problems; (*f*) a diagnosis by *DSM*-IIIR criteria; and (*g*) a treatment plan with specific goals. The use of a problem list in psychiatry has been controversial because some authorities have argued that problems are difficult to measure when they cannot be easily quantitated or objectively verified. This problem is common for many psychiatric problems such as hallucinations, thought disorders, or depression. Others have argued for a more behavioral approach to problem identification that would substitute readily identifiable behaviors such as psychomotor retardation, disorganization, confusion, and agitation in place of internal thoughts and emotions. The patient's psychological functioning is more than a sum of behaviors. Therefore, any system of management and documentation that ignores the patient's internal psychological state will not be acceptable to the field. One possible solution is the use of standardized scales such as the Beck Depression Inventory (BDI), Brief Psychiatric Rating Scale (BPRS), or Global Assessment Scale (GAS) to record the patient's status. These scales combine observations of the patient's behavior and documentation of the patient's reports of internal thoughts and emotions. However, their administration is time consuming and requires additional staff training. Suffice to say that the patient's psychiatric problems must be documented in the medical record even if they seem more subjective than physical problems. Furthermore, there must be a record of the ongoing treatment and its effects on the resolution of these problems.

Psychiatrists also must consider the issue of confidentiality in the documentation of the patient's psychiatric difficulties since these problems incur more stigma in the society than most physical problems. Therefore, psychiatrists are often circumspect in the documentation of these problems, especially in an outpatient record. Sexual, marital, interpersonal, and affective problems and fantasies are often described in a vague fashion to protect the patient should the record ever become public. Attempts to describe the patient's concerns as problems of daily life may belie the serious nature of many psychiatric disorders in an attempt to sanitize them. However, not all vague medical records are a result of the psychiatrist's attempts to protect the patient. Some are due to an imprecise articulation of the patient's problems and treatment. A solution to this problem may depend more on society's enactment of secure confidentiality laws than any attempt to force psychiatrists to compromise their patients' future social well being.

Utilization Review (UR) (QA.2.3.2)

The rising cost of health care makes it imperative that health care organizations improve their efficiency at the same time they maintain the quality of the care they provide. The Joint Commission requires that each organization review its clinical operations to identify any examples of overutilization, underutilization, or inefficient scheduling of resources (46). A delay in the treatment with lithium of a bipolar patient because the necessary baseline thyroid function and renal function tests were not scheduled in a timely fashion is an example of the inefficient utilization of hospital resources. The extended hospitali-

zation of an elderly demented patient awaiting appropriate placement and the hospitalization of a nonsuicidal, depressed patient who could be adequately treated as an outpatient are examples of overutilization. A typical case of underutilization of resources is the treatment of a depressed patient with antidepressant medication at a dose that is too low to maintain an adequate blood level of the medication. The UR process includes (*a*) a preadmission review to assess the appropriateness of entry to the hospital and (*b*) a concurrent review during the patient's stay in the hospital to assess the appropriate progress of treatment. The information collected by the UR process should help develop a program to plan, organize, and control the organization's resources in the most cost-effective manner consistent with high quality care.

Utilization review in psychiatry differs in important ways from that in other medical specialties. Because of the social stigma, the psychiatric UR process must be accomplished in a way that carefully protects the confidentiality of the patient. Utilization review is often based on a comparison of the patient's length of stay (LOS) with the average length of stay of patients in a similar diagnostic grouping. Although this relationship appears to hold in surgery and internal medicine, it does not in psychiatry. There is little consistent relationship between psychiatric diagnosis and the length of inpatient treatment. This means that psychiatric UR must be based on diagnosis-independent, explicit criteria such as homicidal and suicidal ideation, overt psychosis, or agitation.

Review of Accidents, Injuries, and Patient Safety (QA.2.3.3)

Psychiatric patients and staff suffer the same injuries due to falls, exposure to contaminated materials, and unsafe working conditions as patients and staff in other specialties. However, there are two types of injuries that may be more common on a psychiatric service than in other specialties—inappropriate sexual contact and violence. Patients on a psychiatric service are generally intact physically. Therefore, many of the sexual feelings that decrease in intensity or disappear during physical illness remain unaltered during psychiatric illness. In fact, many psychiatric illnesses have a prominent sexual component. Furthermore, the group process on an inpatient psychiatric service attempts to enhance the patient's expression of strong feelings as part of the process of decreasing the patient's feelings of isolation and alienation. Although there are strong proscriptions against the acting out of sexual feeling in the hospital setting, such acts occasionally do occur. They can produce significant injury to both participants but especially to the more impaired or vulnerable partner. Many hospitalized psychiatric patients are not in the position to make a mature, independent, and rational choice about sexual involvement or to resist persistent sexual advances made by other patients. Therefore, such activity may be considered an assault if one partner is unable to understand the nature of the activity or resist it. The situation is obviously even more serious if it involves a mental health professional and a patient.

Violence can occur on many medical services but is more frequent on a psychiatric service. Patients may be suicidal or commit violent acts against staff or other patients. Some patients, such as those with certain personality disorders or substance abuse problems, can control their behavior and should be held responsible for any violence they commit. Other patients may not be able to control their violent behavior because it is a direct consequence of an acute psychosis or an organic brain disorder. These patients cannot be held responsible for their violent behavior and must be controlled by the staff. Violence can be managed by physical methods or by medication. The choice of one or the other management method depends on the etiology of the violence. Antipsychotic medication is often useful in controlling violence caused by psychosis or organic brain disorders. Sometimes a physical method such as restraint or seclusion is necessary. The Joint Commission requires that institutions develop specific guidelines for the use of physical restraint or seclusion to ensure patient safety (2, 25).

Credentialing and Clinical Privileges (QA.2.4 and QA.2.5)

The Joint Commission requires that institutions use the information from the various QA activities to help make decisions about credentialing and privileges for clinicians who can practice independently and those who cannot. The former group generally includes staff psychiatrists, whereas the latter includes house officers and nonphysician mental health professionals. Several different types of QA information can be used in the assessment of the medical staff. Individual patterns of psychopharmacologic drug prescription should be examined. The circumstances under which they prescribe physical methods of control, such as restraints or seclusion, should be explored. Medical records can be surveyed to ensure that they are complete and that the clinical information is entered in a timely and legible fashion. House officers who cannot practice independently are monitored by a process called clinical supervision. Supervision was originally developed to guide psychiatrists and other mental health professionals as they learned to practice psychotherapy. Its use was subsequently extended to provide teaching and monitoring for other aspects of psychiatric treatment including the prescription of psychopharmacologic medication. Supervisory reports are a confidential data source that could, under clearly defined circumstances, be used for credentialing and granting clinical privileges. Information from other nonphysician mental health professionals can be gathered from the QA monitoring of their individual disciplines.

QA Monitoring Using Clinical Indicators (QA.3)

The Joint Commission has described a 10-step process that can be used by practitioners to identify and monitor clinical indicators of important aspects of care. The process identifies opportunities to improve and correct problems in care (QA.3.1). The emphasis is on those aspects of care that affect large numbers of patients, are associated with high risk, or produce problems for patients or staff (QA.3.2). The 10 steps include: the assignment of organizational responsibility for the monitoring process; the delineation of the range of care provided by the institution; the identification of important aspects of care; the identification of indicators for monitoring these aspects of care; the establishment of indicator thresholds that, when crossed, will prompt further evaluation of care; the collection of indicator data; the evaluation of problems with specific elements of care identified when indicator thresholds are reached; the correction of deficits in care; the reassessment of care to determine the effectiveness of corrective actions; and the communication of the results of the monitoring process throughout the organization. The JCAHO has begun to develop standardized indicators for each medical specialty, which every accredited hospital will be required to monitor. Currently there are no pilot indicators for psychiatry. The nonquantitative nature of some psychiatric treatments, such as the psychotherapies, hinders the development of indicators. However, there are objective and quantifiable indicators for several other areas of psychiatry (Table 22.3).

IMPLEMENTING A PSYCHIATRIC QUALITY ASSURANCE PROGRAM

This section presents an outline for the development of a comprehensive psychiatric quality assurance program that includes many of the specific JCAHO QA standards (Table 22.4). The code number for each standard is noted to the right of the applicable line in the table. There are five main stages in the implementation of a psychiatric QA system: (*a*) establish the organizational structure of the QA program; (*b*) educate clinical staff about the QA process; (*c*) establish review systems to identify and collect QA data; (*d*) analyze QA data from all sources and resolve the identified problems in patient care; and (*e*) communicate the results of the QA process. Each of these stages includes several more specific steps.

Psychiatry, more than many other medical specialties, depends on an interdisciplinary team approach to treatment. Therefore, an effective psychiatric QA program requires an organizational structure that integrates the clinical work of the various disciplines and clinical services in the department. A departmental quality assurance committee should be formed with members from each of the disciplines (e.g., psychiatry, social work, nursing, psychology, and occupational therapy) and clinical services (e.g., outpatient, consultation liaison, inpatient, day treatment, emergency, substance abuse). Each representative is responsible for developing and maintaining QA activities in their respective discipline or service. Optimally, the representatives to the QA committee should be the heads of each of the disciplines and services. The various discipline and clinical service QA committees serve as an arena for the discussion of problems and successes in the provision of clinical care. The departmental QA committee provides a forum for integration of quality assurance information from the various components of the department that might not normally communicate routinely.

The departmental, clinical service and discipline meetings are the best setting for quality assurance education. The QA process is alien and somewhat threatening to many clinicians. Their initial reaction is to resist the process and complain that it interferes with the provision of clinical care. It is uncomfortable for anyone to feel that their decisions are constantly under scrutiny. Two techniques help minimize this resistance, humor and an emphasis on the scholarly aspects of patient care. Many of the incidents reported in the meeting can be the basis for jokes that might be seen as insensitive by individuals outside of the profession. They serve a purpose in decreasing tension and allowing the participants to examine their decisions and clinical problems that have a significant effect on the life of patients. The key to educating staff about quality assurance is an emphasis on the scholarly aspects of the process. For example, monitoring results may raise appropriate questions about the limita-

Table 22.4.
Implementing a Psychiatric Quality Assurance Program

1. Organize the QA program	
Appoint a director of QA	QA.1.1
Organize a departmental QA committee	
Organize discipline and clinical service QA committees	
Create a written QA plan	QA.1.3
Establish operational links with risk management	QA.1.4, QA.1.5
2. Educate clinical staff about the QA process	
Organize a monthly departmental staff QA meeting	QA.2.1.1.1
Organize QA meetings for clinical disciplines and services	
Organize QA workshops and seminars	
3. Establish review systems to identify and collect QA data	
Utilization review	QA.2.3.2
Morbidity and mortality (M and M) meetings	
Accident and Incident reports	QA.2.3.3
Medical record review	QA.2.1.1.4
Indicator monitoring (JCAHO 10-step model)	QA.3
Drug usage evaluation	QA.2.1.1.3
4. Analyze QA data from all sources; resolve identified problems	QA.3
Determine cause of serious individual incidents	
Establish formal mechanisms to resolve individual problems	
Search for trends in patient care problems	
Establish formal mechanism to resolve repeated problems	
5. Communicate QA data, analysis, and interpretation	
To clinical staff within the clinical service	
To other clinical services and disciplines	QA.4.2
To the larger institution	QA.4.2

tions of the diagnostic or treatment process. These may lead to searches in the medical literature or the design of studies in an attempt to solve the problem. Generally, if the medical staff feels that the quality assurance process is interesting and intellectually stimulating, they are more likely to participate actively in departmental, clinical service and discipline meetings. Under some circumstances, the monthly meetings must be augmented with seminars and workshops. These are useful to introduce staff to the formal JCAHO QA requirements and to train members of the staff who will be monitoring routine clinical care. The QA educational process is usually slow because clinicians must explicitly identify and investigate important elements of care that they usually perform intuitively. Furthermore, as these elements of care are scrutinized, their rationale often begins to appear less certain than before. For example,

clinical impressions suggesting that some neuroleptic medications are appropriate for paranoid patients whereas others should be used for geriatric patients seem less convincing. The result of the process is often a more critical approach to the field and a reduction in the number of questionable treatment approaches.

The quality assurance process depends on data gathered from two broad systems: (a) ongoing review of previously identified important aspects of care and (b) documentation of individual complications in patient care and adverse incidents involving patients and staff. Many of the components of the former (e.g., utilization review, medical record review, indicator monitoring, and drug usage evaluation) have been discussed previously. It is the responsibility of the various disciplines and clinical services to identify elements of care that will be continuously reviewed in these processes. However, important issues in care cannot always be identified in advance. The components of the latter system, morbidity and mortality (M and M) meetings, and incident reports provide mechanisms to capture unanticipated problems in patient care. Morbidity and mortality meetings, in particular, provide some of the more important and interesting issues for discussion in QA meetings. These may include failures to respond to treatment, unusual severe reactions to medication, episodes of violence, or significant staff discord provoked by particularly provocative patients with personality disorders. Each clinical service should produce M and M reports and present them in the departmental QA meeting. Often M and M reports and incident reports will identify problems in care that should be continuously monitored. These will then become the basis for the development of new clinical indicators.

Quality assurance data must be analyzed for patterns that indicate significant problems or successes in the provision of care. The conclusions of this analysis should be presented to the clinical staff for discussion. The use of this information to improve clinical care is probably the most important part of the process. A formal mechanism must be developed to ensure that problems in the provision of care are resolved and successful clinical processes are broadly applied throughout the department. The results of these interventions should be presented to the clinical staff for discussion during the various QA meetings. This latter process is part of the last step in implementation of the QA program, the communication of QA findings to other components of the department and the health care organization.

FUTURE OF PSYCHIATRIC QUALITY ASSURANCE

During the last 75 years, quality assurance has evolved from the assessment of a few minimal standards, which most clinicians today would find primitive, to extensive programs monitoring the provision and outcome of important elements of care. Despite this progress, many questions remain unanswered. The definition of quality in medicine itself remains uncertain. The public often has one definition whereas members of the profession have another. Debate continues about whether the measure of quality should be the adherence to clinical standards, the successful outcome of care, or another altogether different parameter. Health care providers are devoting significant resources to quality assurance, yet few studies have demonstrated the effectiveness of these programs in producing quality care. Future research must address this question. The continuing work on the development of indicators and criteria shows how difficult it is for professionals to identify or to agree on quality standards. Furthermore, the amount of time and effort necessary to collect quality assurance information means that only a few elements of care can be monitored at the same time. Critics of contemporary quality assurance rightly question whether these few elements are truly representative of the care provided by the entire health care organization. One obvious solution to this problem is to increase the scope that is monitored. If this is to be done without an enormous outlay of additional resources, new methods must be devised to record and evaluate clinical care as it is provided rather than relying on periodic review of medical records. This will require the development of standardized methods of recording clinical information that are sensitive to, but not overwhelmed by, the variation inherent in all disease processes.

If the medical profession has difficulty defining quality care, the public is often just the opposite. To many patients, quality care is equated with a successful outcome. Anything less is often seen as an indication that care was inadequate and redress is appropriate. To a great extent, the profession is responsible for this perception. The news media reports miraculous new treatments, often without a discussion of the likelihood of success or risks inherent in all procedures. Physicians have, in the past, been accustomed to practicing unchallenged and unquestioned. However, current social and political concerns about accountability and the cost of care make it clear that this is a thing of the past. If patients demand accountability, it is only fair that they understand the uncertainties intrinsic to all medical care. The road to quality in medicine is not always straight or free from obstruction. Chance alone will often dictate that some medical processes will go awry in the best of institutions where all appropriate standards have been followed. It is the medical profession's obligation, and perhaps its best defense, to educate patients about these uncertainties so that they have more control over their lives and thereby relieve physicians of responsibilities that are not really their's to shoulder.

References

1. Boerhaave H. Aphorisms: Concerning the knowledge and cure of diseases. London: B. Cowse and W. Innys, 1715.
2. Joint Commission on Accreditation of Healthcare Organizations: Accreditation manual for hospitals. Chicago: Joint Commission on Accreditation of Healthcare Organizations, 1991.
3. American Psychiatric Association. Diagnostic and statistical manual of mental disorders DSM-III-R. Washington, D.C.: American Psychiatric Association, 1987.
4. American Psychiatric Association. Manual of psychiatric peer review. Washington, D.C.: American Psychiatric Association, 1985.
5. Donabedian A. Criteria and standards for quality assessment and monitoring. QRB 1986;12:99–108.
6. Donabedian A. The criteria and standards of quality. Ann Arbor: Health Administration Press, 1982.
7. Fauman MA. Quality assurance monitoring in psychiatry. Am J Psychiatry 1989;146:1121–1130.
8. Lehmann R. Joint Commission forum: Forum on clinical indicator development: A discussion of the use and development of indicators. QRB 1989;15:223–227.
9. Joint Commission on Accreditation of Hospitals. Monitoring and evaluation of the quality and appropriateness of care: A hospital example. QRB 1986;12:326–330.
10. Joint Commission on Accreditation of Healthcare Organizations: Monitoring and evaluating the quality and appropriateness of care. Chicago: Joint Commission on Accreditation of Healthcare Organizations, January 1988.
11. Joint Commission on Accreditation of Healthcare Organizations: Agenda for change update, Vol. 1., No.1. Chicago: Joint Commission on Accreditation of Healthcare Organizations, September 1987.
12. Chambers LW, Sibley JC, Spitzer WO, Tugwell P. Quality of care assessment: How to set up and use an indicator condition. Clin Invest Med 1981;4:41–50.
13. Lane DS, Kelman HR. Assessment of maternal health care quality: Conceptual and methodologic issues. Med Care 1975;13:791–807.
14. Kessner DM, Kalk CE, Singer J. Assessing health quality—the case for tracers. N Engl J Med 1973; 288:189–193.
15. Tischler GL, Astrachan BM. Quality assurance in mental health: Peer and utilization review. Rockville, MD: Unites States Department of Health and Human Services, 1982.
16. Tischler GL, Riedel DC. A criterion approach to patient care evaluation. Am J Psychiatry 1973; 130:913–916.
17. Spiegel JP, Hammersley DW. Peer review: An obligation for psychiatrists. Am J Psychiatry 1974;131:1382–1384.
18. Towery OB, Windle C. Quality assurance for community mental health centers: Impact of P.L. 94-63. Hosp Community Psychiatry 1978;29:316–319.
19. Zusman J. Quality assurance in mental health care. Hosp Community Psychiatry 1988;39:1286–1290.
20. Affeldt JE, Roberts JS, Walczak RM. Quality assurance: Its origin, status and future directions—a JCAH perspective. Eval Health Professions 1983;6:245–255.
21. Roberts JS, Coale JG, Redman RR. A history of the Joint Commission on Accreditation of Hospitals. JAMA 1987;258:936–940.
22. Fauman MA. Monitoring the quality of psychiatric care. Psychiatr Clin North Am 1990;13:73–88.
23. Wells KB, Brook RH. Historical trends in quality assurance for mental health services. In: Stricker G, Rodriguez AR, eds. Handbook of quality assurance in mental health. New York: Plenum, 1988:39–63.
24. McAninch M. Accrediting agencies and the search for quality in health care. In: Stricker G, Rodriguez AR, eds. Handbook of quality assurance in mental health. New York: Plenum, 1988: 363–384.
25. Joint Commission on Accreditation of Healthcare Organizations. Consolidated standards manual/89. Chicago: Joint Commission on Accreditation of Healthcare Organizations, 1989.
26. Goran MJ, Roberts JS, Kellog MA, Fielding J, Jessee W. The PSRO hospital review system. Med Care 1975;13:1s–33s.
27. American Psychiatric Association, Ad Hoc Committee on PSROs. Model criteria sets. Washington, D.C.: American Psychiatric Association, 1974.
28. Drude KP, Nelson RA. Quality assurance: A challenge for community mental health centers. Prof Psychol 1982;13:85–90.
29. American Hospital Association: PRO implementation and medical review requirements. Chicago: AHA, July 1984.
30. Sullivan FW. Professional standards review organizations: The current scene. Am J Psychiatry 1974;131:1354–1358.
31. Liptzin B. Quality assurance and psychiatric

practice: A review. Am J Psychiatry 1974;131: 1374–1377.

32. American Psychiatric Association. Manual of psychiatric peer review. Washington, D.C.: American Psychiatric Association, 1985.

33. Claiborn WL, Biskin BH, Friedman LS. CHAMPUS and quality assurance. Prof Psychol 1982;13: 40–49.

34. Cohen LH, Strickler G. Mental health quality assurance: Development of the American Psychological Association/CHAMPUS program. Eval Health Professions 1983;6:327–338.

35. Claiborn WL, Stricker G. Professional standards review organizations, peer review and CHAMPUS. Prof Psychol 1979;10:631–639.

36. Armstrong B. CHAMPUS and APA join forces to develop a model system of peer review. Hosp Community Psychiatry 1977;28:914–915.

37. Long RS. Third party payment: psychiatric peer review. In: Stricker G, Rodriguez AR, eds. Handbook of quality assurance in mental health. New York: Plenum, 1988:401–419.

38. Shueman SA, Penner NR. Administering a national program of mental health peer review. In: Stricker G, Rodriguez AR, eds. Handbook of quality assurance in mental health. New York: Plenum, 1988:441–453.

39. Cohen LH. Peer review of psychodynamic psychotherapy: An experimental study of the APA/CHAMPUS program. Prof Psychol 1981;12:776–784.

40. Biskin BH. Peer reviewer evaluations and evaluations of peer reviewers: Effects of theoretical orientation. Prof Psychol 1985;16:671–680.

41. Cohen LH, Oyster-Nelson CK. Clinician's evaluations of psychodynamic psychotherapy: Experimental data on psychological peer review. J Consult Clin Psychol 1981;49:583–589.

42. Cohen LH, Nelson DW. Peer review of psychodynamic psychotherapy: Generous versus restrictive reviewers. Eval Health Professions 1982;5:130–144.

43. Vanagunas A. Quality assessment: Alternate approaches. QRB Special Ed. Toward a comprehensive quality assurance program. Chicago: Joint Commission on Accreditation of Healthcare Organizations, 1979:8–11.

44. Joint Commission on Accreditation of Hospitals. Accreditation manual for hospitals. Chicago: Joint Commission on Accreditation of Hospitals, 1980.

45. Joint Commission on Accreditation of Healthcare Organizations: Agenda for change update, Vol. 2, No. 1. Chicago: Joint Commission on Accreditation of Healthcare Organizations, June 1988.

46. Joint Commission on Accreditation of Healthcare Organizations. The Joint Commission guide to quality assurance. Chicago: Joint Commission on Accreditation of Healthcare Organizations, 1988.

47. Roberts JS, Schyve PM, Prevost JA, Ente BH, Carr Maureen. The agenda for change—Future directions of the Joint Commission on Accreditation of Healthcare Organizations. In: Graham NO, ed. Quality assurance in hospitals. Rockville, MD: Aspen, 1990:44–61.

48. Diamond H, Tislow R. Synder T, Rickels K. Peer review of prescribing patterns in a CMHC. American J Psychiatry 1976;133:697–699.

49. Gullick E, King LJ. Appropriateness of drugs prescribed by primary care physicians for depressed outpatients. J Affective Disord 1979;1:55–58.

50. Eastaugh SR. Limitations on quality assurance effectiveness: Improving psychiatric inpatient drug prescribing habits of physicians. J Med Syst 1980;4:27–43.

51. Michel K, Kolakowska T. A survey of prescribing psychotropic drugs in two psychiatric hospitals. Br J psychiatry 1981;138:217–221.

52. Prien RF, Balter MB, Caffey E. Hospital surveys of prescribing practices with psychotherapeutic drugs. Arch Gen Psychiatry 1978;35:1271–1275.

53. Fauman MA. Tricyclic antidepressant prescription by general hospital physicians. AM J Psychiatry 1980;137:490–491.

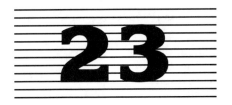

Radiology

Donald L. Renfrew, M.D., Frank H. Weigelt, F.A.C.H.E., and Robert C. Brown, M.D.

DEFINITION

The American Medical Association's Council on Medical Service defines high quality care as that "which consistently contributes to improvement or maintenance of the quality and/or duration of life" (1). The Joint Commission on the Accreditation of Healthcare Organizations (JCAHO) states that "As part of the hospital's quality assurance program, the quality and appropriateness of patient care services provided by the diagnostic radiology department/service are monitored and evaluated . . ." (2). Philip Cascade, writing for the American College of Radiology, states that the charge of the quality improvement program is "to improve patient care by identifying and correcting patient care problems" (3). Thus, the interest in quality health care is clear as is the mandate to provide it in radiology.

In terms of examining the issue of quality care, Donabedian (4) identifies the three major components of medical service as structure, process, and outcome. *Structure*, the environment in which radiology services are provided, includes processor maintenance, imaging equipment calibration, timer checks, and radiation exposure monitoring (5, 6). The evaluation of *process* involves comparing current events against preset criteria and includes such items as evaluation of film repeat rates, conformity with established imaging protocols, and

timeliness of examination performance. In the broadest sense, *outcome* addresses the disposition of the patient, measured, for example, by morbidity, mortality, and quality of life. For evaluation of radiology services, a somewhat more constricted view of outcome may be substituted, namely, evaluation of the accuracy of the radiologic interpretation (5). Cascade (6) also includes evaluation of the appropriateness of examination performance and image quality in this category.

Radiologists and radiology technologists have long been involved in monitoring the quality of the structure and process components of care. An extensive, widely accepted quality control methodology exists. This aspect of quality assurance (QA), once implemented, is largely routine. Evaluation of physician performance, which usually falls into the outcome component of quality assurance, is a considerably more sensitive issue. A relatively extensive literature on this topic exists, however, and while conclusions regarding evaluation of physician performance are not as secure, we will offer some recommendations.

MONITORING AND EVALUATION

The JCAHO has identified a 10-step process for monitoring and evaluation (2).

These steps, along with explanation and some examples drawn from the Department of Radiology at the University of Iowa Hospitals and Clinics (UIHC), follow:

Step 1.   Assign Responsibility for Monitoring and Evaluation Activities

The organization of the quality assurance program within the Department of Radiology at UIHC is highly structured (see Fig. 23.1). The chairman appoints three quality assurance committees.

One of these committees is the technical and administrative quality assurance committee. This committee addresses issues of structure, process, and outcome components regarding technologist and engineer performance. There are separate subcommittees for diagnostic radiology and nuclear medicine. The second committee is the professional radiology quality assurance committee, which reviews mainly physician performance. Finally, the radiation oncology quality assurance committee reviews both physician and technologist performance in that area.

These committees report to the department chairman and are responsible for monitoring, evaluating, and insuring quality care.

Step 2.   Delineate the Scope of Care Provided by the Department

The Department of Radiology at the UIHC is responsible for both the technical and interpretation components of most imaging procedures, as well as those interventional procedures performed by or under the supervision of the staff radiologists. The exceptions include cardiac angiography, cardiac echocardiography, and some obstetrical ultrasound. The department of radiology assumes primary responsibility for patients within the department, unless the patients are accompanied by a responsible physician from outside the department. The department is also responsible for all aspects of radiation therapy.

Step 3.   Identify the Most Important Aspects of Care Provided by the Department

Identifying which aspects of care are most important is perhaps the most difficult decision for those involved in QA. Highest priority obviously should be given to those activities with the greatest impact on patient care. Features that may indicate

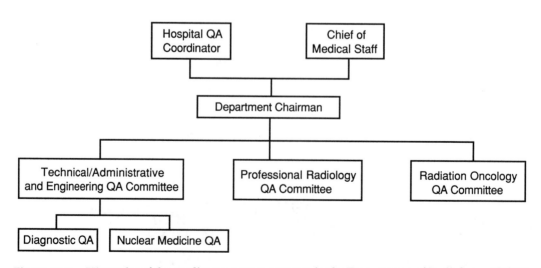

Figure 23.1.   Hierarchy of the quality assurance program in the Department of Radiology at UIHC.

importance to patient care include procedures of high volume or high risk (3). High volume screening mammography has been the focus of many studies, including large-scale evaluations by Bird (7) and Sickles et al. (8). Regarding high risk, Bowyer and Elizabeth (9) reported that, although invasive radiologic procedures accounted for only 5 (17%) of 29 radiology-related losses from closed claims, they represented 71% of the total radiology losses. In identification of important aspects of patient care, it should be remembered that it is necessary to select topics that are known or suspected to be a problem or that may become a problem within the facility (10).

Quality assurance is a dynamic process, and those aspects of care that present problems will undoubtedly change. Thus, the quality assurance committees within the department of radiology identify new problems in a dynamic, ongoing fashion.

Step 4. Identify Indicators (and Appropriate Clinical Criteria) for Monitoring the Important Aspects of Care

Indicators are measurable variables that relate to the important aspects of care identified in step 3.

Step 5. Establish the Thresholds for Evaluation Related to the Indicators

Thresholds may be derived from historical data within the hospital or publications within the medical literature. Problems with using the literature regarding thresholds include systematic and chance population variation between the literature reference and one's own hospital, and the tendency to report positive results. Statistical analysis helps in determining the effect of chance population variation; the other two variables are difficult to estimate. As an example, Higashida et al.'s (11) data regarding complications of percutaneous balloon embolization may be used as a threshold: the investigators report a stroke rate of 9/84 or 11% and a death rate of 15/84

or 18%. The 95% confidence intervals for these figures range from 5 to 13% for stroke and 10 to 26% for death (12). Suppose that stroke rate forms the indicator and that this is measured at 30%. It is unlikely that chance alone accounts for such a high indicator. This rate could still represent: (*a*) systematic patient variation (the QA committee's hospital's patients are "sicker"); (*b*) the tendency for investigators to report, and journals to publish, favorable results; (*c*) possible incompetence by the performing invasive neuroradiologist; or (*d*) small numbers contributing to the 30% rate, that is, wide confidence intervals around the estimate itself.

Regardless of whether a threshold is chosen on the basis of a figure from the literature, prior department experience, or other hospitals' experience, the threshold may undergo revision with time. Complication rates of newly described procedures may be expected to be higher than complication rates of the same procedure following prolonged experience.

Step 6. Monitor the Important Aspects of Care by Collecting and Organizing the Data for Each Indicator

Data come from many sources. Perhaps the most common method of data collection and recording is the creation of forms and assignment of personnel to fill out these forms. While the QA committee may maintain the most control over data collection in this manner, such measures are likely to be perceived as intrusive. Other sources, particularly those outside the department, should be sought. Monitors outside the department may measure variables more accurately, because the collectors of the data are not the same individuals as those being evaluated with the data. Examples of external monitors include records of those emergency resuscitations performed within the department (derived from a database collected by the cardiopulmonary resuscitation committee documenting all code blues within the hospital).

In the future, the centralized risk control

surveillance program at UIHC will provide adverse occurrences and outcomes of radiology care to the department when these occurrences can be attributed to radiology care.

Step 7.   Evaluate Care When Thresholds Are Reached in Order to Identify Either Opportunities to Improve Care or Problems

As data become available, they are compared to the thresholds established by the QA committee. In our division of nuclear medicine, a misadministration rate of 0.01% of total radiopharmaceutical administrations per year serves as the threshold. In 1 year, one misadministration in 8000 procedures would result in a misadministration rate of 1/8000 or 0.013% and thus exceed the misadministration rate.

Step 8.   Take Actions to Improve Care or Correct Identified Problems

An ideal situation exists when a simple cause for exceeding the threshold can be identified. For instance, in the above example of nuclear medicine, a vial may have been mislabeled as a bone agent rather than a renal agent. Alerting all technologists in the department of the error and cautioning against such errors may be all that is necessary to improve quality.

Step 9.   Assess the Effectiveness of Actions and Document the Improvement in Care

Continuing to measure the indicators identified in step 4 provides data to ascertain whether measures taken in step 8 are actually successful. If the initial solution is unsuccessful, step 8 may be repeated. A common error is to assume that, because an action was taken in step 8, the problem shown by indicator data has been solved. This is monitoring the *action* rather than

the problem. Correct procedure reevaluates the indicator data after the action to demonstrate the effectiveness of the action.

Step 10.   Communicate the Results of the Monitoring and Evaluation Process to Relevant Individuals, Departments, or Services and to the Organizationwide Quality Assurance Program

At the UIHC, the minutes of the department of radiology's quality assurance committees are automatically forwarded to the coordinator of the quality assurance support service, who summarizes relevant QA discussion for the professional practice subcommittee, which, in turn, reports to the chief of the medical staff and the University Hospital Advisory Committee. Since the QA committee minutes document steps 1–9 of the above monitoring and evaluation process, communication of relevant information is automatic.

Problem identification forms the key to QA benefit. Radiology departments vary greatly, and the indicators that are meaningless in one department may be vital in another. Within these limitations, we offer the following indicators and thresholds.

STRUCTURE AND PROCESS INDICATORS

The following structure and process indicators and thresholds do not represent all that are used at UIHC, but are rather a representative sample of indicators and thresholds used by the different committees.

Technical and Administrative Quality Assurance Committee: Diagnostic Radiology

Film Repeat Rate.   The threshold is set at 9% for the entire department. Repeat rates are tracked by section and/or service within the division so that management attention can be focused wherever problems develop.

Incident Rate. The incident rate is calculated by dividing the number of incident reports received by the number of procedures performed. The threshold rate for investigation is 0.5% of patient procedures/month. Anyone may file an incident report. The policy requires a report on *any* untoward or unexpected occurrence within the department. Examples of items that are reported in incident reports include falls, contusions or abrasions, lacerations, intravenous line problems, wrong patient examined, wrong date of examination, duplicate examination, examination of a pregnant woman, medication error, and staff injuries. Although a threshold of 0.5% for the incident rate is in place, virtually all incident reports are individually reviewed.

Procedure Reports Awaiting Results More Than 3 Days. The threshold for this indicator is greater than 7% of reports performed per month awaiting results for more than 3 days. Several methods exist whereby clinicians may obtain preliminary results regarding scan findings; this indicator is in place to insure that the final procedure report is rendered in a timely manner.

Late Charge Rate. The threshold for this indicator is 2% of total charge documents submitted late per month. Charges for procedures should be forwarded in a timely manner to the billing office. Late charges form a nuisance not only for the patient and the patient's insurer, but also for the billing office. Furthermore, at UIHC, "charge" is the milestone at which point a report becomes "official." This is thus also a measure of timely results reporting.

Patient Complaints. The threshold for this indicator is 0%; that is, all complaints are reviewed. Patients who complain to secretaries, technologists, or physicians are urged to fill out a complaint form available in the department. The patients are given assistance as necessary for completion of this document.

Technical and Administrative Quality Assurance Committee: Nuclear Medicine

Misadministration Rate. The threshold rate for misadministration is 0.01% of total radiopharmaceuticals injected/year. Since the division of nuclear medicine performs approximately 8000 examinations yearly, a single misadministration will indicate that investigation to identify the problem is indicated.

Wasted Radiopharmaceuticals. The threshold for this indicator is greater than 5% of total products (standing ordered and compounded) wasted per month. A certain amount of waste is inevitable, but the threshold is set to trigger investigation of amounts in excess of expected levels.

Cancelled Charges, Examination Modifications, and Repeat Studies Due to Equipment Failure, etc. The threshold for this indicator is 2% of total procedures per month.

Incident Rate, Procedure Reports Awaiting Final Results for More Than 3 Days, Late Charge Rate, and Patient Complaints. These are all handled in the same manner as described under "Diagnostic Radiology."

Technical and Administrative Quality Assurance Committee: Radiology Engineering

Annual Radiographic Systems Inspection. The threshold is 0%; that is, all problems are dealt with by radiology engineering as they occur; action is reported to the technical and administrative QA committee.

Daily Processor Densitometry Tests. The threshold is 0%.

Down Time for Unscheduled Maintenance. The threshold is 0%.

Preventive Maintenance Performed on Schedule. At least 95% of preventive maintenance should be performed on schedule.

Professional Radiology Quality Assurance Committee

Appropriateness Review (Adequate History, Correct Study, etc.). The policy dictates that the department prospectively review requisitions to determine appropriateness of the examination ordered. All requisitions are reviewed by receptionists, technologists, and physicians, as appropriate, prior to performance of the procedure. A retrospective, postprocedure review is also undertaken. Physicians on the QA committee department complete forms regarding examination appropriateness on randomly selected requisitions and associated interpretations. The forms (see Fig. 23.2) indicate (among other things) whether a correct clinical history was provided and whether the correct examination was performed. Completed forms are entered into a database. An appropriate history must be present on at least 80% of requisitions, and the correct study must have been performed in at least 90%.

Contrast Reactions. The threshold for all adverse reactions is 5%, for intermediate reactions 1%, and for severe reactions 0.05%. Radiologists complete a "Contrast Media Reaction Report" for all contrast reactions of any severity. Data concerning type of contrast media, severity of reaction, and treatment are collected using this form. The department also has available the total number of all contrast injections. Contrast media reaction rates are calculated from these data and monitored.

Angiographic Complications. The Society for Interventional and Cardiovascular Radiology (SCVIR) has taken a leading position regarding quality assurance in interventional radiology. SCVIR outlines in a handout available from the organization the entire 10-step JCAHO process for monitoring and evaluation of care. SCVIR has developed many indicators, including those for appropriateness of diagnostic and therapeutic interventions, aspects of care (e.g., puncture site complications, neurological complications), and efficacy (e.g., technical success rates for angioplasty). The threshold for angiographic complications at our institution is greater than 5%.

Neuroangiographic Complications. The threshold for diagnostic neuroangiographic complications is greater than 5%. For the particular interventional neuroangiographic procedure of balloon occlu-

Radiology Quality Assurance Review

Patient ID   Date of Exam   Staff Radiologist

Diagnosis

Subspecialty	
Ortho	☐
Neuro	☐
Chest	☐
Cardiov	☐
Abdomen	☐
Peds	☐
Nuc Med	☐
Angio-Interv	☐
Ultrasound	☐

Type of Exam	
CT	☐
MRI	☐
Plain film	☐
Ultrasound	☐
Fluoro	☐
Interventional	☐
Mammography	☐
Nuc Med	☐
Other - Specify	☐

A. Case Review	Y	N
diagnosis:		
correct		
proof:		
pathology		
surgery		
consensus		
clinical		
other		
film quality:		
acceptable		

B. Report Review	Y	N
clinical history:		
correct exam:		
report addresses clinical problem:		
conclusion clear and logical:		

Review date:

NOTE: Report either a case review, a report review, or both on this form. Comments may be noted on reverse.

Figure 23.2. Radiology quality assurance review form in use in the Department of Radiology at UIHC.

sion of aneurysms, the threshold is 30% for combined stroke and death (see above discussion under "step 5" of "Monitoring and Evaluation"). In fact, given the infrequency of interventional neuroradiology procedures, the professional QA committee has been reviewing all complications.

Radiation Oncology

Physician Review of Patients on Treatment. At least 95% of the charts of patients on treatment must be signed weekly.

Physician Review of Laboratory and X-Ray Results. At least 95% of reports must be signed by physicians.

Staff Technologists' Credentials for Current Good Standing with the American Board of Radiologic Technologists or Equivalent. 100% of staff technologists must be in good standing.

In-service Training Scheduled between September and April. One in-service training is held per month with no two consecutive months without a scheduled session.

Incident Reports. All incident reports are reviewed.

Patient Complaints. All complaints are reviewed.

Patient Treatment Record and Signed Consent for Treatment. 100% of patients must have a signed informed consent on the chart at the time of treatment.

Dosimetry Parameters and Treatment Calculations. 100% of treatment calculations should be within 1%.

Accuracy of Dose Summations. All treatment doses recorded should fall within 1% of actual dose delivered.

Chart Review for Dosimetry. All charts should accurately document recording dosimetric information.

OUTCOME INDICATORS

Evaluation of diagnostic radiologists, which is the province of the professional radiology quality assurance committee at UIHC, generates considerably more animosity than does evaluation of, for example, film quality. In addition, although the radiology literature contains multiple studies of physician error, most physicians (including radiologists) appear to have fundamental misconceptions regarding errors in radiology. From a QA perspective, these misconceptions may hinder efforts at problem solving. Before discussing specific quality assurance measures, we will review the causes of physician resistance to quality assurance and the literature regarding radiologist error.

Physician Resistance

Most physicians avoid or resist quality assurance. Miller and Flanagan (13) suggest that this follows from physician immaturity. They offer a "growth and development" model wherein physicians pass through infancy, adolescence, young adulthood, and maturity regarding involvement in and support of quality assurance. Denial, anger, and frustration mark early stages of development, whereas acquiescence and finally innovation and creativity form the hallmarks of later stages. While this model offers solace to the quality assurance chairperson, other perhaps less patronizing explanations exist for physician resistance to many formal quality assurance measures.

Physicians are busy people, and time is their currency. If an activity does not capture a physician's attention, the physician will actively avoid the activity, and, if forced to participate, begrudge the time spent. If a physician identifies a problem within his or her practice, it is likely that he or she will implement the solution, and, if satisfied, consider the matter closed. Physicians generally regard documentation of such problem solving as an unnecessary bother.

In addition to being regarded as a waste of time, quality assurance deals with errors. Identification of physician error carries tremendously important medical-legal ramifications, as those physicians who have been required to give depositions or take the witness stand can attest. Although some states (as Iowa) protect quality assurance data from discovery, it is sometimes difficult to convince physicians that such protection is adequate. Creating a registry of mistakes makes little apparent sense in light of settlements and verdicts in certain malpractice cases. Berlin (14), for example, recounts the case of a barely perceptible osteogenic sarcoma—only five of eight radiologists on the medical-legal committee of the American College of Radiology found the lesion without help—resulting in a settlement of $2.25 million.

Given these well-founded concerns, how does one pursue quality assurance without alienating physicians or increasing risk of malpractice suits? The best answer to this difficult question may be that although quality assurance is time consuming, it is better to have control over the process than to allow an external agency such control. In addition, quality assurance, appropriately conducted, will improve our abilities as radiologists via identification of problems and the solutions to those problems.

Studies of Physician Error

If asked to identify the source of radiologists' errors, most physicians imply (more or less diplomatically) that radiologists are ignorant, lazy, or disorganized. That is, radiologists make errors because of: (*a*) lack of knowledge of the disease process; (*b*) lack of time spent reading the examination, comparing the present examination with prior studies, or speaking with the referring physician and/or patient (15); and (*c*) lack of a successful, organized format for interpreting the examination. An indicator such as "percentage correct" may be used regarding diagnostic interpretation (10). Even disregarding the inherent problems with measuring this indicator (see below), corrective action, given that the indicator passes a threshold, depends upon which (if any) of the three factors listed is responsible for the errors.

Lack of Knowledge

Since radiologists, particularly academic radiologists, are interested in unusual, challenging, and interesting cases, emphasis in many conferences during training focuses on specific imaging characteristics of relatively rare disease processes. This emphasis may obscure the fact that few patients have rare illnesses, and that mistakes because of lack of knowledge of rare diseases are infrequent. Smith (16) found that lack of knowledge accounted for only 14 (3%) of 437 identified errors (see Table 23.1). Yerushalmy et al. (17) found that readers missed approximately 30% of positive radiographs when screening for tuberculosis, and that these errors could not be attributed to ignorance regarding the findings of tuberculosis. Garland (18) found that, when comparing two sets of films, there was 30% interobserver variability and 20% intraobserver variability. It is difficult to attribute intraobserver variability to lack of knowledge. Muhm et al. (19) found that most peripheral lung carcinomas detected on serial radiographs were "missed" on the first examination on which the lesion was, in retrospect, visualized. The readers in this study were fully aware of the significance of pulmonary nodules, so, again, it is difficult to attribute the errors to lack of knowledge. Oestmann et al. (20) confirmed a large false-negative rate for reading lung tumors on chest radiographs. Cooley and co-workers (21) found a false-negative rate of 10% regarding malignancy detection on barium enema examination. Few of the errors were attributable to lack of knowledge; most were because of poor technique or what the authors called "momentary lapses."

It is difficult to generalize from the extremely specific studies on tuberculosis screening (a test that is no longer even performed) or indeed any single examina-

Table 23.1.
Distribution of 437 Radiology Errors Collected Over a 2-Year Period.[a]

Error Category	Number	%
Underreading	209	48
Poor communication	66	15
Complacency	60	14
Faulty reasoning	43	10
Unknown	45	10
Lack of knowledge	14	3

Adapted from Smith MJ. Error and Variation in Diagnostic Radiology, 1967. Courtesy of Charles C Thomas, Publisher, Springfield, IL.

tion to the wide field of radiology. Marcus Smith's study (16), perhaps the most comprehensive to date, demonstrates that lack of knowledge accounts for few errors. Smith's study, however, antedated computed tomography, ultrasound, much of nuclear medicine, and magnetic resonance imaging. Since there is so much more to know now, lack of knowledge may play a more important role in errors. Academic institutions, however, perform and publish nearly all such studies. Nevertheless, the results of such studies may not apply to the private sector general radiologist, where the prevalence of disease and frequency of encountering a rare disease are entirely different (22).

In summary, there is little evidence to suggest that lack of knowledge plays a major role in most errors of interpretation in radiology.

Lack of Time Spent Reading

It is not only the accuracy of an experienced subspecialist radiologist that impresses students and clinical colleagues, but also the speed. Recognition and diagnosis are often almost immediate. Although radiologists generally do not rely on such instantaneous impressions, they do frequently work quickly. Does rapidity hinder performance?

Smith (16) suspected that acceleration of reading speed increased false negatives, but stated that he had inadequate data to examine this possibility objectively. Of the group of radiologists that Smith studied, two had roughly equal volumes of work and made almost exactly the same number of mistakes. Smith states, "This similarity existed despite a ten year difference in age and experience, a difference in location of residency training, and a different approach to reading—one observed and dictated rapidly, the other slowly with frequent reviews." Such a single observation, however attractive, must be regarded as anecdotal.

Oestman et al. (20) have demonstrated significant differences in performance when comparing ultrashort reading times for chest radiographs. When holding the false-positive fraction constant, large differences in the false-negative rates appeared when comparing 0.25-, 1-, and 5-second readings with readings of unlimited time. Differences between the unlimited time readings and 5-second readings were considerably smaller. Unfortunately, the clinical utility of this study is limited: it would appear more relevant to have set the time intervals at, for example, 30 seconds and 2 and 5 minutes. In addition, the investigators do not specify how much time readers took when allowed to view the radiographs for an "unlimited" time.

Christensen et al. (23), using a set of films specifically chosen to have subtle abnormalities, demonstrated that experienced readers discontinued their search while they were still making a significant number of true-positive observations and while the true-positive detection rate was higher than the rate for false positives. The results for less experienced readers was not as convincing: inexperienced readers began to have proportionately more false positives during extended observation. Berbaum and co-workers have come to a different conclusion in a similar study, where they demonstrated proportionately more false positives than true positives when search time was increased (Berbaum KS, Franken EA, Dorfman DD et al. Time course for satisfaction of search. Manuscript under review.). The medical care algorithm for the disease process in question determines the utility of trading true positives for false positives. Indeed, such an algorithm is likely to vary from patient to patient with the same disease. Mandating reading times for examination interpretation is unlikely to be productive anyway: a radiologist required to take a certain amount of time to interpret an examination would likely spend the time he or she feels is appropriate to the examination and then cease searching, even if the film is in front of him or her.

Lack of Organization

Lucy Frank Squire's excellent textbook *Fundamentals of Radiology* (24) has long served as the first radiology textbook medical students read. In Chapter 3, "How to Study a Chest Film," Squire encourages a systematic approach to radiographic interpretation. Other texts advise a similar systematic approach to radiographic interpretation for such varied applications as hand films in evaluation of arthritis (25) and temporal bone computed tomography (CT) (26). Most radiologists, at least initially, use a systematic interpretation of radiographs.

Expert radiologists often find, however, that somewhere between the beginning of training and during or after residency they discard systematic search. This appears to be particularly true of those examinations that are frequently read. Kundel et al. (27) found that a random scanner computer model more closely resembled the search patterns in two experienced radiologists than did a systematic scanner. Kinard et al. (28) found that use of a worksheet increased true positives in reporting body-CT images, and Parker et al. (29) found similar findings in detection of pulmonary nodules.

Without more extensive research than is available to date, it is difficult to arrive at a conclusion to enforce systematic search. Regardless of the results of such studies, individual radiologists differ, and externally mandating a systematic search is not possible.

If lack of knowledge, time of reading, and organization have little to do with radiographic errors, what does? Given that radiology has been in existence for nearly 100 years and that errors in radiology have been well recognized and studied for over 40 years, it stands to reason that there is no simple solution to this problem. Yerushalmy et al. (30) proposed that all screening radiographs for tuberculosis be dual read. They further proposed to deal with the false positives generated by the second reading by having yet a third radiologist pass judgment on any case interpreted as positive by either of the first two readers. While such a system might work, Yerushalmy and co-workers make no mention of a very real cost: the time of a second radiologist to reread all of the screening studies and the third to judge all positive cases. A large increase in the number of radiologists would be required to dual-read all films. It should be noted that modified dual reading is in effect in many teaching hospitals, where clinicians, resident radiologists, and staff radiologists all interpret an examination, frequently independently. This probably decreases the likelihood of missed diagnoses in the University setting, but it may also increase false positives.

Creation of indicators for physician performance regarding correct diagnosis may be possible. Correction of lack of knowledge is straightforward: notification of the physician making the error of the necessary information. When the problem is other than a lack of knowledge—most of the cases—it may be difficult to form a solution. Perhaps Marcus Smith's alternate designation for his "miscellaneous" category could apply to many errors in radiology: "Endeavors of Satan."

Problem Case Conference

Paul S. Wheeler (31) first described the "Difficult Diagnosis Conference" in 1982. In this conference, cases of radiologists' mistakes are shown. Wheeler cited four sources for garnering radiographic mistakes: (a) prior reports and films when comparing a present examination with a past one; (b) special imaging procedures (e.g., CT) that better demonstrate abnormalities on plain films, which may be obvious in retrospect; (c) hospital conferences of other specialties; and (d) clinical consultations and pathology reports. At the conference, radiologists present the examination that was misinterpreted and identify the cause of the mistake. Wheeler lists a variety of causes for radiographic errors, and notes that "most missed cases stem from a failure to look at difficult 'hidden zones' on routine diagnostic radiographs." His observation would appear to favor a systematic approach to radiographs and echoes Smith's observation that underreading is the most frequent cause of radiologist error (16). Wheeler also notes that the clinical history provided with the radiographic examination is not always helpful. Eldevik et al.'s (32) study on the value of history in interpretation of computed tomography and myelography supports the notion that clinical history may actually worsen diagnostic performance (32), although other studies demonstrate improved performance with clinical history (33, 34).

At the UIHC we hold a monthly "problem case conference" during which we discuss radiographic errors collected by the various divisions of diagnostic radiology. The causes and remedies of these errors are discussed in group format although, given the nonquantitative nature of the conference, it is speculative as to whether the remedies have the desired effect. As encouraged by Wheeler, we preserve anonymity regarding identification of the erring physician during the conference. We do, however, maintain a confidential record of the physicians and cases.

Overreading of Physician Work (Physician-Specific Data)

Some physicians comply willingly with the charge to bring cases to the problem case conference; others comply reluctantly and others not at all. Tallying the number of errors results more in a quantification of enthusiasm for the conference format than an evaluation of a given radiologist's abilities. Work loads vary and are difficult to calculate, so that even such a simple indicator as "number of errors reported in morbidity and mortality conference/cases read per month" is not readily accomplished. Add to this the fact that the disease prevalence, case difficulty, and work conditions all vary, and it is clear that the problem case conference is a qualitative rather than a quantitative tool. An alternative is to attempt to measure errors of radiologists that occur in a relatively constant environment, that is, errors committed when the same number of a same type of examination is read. The errors could be found, for example, through formal overreading of a set of films.

A difference of opinion exists regarding the utility of formal overreading. Virapongse et al. (35) feel that such overreading is not ideal: "In view of the volume of radiologic interpretations, this is impractical on a percentage basis. Further, the director [the overreading physician] cannot be considered an absolute authority. Frequently, his or her field of expertise is limited." Viraspongse and co-workers offer a problem case conference (such as is proposed by Wheeler and outlined above), pathology correlation in available cases, and evaluation of radiologists by colleagues (both in the radiology department and other services) as better methods to evaluate physicians. Cascade has offered not only a subdivision of interpretation errors, but also a threshold: Serious disagreements should fall within 1 standard deviation of the mean for radiologists with similar responsibilities (3). Not all radiologists will have equal performance (fall on a single mode). Such a threshold will automatically single out about one-third of the department for evaluation. What action should be undertaken? Lack of knowledge appears unlikely to be the problem, so didactic conferences or reading assignments probably will not help. Mandating search time and path are likely to be met with hostility, and there is no clear evidence that they work anyway. If a single radiologist falls far below the mean (or, for that matter, far above the mean), the professional quality assurance committee could act as a detective and try to ascertain the cause of such performance. The committee should prepare for discouragement, however, for it is a fact that variation exists in radiologists' abilities, and there may appear to be no simple method of improving the lowest scores. Perhaps the ultimate answer is a long-term solution wherein radiology systematically favors residency candidates with better aptitude for complex visual tasks, since such abilities are measurable and do not necessarily accompany intellectual ability (36).

At present, the Department of Radiology at UIHC uses a "Radiology Quality Assurance Review" form (Fig. 23.2) to garner physician-specific data. Staff radiologists are encouraged to fill out these forms during the many interesting case conferences, when they obtain feedback from clinicians or pathologists, or whenever they become aware of a radiological error. Although such a method of overreading does provide physician-specific data, there is tremendous bias in the cases reported. For this reason, the professional radiology quality assurance committee is considering more formal evaluation of performance in a controlled setting. The department has an "on-line" reading room, in which all radiologists of the department serve. The denominator would thus be more controlled. Cases may be selected by a film room employee for overreading, generating less biased overreading than is present with voluntary completion of the quality assurance forms.

CONCLUSIONS

Quality assurance measures addressing structure and process are established. The indicators and thresholds presented above provide suggestions for QA programs. Implementation of these suggestions, when supplemented by others deemed appropriate for the institution, should satisfy the JCAHO requirements regarding structure and process.

Evaluation of outcome, or diagnostic radiologists' performance, is more difficult. In the Presidential Address of the Thirty-fourth Annual Meeting of the Radiological Society of North America, L. Henry Garland (37) chose as topic "On the Scientific Evaluation of Diagnostic Procedures." Garland noted the significant number of missed positives in tuberculosis screening, the high inter- and intraobserver variability, and the failure of schemes, both simple and elaborate, to rectify the situation. Garland stated in his conclusion: "When physicians disagree with each other and with themselves on the interpretation of roentgenograms in an appreciable percentage of cases, it is noteworthy. . . . The first reaction of every new observer is: 'This doesn't happen to me.' To these, we suggest: 'Try it systematically.' "

Other investigators have voiced at least some despair when formally evaluating radiologist performance. Cooley et al. (21) noted that "the present report is not flattering to our diagnostic achievements." Of his large study, Smith (16) noted "One unforeseen result of the total effort has been the development of occasional feelings of insecurity about personal ability and resignation to the unhappy prevalence of error."

The JCAHO does not insist that this unhappy prevalence go away. The *Accreditation Manual for Hospitals* mandates, rather, that the QA committee document systematic attempts to improve quality of care. The QA committee controls the indicators, thresholds, and solutions to the problems discovered. The problems may be challenging and there may be as yet little information in the literature for solving them, but with persistence and time, we may find at least partial solutions.

References

1. Council on Medical Service, American Medical Association. Quality of care. JAMA 1986;256: 1032–1034.
2. Joint Commission on Accreditation of Healthcare Organizations. Accreditation manual for hospitals. Chicago: JCAHO, 1990.
3. Cascade P. Diagnostic imaging/radiology quality improvement program. Reston, VA: American College of Radiology, 1989.
4. Donabedian A. Explorations in Quality Assessment and Monitoring, Vol. I: The definition of quality and approaches to its assessment. Ann Arbor: Health Administration Press, 1980.
5. Walczak RM. JCAH QA Standards clarified. In: American College of Radiology: Quality assurance diagnostic imaging and radiation therapy. Reston, VA: American College of Radiology, 1985.
6. Cascade PN. Quality improvement in diagnostic radiology. AJR 1990;154:1117–1120.
7. Bird RE. Low-cost screening mammography: Report on finances and review of 21,716 cases. Radiology 1989;171:87–90.
8. Sickles EA, Ominsky SH, Sollitto RA et al. Medical audit of a rapid-throughput mammography screening practice: Methodology and results of 27,114 examinations. Radiology 1990;175:323–327.
9. Bowyer RN, Elizabeth A. High radiology losses related to invasive procedures. Radiol Management, January 1986;10–12.
10. Cofer J. Introduction. American College of Radiology. In: American College of Radiology: Quality assurance diagnostic imaging and radiation therapy. Reston, VA: American College of Radiology, 1985.
11. Higashida RT, Halback VV, Barnwell SL et al. Treatment of intracranial aneurysms with preservation of the parent vessel: Results of percutaneous balloon embolization in 84 patients. AJNR 1990;11:633–640.
12. Daniel WW. Biostatistics: A foundation for analy-

sis in the health sciences. 4th ed. New York: John Wiley & Sons, 1987:149.

13. Miller ST, Flanagan E. Growth and development of physicians in quality assurance: an ontogeny for quality assurance managers. QRB December 1988;14:358–362.

14. Berlin L. Observer error—Is a "miss" malpractice? In: James AE, ed. Medical/Legal Issues for Radiologists, Chicago: Precept Press, 1987:121–126.

15. Sartoris DJ. Diagnostic imaging interpretation: comprehensiveness means quality. AJR 1987;149:199–200.

16. Smith MJ. Error and variation in diagnostic radiology. Springfield, IL: Charles C Thomas, 1967.

17. Yerushalmy J, Harkness JT, Cope JH, Kennedy BR. The role of dual reading in mass radiography. Am Rev Tuberc Pulm Dis 1950;61:443–464.

18. Garland LH. Studies on the accuracy of diagnostic procedures. AJR 1959;82:25–38.

19. Muhm JR, Miller WE, Fontana RS, Sanderson DR, Uhlenhopp MA. Lung cancer detected during a screening program using four-month chest radiographs. Radiology 1983;148:609–615.

20. Oestmann JW, Greene R, Kushner DC et al. Lung lesions: Correlation between viewing time and detection. Radiology 1988;166:451–453.

21. Cooley RN, Agnew CH, Rios G. Diagnostic accuracy of the barium enema study in carcinoma of the colon and rectum. AJR 1960;84:316–331.

22. Chang PJ. Bayesian analysis revisited: A radiologist's survival guide. AJR 1989;152:721–727.

23. Christensen EE, Murry RC, Hollad K et al. The effect of search time on perception. Radiology 1981;138:361–365.

24. Squire LF. Fundamentals of radiology. 3rd ed. Cambridge, MA: Harvard University Press, 1982.

25. Brower AC. Arthritis in black and white. WB Saunders, Philadelphia: 1988.

26. Hanafee W, Mancuso A. Introductory workbook for CT of the head and neck. Baltimore: Williams & Wilkins 1984.

27. Kundel HL, Nodine CF, Thickman D, Toto L. Searching for lung nodules: A comparison of human performance with random and systematic scanning models. Invest Radiol 1987;22:417–422.

28. Kinard RE, Orrison WW, Brogdon BG. The value of a worksheet in reporting body-CT examinations. AJR 1986;147:848–849.

29. Parker TW, Kelsey CA, Moseley RD et al. Directed versus free search for nodules in chest radiographs. Invest Radiol 1982;17:152–155.

30. Yerushalmy J, Harkness JT, Cope JH, Kennedy BR. The role of dual reading in mass radiography. Am Rev Tuberc Pulm Dis 1950;61:443–464.

31. Wheeler PS. Risk prevention, quality assurance, and the missed diagnosis conference. Radiology 1982;145:227–228.

32. Eldevik OP, Dugstad G, Orrison WW, Haughton VM. The effect of clinical bias on the interpretation of myelography and spinal computed tomography. Radiology 1982;145:85–89.

33. Berbaum KS, Franken EA, El-Khoury GY. Impact of clinical history on radiographic detection of fractures: A comparison of radiologists and orthopedists. AJR 1989;153:1221–1224.

34. McNeil BJ, Hanley JA, Funkenstein HH, Wallman J. Paired receiver operating characteristic curves and the effect of history on radiographic interpretation: CT of the head as a case study. Radiology 1983;149:75–77.

35. Virapongse C, Clore F, Walker R. Setting up a quality-assurance program: Issues with impact on patient care. Appl Radiol February 1987;16:26–33.

36. Smoker WR, Berbaum KS, Leubke NH, Jacoby CG. Spatial perception testing in diagnostic radiology. AJR 1984;143:1105–1109.

37. Garland LH. On the scientific evaluation of diagnostic procedures. Radiology 1949;53:309–328.

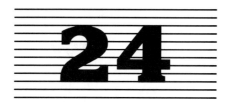

Surgery

Dennis M. Domsic, M.B.A.,
Edward E. Mason, M.D., Ph.D., and Robert J. Corry, M.D.

In a 1933 report of the Committee on the Costs of Medical Care, Lee and Jones noted eight "articles of faith" as the basis for the concept of good medical care:

1. Good medical care is limited to the practice of rational medicine based on the medical sciences.
2. Good medical care emphasizes prevention.
3. Good medical care requires intelligent cooperation between the lay public and the practitioners of scientific medicine.
4. Good medical care treats the individual as a whole.
5. Good medical care maintains a close and continuing personal relation between physician and patient.
6. Good medical care is coordinated with social welfare work.
7. Good medical care coordinates all types of medical services.
8. Good medical care implies the application of all the necessary services of modern, scientific medicine to the needs of all the people (1, 2).

This concept of quality of medical care still holds today and has been stated in such terms as scientific, prevention, partnership with the informed patient, holistic medicine, continuity of care, multidisciplinary approach, comprehensive services, and the "right to care." The ongoing task at hand is not only meeting these goals but also measuring attainment—the focus of quality assurance programs.

QUALITATIVE STUDIES

The classic works of Avedis Donabedian denote three basic forms of qualitative studies. These include studies of structure, process, and outcome of care (Fig. 24.1) (3). *Structure* deals with the resources associated with the provision of care such as staffing, equipment, space, etc. Historically much of the Joint Commission on Accreditation of Healthcare Organizations' (JCAHO) efforts focused on this aspect of care.

Process aims to analyze the practice of care delivery. It involves direct observation of patient care and studies based on the medical record. These studies may be conducted concurrently or on a retrospective basis. Audits need to be structured utilizing explicit or implicit criteria developed and approved by the surgical staff. The emphasis, however, should be on the utilization of explicit criteria that represent at least the standard of practice for the local community but more preferably standards justified by scientifically conducted clinical studies.

Outcome studies emphasize the results of care and the intervention of the health care provider. Avoidable mortality, errors, nosocomial, iatrogenic, and drug-induced

Structure: Resources Committed to Patient
                      Care
                    Personnel
                    Equipment
                    Supplies
                    Space
Process: Practice of Patient Care Delivery
                    Surgical indications
                    Technique
Outcome: Results
                    Morbidity
                    Mortality, early
                    Errors
                    Complications
                    Patient satisfaction
                    Function and productive potential
                    Life expectancy
                    Risk benefit optimized

Figure 24.1. Donabedian's classic forms of qualitative studies applied to surgical services.

complications are the routinely reviewed occurrences in this form of quality assurance. As more and more emphasis is placed on cost containment, outcome studies are becoming the focus of the government and third party payers. Conducting such studies within the hospital not only will assist in meeting JCAHO standards but may also serve as a proactive measure in coping with outside reviews that often oversimplify and misrepresent to the public the caliber of care provided.

In quality assurance parlance, the oversimplified goal of the profession of surgery is ultimately to improve patient outcome. To do this requires not only the study of outcome but the relationship of process and outcome. The latter requires a systematic analysis resulting from clinical research and surgical case audit.

In the long run a longer, better life is the goal of medical care. To evaluate properly, we need data from life-long care to document outcome of productivity, health, and happiness so that competing equations for no care and various options of care can be objectively compared. The discrepancy between available care and the money to pay for that care demands that these equations be developed and used in decisions regarding use of available funds.

JCAHO REQUIREMENTS

In the early years of the JCAHO, the focus of accreditation standards for surgery was on the establishment of a tissue committee reporting on the proportion of normal tissue removed and a credentials committee monitoring staff appointments (4). Today, measurements of functions rather than committees serve as the foundation for ensuring the documentation of the delivery of quality care.

The emphasis of this chapter will be the function of surgical case review as a component of a hospitalwide quality assurance (QA) program. Surgical case review (Standard MS 6.1.2.) must now be accomplished formally on a monthly basis to assure that surgery performed in a hospital is justified and of high quality. Incorporated in this requirement is a review of each case, whether or not a tissue specimen was removed. Sampling of patient cases for review is permissible whenever it is documented that reviews consistently support the justification and quality of individual surgical procedures or the surgical procedures performed by individual practitioners. All records in which a major discrepancy exists between preoperative and postoperative diagnosis must be evaluated (5).

The elements of the quality assurance process as described by the JCAHO are as follows:

1. Assignment of responsibility for monitoring and evaluation activities;
2. Delineation of the scope of care;
3. Identification of the most important aspects of care;
4. Identification of indicators and appropriate clinical criteria for monitoring the important aspects of care;
5. Establishment of thresholds (levels, patterns, trends) for the indicators that trigger evaluation of the care;
6. Monitoring the important aspects of care by collecting and organizing the data for each indicator;
7. Evaluating care when thresholds are

reached in order to identify either opportunities to improve care or problems;

8. Taking actions to improve care or to correct identified problems;
9. Assessing the effectiveness of the actions and document the improvement in care; and
10. Communicating the results of the monitoring and evaluation process to relevant individuals, departments, or services and to the organizationwide quality assurance program (6).

QA PROGRAM ORGANIZATION

Although a hospital's governing body has ultimate responsibility for the quality of surgical care delivered, the true standard setters and monitors are the surgical staff. Recognition by the staff of the necessity for and importance of an effective quality assurance program is the primary ingredient for success. This statement may appear to be trite and too elementary for a text of this nature but all too often a quality assurance program can be simply a collection of paper to keep hospital administration and the JCAHO off the surgical staff's back rather than a critical component of the delivery of high quality care. After all, it involves a commitment of time and energy in an activity that may prove embarrassing to an individual practitioner and has associated legal risks.

The identification of the most important aspects of surgical care, the establishment of indicators, development of clinical criteria, and setting of threshold levels are all in the domain of the surgical staff. One common organizational form utilized in hospitals is to delegate quality assurance for surgical care to a committee composed of surgeons who report periodically to the hospital's medical staff or, in larger facilities, to the surgical department(s). This committee, or representatives thereof, should hold primary responsibility for these functions. However, any criteria or indicators developed should be discussed with the affected surgeons and adopted by the surgical staff as a whole. For the most part, consensus should be reached. In cases where consensus does not result, the appropriate medical staff officer will need to be the decision maker. Conflict can be minimized or adjudicated by use of literature searches and appropriately researched criteria.

For a QA program to be cost-effective and as little of a burden as possible on the physician group, support staff must be provided to do the legwork. Chart reviews to determine whether care of individual patients meets established criteria can be easily and competently conducted by trained registered nurses or medical record technicians. Criteria must be developed with this methodology in mind. All cases not meeting the criteria require physician review. Confidentiality is an absolute necessity if physicians are to be willing participants. Discussion of cases at staff meetings can serve as a forum for education and avoidance of recurrence of similar problems. Individual practitioners should be informed in private of discrepancies, with an opportunity for comment and rebuttal, before definitive corrective action is taken.

Reports of findings in individual cases are helpful in judging the clinical competence of a practitioner; however, the more appropriate methodology is the development of trended data by service and individual surgeon. In this manner, problems are more readily identified and documented. In actuality, trended data may permit early warning signs so as to be able to avert potential problem cases before it is too late for the patients' welfare. Ultimately this is the real intent of QA rather than just to document the presence or absence of problems.

Inexorably linked to quality assurance is cost effectiveness: complications cost money. Furthermore, lengths of stay are extended with limited resources unnecessarily expended; patient suffering occurs; family inconvenience results; work productivity falls; and everybody loses. QA is not only a fiduciary responsibility but also an ethical one.

SURGICAL CARE QUALITY ASSURANCE

Access and Structure

The first level of quality assurance for surgical care is simply whether surgical services are in fact available to the members of the community. At the hospital level, this raises the question as to whether the appropriately trained specialists are on the staff. Are the necessary facilities present: operating rooms, instrumentation, qualified support staff, surgical pathologists, radiologists, etc.? Is this care made available to all members of the community or is it in some way limited?

Indications for Surgery

The next question is whether the surgical services provided are performed for the appropriate indications. This is really the first emphasis of the JCAHO function of surgical case review.

The University of Iowa Hospitals and Clinics' Surgical Case Review Program (7) is utilized in this text as an example of a protocol designed to meet JCAHO survey scrutiny. Surgical indications monitoring was initiated by developing a listing of all inpatient and outpatient procedures performed. A computer-generated list was prepared with procedures classified by current procedural terminology (CPT) codes in descending order of frequency of occurrence. Explicit criteria were established by the appropriate clinical staff in order to evaluate the indications for performing a surgical procedure. As the program was implemented, emphasis was placed on developing criteria for the most frequently performed procedures with the goal of eventually attaining 100% review of all procedures. Once a department is able to document the appropriateness of care for a given surgical procedure, cyclic review of a random sample of cases is permitted.

The explicit criteria developed are of four types (Fig. 24.2). The first is criteria representing evidence of significant pathology. The tissue specimen itself verifies the procedure and its appropriateness. An example of this would be hydrops of the gallbladder (white bile in a gallbladder with stone impacted in cystic duct). Certainly the presence of hydrops of the gallbladder justifies the appropriateness of the cholecystectomy and no further review is necessary.

The second form of criteria is that which represents pathologic evidence that the named procedure was performed. This criteria, however, cannot be used singularly to justify the procedure. Here an example would be the removed specimen being a hernia sac. This is evidence that a herniorrhaphy was performed but not necessarily that it was indicated preoperatively. Indication criteria described below would also need to be present to document justification of the procedure.

The third form of criteria is that which represents pathologic evidence that the procedure was performed adequately. For this criteria, an example would be a specimen which is a segment of a cancerous bowel with adequate margins. The presence of adequate margins indicates an adequate resection but not necessarily that the resection was indicated preoperatively. Thus the indications criteria must be existent in the clinical condition of the patient.

The fourth form of criteria is that which specifies the required preoperative indications. These criteria may be applied in

Tissue alone:	Specimen verifies the procedure and appropriateness (e.g., hydrops of the gallbladder—white bile in the gallbladder with stone impacted in cystic duct)
Confirmatory:	Pathologic evidence that the procedure was performed but not necessarily indicated (e.g., hernia sac)
Adequacy:	Pathologic evidence that the procedure was performed adequately but not necessarily indicated preoperatively (e.g., segment of cancerous bowel with adequate margins)
Indications:	Required preoperative indications (see Appendices A–I for examples)

Figure 24.2. Surgical indications monitoring criteria types.

combination with any of the aforementioned criteria or used alone.

Appendices A–I provide examples of the written criteria utilized for:

A. flexible sigmoidoscopy
B. splenectomy
C. exploratory laparotomy for abdominal trauma
D. renal transplant
E. thyroidectomy
F. cholecystojejunostomy, choledochojejunostomy, or choledochoduodenostomy
G. vagotomy and antrectomy
H. reduction mammoplasty
I. femoral-popliteal bypass

Surgical Process and Outcome

The next aspect of surgical case review is the technical performance of the surgeon and surgical team. Were the appropriate techniques utilized? What errors may have occurred? Were there any complications of a temporary or permanent nature that could have been avoided? And obviously, did a surgical death result?

Traditionally the most thorough form of surgical case review has been the mortality and morbidity conferences that are associated with surgical training programs. In its ideal form, such conferences are held on a frequent enough basis to ensure the review of all cases in a timely fashion so that pertinent facts regarding the patient's condition and treatment are fresh in the presenter's mind. The records of the conference are kept in strict confidence to facilitate complete candor and open discussion. The focus is toward education and not discipline. Disciplinary action of some form may be necessary in extreme cases where repeated errors occur or the performance of a practitioner becomes unacceptable due to some physical or mental limitation or simply incompetency that is not responsive to corrective measures. With such conferences the surgical quality of individual physicians actually becomes common knowledge among peers. Peer pressure will often resolve problems and thus not require direct action by those administratively responsible for the surgi-

cal program. Minutes of meetings that incorporate corrective actions taken can be utilized to meet JCAHO requirements.

As the science of epidemiology has been applied to surgical case review, the recording of pertinent data and statistical analysis now augment the mortality and morbidity conferences. The data can be drawn from the discussions at the conference and through other sources that can be utilized to enhance the analysis of the quality assurance program. Chart reviews by nurses or technicians may be performed to extract data and develop the necessary trended data.

Some typical examples of the latter activity would be the recording of data regarding the incidence of wound dehiscence, anastomosis leaks, presence of temporary and permanent neurological deficits for neurosurgical cases, mortality, etc.

These data should be presented on at least a monthly basis to the quality assurance committee with the reporting of trended data no less than semiannually. Graphic presentation of trended data facilitates interpretation and analysis. The trended data may be used as a basis to trigger further review, to justify the elimination of continued review or conversion to sampling techniques rather than review of all cases, and to document the impact of corrective action.

Nonsurgical Monitors

In addition to the quality assurance monitors specific to surgical case review, other factors indicative of patient care must be monitored and measured. Elements required by the JCAHO include infection rates, transfusion, and drug utilization. Additional factors commonly reviewed are readmissions that occur within some specific time period such as 1 week, prompt completion of operative reports and medical records, unplanned admissions following outpatient surgery, inadequate preparations for diagnostic tests, cancellations of surgical cases, autopsy rates, and Medicare and Medicaid denials and appeals.

Appendix J depicts the typical monthly quality assurance report format presented to the University of Iowa Hospitals and Clinics (UIHC) Department of Surgery quality assurance committee. The report is presented by the quality assurance coordinator for each patient care service. This individual is a senior faculty member who has the reputation of being competent and fair. It is essential that the quality assurance coordinator be respected and trusted by his/her peers.

In addition to the summarized data presented to the committee, a data file is kept on the performance of individual faculty members. Information stored in the file includes such items as major and minor complication rates, surgical errors, mortality rates, and number and types of surgical procedures performed. This is made a part of the clinical privilege renewal process, in the evaluation of a surgeon's competency and performance.

FUTURE TRENDS

What will be the natural progression of the quality assurance activities of hospitals and health care professionals? Implementation of the JCAHO standards results in a performance database of individual practitioners as measured against standards determined by the hospital's medical staff. The future will hold comparisons based on criteria not developed and determined by individual medical staffs but by outside review bodies and insurance carriers. We see this trend already in the utilization requirements of governmental agencies and Professional Standards Review Organizations (PSROs). Utilization studies are crossing over to forms of quality analysis. Examples are Medicare and Medicaid pre-procedural review requirements and readmission reviews. Sanctions for "quality problems" are in the implementation stage by PSROs. Outside review is being forced upon the hospital and individual practitioners. Payments are being denied for services performed when determined not to be justified or the result of a provider error.

The situation has developed where resistance to these efforts is nonproductive or even counterproductive. The only successful response is for the practitioners to

become active participants in the criteria and standards development by serving as PSRO reviewers, volunteering for committee assignments, and generating their own specialty databases.

An example of the latter is the establishment of the National Bariatric Surgery Registry (NBSR). The NBSR is an organization of surgeons in the United States and Canada who surgically treat morbid obesity. The NBSR is directed by Edward E. Mason, M.D., Professor, Department of Surgery, University of Iowa, and originator of gastric bypass (1966) and vertical banded gastroplasty (1980) for treatment of morbid obesity. This registry collects standardized data regarding patient histories, operative procedures, and patient outcomes following surgical treatment. The goal of the NBSR is to promote optimum care for the morbidly obese patient through standardized statistical analyses. Its first focus is to determine and document the medical effectiveness of surgical treatment of morbid obesity through a patient outcome study. Concomitantly, reports are produced comparing the data from individual surgeons versus the pooled data of all participating physicians. Appendix K lists the table of contents of the standardized reports provided quarterly to the NBSR members. The data of individual patients and surgeons are kept confidential.

The analyses are used to determine the efficacy of bariatric surgery in general and the efficacy of the different surgical approaches. The pooled data may eventually be used to set professional standards regarding the indications for surgery, the surgical techniques utilized, acceptable complication types and rates, and the qualifications necessary for the granting of surgical privileges. Individual data can be used for self-evaluation or, with the surgeon's permission, as part of a hospital's quality assurance program. In addition, such pooled data will be available for use in justifying to third party payers what conditions under which reimbursement should be made available for this form of treatment. The approach is scientific and follows established methods of clinical research. This is a prime example of how quality assurance and clinical research do in fact coexist and should be complementary.

PATIENT SATISFACTION

The remaining form of surgical quality assurance and one of the most important from a "business" standpoint is patient satisfaction. This is one the profession so often overlooks.

The "quality" we have discussed thus far is a product defined by the health care profession. Brent C. James, M.D., refers to this as "content quality." It is the technical component of medical care and the resultant outcome (8).

The patient evaluates "delivery quality." James states that "delivery quality refers to all aspects of an organization's interaction with the customer in delivering the output." This form of quality analysis is evaluated by patient expectations and reflects the interpersonal relationships associated with the provision of service (8).

The simplest although gross indicator of patient satisfaction in the current competitive marketplace is growth in caseload. However, surgical departments need to be more formal and exact in evaluating patient satisfaction. Find out what patients think of your surgical staff and the institution in which they practice. This can be accomplished through properly designed surveys or marketing tools such as focus groups. The complicated goal is to strike a balance between patient satisfaction and quality care. The presence of patient satisfaction does not necessarily indicate the existence of quality surgery. It does, however, indicate the presence of a quality service in that the consumer is happy.

Quality is, by definition, a value judgment. Health care quality assurance science attempts to quantify the medical results. The patient, however, is often not interested in quantification except with reference to the hospital and physicians' billings statements and clinic waiting time. In today's age of litigation and informed patient involvement in medical care delivery decisions, the surgeon and hospital must rank patient satisfaction high on their quality analysis list. Failure to do this will lead to malpractice suits and loss of pa-

tients to competing institutions and organizations.

A study of 6000 individuals by Brent Jacobsen (8) to discover factors that determine perceptions of hospital quality within Intermountain Health Care found that there were two major questions determining patient evaluation of quality indicators. These were: Was the health care team able to explain the disease process, the treatment choices, and the likely outcomes in a way that the patient and family could understand? Did the patient and family participate in the medical decision-making process?

One is cautioned to be cognizant of these factors not only for JCAHO review but importantly for the business and financial benefit in addition to the primary ethical responsibilities to the patient. The typical dissatisfied patient does not complain to the surgeon, but to his/her family, friends, and associates. When this takes place, the surgeon is not there to rebut the statements made. The second pervasive method of patient complaint is nonverbal—they walk away and do not return.

References

1. Lee RI, Jones LW. The fundamentals of good medical care. An outline of the fundamentals of good medical care and an estimate of the service required to supply the medical needs of the United States. Publication of the Committee on the Costs of Medical Care: No. 22, Chicago: The University of Chicago Press, 1933:6–10.
2. Kessner DM, Kalk CE, Singer J. Assessing health quality—The case for tracers. N Engl J Med, 1973; 288(4):189.
3. Donabedian A. Explorations in quality assessment and monitoring. Vol. I. The definition of quality and approaches to its assessment. Ann Arbor: Health Administration Press, 1980:79–128.
4. Pollock A, Evans M. Surgical audit. London: Butterworths, 1989:25.
5. Joint Commission on Accreditation of Healthcare Organizations. Medical staff standards. Accreditation manual for hospitals. Chicago: JCAHO, 1990:112.
6. Joint Commission on Accreditation of Healthcare Organizations. Quality assurance standards. Accreditation manual for hospitals. Chicago: JCAHO, 1990:214.
7. The University of Iowa Hospitals and Clinics' Surgical Services Subcommittee Surgical Case Review Protocol Iowa City: University of Iowa, 1990.
8. James BC. Quality management for health care delivery. Chicago: The Hospital Research and Educational Trust of the American Hospital Association, 1989:11–14.

APPENDICES

APPENDIX A

Surgical Case Review Criteria:
Flexible Sigmoidoscopy

Amanda M. Metcalf, M.D., *Assistant Professor of Surgery, The University of Iowa*

Indications "I"
1. Hematochezia (bloody stools), or
2. Hemoccult positive stools, or
3. Evaluation of patients with strong family history of colon carcinoma, or
4. Evaluation of patients with benign or malignant strictures of rectum, sigmoid/descending colon, or
5. Follow-up in patients undergoing ileosigmoidostomy for carcinoma, ulcerative colitis or Crohn's disease (inflammatory disease of colon), or
6. Evaluation of sigmoid diverticular disease, or
7. Evaluation of patients with possible pseudomembranous colitis or ischemic colitis, or
8. Evaluation of proctosigmoiditis (inflammation of rectum or sigmoid), or
9. Biopsy or snare removal of polyp seen in left transverse, descending, or proximal sigmoid on barium enema.

Confirmatory "C"
Tissue "T"
Criteria Required "I"
Data Retrieval Instructions
    Report the following conditions:
        Sigmoidoscopy:
            Gastrointestinal bleeding, or
            Bowel perforation

APPENDIX B

Surgical Case Review Criteria:
Splenectomy

Wilbur L. Zike, M.D., *Associate Professor of Surgery, The University of Iowa*

Indications "I"
History of one or more of the following:
1. History and prior workup of idiopathic thrombocytopenic purpura (depleted platelets and skin bruises), or
2. Hypersplenism—active bone marrow but depleted circulating blood elements, red cells, or white cells, or

3. Staging for Hodgkin's disease or other lymphoma previously diagnosed by lymph node biopsy or exploratory laparotomy, or
4. As part of a total or partial gastrectomy for cancer, or
5. As part of a total or partial pancreatectomy, or
6. Congenital spherocytosis (history of anemia and blood reports of splenocytes), or
7. History and prior workup of splenic cyst, abscess, pseudocyst, hematoma, etc., or
8. Huge spleen (wt 2000 gm): (physical discomfort and evidence by biopsy that bone marrow is active), or
9. Ruptured spleen secondary to trauma thought not amenable to splenorrhaphy.

Confirmatory "C"
Tissue "T"
Criteria Required: "I"
Data Retrieval Instructions

APPENDIX C

Surgical Case Review Criteria:
Exploratory Laparotomy for Abdominal Trauma

Wilbur L. Zike, M.D., *Associate Professor of Surgery, The University of Iowa*

Indications "I"
1. Penetrating wound of abdomen, lower chest, back, or perineum
   a. Perforated viscus
      1) History of gunshot wound, or
      2) History of stab wound with exposure of viscera or leakage of GI contents from wound, or
      3) Stab wound with abdominal tenderness and positive paracentesis or peritoneal lavage or free air, or
      4) Stab wound with signs of sepsis, shock, or peritonitis, or
      5) Injury to urinary tract demonstrated by radiologic examination, or
   b. Massive abdominal bleeding:
      1) History of wound with resistant hypotension, or
      2) Injury of liver or spleen or kidney demonstrated by radiologic examination, or
2. Blunt trauma of abdomen, lower thorax, back, or pelvis
   a. Ruptured viscus
      1) History of injury with abdominal tenderness and abdominal paracentesis or free air determined by radiologic examination or sepsis, or
      2) Injury of urinary tract demonstrated by radiologic examination, or
   b. Massive abdominal bleeding
      1) History of injury with resistant hypotension, or
      2) Injury of spleen, liver, or kidney as demonstrated by radiologic examination

Confirmatory "C"
Tissue "T"
Criteria Required "I"
Data Retrieval Instructions

APPENDIX D

Surgical Case Review Criteria:
Renal Transplant

John L. Smith, M.D., *Assistant Professor of Surgery, The University of Iowa*

Indications "I"
1. Irreversible chronic renal failure secondary to one of the following:
    a. Diabetes, Type I or II (DM), or
    b. Chronic glomerulonephritis (CGN), or
    c. Membranous proliferative glomerulonephritis (MPGN), or
    d. Polycystic kidney disease (PCD), or
    e. Alports, or
    f. Lupus or other active systemic illness, or
    g. Hypertension (HTN), or
    h. Pyelonephritis, or
    i. Obstructive nephritis, and
2. Patient is uremic as documented by the physician, or on hemodialysis or peritoneal dialysis, or
    *a. Creatinine clearance <20 cc/min, or
    *b. Total urine protein >1.0 gm, or
    *c. Serum creatinine >4.5 and BUN >50, and
3. Adequate bladder or conduit for transplant as documented by the physician, or
    a. Indicated by delayed voiding cystourethrogram (DVCG), or
    b. Loopogram, or
    c. Urology consult, and
4. Patient is free of active infection/communicable disease, and
5. Patient is considered a reasonable risk for surgery by the physician, and
6. Patient psychosocially suitable for transplant, and
7. Age newborn to 65 years; patient >65 considered on individual basis.
Confirmatory "C"
Tissue "T"
Criteria Required "I"
Data Retrieval Instructions
1. Irreversible—end-stage renal disease (ESRD), no function, etc.
2. Presence of ESRD would indicate that a patient is uremic.
3. If any questions, check for appropriate consults and their conclusions and recommendations.
4. Psychosocially suitable—see social worker's notes. Patient is able to care for self or is a dependent of a capable adult, must be psychosocially sound, i.e., able to adjust to new organ and medication side effects.

---

*Liberal variation established at UIHC in order to accommodate diabetic patients receiving combined pancreas and renal transplant.

APPENDIX E

Surgical Case Review Criteria: Thyroidectomy

Nelson J. Gurll, M.D., *Professor of Surgery, The University of Iowa*

Indications "I"
1. For hyperthyroidism
   a. Elevated serum concentration of thyroxine (T4) or triiodothyronine (T3), decreased TSH (by sensitive assay), or
2. For thyroid cancer
   a. On physical examination the presence of one or more findings:
      1) Thyroid nodule, or
      2) Goiter, or
3. For thyroid nodule
   a. On physical examination the finding of:
      1) Thyroid nodule, or
   b. Laboratory evaluation which shows one of the following:
      1) Cold uptake in nodule on nuclear medicine scan, or
      2) Cellular material on fine needle aspiration for biopsy cytology (FNABC), or
      3) Recurrence after aspiration of cyst (initially determined by sonography or aspiration) or
4. For goiter
   a. History of one or more of the following:
      1) Dyspnea, or
      2) Dysphagia, or
      3) Hoarseness, or
      4) Worry about the possibility of cancer, or
      5) Concern about cosmetic appearance of neck, or
   b. Physical examination with findings of one of the following:
      1) Enlarged thyroid, or
      2) Substernal location of goiter, or
      3) Substernal goiter on chest x-ray
Confirmatory "C"
Tissue "T"
Criteria Required "I"
Data Retrieval Instructions

APPENDIX F

Surgical Case Review Criteria: Cholecystojejunostomy, Choledochojejunostomy, or Choledochoduodenostomy

Wilbur L. Zike, M.D., *Associate Professor of Surgery, The University of Iowa*

Indications "I"
Special Note: Procedures for cancer require criteria 1 and 2.
1. Obstructive jaundice, and/or
2. Biopsy-proven cancer or pancreatitis, or
3. Obstruction of distal common bile duct stone, stricture or external compression: recurring bilirubin common bile duct stones, or
4. As part of a larger operation requiring partial or total pancreatectomy.
5. Poor risk patient requiring operation for common duct stone.
Confirmatory "C"
Tissue "T"
  2) Pancreatitis, or
    cancer of bile ducts, gallbladder, liver, ampullary papilla, or duodenum, or
    metastatic cancer to porta hepatis
Criteria Required "I" or "T" & "I" in case of carcinoma
Data Retrieval Instructions
1. Obstructive jaundice, elevation in direct bilirubin (>1.0) *and/or* alkaline phosphatase (>115), or
Percutaneous cholangiogram or ERCP (endoscopic retrograde cholangiopancreatography) showing obstruction in the extrahepatic biliary tree.
2. Preoperative biopsy *or* from tissue removed at time of operation.

APPENDIX G

Surgical Case Review Criteria: Vagotomy and Antrectomy

Wilbur L. Zike, M.D., *Associate Professor of Surgery, The University of Iowa*

Indications "I"
1. Documented peptic ulcer disease unresponsive to nonoperative therapy or complicated by bleeding, perforation, posterior penetration, or obstruction, or
2. Distal gastric tumors or polyps, malignant or benign, which require resection because of malignancy, or bleeding, or for diagnosis, or
3. As part of a greater resection, i.e., Whipple operation for carcinoma of the pancreas, or
4. As necessary to control bleeding or perforation or tissue devitalization secondary to trauma, gastritis, or "stress ulceration."

Confirmatory "C"
1. Peptic ulcers or tumors documented by barium upper GI study or UGI endoscopy (lesion shiny white blur) or
2. Tumors biopsied (unless submucosal), gastritis, and gastric ulcers.

Tissue "T"
1. Carcinoma or other tumor (benign or malignant)

Criteria Required:
1. "I" + "C" + "T" for tumor
2. "I" + "C" for remainder

Data Retrieval Instructions

APPENDIX H

Surgical Case Review Criteria:
Reduction Mammoplasty

Peter R. Jochimsen, M.D., *Professor of Surgery, The University of Iowa*

Indications "I"
1. Clinically diagnosed enlarged breasts with at least one or more of the following signs or symptoms:
   a. Neck or back pain
   b. Breast pain
   c. Shoulder grooving from bra strap
   d. Intertriginous dermatitis
   e. History indicating psychological stress secondary to enlarged breasts.

Confirmatory "C"
1. Photographs secured where possible.
2. Tissue removed at operation exceeding 200 gm per breast.

Tissue "T"
1. Operating room or pathology report indicating weight of specimen removed from each breast.

Criteria Required "I" + "C" + "T"
Data Retrieval Instructions

APPENDIX I

Surgical Case Review Criteria:
Femoral-Popliteal Bypass

Timothy F. Kresowik, M.D., *Assistant Professor of Surgery, The University of Iowa*

Indications "I"
1. One of the following:
   a. Intermittent claudication, or

    b. Ischemic skin changes, or

    c. Rest pain in affected leg, or

    d. Presence of aneurysm in femoral or popliteal artery

       and

    e. Arteriography demonstrating blocked or narrowed artery (femoral or popliteal), or

    f. Duplex scan defining diseased area, or

    g. Noninvasive lab study indicating diminished blood supply to affected leg, or

    h. Femoral or popliteal aneurysm by ultrasound, CT or MRI scan or seen on arteriogram .

Confirmatory "C"

Tissue "T"

Criteria Required: "I"

Data Retrieval Instructions

    b. *Ischemic skin changes:* skin changes or breakdown from impaired vascularization.

    g. *Noninvasive lab studies:* limb pressure studies.

APPENDIX J

University of Iowa Hospitals and Clinics
QUALITY ASSURANCE PROGRAM
MONTHLY MONITORING REPORT—CLINICAL DEPARTMENT

For the Month of: <u>NOVEMBER 1990</u>
Clinical Department: <u>SURGERY</u>
Department Head Responsible: <u>Robert J. Corry, M.D.</u>

This material has been prepared for use by a University Hospitals Staff Committee investigating ways to reduce morbidity and mortality.

1	2	3	4	5	6	7	8
Brief Description of Monitor or Routine Data Collected	Threshold Rate/Range Requiring Further Investigation	Results of Monitoring or Data Analysis (Report Positive *and* Negative Results)	Did Data in col. 1 Indicate a Problem? If "No", do not complete cols. 5–8 OR Statement of Problem	If a Problem, Corrective Action Taken or Changes Implemented	Evidence of Resolution	Other Departments or Subcommittees Involved	Date of Problem Resolution
1. Infection rates							
a. General Surgery			No problem. However, now that two years trend data have been developed the QA Committee will reestablish threshold levels at a lower rate				
Clean	>3%	2.9%					
Clean contaminated	>10%	8.1%					
Contaminated	>15%	9.7%					
Dirty	>20%	5.0%					
Urinary tract with Foley catheters	>7%	3.7%					
Respiratory tract infection—lower	>7%	3.7%					
Skin—IV inflamm reaction	>3%	1.2%					
b. Neurosurgery			*Per ops performed*	Clean infection rate above threshold. This is the first month this has occurred. Review of cases indicates no major problem; however, we will continue to monitor for significant trend. Review of cases at conference indicated different organisms with no common etiology found.			
Clean	>2.5%	4.5%	3/67				
Clean contaminated	>8.0%	0.0%	0/4				
Contaminated	>15%	0.0%	0/4				
Dirty	>15%	0.0%	0/3				

Data and threshold levels not actual. Presented for information and as example of report format and content.

APPENDIX J—*continued*

University of Iowa Hospitals and Clinics
QUALITY ASSURANCE PROGRAM
MONTHLY MONITORING REPORT—CLINICAL DEPARTMENT

For the Month of: <u>NOVEMBER 1990</u>

Clinical Department: <u>SURGERY</u>

Department Head Responsible: <u>Robert J. Corry, M.D.</u>

This material has been prepared for use by a University Hospitals Staff Committee investigating ways to reduce morbidity and mortality.

1	2	3	4	5	6	7	8
Brief Description of Monitor or Routine Data Collected	Threshold Rate/Range Requiring Further Investigation	Results of Monitoring or Data Analysis (Report Positive *and* Negative Results)	Did Data in col. 1 Indicate a Problem? If "No", do not complete cols. 5–8 OR Statement of Problem	If a Problem, Corrective Action Taken or Changes Implemented	Evidence of Resolution	Other Departments or Subcommittees Involved	Date of Problem Resolution
2. Transfusion subcommittee noncompliance report	<100% justified	All transfusions met indicated criteria					
3. Wound dehiscence	>0%	0 of 225 cases	No problem				
4. Anastomosis leaks	>0%	1 of 47 cases = 2.1%	*Complication:* esophageal aspiration occurred during operation of fundoplication and placement of gastrostomy tube. Laceration was surgically closed during operation. Case reviewed with involved staff. Trend data does not indicate need for other corrective action.				
5. Complication rate for craniotomy, tumor	>0%	1 of 11 cases = 9%	*Temporary complication:* partial rt CN-III palsy, CN-IV palsy, CN-V palsy and mild left hemiparesis. Case reviewed at Neurosurgery Mortality and Morbidity Conference.				
6. Complication rate for stereotactic intracranial surgery	>0%	0 of 2 cases = 0%	No problem				

Data and threshold levels not actual. Presented for information and as example of report format and content.

APPENDIX J—*continued*

University of Iowa Hospitals and Clinics
QUALITY ASSURANCE PROGRAM
MONTHLY MONITORING REPORT—CLINICAL DEPARTMENT

For the Month of: <u>NOVEMBER 1990</u>
Clinical Department: <u>SURGERY</u>
Department Head Responsible: <u>Robert J. Corry, M.D.</u>

This material has been prepared for use by a University Hospitals Staff Committee investigating ways to reduce morbidity and mortality.

1	2	3	4	5	6	7	8
Brief Description of Monitor or Routine Data Collected	Threshold Rate/Range Requiring Further Investigation	Results of Monitoring or Data Analysis (Report Positive *and* Negative Results)	Did Data in col. 1 Indicate a Problem? If "No", do not complete cols. 5–8 OR Statement of Problem	If a Problem, Corrective Action Taken or Changes Implemented	Evidence of Resolution	Other Departments or Subcommittees Involved	Date of Problem Resolution
7. Complication rate for transsphenoidal resection of pituitary tumor	>0%	0 of 2 cases = 0%	No problem				
8. Endovascular procedure (embolization) complications	>0%	0 of 1 case = 0%	No problem				
9. Head trauma surgery							
a. Complication rate	>0%	0 of 6 cases = 0%	No problem				
b. Death rate	>0%	0 of 6 cases = 0%	No problem				
10. Readmission within one week	>0%	1 of 300 cases = 0.003%	Renal transplant patient admitted due to rejection. No corrective action necessary.				
11. Operative report dictation	Threshold rate = >0% for *missing, insuff.* or *no sign.*	# of discharges analyzed = 400 Missing = 2 (0.5%) Insuff. = 2 (0.5%) No sign. = 3 (0.75%)	Above thresholds. Will continue to monitor for significant trends.	Noncompliant physicians notified and delinquencies corrected.	Dictation completed within 48 hours of physicians being notified.		
12. Unplanned admissions following same-day surgery	>0%	1 of 15 cases = 6.7%	Admission was due to nausea and vomiting. Review of case indicates patient properly handled. No corrective action necessary.				

Data and threshold levels not actual. Presented for information and as example of report format and content.

APPENDIX J—*continued*

University of Iowa Hospitals and Clinics
QUALITY ASSURANCE PROGRAM
MONTHLY MONITORING REPORT—CLINICAL DEPARTMENT

For the Month of: <u>NOVEMBER 1990</u>
Clinical Department: <u>SURGERY</u>
Department Head Responsible: <u>Robert J. Corry, M.D.</u>

This material has been prepared for use by a University Hospitals Staff Committee investigating ways to reduce morbidity and mortality.

1	2	3	4	5	6	7	8
Brief Description of Monitor or Routine Data Collected	Threshold Rate/Range Requiring Further Investigation	Results of Monitoring or Data Analysis (Report Positive *and* Negative Results)	Did Data in col. 1 Indicate a Problem? If "No", do not complete cols. 5–8 OR Statement of Problem	If a Problem, Corrective Action Taken or Changes Implemented	Evidence of Resolution	Other Departments or Subcommittees Involved	Date of Problem Resolution
13. Allergic reactions to medications in Surgery Outpatient Clinic (SOC)	None	None	No				
14. Inadequate preparation for diagnostic tests	None	None	No				
15. Same-day surgery cancelled on the day of surgery	None	9/17/90: #84-97612 Breast biopsy after needle localization cancelled—no lesion identified	Case pending—chart review and radiographic reports to be analyzed and reported at next Mortality and Morbidity Conference.				
16. Autopsy report summary: *month/year*	N/A		No problem				
a. # deaths		9					
b. # (%) autopsy		4 (44.44%)					
c. Autopsy reports completed		2					
d. # (%) of cases with additional pathological findings*		0 (0%)					
e. Monthly hosp. autopsy rate		40.38%					
f. Yearly hosp. autopsy rate		40.38%					

Data and threshold levels not actual.
Presented for information and as example of report format and content

*Reports indicate that major clinical diagnoses and major autopsy diagnoses were not identical or that there were major additional diagnoses. See autopsy reports for detailed information.

APPENDIX J—*continued*

University of Iowa Hospitals and Clinics
QUALITY ASSURANCE PROGRAM
MONTHLY MONITORING REPORT—CLINICAL DEPARTMENT

For the Month of: NOVEMBER 1990

Clinical Department: SURGERY

Department Head Responsible: Robert J. Corry, M.D.

This material has been prepared for use by a University Hospitals Staff Committee investigating ways to reduce morbidity and mortality.

1	2	3	4	5	6	7	8
Brief Description of Monitor or Routine Data Collected	Threshold Rate/Range Requiring Further Investigation	Results of Monitoring or Data Analysis (Report Positive *and* Negative Results)	Did Data in col. 1 Indicate a Problem? If "No", do not complete cols. 5–8 OR Statement of Problem	If a Problem, Corrective Action Taken · or Changes Implemented	Evidence of Resolution	Other Departments or Subcommittees Involved	Date of Problem Resolution
17. Quarterly summary of resolved Medicare and Medicaid denials	N/A	Appeal case overturned. Admission determined to be justified					
18. Medicare and Medicaid pending report of appeals in process	N/A	3 cases are pending report					

Data and threshold levels not actual. Presented for information and as example of report format and content.

APPENDIX K

National Bariatric Surgery Registry Report Summary

I. Introduction: Patient population summary	Description of study universe
II. Patient History: Patient age and gender	Patient age and gender by weight category
Operative patient weight	Operative weight and body mass index by weight classification and procedure type
Waist and hip ratios	Waist to hip circumference ratio at initial visit
III. Operative Information: Primary bariatric procedure	Frequency of various procedure types and obesity category by operative type
Gastric stoma	Reinforcement utilized and external circumference
Pouch volume measurements	Measurement method and pouch volume by procedure category
Operative length	Time of procedure by weight category
Postoperative hospital stay	Hospital days by weight category
Operative complications	Overall complication and wound infection rates by procedure category
	Complication specific rates by weight classification: Wound infection Deep venous phlebitis GI leak Subphrenic abscess Wound dehiscence Evisceration Pulmonary embolus Respiratory Cardiac Renal Hepatic Neurologic Other
IV. Reoperation Information:	Gastric banding, gastric sling, Silastic ring vertical gastroplasty, vertical banded gastroplasty and distal Roux-en-Y gastric bypass
	Reoperation performed

V. Mortality:	Deaths by operative type, diagnosis, and days postop
VI. First Follow-up Information:	Disease present
	Summary of hypertension, diabetes, vomiting, and heartburn at initial visit and first follow-up visit post surgery
VII. Data Completion Rates:	Physician's rate of compliance for completion of data submittal requirements

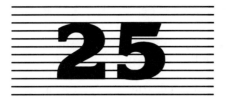

Urology

Bernard Fallon, M.D.

United States society increasingly expects a health care system that will correct all illness perfectly. The payers of the health care bill have noted that national health care spending has increased from $42 billion in 1965 to $600 billion in 1990, a 14-fold increase. Stated another way, it has gone from 6.7% of gross national product (GNP) in 1965 to 11.4% of GNP in 1990. Employers' contributions to health care insurance has increased from 8% of corporate profits in 1961 to 60–80% of corporate profits in 1990 for Fortune 500 companies. Yet, 37 million Americans are uninsured and an estimated 20 million more are underinsured. What would the cost be if all had adequate insurance?

In the Canadian and British health care systems, total cost is about 6–7% of GNP, yet average life span in these countries is the same as America's 74 years. Studies of various medical and surgical procedures indicate that as much as 30% of medical care may be performed for inappropriate indications.

All of the above points were discussed in a recent opinion page of a prominent daily newspaper (1), and the article concluded with a plea for funding research on the outcomes of medical care to a much greater extent than exists at present.

A potential need for rationing or at least prioritizing health expenditures is also under discussion in the lay press (2), as the state of Oregon seeks a waiver from federal Medicaid regulations requiring that "all medically necessary services" be funded. *Newsweek* magazine has also published an article by a physician, discussing the multiple dilemmas in which he finds himself, attempting to render good medical care in an environment that simultaneously demands cost-consciousness and perfection of outcome (3).

The Joint Commission on Accreditation of Healthcare Organizations (JCAHO) is a private body that sets standards and guidelines for hospitals, which may voluntarily seek its accreditation. Nonaccreditation may injure a hospital in respect to its teaching programs and place it in jeopardy for state and federal funds (4). The JCAHO has traditionally set criteria for hospitals which address the structure of medical care—the physical facility, available technology, safety requirements, and credentialling procedures for staff. In the past several years, JCAHO guidelines have extended into the area of the process of care and recently have begun to address outcomes issues, in parallel with payers' questions regarding quality of care and outcomes, with increasing expenditure.

UROLOGY DEPARTMENTS

JCAHO outcomes indicators are already being applied in several areas hospitalwide, including anesthesia and obstetrics departments. In the next few years, outcomes indicators will be forthcoming for at least 22 other areas of medical activity, including urology (5). Hospital accreditation will be based on the results of those indicators, combined with on-site visits that will analyze the traditional structure and process of care (6).

At this time, there are no JCAHO standards addressed specifically to urology departments, including urology, a quality assurance program that complies with the JCAHO standard for hospitals (7). The departmental program in urology therefore is a part of, and has the same goals and characteristics as, the hospital program. These include a written quality assurance plan, coordination with risk-management activities, and monitoring the quality and appropriateness of patient care and the performance of those with clinical privileges in urology. Data are gathered from within the urology department and from external sources such as the pathology department, blood bank, pharmacy and therapeutics committee, and particularly from the epidemiology department.

A 10-step process has been outlined by the JCAHO for monitoring and evaluating the quality of medical care, and this process can be applied within a urology department. The process is composed of the following 10 steps:

1. Assign responsibility for monitoring and evaluation activities;
2. Delineate the scope of care provided by the organization;
3. Identify the most important aspects of care provided by the organization;
4. Identify indicators (and appropriate clinical criteria) for monitoring the important aspects of care;
5. Establish thresholds (levels, patterns, trends) for the indicators that trigger evaluation of the care;
6. Monitor the important aspects of care by collecting and organizing the data for each indicator;
7. Evaluate care when thresholds are reached in order to identify either opportunities to improve care or problems;
8. Take actions to improve care or to correct identified problems;
9. Assess the effectiveness of the actions

and document the improvement in care; and
10. Communicate the results of the monitoring and evaluation process to relevant individuals, departments, or services and to the organizationwide quality assurance program.

ESTABLISHING A DEPARTMENTAL QUALITY ASSURANCE PROGRAM

Costs

No studies have heretofore been published that document the effectiveness or productivity of any quality assurance program, either on a departmental or a hospital level. Nevertheless, such programs are being mandated and will themselves involve cost. The JCAHO is now recommending that 1% of a hospital's operating budget should be devoted to quality assurance activities. With an estimated 1989 national hospital expense of $175 billion, the cost nationally in hospitals of quality assurance activities should therefore be approximately $1.75 billion per annum, which translates to $44 for each of an estimated 40 million admissions. The proportion and amount spent would vary greatly among hospitals, as there obviously may be a great difference between 1% of the budget in a 100-bed hospital and that in a 600-bed hospital.

Within the University of Iowa Hospitals and Clinics (UIHC), the cost per admission, based upon annual budget and admissions, would be $57. Actual costs of quality assurance (QA) programs are extremely difficult to determine, as accounting depends to a large extent on many individuals' estimates of time spent in QA activities, estimates of the value of such individuals' time, and estimates of relatively uncontrollable expenses such as printing, paper, and computer time. The UIHC, however, has attempted such an actual cost study, but as QA activities are so diffuse, the best conclusion that could be achieved was that QA costs a very indefinite $45 per admission. With QA activities expanding, the cost will increase.

Within our hospital, approximately two-thirds of the cost is associated with the quality assurance department, a facet of hospital administration, and approximately one-third ($15 per admission) of the cost is borne by the clinical departments. These figures may give some guidance to departmental administrators in urology in estimating present and future expenses.

Personnel

The ultimate responsibility for QA lies with top management (8). Within a urology department, therefore, the department head bears responsibility at least to review all QA information and to stimulate its development. This can best be done within the structure of a QA committee (9), which preferably is composed of all staff physicians in the urology department and the one or two nonphysician personnel who may be responsible for most of the data gathering. The direct administrative approach will ensure that the medical staff will be exposed to, learn from, and perhaps influence and stimulate, departmental QA activities. The QA committee should be chaired either by the department head or by a designated senior staff physician.

In smaller departments, a lay administrator may be given the responsibility of collecting and collating the QA information derived from various sources. In larger departments, it may be advisable to employ a part-time or full-time QA coordinator, who should preferably have a medical background, and perhaps, ideally, should be a registered nurse with urological or research experience. Facility in use of computers, data gathering, storage, retrieval, and analysis are highly desirable in such an individual. The initiative and skills required of this ideal person will not be cheap.

Other departmental personnel who will participate in a QA program include inpatient and outpatient nursing staff. While the nursing department in each hospital should have its own QA program, urology nurses can contribute in a variety of ways to the urology department's program and certainly bear significant responsibility for the quality of care within the department.

The departmental head and/or the QA chair need to demonstrate a cooperative and sensitive attitude to the nursing department that will permit the integration of urology nurses into both departments' QA plans. In a situation where data are being gathered and analyzed by two independent groups, the possibility exists that suspicions of hostility or accusatory attitudes may arise. Such feelings will be to the detriment of both groups and will detract from the overall QA effort. The QA manager in each department must be aware of any such problems that may arise and attempt to avoid and resolve them by appropriate interdepartmental consultation and open communication.

Another group within the urology department that should and can play a role in the QA program is the secretarial and chart control staff. Coding and abstracting of chart data constitute major elements of a QA program, and these personnel must be aware of the program and the need for utmost accuracy in their work. Their integration and participation in the program is best achieved through having an administrative representative on the QA committee.

Within an academic urology department, the resident physician staff must be involved in at least some extent in the QA effort. Although the primary function of residents and fellows within a department is a learning one, they obviously participate to a great extent in the service functions and thus play a direct part in the quality of care within their department. They must be aware of, and participate in, the QA efforts of the department, both to assist in that effort and to further their own education within the area. While the faculty can relay QA information to a large extent to residents and fellows, it is advisable to include a resident on the QA committee, to transmit such information, and to encourage and coordinate resident QA activities.

Written Plan

The chair of the QA committee is responsible for a departmental QA plan. This must be written in such a way as to describe the full scope of departmental activities in the clinical and medical record fields. It is best begun by assessing and tabulating the department's inpatient and outpatient care in statistical fashion. Numerical descriptions of the department's activities are usually relatively easy to obtain. Sources include the departmental administration, hospital administration, operating room administration, nursing, and epidemiology.

Descriptors of activity (Table 25.1) provide a good estimate of the department's overall significance within the hospital and, in our case at UIHC, indicate that the urology department is responsible for approximately 2–3% of the hospital's activities, a somewhat humbling piece of knowledge.

Once the major numerical descriptors have been obtained, the plan should proceed to describe the most important aspects of care. Again, numerical descriptors are important and the most frequent operating room and office procedures in our department in fiscal year 1989–1990 are listed in Table 25.2.

Table 25.1.
Major Numerical Descriptors of Clinical Activity in a Urology Department

Inpatient
  Annual admissions
  Annual discharges
  Average daily inpatient census
  Annual number of deaths
Outpatient
  Total annual outpatient visits
  Daily average of outpatient visits
  Annual number of office procedures
  Annual number of radiological examinations
    requested
Surgical
  Annual number of open surgical procedures
  Annual endoscopic surgical procedures
  Other surgical procedures, e.g., ESWL
  Total annual inpatient surgical procedures
  Total annual outpatient surgical procedures
Personnel
  Total number of physicians—faculty and residents
  Total number of administrative and secretarial personnel
  Total number of nursing personnel, both inpatient and outpatient

Table 25.2.
Most Frequent Procedures in UIHC Urology Department 1989–1990

Operating room procedures
  Extracorporeal shock-wave lithotripsy
  Transurethral prostatectomy
  Ureteroscopy with or without stone extraction
  Transurethral resection of bladder tumor
  Circumcision
  Bladder biopsy
  Inflatable penile prosthesis insertion
  Bilateral orchiectomy
  Transperineal insertion of Au[198] seeds
  Urethroplasty for hypospadias
  Radical nephrectomy
  Radical retropubic prostatectomy
Office/clinic procedures
  Cystoscopy
  Urinary flow study
  Cystoscopy with stent placement
  Cystometrogram
  Transrectal ultrasound, with or without prostate biopsy
  Intravesical instillation of chemotherapeutic agent
  Cystoscopy with retrograde pyelogram
  Intracorporeal injection of pharmacologic agents

Such quantitative data provide part of the basis for a variety of monitors of quality of care, as the JCAHO has requested that the most frequently performed procedures be analyzed in regards to quality. A second factor, however, in constructing QA monitors is the importance of procedures, and thus clinical judgment and experience must be used to place emphasis upon the monitoring of those procedures that are the most intrinsically difficult and/or carry the most risk for the patient. In urological practice, the most complication-prone procedures are radical operations, such as for cancer of the bladder, prostate, kidney, and testis, particularly those in which a concomitant urinary diversion is carried out. Procedures involving microscopic anastomoses such as penile revascularization or vasovasostomy are also characterized by intrinsic difficulty requiring specialized surgical skills, although they involve less risk to the patient. Such procedures should also be included in the QA plan, particularly as they lend themselves rather well to early outcomes monitoring.

Most of the procedures thus far suggested for monitoring are performed on an inpatient basis, and care must also be taken in the construction of a QA plan to construct monitors of outpatient care. It may be somewhat more difficult to construct meaningful outpatient monitors because of the relatively brief contact with patients, low volume of chart work, and sometimes incomplete follow-up, which hinders the development of outcomes data (9, 10). Nevertheless, as we have many more patient contacts and perform many more procedures in the office or clinic than in the inpatient area, efforts must be made to assess quality of care rendered to outpatients.

The QA plan, then, should contain written descriptions of proposed monitors covering various areas of the department's activities. It must, however, be flexible, so that new monitors can be introduced periodically as practice changes, and old monitors may be dropped out if they are somehow unsatisfactory, or if performance in that particular area is consistently demonstrated to be of highest quality. The introduction of new monitors will also reduce any tendency toward stagnation in the QA committee's activities and attitudes. Likewise, periodic rotation of membership on the committee will assist in this regard.

Data Gathering

Much of the data accrued by the QA committee will come from sources outside the urology department, such as the pathology department, epidemiology department, pharmacology committee, etc. Such data can be funnelled to the QA committee chair or coordinator. Quantitative and qualitative data regarding departmental structure and personnel should be the responsibility of the department head or lay administrator. Secretarial and chart control personnel can gather and collate much of the information that comes from chart auditing.

The physicians in the department must be involved in the data-gathering process to some extent. Without this activity, the QA program will tend to be regarded by them as another bureaucratic nuisance that is impeding their free decision making. A major benefit of physician involvement in the auditing process is an improvement in their own performance in the areas that are being audited. In one study, passive receipt by physicians of information regarding their own performance of selected preventive health measures (routine mammography and influenza vaccination) improved their rate of ordering or performing such procedures to a slight degree, while active involvement in the auditing process improved their performance more significantly (11).

Data Management

Data are best collected in some instances on an annual basis, but in most instances on a monthly basis. Computer entry of data is perhaps the most efficient method of storage and certainly facilitates the recognition of trends and the establishment of thresholds in various monitors, which may help in the early identification of problems or ways to improve the delivery of care in the department. All significant information should be presented by the QA chair to the QA committee at mandated monthly meetings.

The QA chair must keep detailed minutes of these meetings in which the data and problems discovered are fully described. State statutes have granted immunity to the peer review process (4), of which QA programs are a part, and thus specific identification in the minutes of problems in the delivery of care by the department as a whole or by individual physicians will not be legally discoverable. Such detailed minutes have in our recent experience assisted greatly in accreditation of the UIHC by the JCAHO.

Communication of Results

A great deal of sensitive information will be accumulated by and discussed in a QA committee. The committee, its chair, and the department head obviously bear major responsibilities in their handling of this information. For improvement of medical care within the department, some of the information, probably in selected or summarized fashion, will need to be transmitted to all departmental personnel or to relevant groups or individuals. In such transmission, emphasis must be placed on the educational nature of the material and on ways in which it can be utilized for future performance enhancement. The mode of transmission of information is particularly important in any instance where criticism of an individual or group might be inferred. Letters or memos are susceptible to misinterpretation, or they may generate emotions that will lead to an undermining of the QA program. It is vitally important for departmental morale, therefore, that sensitive information or criticisms be discussed by one of the QA administrators face to face with the involved personnel. This will allow for better communications, bilateral suggestions for improvement, and a more willing acceptance of the need for correction of problems discovered.

The departmental QA committee is also responsible to the hospital QA program and must transmit its findings and the results of its actions to the central hospital QA department or committee. The monthly tabulation of monitor results must be sent to the hospital committee, along with minutes of the meetings. The department head may choose to withhold certain particularly sensitive findings regarding individuals and indeed may have a responsibility to attempt to resolve major problems in a private and confidential fashion.

A strong and reliable sense of discretion is obviously a mandatory characteristic for any personnel involved in QA activities, either on a departmental or hospital level. Great care must be taken to avoid injury to any individual's or group's reputation, to avoid back biting, gossip, and possibly libelous statements, and to emphasize continually the positive intent of QA activities, that is, the goal to improve the department's delivery of medical care to its patients.

Problem Resolution

A necessary element of any QA program is a method to attempt to resolve identified problems and later to restudy and confirm that improvement or resolution has, in fact, occurred. The method of resolution has been the subject of much debate, particularly in relationship to problems associated with physicians. Physicians' attitudes may be affected by time constraints, reimbursement incentives, and a bias toward active treatment rather than preventive or administrative medicine (12).

The effect of continuing medical education (CME) in changing physician behavior or patient outcome is equivocal at best, and most studies find it produces little improvement (13). The use of packaged educational materials has been studied in randomized trials and found to improve physician behavior or performance in those who were already performing at a higher level, but to have little effect on the behavior of those who were deficient (14). An innovative attempt to affect physicians' prescribing of overused drugs was instituted in one randomized study in which the trial group of physicians were subjected to academic "detailing," modeled on pharmaceutical representative activities. A statistically significant and long-lasting decrease in the prescribing of these drugs occurred in the study group compared to control physicians, who received only printed educational materials (15).

Feedback regarding physicians' compliance rates with certain criteria of medical care, particularly when combined with information regarding their peers' or group performance, has been found to improve the individual's compliance. Superior performance has been noted when the individual is first asked to estimate his or her own compliance rate before the feedback regarding actual compliance is provided (16). Such a method may help to expose a "perception-reality gap."

Reminder systems, such as notes attached to the chart, checklists that the physician annotates during the visit, or follow-up notes sent to the physician have been found in multiple studies to improve physician compliance with a variety of medical care criteria (17–19), especially follow-up on abnormal test results, which is obviously a very critical area.

One major problem with feedback and reminder systems, particularly in academic institutions, is that the health care provider may not be treating a well-defined population on a continuing basis. This is less true in surgical departments than in medical departments, but absences from clinical service due to research activities or travel commitments increase the likelihood that important information will not reach, or be acted upon, by the appropriate staff member.

On occasion, QA activities may uncover a physician-associated problem of such magnitude that administrative action is required for its resolution. Whether this is a single incident, or a pattern of events, the rate-limiting step at this level is the reluctance of the medical staff or department head to restrict or sanction one of their colleagues (9). This major barrier must be removed for the effective QA program to function. Public recognition of its removal will also reduce the perception of physicians as a self-protective group.

The main thrust of medical QA programs is identification of problems, corrective action, and restudy until problem resolution is documented. A somewhat more positive attitude might be created if we applied lessons from industrial quality control systems in which the major goal is to achieve continual improvement rather than seeking to identify individual flaws (20). Industry has long recognized that improved quality may be the best method of controlling cost and that quality control requires the attention of high management. Analysis and improvements in systems design or the production process may be more effective than tinkering with the final product. The quality control cycle is a never-ending one in which continual improvement in performance is sought rather than achievement of a preset standard. In industry, it has been recognized that the greatest quality improvements are achieved when all employees receive information based upon high values and a sense of pride, in a trusting and cooperative atmosphere, rather than an environment of fear.

Respect for the worker, who must be presumed to be trying hard, is critical.

Investments of time and money in education and in study should be substantial. Leaders should promulgate a shared vision of continuous improvement in health care delivery rather than a negative, punitive attitude directed at finding fault and assigning blame (21).

EPIDEMIOLOGY CONSIDERATIONS

Individual departments within a hospital, including urology, may not have the facilities for QA activities of the extent desired by the JCAHO. Certainly, in view of the relatively recent emphasis on departmental programs, the long-term experience is not present for collecting and summarizing large data bases. For certain monitors, such as infection rates, it is valuable for each department to compare its results with hospital wide rates. Statistical and analytical expertise of the type required for a QA program may not be available within the department.

Within a hospital, the epidemiology department traditionally has been the repository of much longitudinal data required for JCAHO accreditation, and as hospital QA programs have developed, they have maintained a close relationship with, or have been administered from, the epidemiology department.

It has been suggested that quality assurance is the new epidemiology. Epidemiologists have embraced risk management, drug use review, surgical case review, and other QA elements (22). Their willingness to do this, and their expertise in continuous monitoring techniques, along with the availability of trained personnel can be of great assistance at the clinical departmental level. Friendly cooperation with the epidemiology department will assist each department greatly in developing and refining monitors or measures of quality care. For many departmental monitors, epidemiology is already collecting the data and has established norms of performance on a hospital wide and departmental basis. Epidemiological methods in the past have focused on access to medical care, methods and process of delivery, and in several areas on outcomes of care (23). As those methods are the basis for QA activities, it seems logical that we should learn from and gain assistance from the epidemiologists.

Within urology departments, however, we must take responsibility for our own QA activities. Cooperation with the epidemiology department does not mean handing over what we may regard as an unpleasant bureaucratic task. This will result in an unpleasant "us versus them" attitude.

We, as urologists, also have an understanding of our own field and an appreciation of significant or important events and trends that even the experienced epidemiologist cannot be expected to develop. Urologists can best appreciate which monitors are most valuable and should be emphasized and can most quickly recognize those that may have little significance for patient care and can be discarded or reviewed less intensively. We will be most familiar with changes in urological practice as they develop and most quickly recognize the new areas that need research.

The two departments must therefore work in concert to continue to develop the QA program in its most effective fashion. Personal contacts at reasonable intervals between the departmental QA chair and the hospital epidemiologist will be invaluable in this effort, and potential quality concerns recognized by one or the other may be discussed and acted upon.

RISK MANAGEMENT EFFORTS

The aims of a risk management program are to minimize injury to patients as a result of medical care delivered, to identify cases of injury that might result in tort claims, and to minimize the negative outcomes and costs associated. It is an area of medical endeavor that falls naturally under the aegis of QA programs and epidemiology departments. Risk management programs are widely felt (with little documented evidence) to reduce the number and size of medical malpractice claims. The interest in such programs is illustrated in the results of a questionnaire sent to medi-

cal schools, which documented that 45% of 69 responding schools had recently sponsored continuing medical education programs related to risk management. Likewise, 68% of 31 responding state medical societies had recently sponsored such a program (24).

In Michigan, data accumulated from 1976 to 1989 indicated that urology was not among the 10 most-sued specialties (25). During that period, the Michigan Physicians Mutual Liability Company paid a total indemnity of $232 million. The two major maloccurrences, accounting for 34 and 26.5%, respectively, of the total sum were "errors in diagnosis" and "procedure improperly performed."

In Illinois, from 1976 to 1988, the closed-claim frequency for urologists was 421, with 16% of these cases being "closed with indemnity" (26). Nationally, the most common cases in which errors in diagnosis by urologists resulted in files closed with indemnity were torsion of the testis, cancer of the prostate, cancer of the testis, and lung cancer (missed lesion on chest x-ray). The highest average settlement per case was $758,000, for testis cancer, with the others all less than $100,000 average (27). The most frequent "procedure improperly performed" diagnoses were calculus of kidney, hyperplasia of the prostate, cancer of the prostate, and male sterilization.

These and similar data should be available to the QA committee and will be valuable in planning monitors that will help in the risk management and QA effort.

SELECTING QA MONITORS

The quality of health care has been said to reflect the proportion of achievable improvements in health actually attained (28). It may be alternatively stated as effectiveness of care, and a variety of methods have been used to assess it, which may be broadly stated as structure, process, and outcomes analysis.

Monitors of Structure

In the past, the JCAHO has emphasized the structure of the health care organization in accreditation inspections. Thus, physical facilities, departmental organization, safety, and credentialling of staff have been important aspects of hospital accreditation. Such monitors of structure should be included in the initial efforts of a departmental QA program.

Within our urology department, a file is maintained on each physician in which continuing documentation is kept regarding medical licensure, graduate education, specialty certification, and health problems. Annual review of each physician's competence in clinical judgment and in surgical performance is carried out by the QA chair and department head. A letter of recommendation is then sent to the credentialling committee of the hospital regarding renewal of each physician's clinical privileges, and a copy is inserted in the individual's file.

The statistics of the department morbidity and mortality conferences are reviewed annually. The total numbers and types of complications associated with each physician are reviewed and a relevant entry made in the physician's file. Great care must be taken to correlate these comments with the individual physician's case load and case mix, as there may be very large variations among staff members in these respects in this era of subspecialization. Severity of illness and comorbidities may vary greatly among different physicians' patients, and these must be taken into account, although their analysis and quantification may be exceedingly difficult.

These monitors of physician capabilities will ensure that the department and the hospital are providing appropriate medical staff to render high quality care.

Periodic evaluation of other facilities, such as office space, number of examining and procedure rooms, availability of and access to laboratory and radiological services, and allotment of adequate operating room time should be carried out. These should be related to total outpatient and inpatient numbers and documented in the department's QA files.

A variety of other structural criteria regarding personnel and facilities in the department can be created which will illustrate and document that the organization is suitably equipped to deliver high quality medical care.

MONITORS OF PROCESS OF CARE

The process of care is the actual performance of, or delivery of, medical care. QA monitors of process have traditionally been of a chart auditing variety, basically looking at the quality of specific items in the chart, such as allergy labeling, history and physical examinations, and discharge summaries. More recently, emphasis is being placed on the decision making prior to the actual delivery of care, with the assumption that decision analysis will produce guidelines that ultimately will lead to more appropriate and better quality use of available medical techniques and technology, both diagnostic and therapeutic.

Chart Auditing

Medical Record Review

Within our department of urology each month, we select a different surgical procedure, such as radical prostatectomy, hypospadias repair, extracorporeal shock-wave lithotripsy (ESWL), etc., for a medical record review. The procedure selection attempts to analyze the frequent and the difficult operations, and it is based also on the various specialty areas in urology, so that all staff physicians are involved in the scrutiny. Each month, we review the charts of the 10 patients who have most recently undergone that operation, and the analysis is performed by both the clinical faculty and the QA coordinator. The analysis is based upon a form designed to summarize the completeness of medical record keeping (Appendix A). Results are communicated to faculty and residents.

In general, this review has revealed the record keeping to be quite good for inpatient procedures, with occasional inadequacies being found both in resident and faculty performance. Major problems were initially found in the outpatient procedures analyzed, such as ESWL, ureteroscopy, and bladder biopsy. Frequently, operative notes were dictated, but no notes were written or dictated summarizing the visit, or the recovery period, or condition on discharge. Often, no clear plan for follow-up was evident from the chart, and no record of medications prescribed was kept. A form was therefore designed to attempt to facilitate this type of record keeping (Appendix B), and restudy of the problem procedures and other outpatient procedures has demonstrated a dramatic improvement in the deficient areas.

Surgical Case Review

Surgical case review (SCR) is now a JCAHO-mandated activity in all hospitals, and at UIHC it is carried out within each department by QA personnel. Following JCAHO guidelines, all procedures undergo review, initially at the 100% level, and if review proves satisfactory, this is reduced to the 25% level for most procedures. While most physicians dislike the idea of guidelines, they really represent the indications for a procedure, be it diagnostic or therapeutic, and incorporate an attempt to confirm that the procedure was properly performed and that the preoperative diagnosis was accurate by using information from the pathology report. Figure 25.1 represents the results of our continuous monitoring in this area from January 1989 to April 1990. One can easily see that our urology department has an excellent record of compliance with SCR criteria and that there has been some improvement in compliance with the passage of time. This is not really surprising considering that we designed our own criteria, as do other departments. Certainly, our effort in this direction fulfilled the main objectives, which was to comply with JCAHO regulations and to continue hospital accreditation.

Outpatient Surgery Cancellations

As outpatient surgery increases in volume in all surgical specialties, monitoring of the cancellation rate can be used as a criterion of quality of care. Cancellations are due to unavoidable factors related to the patient in approximately 50% of cases (travel difficulties, unexpected viral illness, a change of mind). The rest are usually due to failures in the preoperative evaluation process, discovered on the day of surgery, such as an abnormal laboratory value, chest radiograph, or electrocardiogram. Failure to discover that the patient is

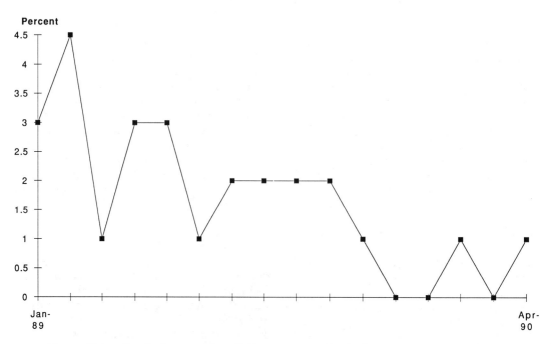

Figure 25.1.   Surgical case review: Failure to meet criteria, January 1989 to April 1990.

Percent

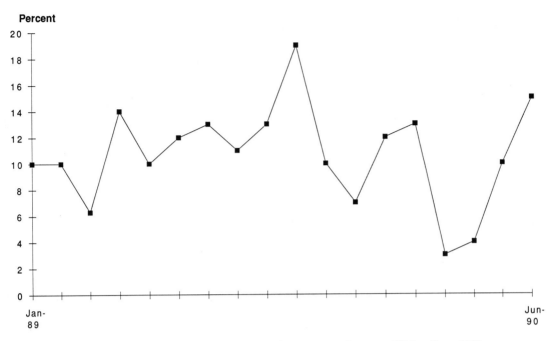

Figure 25.2.   Cancellation rate: Same-day surgery, January 1989 to June 1990.

being treated with anticoagulants or aspirin is also relatively frequent and could be disastrous.

Our average cancellation rate (avoidable plus unavoidable) is 10%, and 18 months of data are presented in Figure 25.2. In spite of numerous discussions at QA meetings and numerous reminders to resident and faculty physicians, there is no downward trend. This may mean that our 10% average cancellation rate (5% avoidable) is a reasonable standard or threshold.

APPROPRIATENESS AND VARIATIONS IN PATTERNS OF MEDICAL CARE

Obviously, looking at our data, one needs to ask why 98–99% of our procedures are appropriate, and only 1–2% inappropriate, while large volumes of literature conclude that up to one-third of hospitalizations and medical interventions are performed for inappropriate reasons.

A study of carotid endarterectomy concluded that 35% were done for appropriate reasons, while the other 65% were inappropriate or equivocal (29). A similar study

of coronary artery bypass grafts concluded that 56% of the operations were done for appropriate reasons, and 44% for equivocal or inappropriate reasons (30). Using similar techniques, another study found that 44% of cardiac pacemakers were definitely indicated, 36% possibly, and 20% not indicated (31).

Many studies have examined the rate of hospitalization for various diagnoses, and the rates of performance of medical interventions in small and large areas of the United States. For some diagnoses and procedures, the rates of admission are consistent within and across areas, but other diagnoses and procedures fall into a category of "high variation," with as much as 3-fold differences in their use (32–34). Variations in admission rates for many diagnosis-related groups (DRGs) have been demonstrated also for pediatric hospitals (35), Canadian hospitals (36), and university-owned teaching hospitals (37). High variation and low variation DRGs are relatively consistent in different areas. Differences in appropriateness probably do not explain the variations (38). Variations are similar with insurance plans that provide free care and those that include cost sharing by the patient (39), indicating that cost sharing causes patients to reduce consumption of both inappropriate *and* appropriate care, which is not desirable.

The major reason behind these variations seems to be physicians' practice habits (33, 40). For many technologies and medical interventions, the indications are somewhat uncertain, particularly in fields with rapid scientific advances. Where an intervention may be somewhat optional or an application of technology indefinite, some physicians will be "aggressive," and some "conservative." Experience seems to lead to greater conservatism (41).

It must be noted that much of the information regarding inappropriate use of medical care and inappropriate hospitalization is garnered from studies which use "the Delphi technique," a technique with which many clinically oriented physicians may have violent disagreement. Panels of experts, health care researchers, economists, and physicians (who are mostly not in the medical specialty under study) review the literature and use their own expertise to compose a list of "appropriate and inappropriate" indications for a particular medical intervention. The indications are weighted for importance and significance and then applied in chart reviews (42). The findings with such a technique are heavily dependent on complete charting by treating physicians of the rationale and indications for their decisions. One might also assume that the researchers may have a cost control-oriented bias toward finding high rates of inappropriate care, just as we in our urology department have a self-justifying bias toward finding low rates of inappropriate care.

Variations in Care in Urology

There is little literature on variations in urological practice. Transurethral prostatectomy (TURP) has been investigated, and, as with other surgical procedures, has been noted to have significantly different rates both in small and large and in urban and rural areas (43, 44). Even in the case of TURP, an operation with which we have more than 50 years of experience, the indications for its performance are not

clearly defined, and variations seem to depend mostly on whether we are "interventionists" or "observationists." Within Iowa, the lifetime probability of a man undergoing TURP varies between 15 and 45% in different small areas (JW Wennberg, personal communication). Recent attention to this topic, coupled with newer approaches to the treatment of benign prostatic hypertrophy (BPH), whose indications and outcomes are also unclear, have led to the initiation of randomized clinical trials by both the Veterans Administration and the American Urological Association. Whether these trials will resolve the problem of indefinite indications for prostatectomy is debatable. One side effect of these, as of many clinical trials, is that they lead to increased use of diagnostic testing, such as prostatic ultrasound and urodynamic and flow studies. Use of these tests, which are not proven to be truly beneficial in the evaluation of the condition or the decision to treat, tends to become routine, even among urologists who are not involved in the clinical trials.

Another example of technology with widespread variations in use is transurethral prostatic ultrasound, a relatively new urological tool, the indications for which are not at all clear, even to a panel of alleged experts (45). Nevertheless, with encouragement from industry, and with a turf-protecting desire to circumvent radiologists, urologists are purchasing the equipment in large volume, and using it widely in the evaluation of benign and malignant prostatic disease. Another widespread use is in screening for early prostatic cancer, an effort of uncertain value to either the individual or group with that diagnosis, but which seems to have resulted in a nationwide increase in radical prostatectomy.

Even in the case of old and familiar diagnostic techniques, such as the excretory urogram and the cystogram, large variations in frequency of use occur. Urologists who own radiological equipment perform these tests 4 to 4.5 times more frequently in patients with voiding symptoms than urologists who must refer the patient to a radiologist for the examination (46). Urologists also charge more than radiologists, resulting in imaging charges per episode that are 4–7 times higher for those owning the equipment.

Considering the multiple reasons that lie behind the variations in use of care and the lack of scientifically reliable data to guide us, it becomes extremely difficult within a urology QA program to construct criteria that are highly valid for many diagnostic tests or operations. A combination of explicit criteria (lists of indications, which can be used by a nonexpert to perform review) and implicit review (performed without lists by an expert using his or her best judgment) can be used. In uncertain areas, further research is necessary—a trite and commonly used solution to many problems, which defers the need for action.

OUTCOMES MONITORS

The last major area of QA monitoring is the assessment of outcomes. This area is slowly developing both on a small, departmental level and on a national level. A negative summary of possible outcomes is given in the five Ds—death, disability, disease, discomfort, and dissatisfaction (47).

Death

The first and worst of these, death, is the most easily and reliably extracted from a medical chart, and is now being used by the Health Care Financing Administration (HCFA) as part of a publicly available data base of hospitals' performance (48). Interestingly, death rates for particular DRGs vary widely among hospitals, due possibly to differences in quality of care or severity of illness (49).

Fortunately, in urology practice, death is infrequent, but as all deaths will inevitably be discussed in morbidity and mortality (M&M) conferences, it becomes a monitor in the QA program. M&M discussion is an implicit review by experts, but each death should also be discussed at QA committee meetings to confirm the existence or lack of existence of a quality of care problem. Autopsies are encouraged by the JCAHO, and an autopsy rate of approximately 35% for inhospital mortalities is suggested for

accreditation. Although the value of autopsies is frequently questioned in this age of supposed diagnostic accuracy, a review of published results in the 1980s revealed approximately a 30% rate of major unexpected findings, of which one-third were treatable (50). The most frequently missed diagnoses were pulmonary embolus and myocardial infarction.

Nosocomial Infections

Our epidemiology department does an excellent job of surveillance for nosocomial infections, and the urology department's monthly rate averages seven infections per 1000 patient days (Fig. 25.3). This includes urinary infections, respiratory infections, wound infections, and infections at intravenous catheter sites. When the rate exceeds a threshold of 11 infections per 1000 patient days, the QA committee investigates for patterns of personnel involvement and possible cross-contamination of inpatients. Our wound infection rate (all types of wound) consistently runs at 0–4% and has not posed a problem.

Unscheduled Admissions

All admissions that occur after an outpatient surgical procedure are reviewed for appropriateness. Our average monthly rate is 10% (Fig 25.4). Most admissions occur in stone disease cases, after ESWL or ureteroscopic stone extraction. Pain, nausea, vomiting, or fever are invariably documented as the reason for admission. Most are justified admissions, but on occasion the QA committee will feel that the admission was too precipitous and that the patient showed no sign of problems following the admission. Discharge the following day is a suspicious sign, but not by any means a definite indicator, of unnecessary admission.

Confirmed ESWL Success Rate

The status of each patient undergoing ESWL in our department is investigated 3 months after treatment. This allows for passage of stone fragments and radiologi-

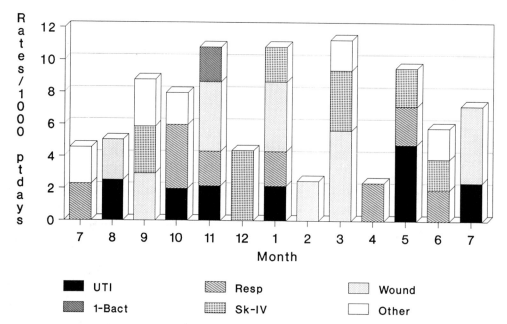

Figure 25.3.   1989–1990 urology department nosocomial rates. *1-Bact,* primary bacteremia; *Resp,* respiratory (upper and lower): *Sk-IV,* skin, intravenous site. This material has been prepared for use by a University of Iowa Hospitals and Clinics staff committee investigating ways to reduce morbidity and mortality.

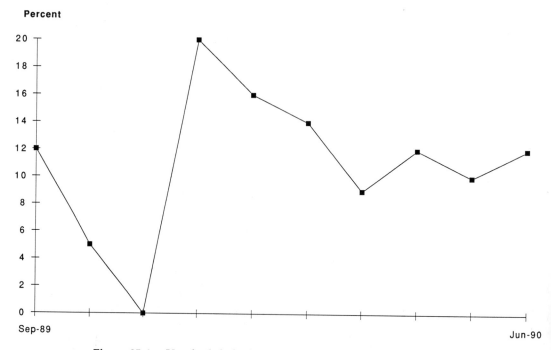

Figure 25.4.   Unscheduled admissions, September 1989 to June 1990.

cal confirmation of stone-free status. If less than 75% of patients are rendered stone free, the QA committee investigates (Fig. 25.5). Failures are usually due to the complexity of the stone disease. Many patients obtain follow-up studies by referring physicians, and it is often difficult for us to confirm success in these cases.

Patient Satisfaction Questionnaire

A six-item questionnaire regarding satisfaction with inpatient care is given to all inpatients on the day of discharge. The patient's faculty and resident physicians are named on the questionnaire (Appendix C). Patients are guaranteed anonymity. Comments are invited. Inpatient satisfaction rates are consistently very high, and most complaints refer to hospital food, poorly functioning television sets, and nocturnally noisy roommates. The most common physician-related complaint is inadequacy of preoperative counseling, and the involved physicians are always informed by the QA personnel. Longitudinal

results of this questionnaire are presented in Figure 25.6.

Randomly selected outpatients (20 per month) are asked to complete a questionnaire regarding their office or clinic visit (Appendix D). Results are more frequently negative. Approximately 30% of patients register some complaint, usually about waiting time, and frequently about the hurried manner that they perceive in some physicians they encounter. These results spur us on to better efforts in these areas.

Patient questionnaires are often criticized as QA monitors. However, there is considerable evidence that their results relate to the humaneness and technical competence of the caregiver (51). These qualities and outcome satisfaction are usually rated highly by patients, whereas dissatisfaction is most often expressed in regards to cost, bureaucracy, and inadequacy of counseling or information given (52). Certainly humaneness, compassion, and commitment to the patient are necessary characteristics in a physician (53) and are rarely addressed in critical health research literature. Questionnaires allow us to demonstrate that these vital qualities

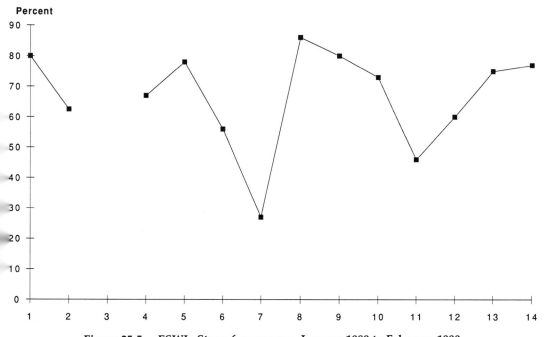

Figure 25.5.   ESWL: Stone-free success, January 1989 to February 1990.

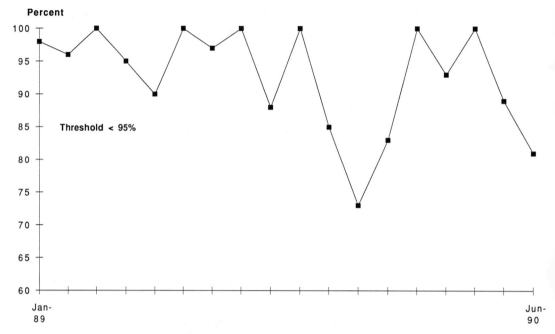

Figure 25.6. Satisfaction questionnaire, January 1989 to June 1990.

still are widely prevalent in medical caregivers. They also may help us to discover unsuspected problems at low cost.

Adverse Occurrences

One of the most interesting, useful, and certainly controversial monitors in our departmental QA program is the reporting of adverse occurrences in patient care. The term itself generated sufficient hostility that it has been changed to risk control surveillance. The surveillance is carried out by epidemiology nursing personnel who audit inpatients' charts on a daily basis. The data are reported monthly to our QA chair and discussed in committee. Each occurrence is referenced with a code number indicating faculty physician responsibility. Adverse events are subclassified into new conditions, accidents, patient complaints, medication-related, and procedure-related events. The first three of these are of very low incidence and rarely signify a QA problem.

Medication-related events are due to nursing errors in approximately 70% of cases. These consist mostly of missed dosage administration, wrong dose, and occasionally wrong patient, and have rarely given rise to problems. Physicians feel that responsibility is unjustly being assigned to them for what they see as a nursing problem. Medication error analysis has indicated that errors are physician-related in about 25% of instances, with prescription and transcription errors being predominant (54). About 20% of these errors have the potential for major impact. The prevailing medication error rate in United States hospitals is 0.6 to 3.5% and can be significantly reduced by QA activity.

Our monthly discussion of the procedure-related adverse events also gives rise to considerable controversy, principally because urologists do not fully agree with what is perceived by the epidemiologists to be an adverse event, and secondarily because the epidemiology program may note several different adverse events in the hospital course of a single patient. The urologist will tend to look upon this as a single bad outcome. The sensitivity of urologists is related to the implication that the procedure may not have been properly performed, which as previously noted, is a common cause of law suits (25, 26). Also, the urologist is (probably unnecessarily) nervous that records of his or her adverse occurrence data may some day become available to lawyers or to the national practitioner data bank (55). Dialogue between epidemiology and urology is necessary to modify any imperfections in this area and to render the information obtained as useful as possible. Undoubtedly, the epidemiology review discovers more maloccurrences than are reported at our monthly M&M conference. This is partly a matter of semantics, and partly due to the differences in perception of the two specialties. Regardless, "sentinel event" assessment has arrived as a QA tool both on a local level through chart auditing (56) and on a national level using administrative data bases (57).

Other Outcomes Monitors

Many other outcomes monitors can be easily constructed in urology, and comparative data can be obtained from the literature to establish standard or threshold results. Most procedures will be performed with a frequency that warrants only annual review. Examples of procedures that produce rapid information on desired or undesired outcomes are penile prosthesis insertion, vasectomy, vasovasostomy, varicocele ligation, and hypospadias repair. Outcomes data for the treatment of malignancies or other complex diagnoses are not as easily obtained, as the necessary follow-up period is considerably longer.

Within an academic department, clinical research papers or abstracts can be filed as QA information. Such data and results from the urological literature must be interpreted cautiously, in light of the previously discussed variations in medical decision making. Also, outcomes data in the literature are primarily from academic centers and should not necessarily be broadly applied in comparisons with private practice hospitals, as there may be significant and unpredictable differences in hospital structure, socioeconomic base, case mix, severity of illness, and other unmeasured confounding variables.

Benign Prostatic Hyperplasia

The most interesting area in which outcomes research in currently impacting urology is in the treatment of benign prostatic hyperplasia (BPH) and, in particular, in the performance of TURP, which is second on the list of frequency of Medicare operations (cataract repair is first). The operation has a major national economic impact, is performed in a degenerating age group, and is now being performed at a rate 150% greater than 20 years ago (58). Major geographic rate variations are known to occur. Outcomes research using large, international, administrative data bases suggest that unfavorable outcomes such as death and reoperation occur 1.45 times and 3 times, respectively, more frequently following TURP than following open prostatectomy for BPH (59). Decision analysis techniques have concluded that there is no significant difference in life span or in quality adjusted life months between men who undergo TURP and those who undergo watchful waiting for moderate symptoms of prostatism (60). The most sensitive index of success of TURP in these patients is the patient's perception of disability due to his symptoms. This has led to a suggestion that the patient should be the major decision maker in whether to undergo the operation, after first reviewing, and being instructed on, extensive educational materials (61).

As previously mentioned, the Veterans Administration and the American Urological Association have separately sponsored major outcomes projects in the treatment of BPH. As the potential outcomes are somewhat ill defined, subjective, and not always reliable and reproducible, the results and recommendations of such studies are likely to be vague and subject to much criticism.

CONCLUSION

This chapter has attempted to describe QA efforts in one urology department and relate the effort both to JCAHO requirements and to the burgeoning discipline of health services research. QA is often viewed as a bureaucratic tool to discover "bad physicians." However, there are not many bad physicians (62). Although physicians' practices are motivated by multiple factors, the desire to perform well and in compassionate fashion remains highly valued both by us and our patients. The concept of continual improvement in performance has long been embraced by physicians, as witnessed by postgraduate and continuing medical education activities.

Evidence of variations in patterns of care render us liable to the accusation of performing unnecessary procedures, but the methodology of these studies is subject to significant debate. Such evidence, combined with spiraling costs, have inevitably led to scrutiny by payers, which will become more intense in the future (63). A new government agency was established in 1989, the Agency for Health Care Policy and Research (AHCPR), whose goals are "to promote the quality, appropriateness, and effectiveness of health care services, and access to such services" (64). This agency will undoubtedly cause more pressure on hospitals and physicians in the QA and cost-control areas.

We need to cooperate with these efforts. We need to become more familiar with the evaluative sciences, statistics, mathematical modeling, and psychometrics to justify or modify what we are doing. In areas of medical uncertainty, we need to reduce intervention rates. We need to evaluate properly the utility of new technology before applying it broadly. We need to emphasize the preventive aspects of medicine, which are usually less costly and contribute more significantly to increases in duration and quality of life. These aspects must be communicated more extensively to the public and the government whose habits and policies certainly contribute to the problems that we address in quality assessment of medical care.

References

1. Ray R. The challenge for a quality health policy. Des Moines Register, May 23, 1990:9A.
2. Anonymous. Not enough for all. Newsweek, May 14, 1990:53.
3. Rahman F. A doctor's remedy. Newsweek, April 9, 1990:10.
4. Hirsh HL. Hospital and medical staff relations in the USA. Med Law 1988;7:33–39.
5. Graham J. Quality gets a closer look. Mod Healthc 1987;7:20–31.
6. Robinson, ML. Sneak preview: JCAHO's quality indicators. Hospitals 1988;62(13):38–43.
7. Joint Commission on Accreditation of Healthcare Organizations. Quality assurance. Accreditation manual for hospitals. Chicago: JCAHO, 1990;51–57.
8. Skillicorn SA. Quality and accountability. San Francisco, CA: Editorial Consultants, Inc. 1980.
9. Bennett WG, Delafield JP, Mishra SK, Tyler R. Quality assurance in ambulatory care. Acad Med 1989;64(Suppl 2):S22–S27.
10. Norman LA. Evolving principles of office quality assurance. West J Med 1988;149:230–233.
11. Brady WJ, Hissa DC, McConnell M, Wones RG. Should physicians perform their own quality assurance audits? J Gen Intern Med 1988;3:560–565.
12. Pels RJ, Bor DH, Lawrence RS. Decision making for introducing clinical preventive services. Annu Rev Public Health 1989;10:363–383.
13. Haynes RB, Davis DA, McKibbon A, Tugwell P. A critical appraisal of the efficacy of continuing medical education. JAMA 1984;251:61–64.
14. Cohen SJ, Weinberger M, Hui SL, Tierney WM, McDonald CJ. The impact of reading on physicians' nonadherence to recommended standards of medical care. Soc Sci Med 1985;21:909–914.
15. Avorn J, Soumeri SB. Improving drug-therapy decision through educational outreach. N Engl J Med 1983;308:1457–1463.
16. Rosser WW. Using the perception-reality gap to alter prescribing patterns. J Med Educ 1983;58:728–732.
17. McDonald CJ. Protocol-based computer reminders, the quality of care and the non-perfectability of man. N Engl J Med 1976;295:1351–1355.
18. McDonald CJ, Hui SL, Smith DM, Tierney WM, Cohen SJ. Reminders to physicians from an introspective computer medical record. A two-year randomized trial. Ann Intern Med 1984;100:130–138.
19. McPhee SJ, Bird JA, Jenkins C, Fordham D. Promoting cancer screening—A randomized, controlled trial of three interventions. Arch Intern Med 1989;149:1866–1872.
20. Berwick DM. Measuring health care quality. Pediatr Rev 1988;10:11–16.
21. Berwick DM. Continuous improvement as an ideal in health care. N Engl J Med 1989;320:53–56.
22. Wenzel RP, Carlson BB. Hospital epidemiology beyond infection control and toward quality assurance. Clin Microbiol Newsl 1988;10:60–62.
23. Wenzel RP. Quality assessment—An emerging component of hospital epidemiology. Diagn Microbiol Infect Dis 1990;13:197–204.
24. Kapp MB. Survey of continuing medical education programs in legal liability and risk management. South Med J 1990;83:37–38.
25. Berglund TR. Risk management key to reducing liability and promoting quality, says MPMLC. Mich Med September 1989;16–17.

26. Sohn H. Risk management issues in the 1990s—Part I. Clin Urol Forum 1989;2(1):6–12.

27. Sohn H. Risk management issues in the 1990s—Part II. Clin Urol Forum 1989;2(2):5–11.

28. Donabedian A. Quality assessment and assurance: Unity of purpose, diversity of means. Inquiry 1988;25:173–192.

29. Winslow CM, Solomon DH, Chassin MR, Kosecoff J, Merrick NJ, Brook RH. The appropriateness of carotid endarterectomy. N Engl J Med 1988;318:721–727.

30. Winslow CM, Kosecoff JB, Chassin MR, Kanouse DE, Brook RH. The appropriateness of performing coronary artery bypass surgery. JAMA 1988;260:505–509.

31. Greenspan AM, Kay HR, Berger BC, Greenberg RM, Greenspon AJ, Gaughan MJS. Incidence of unwarranted implantation of permanent cardiac pacemakers in a large medical population. N Engl J Med 1988;318:158–163.

32. Braveman P, Oliva G, Miller MG, Reiter R, Egerter S. Adverse outcomes and lack of health insurance among newborns in an eight-county area of California, 1982 to 1986. N Engl J Med 1989;321:508–512.

33. Keller RB. Maine program analyzes small area variations. AAOS Bull 1987;July, 9–12.

34. McMahon LF, Wolfe RA, Tedeschi PJ. Variation in hospital admissions among small areas—A comparison of Maine and Michigan. Med Care 1989;27:623–631.

35. Perrin JM, Homer CJ, Berwick DM, Woolf AD, Freeman JL, Wennberg JE. Variations in rates of hospitalization of children in three urban communities. N Engl J Med 1989;320:1183–1187.

36. Roos NP, Flowerdew G, Wajda A, Tate RB. Variations in physicians' hospitalization practices: A population-based study in Manitoba, Canada. Am J Public Health 1986;76:45–51.

37. Wennberg JE, Freeman JL, Culp WJ. Are hospital services rationed in New Haven or over-utilised in Boston? Lancet 1987;1:1185–1189.

38. Chassin MR, Kosecoff J, Park RE, et al. Does inappropriate use explain geographic variations in the use of health care services? JAMA 1987;258:2533–2537.

39. Siu AL, Sonnenberg FA, Manning WG, et al. Inappropriate use of hospitals in a randomized trial of health insurance plans. N Engl J Med 1986;315:1259–1266.

40. Smits HL. Medical practice variations revisited. Health Aff (Millwood) 1986;5:91–96.

41. Young MJ, Fried LS, Eisenberg J, Hershey J, Williams S. Do cardiologists have higher thresholds for recommending coronary arteriography than family physicians? Health Serv Res 1987;22:623–635.

42. Wennberg JE. Improving the medical decision-making process. Health Aff (Millwood) 1988;7:99–106.

43. Wennberg JE, Gittelsohn A. Health care delivery in Maine I: Patterns of use of common surgical procedures. J Maine Med Assoc 1975;66:123–130, 149.

44. McPherson K, Wennberg JE, Hovind OB, et al. Small-area variation in the use of common surgical procedures. An international comparison of New England, England, and Norway. N Engl J Med 1982;307:1310–1314.

45. Diagnostic and therapeutic technology assessment (DATTA): Transrectal ultrasonography in prostatic cancer. JAMA 1988;259:2757–2759.

46. Hillman BJ, Joseph CA, Mabry MR, Sunshine JH, Kennedy SD, Noether M. Frequency and costs of diagnostic imaging in office practice—A comparison of self-referring and radiologist-referring physicians. N Engl J Med 1990;323:1604–1608.

47. Lohr KN. Outcome measurement: Concepts and questions. Inquiry 1988;25:37–50.

48. Blumberg MS. Comments on HCFA hospital death rate statistical outliers. Health Serv Res 1987;21:715–739.

49. Chassin MR, Park RE, Lohr KN, Keesey J, Brook RH. Differences among hospitals in Medicare patient mortality. Health Serv Res 1989;24:1–31.

50. Landefeld CS, Goldman L. The autopsy in quality assurance: History and current status, and future directions. QRB 1989;15:42–48.

51. Davies AR, Ware JE. Involving consumers in quality of care assessment. Health Aff (Millwood) 1988;7:33–48.

52. Hall JA, Dornan MC. What patients like about their medical care and how often they are asked: A meta-analysis of the satisfaction literature. Soc Sci Med 1988;27:935–939.

53. Spencer FC. Commitment to the patient. ACS Bull 1990;75:6–19.

54. McElroy J, Martin RD, Kreamer S. Medication error analysis: The road to constant improvement. VA Practitioner 1990;7(11):51–58.

55. Berman S. National practitioner data bank highlights risk management meeting. QRB 1989;15:392–397.

56. Brennan TA, Localio AR, Leape LL, et al. Identification of adverse events occurring during hospitalization. Ann Intern Med 1990;112:221–226.

57. Berwick DM, Knapp MG. Theory and practice for measuring health care quality. Health Care Financ Rev (Annual Suppl) 1987;49–55.

58. Birkhoff JD. Natural history of benign prostatic hypertrophy. In: Hinman F, ed. Benign prostatic hypertrophy. New York: Springer Verlag, 1983:5–9.

59. Roos NP, Wennberg JE, Malenka DJ, et al. Mortality and reoperation after open and transurethral resection of the prostate for benign prostatic hyperplasia. N Engl J Med 1989;320:1120–1124.

60. Fowler FJ Jr, Wennberg JE, Timothy RP, Barry MJ, Mulley AG Jr, Hanley D. Symptom status and quality of life following prostatectomy. JAMA 1988;259:3018–3022.

61. Barry MJ, Mulley AG Jr, Fowler FJ, Wennberg JW. Watchful waiting vs immediate transurethral resection for symptomatic prostatism. JAMA 1988;259:3010–3017.

62. Spencer FC, Halley MM. The harmful effects of the "bad doctor" myth. ACS Bull 1990;75:6–12.

63. Roper WL, Winkenwerder W, Hackbarth GM, Krakauer H. Effectiveness in health care. N Engl J Med 1988;319:1197–1202.

64. Stombler RE. New agency will promote quality of care. ACS Bull 1990;75:20–21.

APPENDICES

APPENDIX A

Guidelines for Medical Records Review by Faculty

Please answer "yes" or "no" to all questions. Add any written comments at the bottom of the sheet.

1. Is the history and physical adequate and appropriate?
2. Is there an adequate informed consent note written by resident or staff?
3. Is the reason for the patient's admission obviously and clearly stated?
4. Are allergies (or lack thereof) clearly noted?
5. Are the progress notes informative regarding patient's daily condition (not simply a tabulation of intake, output, and temperature)?
6. Can you easily tell what, if any, procedures were performed, and whether they were deemed immediately to be successful?
7. Are intraoperative or postoperative complications clearly noted?
8. Is there a management plan for such complications stated and its outcome noted?
9. Is the condition on discharge day clearly described?
10. From this description, can you agree the discharge was appropriate?
11. Were there any contraindications to discharge (e.g., high temperature, elevated WBC), and if so, were they addressed in discharge note, or summary?
12. Is there clear evidence of residents' participation in the patients' care (not simply countersigning students' notes)?
13. Is there clear evidence of participation by staff in the patients' care (not simply countersigning resident notes)?
14. Can you tell if homegoing instructions were given by physicians?
15. Is there clearly a follow-up plan?
16. Overall, do you believe the record of this admission would pass scrutiny by an outside agency?

Comments:

APPENDIX B

B-1b CLINICAL NOTES	DATE
	HOSP. NO.
	NAME
	BIRTHDATE
	ADDRESS
• File most recent sheet of this number ON TOP •	IF NOT IMPRINTED, PLEASE PRINT HOSP. NO., NAME AND LOCATION

DATE (month, day, year) & SIGN EACH ENTRY. Affix to signature: R = resident, S = staff, MS = med. student, N = nurse

UROLOGY CLINIC OUTPATIENT DISCHARGE NOTE
IN LIEU OF THIS FORM, A BRIEF DISCHARGE NOTE MAY BE DICTATED.

ADMITTING DIAGNOSIS:

OPERATION PERFORMED:

POSTOPERATIVE DIAGNOSIS:

OUTCOME OF OPERATION:

POSTOPERATIVE CONDITION:

DISCHARGE CONDITION: Within Normal Limits   If Not, Explain:

VITAL SIGNS:

PATIENT ALERT:

PATIENT TAKING P.O.

PATIENT WALKING

DISCHARGE INSTRUCTIONS GIVEN: Yes   No

RELATIVE PRESENT: Yes   No

DISCHARGE MEDICATIONS:

FOLLOW UP PLAN: UIHC/LMD (IDENTIFY):

DATE: TIME:

FUTURE PROCEDURES PLANNED/INDICATIONS:

PATH/LABS PENDING:

PHYSICIAN'S SIGNATURE: _____ , M.D.   DATE: _____

(continue on other side)

94124/6-89   THE UNIVERSITY OF IOWA HOSPITALS AND CLINICS

Side tabs: B-1b | C LABORATORY | D X-RAY EXAM | E CONSULTATION | F SPEC. EXAM | G THERAPY | H PATHOLOGY | I DIAGNOSIS

APPENDIX C

Patient Discharge Questionnaire

The purpose of this questionnaire is to try to improve the quality of care for patients in the Urology Department. Please answer all questions and feel free to make comments. Your name will not be known to the physicians.

Staff Physician: Dr. _____   Senior Resident: Dr. _____

---

1. Were you well informed about your diagnosis and treatment plan before you were admitted?

   Yes ( )   No ( )

   Comments:

---

2. Do you feel that you received good medical care during your hospital stay?

   Yes ( )   No ( )

   Comments:

---

3. Could your hospital care have been better?

   Yes ( )   No ( )

   Comments:

---

4. Who gave you discharge instructions?

   Physician ( )   Nurse ( )   Both ( )

   Comments:

---

5. Do you know who to contact if you have medical problems after discharge?

   Yes ( )   No ( )

   Comments:

---

6. Would you return to this urology department if you develop a new urology problem in the future?

   Yes ( )   No ( )

   Comments:

APPENDIX D

Urology Clinic Patient Satisfaction Questionnaire

For each question please check YES or NO box and add any comments you may have.

---

1. Do you feel you got good care during your visit to the clinic?

YES ☐   NO ☐

    Comments:

---

2. Did your doctors explain your condition well?

YES ☐   NO ☐

    Comments:

---

3. Did you have to wait too long at any point?

YES ☐   NO ☐

    Comments:

---

4. Do you have any helpful suggestions to improve our clinic service?

26

The Clinical Laboratory

Peter J. Howanitz, M.D., and Joan H. Howanitz, M.D.

Laboratorians have been on the forefront of medical practice improvement for 40 years because of the classic work of Belk and Sunderman. Their studies, comparing performance among laboratories, have served as a nidus for development of programs for performance improvement which by now have become common place for all analytes measured by clinical laboratories (1). Such performance improvement programs, commonly referred to as proficiency programs, for routinely surveying analytical practices in clinical laboratories are about to undergo expansion to all laboratory tests, regardless of the site where they are performed. Extending proficiency testing programs to anatomic pathologists, cytopathologists, and cytotechnologists probably will occur within the next few years. Other quality assurance practices widely used in clinical laboratories include use of biological standards for many analytes measured, preventative maintenance programs for all equipment, and personnel qualifications for laboratory directors, medical technologists, and phlebotomists.

Until the mid-1980s, quality assurance practices in laboratory medicine were aimed at process control with almost all emphasis on the analytical step of the laboratory test. At this step, laboratorians placed almost all their efforts, producing national programs for quality control, developing programs for proficiency testing, constructing large data bases that defined current practices and monitored improvements, agreeing on analytical goals for many procedures, implementing use of biological standards, and improving precision and accuracy. Because of the importance of these activities in good patient care, many laboratory quality assurance practices including quality control, personnel standards, and proficiency testing have been endorsed by federal and state legislative regulations.

With the Agenda for Change, the Joint Commission on Accreditation of Healthcare Organizations (JCAHO) caused a refocusing on activities other than the analytical process performed in clinical laboratories (2). Such activities have been the scope of most of the newly introduced quality assurance measurements required in the clinical laboratory by many of the groups responsible for regulations.

In the United States in 1990, the long-awaited Clinical Laboratory Improvement Amendments of 1988 (CLIA '88) were published (3). These amendments updated, consolidated, and modified the requirements of laboratories licensed under Clinical Laboratories Improvement Act of 1967 (CLIA '67) and of laboratories in the Medicare and Medicaid programs. Much of CLIA '88 was aimed at uniform proficiency testing programs for 12,000 hospital, independent, and nursing home laboratories. Early in 1991, Health Care Financing Administration (HCFA) approved a number of proficiency testing programs, which laboratories could use to fulfill the standard that went into effect in early September 1990. Beginning in the summer of 1991, we will experience these strict new rules and tough penalties, which may threaten the existence of some clinical laboratories or entire hospitals. Also in CLIA '88 were a number of requirements for laboratory quality assurance (QA) programs with specific attention to QA programs involving computers.

THE LABORATORY TEST

The product of the clinical laboratory is the laboratory test result. A laboratory test consists of preanalytical phase, analytical phase, and a postanalytical phase. Each of these three phases contains numerous steps, causing some to call all the steps "the total testing process." As in Figure 26.1, the total testing process begins with the clinician considering indications for ordering a test, then involves a loop of activities extending through the measurement process back to the clinician who interprets the result and decides which action is most appropriate for circumstances under consideration (4). Because this process begins and ends with the physician and his or her thought pro-

cesses, these activities also have been described as the "brain-to-brain" transmission of laboratory information.

After considering indications for a procedure, the physician commonly writes the order in a patient's medical record. In other circumstances, a verbal order or telephone order is given to a nurse who carries out the physician's request. This order may be transmitted to the clinical laboratory in the form of a paper requisition or an electronic request. In some circumstances, the order requires the patient to be adequately prepared for the procedure including restricting or requiring eating, a certain posture prior or during specimen collection, or specific activities such as exercising. The ingestion of food, posture, and exercise all have been shown to have major influences on some laboratory procedures. Usually a blood specimen is procured from the patient by phlebotomy and the specimen placed in the proper container and transported to the clinical laboratory within a preset period of time.

Within the clinical laboratory, a patient specimen undergoes accessioning into the clinical laboratory record keeping system, and blood cells are removed by centrifugation if a serum or plasma specimen is

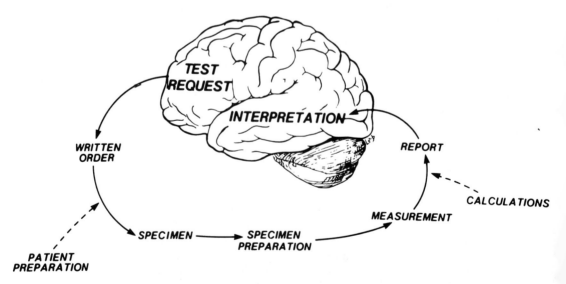

Figure 26.1 Outline of steps from the time the laboratory test is requested until the result is interpreted (4).

required. The specimen then is stored under appropriate conditions until assay. The analytical process usually involves measurements made by large laboratory instruments operated by trained and certified medical technologists who may produce as many as 3600 patient results per hour. Depending upon the instrumentation, result calculations are either performed automatically by the instrument or manually by the technologist, who then also verifies that the results are correct. These results are dispatched to the appropriate patient care area for the patient's medical record and for physician interpretation. Occasionally if the result represents a life-threatening circumstance or if the result is required for an emergent decision, the result may be phoned directly to the physician.

Based on these results, the physician takes appropriate action, which may include ordering another test, changing or continuing the patient's current therapy, seeking consultation, or deciding on a surgical procedure. Quality assurance occurs in a variety of ways at each of the steps in this total testing process.

QUALITY ASSURANCE REQUIREMENTS
Laboratory Licensure and Accreditation

In contrast to other areas of the hospital, compliance with standards of the JCAHO is a minor part of the quality assurance activities performed in the clinical laboratory. A variety of regulatory and voluntary programs designed to establish and maintain *minimum* standards for clinical laboratories have been developed. Standards for laboratory performance are developed by a consensus process and usually are evaluated during on-site inspections by inspectors with preprinted checklists. Those areas that have been subject to monitoring include those listed in Table 26.1. Although appropriate procedures may have been performed, if results are not recorded, that is, if written documentation does not exist, inspectors assume that the

procedure in question has not been performed.

The major groups responsible for licensing or accrediting the clinical laboratory or a discipline within the clinical laboratory in the United States are listed below.

I. Voluntary Accreditation Programs
    1. College of American Pathologists (CAP)
        The CAP developed its laboratory accreditation program over 30 years ago. Approximately 4000 laboratories are accredited and include hospital and independent outpatient facilities in the private sector, the military, the Department of Veterans Affairs Hospitals, the Indian Health Service, and university settings. Accredited laboratories are located in all 50 states, Central America, Europe, the Middle East, and the

Table 26.1.
Key Areas for Licensure and Accreditation[a]

Administrative
    Director qualifications and responsibilities
    Qualifications of personnel
    Safe working environment
    Computers
    Records
    Physician facilities
    Space
    Supplies and inventory
    Continuing education
    Communications
    Reference laboratory referrals
    Laboratory reports
Analytical
    Quality control
    Equipment maintenance (preventive maintenance/function)
    Proficiency testing (surveys)
    Reagents, stains, and media
    Controls and standards
    Procedure manuals
    Validation of methods and instruments
Quality assurance activities
    Personnel
    Total Testing Process

[a]Modified from Duckworth JK. Laboratory licensure and accreditation. In: Howanitz PJ, Howanitz JH, eds. Laboratory quality assurance. New York: McGraw-Hill, 1987:334–353.

Far East. After a laboratory is inspected and accredited, it is reaccredited by on-site inspection every 2 years, self-inspection on alternate years, and a laboratory proficiency program.

Volunteer inspectors, who are peers of the individuals working in the laboratory undergoing inspection, use check lists organized by laboratory sections. These inspectors record the response to each numbered question with a N/A (for nonapplicable), yes, or no. Questions are divided into phase O, I, and II, with phase O questions for information only. Phase I questions represent items that are considered important in the management of a laboratory and any Phase I deficiencies should be corrected. Phase II questions are of major importance and any Phase II deficiencies must be corrected before accreditation is granted. In the course of an inspection, documentation is evaluated in response to 2000 to 5000 questions, depending on the laboratory size.

Although this is a voluntary program, laboratories denied accreditation are reported to the JCAHO (if in a JCAHO accredited hospital) or to HCFA if an interstate laboratory (see below). This program is accepted in lieu of part or all of the requirements of the JCAHO, HCFA, and Centers for Disease Control (CDC) as well as 24 states. We believe these requirements are the most stringent, and laboratories accredited by this program are of the highest quality. A general list of CAP requirements for laboratory accreditation are seen in Appendix A (6).

2. JCAHO

Approximately 5000 acute care and general hospitals currently hold JCAHO accreditations. The standards that applied to laboratories are included in the *Accredi-*

tation Manual for Hospitals in the section entitled "Pathology and Medical Laboratory Services" (7). Standards are similar to those described in Table 26.1. Some of the over 300 specific requirements for laboratory medicine are seen in Appendix B to this chapter. Specific requirements for decentralized laboratory testing as listed in Table 16.13 demonstrate the extent of details specified in these requirements. During the past 15 years, the JCAHO has formally recognized laboratories accredited by the CAP so that additional JCAHO review is not required.

3. American Association of Blood Banks (AABB)

For the past 35 years the AABB has been inspecting and accrediting blood banks and transfusion services. An inspection check list and minimal performance guidelines have been used, and approximately 1200 blood banks are accredited. The AABB also has a program for parentage testing laboratories. Laboratories inspected and accredited by the AABB are usually accredited by other groups as well.

4. American Society of Cytology (ASC)

The ASC has been accrediting cytology laboratories for approximately 20 years. By 1985 approximately 50 laboratories had been accredited.

II. Governmental Agencies

1. HCFA/CDC

In 1965 the Social Security Act established payment benefits for Medicare and Medicaid and regulated laboratories receiving Medicare/Medicaid funds. The Department of Health and Human Services (DHHS) through its agency, the HCFA, has responsibility for promulgating, implementing, and enforcing applicable regulations. Usually HCFA contracts with state Medicare agencies to survey or inspect laboratories. Two voluntary programs, those sponsored by JCAHO and the American Osteopathic Association (AOA), can substitute for on-site surveys by HCFA. Because they can act as substitutes, they are considered equivalent and said to have "deemed status." Approximately 5000 hospitals are accredited by JCAHO and the AOA.

In 1967, laboratories involved in interstate commerce were regulated under the Clinical Laboratory Improvement Act of 1967 (CLIA '67). A number of regulatory requirements including proficiency testing, personnel standards, and accrediting agencies required are different between CLIA and Medicare/Medicaid accredited laboratories. Although CLIA '67 requires inspection of laboratories involved in interstate commerce, it does not provide requirements for those furnishing care for Medicare/Medicaid. Under CLIA '67, the CAP Accreditation Program is an acceptable alternative and has "equivalency." New York state is the only state program that has "equivalency." Differences in Medicare/Medicaid and CLIA '67 have led to CLIA '88, which is scheduled for finalization in mid-1991 (3).

2. Food and Drug Administration (FDA)

The FDA has direct authority for scrutinizing and regulating facilities engaged in testing and providing blood and blood products and inspects these facilities regularly. Approximately 1000 facilities are regulated in this manner. Currently, HCFA investigates fatal transfusion reactions reported to the FDA. The FDA also operates programs that approve laboratory equipment and reagents.

3. Nuclear Regulatory Commission (NRC)

The NRC requires a general license for physicians, clinical laboratories, and hospitals using radioactive material. One license usually suffices to cover an institution's entire radioisotope needs.

4. States and Cities

Approximately one-half of the states regulate clinical laboratories with most requiring on-site surveys (usually annually) and proficiency testing. For those states without laws, agreements are to accept voluntary programs such as the JCAHO, AABB, and CAP in lieu of a state program. New York City is the only city with its own regulatory program for clinical laboratories.

III. Voluntary Standards

1. National Committee on Clinical Laboratory Standards (NCCLS)

This organization is composed of professional organizations, government agencies, and the medical industry and provides the standards generally accepted by the entire clinical laboratory industry. Standards and guidelines are developed by a consensus process and are offered for voluntary compliance, not accreditation or licensure.

2. National Fire Protection Association (NFPA)

This organization is a voluntary organization that publishes standards and codes on clinical laboratory safety. However, NFPA 99 "Standards for Healthcare Facilities" is a primary document containing operational safety requirements for laboratories (8).

IV. Other Agencies and Standards

Occupational Safety and Health Agency (OSHA) protects safety and health of employees in their work place. Standards developed cover such specific occupations as construction work, ship building, and saw mills and clinical laboratory personnel. Environmental Protection Agency (EPA) is responsible for implementing regulations pertaining to hazardous waste management and toxic substances. These standards provide guidelines for regulation of laboratory waste. Compliance with these standards is evaluated by on-site inspections for the laboratory's licensure and accreditation program.

LABORATORY QUALITY ASSURANCE PROGRAMS
Laboratory Process Control

Over the past 40 years, laboratorians have participated in programs that measure and compare analytical performance for almost every analyte measured in the clinical laboratories. Performance is monitored and program participants receive reports that compare their performance to peers. These programs are two general types: interlaboratory quality control programs and interlaboratory proficiency testing programs.

Quality Control Programs

Quality control programs in chemistry are the model for other areas of the clinical laboratory. Because chemistry makes up over one-half of the entire laboratory, programs in this discipline are most important and representative of most of the laboratory. Hematology programs are very similar to chemistry, whereas blood banking and microbiology have some minor differences. Interlaboratory quality control programs require participants to purchase quantities of control materials for extended periods, i.e., 12–18 months in chemistry but as for some hematology measurements, controls are stable for only about 3 months. The number of laboratories that can participate in a program is limited by the quantity of control materials that can be produced as a batch. These materials are packaged in small quantities so that for each day a fresh container may be opened. For chemistry and hematology, quality control materials approximate patient specimens, although they may have a matrix that is human, bovine, mixtures of human and bovine, or ethylene glycol based.

With each analytical run for each analyte, the technologist measures the controls for the analyte in question and plots results on a quality control chart (Fig. 26.2). These charts frequently are called Levey-Jennings charts after the individuals responsible for their introduction into laboratory practice (9). If the results are within defined limits, the analytical run is accepted and patient results are released. If results exceed preset limits, the technologist rejects the analytical run, troubleshoots the procedure, and then repeats the analytical run. Laboratory procedures require two to three quality control specimens throughout the measurement range. When two control samples are used, usually one target value is within the reference interval and the other in the abnormal range. When three samples are used, such as in immunoassay procedures, one sample is within the reference interval and the other two are within the abnormal ranges. Usually abnormal values are chosen at "decision points," levels at which physicians make choices on patient management.

Laboratory practice has been to use quality control rules, which express run acceptance and rejection statistically about a mean. Many of the rules currently used are summarized in Table 26.2 and are divided into those that use control specimens or patient specimens from the laboratory's routine workload. In our experience, most laboratorians use CAP modified rules (10), many still use ± 2 S.D. (from the mean), a few use Shewhart multirules (11), a few now are beginning to use medically useful limits, and a few use a variety of other procedures. Tables 26.3 and 26.4 show the CAP modified rules and Shewhart multirules for run rejection. Both these procedures allow for more than one quality control sample and base decisions on within- and between-run performance. Recently, medically useful limits have been advocated using an automated procedure and a large chemistry analyzer with flexible computer software (12). Such an example is seen in Table 26.5 where the total analytical error for each test can be determined, the imprecision of each measurement procedure (the S.D.) obtained

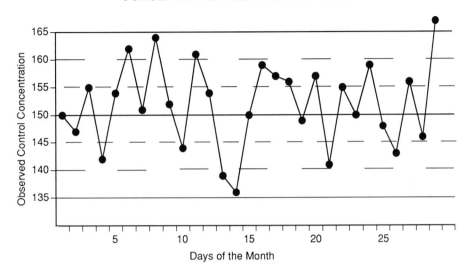

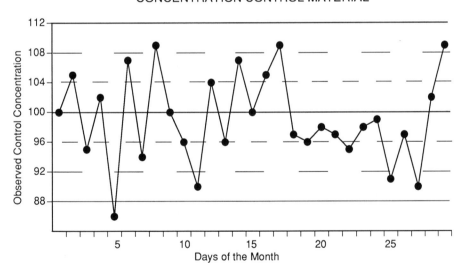

Figure 26.2.   A Levey-Jennings chart of daily quality control results at two levels. Laboratorians plot daily results in relation to the mean and S.D. for every analyte measured.

from past experience, and the medically important systematic and random errors calculated. Such a procedure allows for different limits and a different number and different frequency of quality control samples for each analyte. A recent innovation has been the introduction of quality control grids as part of a chemistry analyzer's software so that the operator can easily select appropriate procedures for each measurement (13).

In North America, many of the quality control programs are offered by one or a group of pathology societies. Figure 26.3

Table 26.2.
Proposed Quality Control Run Rejection Procedures

Criteria	Use	Comment
A. Control samples (statistical)		
±3 S.D.	Rarely	First limits recommended
±2 S.D.	Many laboratories	Easy to implement
±2.5 S.D.	Few laboratories	Easy to implement
CAP modified	Most laboratories	Easy to implement
Shewhart multirule	Rarely	Requires computer
Medical usefulness	Rarely	Requires computer
CUSUM	Rarely	Trend analysis
Triggs' technique	Rarely	Trend analysis
Other multirule schemes	Rarely	Requires computer
B. Patient specimens		
Bull's algorithm	Widely	Used in hematology only
Koepke's algorithm	Rarely	Modified Bull's algorithm
Average of normals	Not used in chemistry	Impractical because of the large number of required specimens

Table 26.3.
CAP Modified Rules

Run rejected when:
 One control in use
  One observation $> \bar{x} \pm 3$ S.D.
  Two consecutive observations $> \bar{x} \pm 2$ S.D.
  Or whenever patient results appear unlikely
 Two controls in use
  One observation $> \bar{x} \pm 3$ S.D.
  Two observations $> \bar{x} \pm 2$ S.D.
  (same control, two consecutive runs, or both controls, same run)
  Or whenever patient results appear unlikely

shows results from the New York State Society of Pathologists' quality control program, which currently uses ethylene glycol-based control materials prepared by Beckman (BKMN) Instrument Company (14). This program offers three levels of control materials and is used in over 300 laboratories for 12–18 months. At the end of each month, results from laboratories are sent to a central computer center, in the case of the New York State Society of Pathologists, the CAP, where data are manipulated and interlaboratory comparisons prepared. Laboratory performance is expressed in terms of a mean, standard deviation (S.D.), and coefficient of variation (CV) for each analyte measured. Laboratorians use such comparisons to monitor their monthly performance in relationship to other participants and to select instrumentation and methods that are more precise (as measured by a lower CV) than they currently use. The scope of such programs includes general chemistry, ligand assay, therapeutic drug monitoring, blood gas analyses, general hematology, coagulation, and physician office laboratories. Occasionally a few new or emerging analytes are not included in a program of this type.

Other Types of Quality Control Procedures Used in the Clinical Laboratory

Hematology. Quality control procedures in hematology most commonly use commercial control materials and quality control rules as described for chemistry. In some laboratories the weighted moving-averages method as described by Bull (15) and refined by Koepke and Protextor (16) are used.

The weighted moving-averages method is used only in hematology quality control and is based upon the empirical observation that averaged red cell indices from patient populations in acute care general hospitals show an approximate Gaussian distribution, are considerably stable, and are similar in all institutions studied for mean cell volume (MCV), mean cell hemoglobin concentration (MCHC), and mean cell hemoglobin (MCH). By use of a com-

Table 26.4.
Shewhart Rules

Warning rule (if exceeded, then data require further inspection):

1_{2s} One observation $> \bar{x} \pm 2$ S.D.

Rejection rules (used if warning rule exceeded; run rejected if any of the rules are violated)

1_{3s} One observation $> \bar{x} \pm 3$ S.D.
2_{2s} Two observations $>$ same limit; that is, $\bar{x} + 2$ S.D. or $\bar{x} - 2$ S.D. (same control, two consecutive runs, or two different controls, same run)
R_{4s} Difference between two observations within run > 4 S.D. (two different controls, one $> \bar{x} + 2$ S.D. and the other $> \bar{x} - 2$ S.D.)
4_{1s} Four consecutive observations $>$ same limit; that is, $\bar{x} + 1$ S.D. or $\bar{x} - 1$ S.D. (same control, four consecutive runs, or two different controls, two consecutive runs)
10_x Ten consecutive observations on same side of mean (same control, ten consecutive runs, or two different controls, five consecutive runs)

Table 26.5.
Medical Usefulness Criteria on a Hitachi 737

Test	Units	Total Error	Observed Precision, S.D.	Systematic Error	Random Error
Sodium	mmol/L	4.0	0.67	4.32[a]	3.05[a]
Potassium	mmol/L	0.3	0.035	6.92	4.37
Chloride	mmol/L	4.0	1.04	2.20	1.96
Total CO_2	mmol/L	3.0	0.75	2.35	2.04
Glucose	mg/dl	8.0	1.20	0.502	0.340
Urea nitrogen	mg/dl	3.0	0.40	0.585	0.338

[a]Systematic and random errors are expressed in multiples of the S.D.; a systematic error of 2.0 corresponds to a 2 S.D. shift: a random error of 2.0 corresponds to a doubling of the S.D.

plex statistical algorithm to evaluate and incorporate successive batches of patient specimen indices into a continually updated mean, daily means are "trimmed and smoothed" (outlier eliminated), thereby deleting the effect of random error and abnormal results. Deviations of these means from specified limits indicate either loss of calibration or a shift in the population tested. Specific patterns of change involving the monitored indices (MCV, MCHC, and MCH) are diagnostic of specific types of instrument malfunctions. Weighted moving averages have been evaluated in comparison with conventional control-based protocols. These studies have identified deficiencies in the weighted moving averages, showing that stabilized whole blood controls could better separate calibration errors from patient variation (17). The continued use of control preparations in conjunction with weighted moving averages therefore was recom-

mended. In a recent study, it was shown that quality control by averaging patient red cell indices does not offer as good error detection as available from conventional charting techniques using stable control materials (18).

Because of the large physiologic variability of white blood cells (WBC) and platelet counts, weighted moving averages cannot be used for daily quality control, and commercial controls are used. Most manufacturers utilize either fixed or unfixed human red blood cells (RBCs), mammalian or human platelets, and avian erythrocytes to simulate human white blood cells, although use of stabilized and unfixed red cells is popular. Sources for control platelets include human, equine, porcine, and bovine platelets.

Quality Control in Blood Banking. Providing patients with safe therapeutically effective units of blood and components is a goal of transfusion therapy.

CONSTITUENT UNIT OF MEASURE METHOD PRINCIPLE INSTRUMENT/SYSTEM	M805101/BKMN/L1						M805102/BKMN/L2					
	AVG. MEAN	SD OF MEANS	AVG. S.D.	AVG. C.V.	NO. FLS	NO. LABS	AVG. MEAN	SD OF MEANS	AVG. S.D.	AVG. C.V.	NO. FLS	NO. LABS
ALBUMIN **G/L**												
DYE BINDING-BCG												
ABBOTT VP							34.6		1.4	4.0	3	3
BECKMN ASTRA 4/8 IDEAL	25.8	0.4	0.6	2.5	41	39	31.9	0.8	0.8	2.5	33	31
GILFORD IMPACT 400,ETC	27.4		1.0	3.8	4	4						
HITACHI 704 BMD	26.0	1.3	0.6	2.5	7	7	33.1	0.7	0.7	2.1	7	7
HITACHI 705 BMD	25.2	1.0	0.9	3.5	19	19	31.8	1.3	0.9	2.9	11	11
HITACHI 717 BMD	27.7		0.6	2.8	5	4	33.1		0.7	2.0	3	3
HITACHI 737 BMD	26.1	0.4	1.0	3.6	8	8	33.2		0.9	2.7	4	4
ROCHE COBAS												
ROCHE COBAS MIRA	26.0	0.6	1.4	5.2	17	16	32.4	0.8	1.6	4.9	15	14
TECHNICON SMA 12/60	25.7		1.1	4.1	6	6	31.1		1.2	4.0	6	6
ALL AUTO CHEM INSTR	26.1	1.0	0.9	3.5	160	144	32.3	1.2	1.1	3.4	121	109
DYE BINDING-BCG W/RA												
IL MONARCH	28.0		1.1	3.8	1	1	33.8		1.1	3.2	1	1
TECHNICON RA 1000	28.6		1.3	4.4	2	2	34.7		1.6	4.6	2	2
ALL AUTO CHEM INSTR	26.2	2.5	0.9	3.3	10	8	32.9	1.4	1.4	4.2	9	7
DYE BINDING-BCP												
ABBOTT SPECTRUM	26.0		1.5	5.9	5	4	31.1		1.7	5.5	5	4
HITACHI 737 BMD	25.7		0.7	2.8	4	4	31.0		0.7	2.3	2	2
ALL AUTO CHEM INSTR	25.2	1.0	1.1	4.1	64	58	30.8	1.2	1.3	4.2	43	39
ALL METHOD PRINCIPLES												
ALL AUTO CHEM INSTR	25.9	1.2	1.0	3.7	234	200	31.9	1.4	1.2	3.6	173	149

Figure 26.3.   A printout of albumin results from an interlaboratory comparison program for daily quality control (14).

Internal programs established within the blood bank are aimed at assuring that procedures, reagents, and instruments are functioning appropriately, that products are safe for use, and that these products are used efficiently and effectively.

Quality assurance in blood banking begins with recruitment and selection of appropriate blood donors. To evaluate recruitment, one needs to monitor the frequency with which blood components are unable to fill the needs and to contrast the shortages with the amount of outdating that occurs (19). Several published studies have shown that low hemoglobin and elevated hepatic enzymes account for about 15 and 30%, respectively, of rejected donors and that the overall rates of rejection are between 7 and 10% of those attempting to donate. If a donor facility has a rejection rate of 20%, it is likely that the staff is not evaluating donors properly and rejecting too many potential donors because of small veins, as this is the most common cause for deferment. Another QA parameter is the incidence of reactions occurring during and following donations. If the donor phlebotomy staff is properly

trained, the donor reactions should be infrequent (less than 1%) and an incomplete or unsuccessful draw should be rare.

The most common analytical procedure performed by blood bank personnel is testing of both donor and patient specimens. Quality control procedures require that antiserum and reagent red cells must react as expected on each day of use. Although reagents used in blood banking are licensed by the FDA, it is necessary to document that the antibody does react with the cells known to be positive for a given antigen and not with cells that are negative. Antibodies chosen for quality control or reagent red cells used in antibody testing should be weakly reactive (1–2+) so that minimum loss of reactivity of the test cells will become apparent. There are no specific requirements for testing of the panel of cells used for antibody identification.

The most important aspect of blood banking quality assurance is a comparison of the patient's current results with previous tests. This can be done by reviewing the patient's blood type with findings previously recorded. In this step, the assumption is that each specimen submitted for typing is correctly identified as to the person from which it was drawn. If such findings indicate the person has not been previously tested, the common practice is to assume that blood typing has been done accurately on the correct specimen. Only a few institutions have implemented a "check type" system in which all patients from whom a specimen has been received for typing for the first time are required to have a second specimen obtained at another time for repeat typing. When the results of the typing on the first specimen are compared with the second, the errors recorded may occur in as many as 0.3% of patients tested (Table 26.6) (20). Findings such as these point to the need for programs to identify patient specimens erroneously drawn, labeled, or typed.

To assure that all blood products are safe for use, all products undergo testing for transfusion-transmitted disease. Currently, all donor units must be negative for hepatitis-B surface antigen (HBsAg), hepatitis-C virus antibody (HCV), antibodies against human immunodeficiency virus I (anti-HIV-I) and human T-cell lymphotrophic virus I/II (HTLV-I/II), a serologic test for syphilis, and show absence of an elevated alanine amino transferase (ALT) level. Because positive findings in tests for HBsAg, HCV, and anti-HIV may have implications for a "healthy" donor, another important part of quality assurance of these tests is that reactive specimens are confirmed as positive with a more specific test. To assure

Table 26.6.
Detection of Mislabeled Blood Bank Specimens

	Years	
	1976–1979	1980–1990
Check type used	No	Yes
Number of errors detected	18	161
Number of units transfused	71,000	220,000
Errors detected/units transfused	1/3944	1/1679
Errors detected/ patients transfused	1/1100	1/280

the safety of the blood supply, all units that are reactive by screening methods for HBsAg and HIV must be destroyed.

Almost all donor blood is converted into two or more components before it is used for transfusion. The method used to prepare components (to remove the plasma or platelets) should result in red cells with a hematocrit not exceeding 80%. If red cells are modified to remove white cells, the method of removal should reduce the total white count by 70% without losing more than 30% of the red cell volume. If frozen, thawed, deglyceralized red cells are prepared, the amount of glycerol remaining should be less than 1%. This can be determined by finding osmolality of less than 500 mosm/kg in units considered ready for transfusion. All units should be visually inspected for hemolysis, and the amount of supernatant hemoglobin should be less than 200 mg/dl. For further information see Polesky (19).

At the time of storage, platelet concentrates must have a minimum number of platelets in a volume of plasma adequate to maintain a pH of ≥ 6.0. When platelets are prepared from whole blood units, 75% of the tested units shall contain at least 5.5×10^{10} platelets/mm^3, with no grossly visible platelet aggregates. In general, platelet concentrates should have minimal red and white cell contamination. Granulate concentrates are prepared usually by cytapheresis and must contain at least 1×10^{10} granulocytes/mm^3 in 75% of the units tested.

Quality Assurance in Microbiology. A comprehensive quality assurance program is necessary to insure reliability and effective use of microbiology results. Like other disciplines, in the clinical laboratory, quality assurance in medical microbiology was proposed in the early 1960s and quickly adopted by regulatory groups. In some ways, quality assurance and quality control activities are similar to activities in other laboratory medicine disciplines and have focused on monitoring the performance of equipment, media, reagents, and susceptibility testing. For example, all reagents and stains are checked with each day of use and results recorded. In other ways, microbiology quality assurance differs from that performed in other disciplines in that some activities are performed at less frequent intervals. For example, microbiologic media now is evaluated on a weekly basis rather than on a daily basis for reagents used in other disciplines of the clinical laboratory. Circumstances surrounding collection and transport of the specimen have received the most attention and have been the most difficult to assure. The most challenging aspect is to evaluate specimen quality and accompanying information and to use this information correctly in the interpretation of these test results. For further information on microbiology quality assurance see Chapter 27.

Proficiency Testing Programs

Proficiency testing is required for almost all tests performed in clinical laboratories. Samples resembling human specimens are prepared in a similar manner to quality control samples, and sent to participants of proficiency programs at regular intervals. Following the same protocols as for patient specimens, proficiency testing samples are measured and results then sent to a central computer facility where interlaboratory comparisons are made. Good laboratory performance is defined in terms of current analytical standards of practice. Some of these standards are based on statistical limits (within $\pm$ 3 S.D. of the mean of participant practices) or a fixed limit (within 2 mmol/L of participant mean sodium concentrations). Each of the samples is graded as "pass" or "fail" in relation to these standards, and according to CLIA '88, failure to score above a certain limit during the year for one test causes loss of certification for that entire discipline.

For most analytes, two sample challenges are sent to participants four times a year. However, changes in laboratory regulations by CLIA '88 will increase these challenges to 20 per year (5 challenges, 4 times a year) beginning in 1991. The largest proficiency program operated by the CAP provides 19 programs for 394 analytes. A list of the programs offered by the CAP for clinical laboratories is seen in Table 26.7. Other programs have a menu that is less extensive.

Figure 26.4 shows participant Comprehensive Chemistry survey results from the College of American Pathologists program in 1990 for specimen C-07 and C-08. As in quality control, laboratory performance data are summarized by a mean and standard deviation (S.D.). For example, an albumin sample measured in 4798 laboratories gave a mean of 4.19 g/dl, a standard deviation of 0.28 g/dl, and a CV of 6.7%. For the albumin method using dye binding and bromcresol green (BCG), performance is identified for each of the instruments used. Although not shown, performance of other methodology-instrument combinations such as bromcresol purple dye binding also are listed. For a laboratory to have unsatisfactory performance for albumin, for example, a laboratory using dye binding BCG (the method) and an Abbott Spectrum (the instrument), performance must fall more than 3 S.D. (0.26 g/dl $\times$ 3 S.D. = 0.72 g/dl) from the mean value (4.30 g/dl). For each analyte measured in clinical laboratories, similar listings of the instrument-method combinations are provided.

Occasionally a few new or emerging analytes are not included in programs of this type. A few representative analytes are listed in Table 26.8 to document the marked improvement in analytical performance over many years of testing.

Other Types of Quality Assurance Programs

The JCAHO's Agenda for Change has required focusing efforts for improvement on steps in the total testing process outside the measurement process itself (2). Emphasis has been placed on patient outcomes, which have been described as the five Ds (death, disease, disability, discomfort, and dissatisfaction) (23). Patient outcomes are easy to identify for medical specialists who have direct patient care requirements, but for laboratorians opportunities for direct patient care are limited as are the identification of laboratory activities that can be directly related to patient outcomes. For this reason, quality assurance activities in the clinical laboratory

Table 26.7.
CAP Proficiency Testing Program

I. Laboratory, general Basic—Series 1, 2	Bacteriology Mycology
II. Hematology/clinical microscopy Comprehensive hematology Comprehensive coagulation module Hemoglobinopathy Clinical microscopy	Yeast Parasitology Mycobacteriology Virology Herpes simplex/chlamydia antigen detection
III. Clinical chemistry Comprehensive chemistry Electrophoresis/chromatography Enzyme chemistry	Rapid microbial detection Acid-fast bacilli smears V. Immunohematology Comprehensive blood bank

Linearity
Lipids
Cerebrospinal fluid chemistry
Urine chemistry—series 1, 2
Critical care (stat) lab
Blood gas
Blood oximetry
Trace metals
Instrumentation
Therapeutic drug monitoring—series 1A,
    1B, 2A, 2B, 3A, 3B
Whole blood cyclosporine
Serum cyclosporine
Urine toxicology
Toxicology
Forensic urine drug testing—screening
Forensic urine drug testing—confirmatory
Blood alcohol
Serum alcohol
Blood lead
	Viral hepatitis markers
	Western blot survey
	Donor center survey
	VI. Diagnostic immunology and syphilis
	    serology
	Diagnostic immunology—series 1, 2
	Syphilis serology
	Rubella
	Diagnostic allergy
	Flow cytometry
	VIIA. Nuclear medicine (in vitro)
	Ligand assay—series 1A, 1B, 2A, 2B
	Maternal α-fetoprotein screening
	Hormone receptor assay
	VIIB. Nuclear medicine (in vivo)
	Transmission imaging—series 1, 2
	VIII. Cytogenetics
	Cytogenetics
	IX. Histocompatibility
	Histocompatibility

IV. Microbiology Comprehensive Microbiology—Immu- nology	HLA-DR testing Peripheral blood lymphocytes

involve mostly structure or process with only a few opportunities addressing outcomes.

The JCAHO has developed a process for implementing a quality assurance program. Table 26.9 lists the 10 steps for Monitoring and Evaluation developed by the JCAHO (24). Responsibility for operation of the clinical laboratory lies with the laboratory director who delegates many operational activities to others. Some of the activities delegated may include the day-to-day operation of the laboratory quality assurance plan; however, the director is required by those responsible for laboratory licensure to serve on the hospital committees where the laboratory quality assurance findings routinely are dis-

cussed. The products of the clinical laboratory are the laboratory test results and the blood bank products available for patient care. The third step in the JCAHO's Monitoring and Evaluation process, the identification of important aspects of service, requires consideration of high risk, high volume, problem-prone activities. These aspects of service for investigation should include each of the steps in the total testing process. The development of proper indicators for quality are important, as efforts for quality assurance need to focus on important aspects of patient care. To gather information that offers little opportunity for improving patient care wastes valuable resources. Table 26.10 shows a list of 32 indicators that over 300 participants

CONSTITUENT METHOD/INSTRUMENT	--------SPECIMEN C-07-------				--------SPECIMEN C-08-------			
	NO. LABS	MEAN	S.D.	C.V.	NO. LABS	MEAN	S.D	C.V.
ALBUMIN - G/DL								
ALL METHOD PRINCIPLES								
ALL INSTRUMENTS	4798	4.19	0.28	6.7	4803	2.98	0.23	7.8
DYE BINDING-BCG								
ABBOTT SPECTRUM	131	4.30	0.26	6.1	132	3.06	0.19	6.1
AM. MON. PERSPECTIVE	23	4.12	0.18	4.3	22	2.96	0.09	3.0
AMERICAN MON. PARALLEL	24	4.24	0.13	3.2	24	3.05	0.14	4.6
BAXTER PARAMAX	465	4.14	0.18	4.3	466	2.90	0.14	4.7
BECKMN ASTRA 4/8 IDEAL	57	4.22	0.09	2.1	59	3.02	0.07	2.2
CIBA CORN. 550 EXPRESS	69	4.08	0.22	5.4	69	2.99	0.17	5.8
COULTER DACOS	54	4.11	0.14	3.3	53	2.93	0.10	3.5
HITACHI 704 BMD	60	4.32	0.11	2.6	59	3.09	0.08	2.5
HITACHI 705 BMD	90	4.17	0.09	2.1	92	3.00	0.08	2.6
HITACHI 717 BMD	110	4.36	0.12	2.9	110	3.11	0.09	2.8
HITACHI 736 BMD	54	4.26	0.13	3.1	54	3.02	0.10	3.2
HITACHI 737 BMD	106	4.33	0.11	2.5	106	3.09	0.10	3.2
IL MONARCH	194	4.03	0.17	4.3	193	2.96	0.12	4.0
KODAK EKTACHEM 400,700	805	3.82	0.13	3.4	801	2.64	0.10	3.9
KODAK EKTACHEM 500	21	3.86	0.14	3.7	21	2.65	0.12	4.7
OLYMPUS AU 5000	51	4.25	0.17	4.0	51	3.16	0.13	4.0
OLYMPUS DEMAND	100	4.27	0.14	3.2	101	3.13	0.11	3.6
ROCHE COBAS MIRA	112	4.23	0.20	4.8	110	3.04	0.15	4.9
TECHNICON RA XT	20	4.38	0.22	5.0	20	3.13	0.17	5.3
TECHNICON RA 1000	60	4.37	0.25	5.7	61	3.14	0.19	6.0
TECHNICON SMA 12/60	31	4.11	0.20	4.9	32	3.04	0.15	4.9
TECHNICON SMAC	135	4.29	0.13	3.0	135	3.08	0.09	3.0
ALL AUTO CHEM INSTR	2979	4.10	0.26	6.3	2977	2.91	0.22	7.7

Figure 26.4. A printout of albumin results from the College of American Pathologists Proficiency Program (21).

at a quality assurance conference indicated as used for their laboratories (25). Many of these indicators have been developed by laboratory staff in consultation with those who work in other hospital departments or are physicians.

Indicators can be developed in-house or those used successfully by others can be implemented into the QA plan of the laboratory. Advantages to the development of indicator studies in-house is that the self-designed studies reflect local practice patterns and can be tailored to accommodate laboratory staffing patterns. However, frequently resources are not available to design meaningful studies, expert opinion is not available on what constitutes an appropriate indicator of quality, and the thresholds for action are poorly defined. Common problems include undertaking corrective action when little chance of improvement occurs or the failure to take corrective action when opportunity for improvement exists. Frequently laboratorians have turned to the scientific literature

for help, but to date the information published about findings from quality assurance programs is limited.

To alleviate these problems, the CAP appointed a committee of experts who developed a list of indicators of laboratory quality by a consensus process and provided these indicators in the form of a series of discreet studies as part of an overall CAP quality assurance program called "Q-Probes." This program is made available yearly on a modest subscription basis. Participants in this program collect information during the same specified time period on preprinted forms, return these forms to the CAP's computer facility where an interinstitutional comparison based on peer groups is developed, and each participant is ranked according to performance. These rankings are returned to participants with a study critique and suggestions for improvement written by the same volunteer experts who identified the indicator and designed the study. This voluntary program began in 1989 and by

Table 26.8.
National CAP Surveys (Average % CV)[a]

	1949	1969	1983	1990
Glucose	16.3	8.0	5.3	3.6
Urea nitrogen	63.5	13.3	8.2	5.8
Chloride	16.4	5.2	2.7	2.6
Calcium	27.6	11.1	3.9	3.0
Cholesterol	23.7	18.5	6.4	5.2

[a]Modified from College of American Pathologists. Comprehensive chemistry survey set C-A. 1990 CAP surveys. Northfield, IL: College of American Pathologists, 1990; and Ross JW, Lawson NS. Performance characteristics and analytic goals. In: Howanitz PJ, Howanitz JH, eds. Laboratory quality assurance. New York: McGraw-Hill, 1987:124–165.

Table 26.9.
10 Steps in Monitoring and Evaluation

1. Assign responsibility. (Who is in charge?)
2. Delineate scope of care/service. (What do we do?)
3. Identify important aspects of care/service. (What is most important, e.g., high risk, high volume, problem prone?)
4. Identify indicators. (What do we measure?)
5. Establish threshold for evaluation. (When do we evaluate?)
6. Collect and organize data. (What are the numbers?)
7. Evaluate. (What is happening?)
8. Take action to improve care. (Fix it!)
9. Assess actions and document improvement. (Did we fix it?)
10. Communicate information to organizational QA program (Does everyone know?)

1990 over 1100 institutions were registered. By the end of 1990, 21 studies have been conducted for pathology and laboratory medicine, and an impressive data base describing practice patterns developed. Table 26.11 shows the indicators used in this program for the clinical laboratory.

Each study usually is conducted for 2–3 months or until enough data is collected from each participant to make statistically significant conclusions. Advantages of this program include the development of indicators by experts, participation in studies that have been refined by field evaluation, receiving preprinted study directions and forms, ranking of performance with peers so that the need for performance improvement can occur, opportunities for remeasurement either alone or with all other participants to document improvement, and the development of a data base of practice patterns of participants.

Use of Indicators in the Clinical Laboratory

In the fall of 1990, a module of the Q-Probes program was aimed at assessing the use of indicators in departments of pathology and laboratory medicine (26). Although the data demonstrate a wide variation in the number of types of indicators in use, some broad trends were identified. The average number of indicators used was dependent on the bed size and hospital type. In those hospitals with more than 500 beds, a median of 17 indicators

were used, whereas those with 100 beds or less reported a median use of 10 indicators. Teaching hospitals reported a median of 15 indicators compared to nonteaching hospitals where 12 indicators were the median. This difference may be partially related to the larger bed size of teaching hospitals. Inspection and accreditation standards also affect quality assurance programs. In the same study, the median hours to comply with the laboratory quality assurance plan was 40 hours in a CAP-accredited laboratory and 28 hours in a non-CAP-accredited laboratory.

When the type of action taken to correct problems was investigated, participants reported they most frequently continued monitoring (98%), followed by written communication (94.9%), counseling of the staff (94.7%), education (94.5%), and system redesign (80.3%). Although this may appear to indicate that the appropriate corrective action has not been taken because most errors are "systems problems" rather than "people problems," it is far easier to provide staff counseling than system redesign. System redesign requires much more effort, some of it in the form of an extensive time commitment of management and staff involved, although it is more effective. For these reasons, we think it was not used as frequently as counseling.

Table 26.10.
Quality Indicators Used in Pathology and Laboratory Medicine

Laboratorywide
   Specimen adequacy and labeling
   Duplicate test order identification
   Delta check follow-up
   Error detection in patient reports
   "Panic value" communication confirmation
   Assessment of standing orders
   Confirmation of physician awareness of laboratory reports issued after patient discharge
   Test turnaround times
Blood bank
   Blood utilization
   Transfusion reactions
   Indicators for platelet transfusion
   Fresh frozen plasma use
Coagulation
   Inappropriate ordering of PT or PTT in anticoagulated patients[a]
   Coagulation factor determinations in patients with normal PT and PTTs
Clinical microscopy
   Microscopic examination of urine specimens with negative dipstick results
Clinical microbiology
   Collection times on submitted specimens
   Solitary blood or acid-fast bacilli cultures
   Inadequate (rejected) specimen submissions
Therapeutic drug monitoring
   Time of specimen collection
   Nondetectable drug levels
   Indications for theophylline or digoxin assays
Clinical chemistry
   Repeat requests for multiphasic analyses within a specified time period
   Preoperative test assessment
   Indications for quantitative β-hCG determinations
   Indications for neonatal bilirubin measurements
   Indications to repeat lactic acid determinations in patients without evidence of acidosis
   Use of thyroxine (T_4) determinations as a screening test
   Feedback of precision of rapid glucose testing
   Adherence to CK protocols
Hematology
   Repeat requests for complete blood counts within a specified period
   Indications for platelet determinations
Clinical immunology
   Indications for syphilis testing in asymptomatic patients

[a]PT, prothrombin time; PTT, partial thromboplastin time; hCG, human chorionic gonadotropin; CK, creatine kinase.

Description of Data from Quality Assurance Programs

Unfortunately for laboratorians, data collected from quality assurance programs and then plotted do not follow usual Gaussian distributions with which laboratorians are most familiar (27). Usually the plotted data have a longer tail toward poorer performance and a shorter tail toward better performance. This is because in a certain number of occurrences a major problem or a number of small problems occur, thereby degrading performance. An implication of the non-Guassian distribution occurs when using statistical approaches to express gathered data. Laboratorians are most familiar with the mean and S.D.s from the mean from daily QC programs, but these statistical terms usually are inappropriate for data obtained from QA programs. Here the median is the preferred term to the mean, with a percentile ranking around the median as seen in Figure 26.5. When discussing the distribution, we recommend using the central 90 percentile, thereby eliminating outliers at the upper and lower 5% of the distribution. Westgard et al. (28) recommend that use of higher limits (e.g., 99%) tends to focus attention on a few extraordinary problems, rather than performance to be expected in routine daily operation.

When following improvement, we recommend that the upper limit (the 95th) percentile be used to chart improvement, as it is more sensitive to change than the mean, median, or mode. As performance improvement occurs, the distribution should become more Gaussian, as the median approaches the mean. For example, laboratorians should describe turnaround times (TAT) goals in terms of 95% of stat tests being completed in a certain period of time, rather than describing TAT as the mean or median of this distribution. As in Figure 26.5, describing 95% of tests complete in 98.5 min is preferable to identifying the median TAT as 45 min for the reason stated above.

Frequently, quality assurance data are expressed without regard to a proper denominator, or sometimes even without a denominator. When the proper denominator is not used, it is impossible to relate the change found to workload, staffing, or any other cyclic event. For example, when phlebotomists identify 133 patients without identification bands during the morning phlebotomy rounds in 1 month and relate this to 83 patients without bands months later, they may incorrectly de-

Table 26.11.
Indicators of Quality Monitored by Q-Probes

Appropriate test utilization (many examples)
Appropriate blood utilization
Autologous blood utilization
Transcription accuracy of test requests
Patients without identification bands
Complications of phlebotomy
Timing of specimen procurement for therapeutic drug monitoring
Specimen adequacy
Antimicrobial susceptibility
Proficiency testing
Error detection in laboratory report
Use of the laboratory result
Quality of blood glucose bedside testing
QA program adequacy
Customer satisfaction
Result turnaround times (many examples)
Nosocomial infection rates

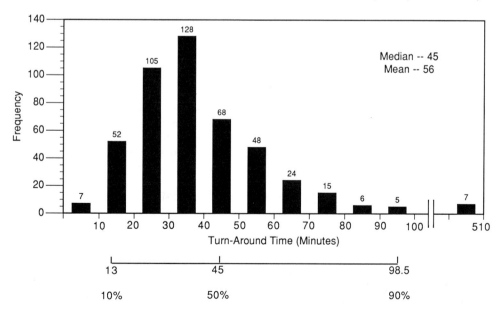

Figure 26.5.   Distribution of turnaround times for glucose results in increments of 10 min.

scribe improvement. The hospital bed occupancy rate during the first month may be twice as great as any succeeding month and twice as many patients may have been seen, thereby increasing the opportunities to detect errors. For these reasons, we recommend much care be given to the consideration of a denominator for the data, and that a denominator always be used.

Appropriate Blood Products and Test Use

There is a great concern that a large proportion of all medical services—as much as 20% or more—provided in the United States are unnecessarily performed for inappropriate reasons. Because the laboratory tests and products account for approximately 20% of all inpatient hospital bills, appropriate use of laboratory tests and products represents a way to improve the quality of health care and at the same time eliminate waste. For this reason, two of the most important aspects of a laboratory quality assurance plan are the blood utilization and test utilization components.

The evolution of quality assurance has had a major impact on blood utilization review. In 1985, the JCAHO introduced a requirement that blood usage review include the evaluation of appropriateness of all transfusions, until blood usage review consistently supports the justification and the appropriateness of blood use. The classic paper by Renner et al. (29) describes how such a program can be developed to identify problems and how practices and blood usage can be improved with the help of the medical staff. At their large tertiary care institution, which provides teaching experiences for medical students and housestaff, the challenge to change blood usage practice patterns was great. A successive program begins with criteria for appropriate use of red blood cells, fresh frozen plasma, platelets, cryoprecipitate, and whole blood, and then details specific blood usage requiring review. Those criteria which Renner et al. recommend are seen in Table 26.12.

Marked improvement in blood usage

Table 26.12.
Specific Blood Use Requiring Reviews

Transfusion of more than 12 platelet concentrates in a 24-hour period
Transfusion of platelet concentrates onto patients with a diagnosis of immune thrombocytopenia purpura (ITP)
Mortality associated with transfusion
Adverse effects associated with transfusion
Transfusion of radiated blood components

occurred such that, during the first year, the number of units transfused that did not meet criteria dropped by over 90%, and within 6 months of beginning the program, no units of blood were given inappropriately to patients. With continued monitoring, appropriate blood utilization has remained at these low levels.

A novel approach to test utilization improvement has been introduced by Schifman (30) who has worked with his medical staff at an academic institution to develop volume indicator criteria for test utilization. For each test requested for patients, the maximum number of times the test can be ordered per week has been determined by the initial result: abnormal or within the reference interval. For example, guidelines for serum creatinine or urea nitrogen allow ordering no more than three times per week if the initial result is with the reference interval, and seven times per week if the initial result is abnormal. If a test is ordered more frequently than specified, the attending physician responsible for the patient's care receives a letter asking for justification for the additional testing. Physicians are assured that these inquiries are not meant to judge the use of laboratory tests, but to examine the reason and circumstances certain tests are ordered and how the test ordering system can be improved. With this approach, unnecessary testing has been decreased by over 80% in just a few years. Of course, differences of opinions did occur, but compromises and adjustments were made openly with the knowledge and consideration of everyone's need. Such a program can succeed only if there is widespread support and cooperation by all members of the medical staff.

A third model of test utilization is that used for the appropriate ordering of solitary blood cultures by the Q-Probes program of the College of American Pathologists (31). In this study the incidence of solitary blood cultures was identified using approximately 125,000 inpatient cultures at 600 institutions. For inpatients the median was 9.8%, with teaching institutions having a higher percentage of solitary blood cultures than nonteaching institutions. Collection by nonphlebotomy personnel was responsible for rates twice as high compared to collection by phlebotomy staff, and the rates when collected by housestaff more than twice as high as when collected by nonhousestaff. This study also identified reasons for collections of solitary cultures with failure to follow up on the diagnostic plan and ignorance the most common reasons given. A few months later, a follow-up study was undertaken beginning with educational materials circulated about appropriate reasons for collection and causes for inappropriate collections of solitary blood cultures. With this educational effort and subsequent remeasurement, marked improvement in the ordering practices were shown.

A variety of professional groups for a number of years have had major efforts underway to develop practice parameters. Over 700 practice guidelines have been developed by 24 physician organizations including many on inappropriate test utilization. One of the most widely known is the effort by the American College of Physicians who developed Blue Cross/Blue Shield Association guidelines for 12 tests (32). These Blue Cross/Blue Shield guidelines were poorly received by pathologists, who were not consulted in their development and who pointed out numerous scientific errors in their recommendations. Both groups recognized this major omission and vowed to work together in the future to develop practice guidelines on test utilization. Such experiences indicate that successful efforts can occur only when individuals from a variety of specialties work together toward a common goal. Currently, many groups within organized medicine are attempting to write guidelines and the American Medical Associa-

tion (AMA) is working cooperatively with these groups including the American Society of Clinical Pathologists (ASCP) and the CAP to guide the development and implementation of practice parameters (33). Properly developed test utilization parameters present a promising strategy to define appropriate care, provide a rational foundation for examining the appropriateness of medical care provided, establish a means to assure appropriate utilization of health care services, and simplify the implementation and the use of developed guidelines as part of a quality assurance program.

EPIDEMIOLOGY OF QUALITY ASSURANCE

A large number of quality indicators are used in laboratory medicine as indicated in Tables 26.10 and 26.11. Each of these indicators may identify important aspects of care that are specific to laboratory medicine and in turn are specific to that indicator alone. Although it is interesting to reflect upon causes of problems identified by studying one indicator and relating those specific causes to another indicator, little useful information can be gathered by this approach. For example, in a study when test turnaround time in 722 emergency room departments was considered, a number of findings impacting the laboratory TATs were found (Table 26.13). The TAT depends on the bed size of the institution, the method of specimen transport, the priority of test (i.e., stat), if a computer is used, the type of specimen, the effect of regularly measuring TAT, the analyte measured, and a host of other factors (34). Although each of these factors has influence on lengthening or shortening the TAT, they have little influence on, for example, the percentage of solitary blood cultures that are collected in an institution.

Specific recommendations, however, can be made about factors that affect the quality and the improvement of quality in clinical laboratories. Leadership is the most important, and without leadership and a commitment by the leaders to quality, the communication of quality goals to

Table 26.13.
Median Potassium TAT in 722 Institutions

	Median TAT
	min
Bedsize	
1–250	32
251–500	36
>500	44
Phlebotomist	
Laboratory personnel	33
Emergency department nurse	45
Emergency department physician	60
Other	40
Method of specimen transport	
Laboratory within emergency department	18
Mechanical transport	30
Courier	36
Clinical staff	24
Stat laboratory measurement	
Yes	35
No	36
Computerization for stat test	
Hospital information system	32
Laboratory information system	35
Computerization of stat results	39
Specimens type	
Serum	38
Plasma	31
Whole blood	23
Effect of regularly monitoring TAT	
Monitor	37
No monitor	34
Analyte measured	
Potassium	44
Hemoglobin	33

others is futile. An important aspect of leadership is to provide follow-up to individuals charged with the operational program; without frequent follow-up, quality assurance will flounder and fail. Leadership should extend to all levels, involving others in the process, providing ownership and, offering opportunities for others to provide suggestions. It is essential that all levels of personnel are involved and have a role.

A good quality assurance plan is essential. Following the 10-step Monitoring and Evaluation process of the JCAHO as in

Table 26.9 provides a structure around how a program should work. The choice of indicators currently used in clinical laboratories is seen in Tables 26.10 and 26.11. For an off-the-shelf complete laboratory QA program, we know of one program, the Q-Probes program of the College of American Pathologists and recommend that program highly. One can customize this program to one's own needs, choosing only those indicators that fulfill appropriate needs, extending monitoring of indicators well beyond the length of time peers monitor, and reinstituting monitors demonstrating previous poor performance.

Although there are many models and approaches that work, the KISS (keep it simple, stupid) principal applies. A simple study design allows easy implementation, quick and thorough execution, meaningful conclusions, and a quantifiable payoff. Many programs have failed because of the associated complexities. For example, to obtain the same information, a prospective study is much easier to do than a retrospective chart review. Data gathering by one individual under your direction is more likely to occur rapidly than done by a committee representing multiple disciplines. A single important conclusion is more valuable to direct improvement than five to ten minor conclusions. The complexity of the quality assurance program also is influenced by the number of indicators used. Laboratorians should choose a few important indicators, then expand that number as staff experience and enthusiasm increases. Quality assurance studies require valuable resources, and an over-commitment of resources leads to little hope for improvement and a disillusioned staff.

Efforts should be directed to monitor "hand-offs"—either the transfer of patients, patient specimens, or information from one individual to another, or from one department to the next. Hand-offs represent changes from one system to the next, and usually each system operates well independently. Where these systems meet represents circumstances where neither system has jurisdiction. It is this interface where most problems originate and where the greatest challenge and opportunity for improvement lies. Obviously the inverse relationship is important, as systems with no to few hand-offs have a lower chance of error than ones with many steps.

QUALITY ASSURANCE PRACTICE PATTERNS

If quality assurance practices are to guide improvements efficiently, their findings must be evaluated in relation to a standard. For most programs, improvement is sought in relation to findings from previous periods of time, so that over long periods, significant improvements are found. Occasionally, situations occur when improvements may not be possible. In response to these circumstances, the JCAHO has recommended establishing a threshold, and if errors exceed this threshold then corrective action can occur. When errors fail to exceed this threshold, then no corrective action is needed and the process is considered appropriate.

However, difficulty arises in setting thresholds. Some have set thresholds so high, thereby assuming that many errors can occur before there is a need for corrective action. In the laboratory this is commonplace because many laboratory activities in a total testing process are not linked directly to patient outcomes and their effect is difficult to document. Others set thresholds so low that every occurrence of an error is evaluated as a sentinel event, and corrective action is associated with no improvement because improvement is impossible.

A national data base such as that developed by Q-Probes is essential in efficiently using resources for quality improvement. Because each participant is given a percentile rank in relation to peers, the current standard of practice can be defined and participants statistically rated in relationship to that standard. Because the number of indicators associated with the quality of laboratory services are finite, and a list covering proposed studies within the next 2 years in the Q-Probes program is almost complete (see Table 26.11), it is reasonable to expect that by 1993, practice patterns in

the form of a large data base will be available for almost all quality indicators in laboratory medicine. As each of these indicators is evaluated and used independently, and then as part of a nationwide program, performance will improve and laboratorians will be able to identify where improvement is possible.

Seen in Table 26.14 are some of the data obtained from the Q-Probes program for five of the 21 studies completed in 1989–1990. Many more percentile rankings for important characteristics of care for each study have been generated than shown here. Each ranking allows defining performance according to peers easily, as well as overall performance at 10th, 50th, and 90th percentile. Those participants whose percentile rank is in the bottom 25% are urged to evaluate and improve performance quickly, whereas those who are between 25 and 50% are urged to seek improvement, but at a more leisurely pace. Those who are in the top 25% are judged to have superior performance and urged not to waste valuable resources now on achieving further improvements. It is our experience that even those in the top 25%, when reviewing the study including their performance data, peer ranking, and critique find easy solutions to improving performance even further.

The development of such a national data base should be able to drive improvement because laboratories with poorest performance are urged to improve immediately and their improvement occurs at the greatest rate, thereby improving median and overall performance remarkably. Such an approach will raise standards in the practice of laboratory medicine very quickly.

CONCLUSIONS: BENEFITS OF QUALITY ASSURANCE PROGRAMS

The benefits of quality assurance programs in laboratory medicine have been questioned (35). We are aware of many anecdotal cases in which quality assurance programs have identified potential problems and avoided patient calamity, and serious consequences have occurred be-

Table 26.14.
Practice Patterns Established by Q-Probes

Study	Number of Institutions	Data Base	All Institutions' Percentiles			Units
			10%	50%	90%	
1. Complications of phlebotomy (35)	613					
a. Median size of bruise		4,048 bruises	20.5	11.0	5.0	mm
b. % of bruised patients		4,048 patients	32.0	16.7	7.1	
c. % of patients identifying an outstanding employee		11,107 patients	25.6	46.7	69.8	
d. Median wait time		23,783 patients	4.0	6.0	15.0	min
2. Autologous blood utilization (36)	612					
a. Transfusions as a % of all red cell transfusions in 1989		2,612,081 RBC units	0.35	2.52	8.43	%
b. Donors who avoided homologous transfusion		11,923 RBC units	78.33	92.31	100.00	%
c. Donor who did not require transfusion		8,351 RBC units	10.00	40.00	66.67	%
d. Units discarded		15,443 RBC units	66.67	40.00	15.15	%
3. Solitary blood culture utilization (31)	538					
a. Inpatient		127,053 cultures	85.9	12.1	2.5	%
b. Total		173,093 cultures	54.5	16.0	4.7	%
4. Interlaboratory stat CSF (37)	492					
a. Cell count		14,760 tests	64	32	15	min
b. Glucose		14,760 tests	63	34	18	min
c. Protein		14,760 tests	68	37	20	min
d. Gram stain		14,760 tests	87	45	24	min
5. Emergency department test TAT (34)	713					
a. Potassium		39,105 tests	41	25	15	min
b. Hemoglobin		42,922 tests	54.3	35.0	22.2	min

Table 26.15.
Benefits of QA Plan in 756 Laboratories

Degree of Benefit	For Patient Outcome	For Management Tool	For Risk Management
No benefit	0.5%	0.5%	1.0%
Limited benefit	12.5%	10.5%	20.4%
Moderate benefit	38.3%	44.2%	37.4%
Considerable benefit	33.0%	33.5%	29.2%
Very beneficial	15.7%	11.3%	12.0%
Total	100%	100%	100%

cause of a lack of a particular program. When laboratories with a quality assurance program for detection of erroneous laboratory reports were compared with those without such a program, those laboratories with a program had a higher likelihood of error detection than those without such a program (27). Such information indicates that each error detected is an opportunity to identify systematic errors, and that each error identified should be considered as an opportunity for improvement. Those who do not look for errors will not find them and will not have opportunities for improvement.

When laboratorians were asked if in their experience quality assurance programs were beneficial, approximately 80–90% thought that the efforts expended were associated with better patient outcomes, risk management, and laboratory management (Table 26.15) (26). Although we are unaware of any systemwide study of the value of quality assurance programs directly affecting patient outcomes, we are convinced that when such studies are formulated, clinical laboratory quality assurance programs will be shown to play a major role in defining, maintaining, and improving quality in the practice of medicine.

References

1. Belk WP, Sunderman FW. A survey of the accuracy of chemical analyses in clinical laboratories. Am J Clin Pathol 1947;17:853–861.
2. O'Leary DS. The Joint Commission looks to the future. JAMA 1987;258:951–952.
3. Medicare, Medicaid and CLIA Programs; Regulations implementing the clinical laboratory improvement amendments of 1988 (CLIA '88). United States Department of Health and Human Services, Fed Reg 55; No. 98, May 21, 1990:20896–20959.
4. Howanitz JH, Howanitz PJ. Introduction to quality assurance. In: Howanitz PJ, Howanitz JH, eds. Laboratory quality assurance New York: McGraw-Hill, 1987:1–19.
5. Duckworth JK. Laboratory licensure and accreditation. In: Howanitz PJ, Howanitz JH, eds. Laboratory quality assurance. New York: McGraw-Hill, 1987:334–353.
6. Commission on Laboratory Accreditation. Standards for laboratory accreditation. Northfield, IL: College of American Pathologists, 1987.
7. Joint Commission on Accreditation of Healthcare Organizations. Accreditation manual for hospitals. Vol I. Oak Brook Terrace, IL: Joint Commission on Accreditation of Healthcare Organizations, 1990:141–164.
8. Codes and standards. Quincy, MA: National Fire Protection Association, 1984.
9. Levey S, Jennings ER. The use of control charts in the clinical laboratory. Am J Clin Pathol 1950; 20:1059–1066.
10. Haven GT, Lawson NS, Ross JW. QAS notes. Pathologist 1980;34:619–621.
11. Westgard JO, Groth T, Burnett RW, et al. A multi-rule Shewhart chart for quality control in clinical chemistry. Clin Chem 1981;27:493–501.
12. Koch DD, Oryall JJ, Quam EF, et al. Selection of medically useful quality-control procedures for individual tests done in a multitest analytical system. Clin Chem 1990;35:230–233.
13. Westgard JO, Quam EF, Barry PL. Selection grids for planning quality control procedures. Clin Lab Sci 1990;3:273–280.
14. College of American Pathologists. New York VII Regional Chemistry 1988 Q/C Program. Group Summary. Northfield, IL: College of American Pathologists; 1990:2.
15. Bull BS. The use of patient values, calibrator, and control materials in the routine laboratory. In: van Assendelft OW, England JM, eds. Advances in hematological methods: The blood count. Boca Raton, LA, CRC Press, 1982:217–227.
16. Koepke JA, Protextor TJ. Quality assurance for multichannel hematology instruments. Am J Clin Pathol 1981;75:28–33.
17. Cavill I, Ricketts C, Fisher J, et al. An evaluation of two methods of laboratory quality control. Am J Clin Pathol 1979;72:624–627.
18. Cembrowski GS, Westgard JO. Quality control of multichannel hematology analyzers: Evaluation of Bull's algorithm. Am J Clin Pathol 1985;83:337–345.
19. Polesky HF. Quality control in the blood center and transfusion service: Current products. In: Howanitz PJ, Howanitz JH, eds. Laboratory quality assurance. New York: McGraw-Hill, 1987:270–286.
20. Lizza CR. Sample integrity—Quality assurance. American Association of Blood Banks. ISBT & AABB 1990 Joint Congress Program. Arlington, VA: American Association of Blood Banks, 1990:100.
21. College of American Pathologists. Comprehensive chemistry survey set C-A. 1990 CAP Surveys. Northfield, IL: College of American Pathologists, 1990.
22. Ross JW, Lawson NS. Performance characteristics and analytic goals. In: Howanitz PJ, Howanitz JH, eds. Laboratory quality assurance. New York: McGraw-Hill, 1987:124–165.
23. Lohr KN. Outcome measurements: Concepts and questions. Inquiry 1988;25:37–50.
24. Fromberg R. Monitoring and evaluation. Chicago, IL: Pathology and Medical Laboratory Services, Joint Commission on Accreditation of Health Care Organization, 1987.
25. Bachner P. College of American Pathologists Conference XVII on quality assurance in pathology and laboratory medicine: Summary. Arch Pathol Lab Med 1990;114:1175–1177.
26. Bachner P, Lent WR. Laboratory quality assurance programs: (Q-Probes). Data analysis and critique. Northfield, IL: College of American Pathologists, 1990:90–18A.
27. Howanitz PJ. Quality assurance measurements in departments of pathology and laboratory medicine. Arch Pathol Lab Med 1990;114:1131–1135.
28. Westgard JO, Burnett RW, Bowers GN. Quality management science in clinical chemistry: A dynamic framework for continuous improvement of quality. Clin Chem 1990;36:1712–1716.
29. Renner SW, Howanitz JH, Fishkin BG. Toward meaningful blood usage review: Comprehensive monitoring of physician practice. QRB 1987; 13:76–80.
30. Schifman RB. Quality assurance goals in clinical

pathology. Arch Pathol Lab Med 1990;114:1140–1144.

31. Schifman RB, Bachner P. Blood culture utilization (Q-Probes). Northfield, IL: College of American Pathologists, 1990:90–05A.

32. Sox HC. Common diagnostic tests. Use and interpretation. Philadelphia: American College of Physicians, 1987.

33. Speicher CE. Practice parameters. Arch Pathol Lab Med 1990;114:823–824.

34. Cembrowski GS, Steindel S. Emergency department turn-around-time. (Q-Probes). Data analysis and critique. Northfield, IL: College of American Pathologists, 1990:90–13A.

35. Howanitz PJ, Cembrowski GS, Bachner P. Labo-ratory phlebotomy: College of American Pathologists Q-Probe study of patient satisfaction and complications in 23,783 patients. Arch Pathol Lab Med Sept. 1991, in press.

36. Renner SW. Autologous blood utilization (Q-Probes). Northfield, IL: College of American Pathologists, 1990:90–11A.

37. Howanitz PJ, Steindel SJ. Intralaboratory performance and laboratorians for stat turnaround times. A College of American Pathologists Q-Probe Study of 4 Cerebrospinal fluid determinations. Arch Pathol Lab Med Oct. 1991, in press.

38. Batsakis JG. Quality assurance: Sissyphean or Sibylline? Arch Pathol Lab Med 1990;114:1173–1174.

APPENDICES

College of American Pathologists Standards for Laboratory Accreditation[a]

STANDARD I: DIRECTOR AND PERSONNEL REQUIREMENTS

The pathology service shall be directed by a physician who is qualified to assume professional, scientific, consultative, organizational, administrative, and educational responsibility for the facilities or services. Whenever possible, the director shall be a pathologist, preferably one certified by the American Board of Pathology. The director shall assume full responsibility for the operation and administration of the laboratory.

In the exceptional circumstances when a physician is not available, a doctoral level clinical scientist may serve as director. Such an individual must be qualified by virtue of documented special training, expertise, and experience in the areas of analytical testing offered by the laboratory. In such cases, the services of a qualified consulting pathologist shall be retained. In all facilities where anatomic pathology services are provided, a pathologist shall perform such services.

Special function laboratories shall be directed by either a physician who is qualified to assume professional responsibility for the special function laboratory or a qualified doctoral level clinical scientist with documented special training, expertise, and experience in the appropriate specific clinical discipline.

The location, organization, or ownership of the laboratory shall not alter the requirements of this Standard, its interpretation, or its application.

STANDARD II: RESOURCES AND FACILITIES

The pathology service shall have sufficient and appropriate space, equipment, facilities, and supplies for the performance of the required volume of work with accuracy, precision, efficiency, and safety. In addition, the pathology service shall have effective methods for communication to ensure prompt and reliable reporting. There shall be appropriate record storage and retrieval.

STANDARD III: QUALITY ASSURANCE

There shall be an ongoing quality assurance program designed to monitor and evaluate objectively and systematically the quality and appropriateness of the care and treatment provided to patients by the pathology service, to pursue opportunities to improve patient care, and to identify and resolve problems.

STANDARD IV: QUALITY CONTROL

Each pathology service shall have a quality control system that demonstrates the reliability and medical usefulness of laboratory data.

---

[a]Commission on Laboratory Accreditation. 1988 College of American Pathologists Standards for Laboratory Accreditation. Northville, IL: College of American Pathologists, 1988.

STANDARD V: INSPECTION REQUIREMENTS

A pathology service which desires accreditation shall undergo periodic inspections and evaluations as determined by the Commission on Laboratory Accreditation of the College of American Pathologists.

APPENDIX B

JCAHO Accreditation Standards

PA.1   Pathology and medical laboratory services and consultation are regularly and conveniently available to meet the needs of patients, as determined by the medical staff.
PA.1.1   The pathology and medical laboratory services are directed by a physician who is qualified to assume professional, organizational, and administrative responsibility for the facilities and for the services rendered.
PA.1.2   There are sufficient qualified personnel with documented training and experience to supervise and conduct the work of the laboratory.
PA.1.3   There are sufficient number of qualified laboratory technologists and supportive technical staff to perform, promptly and proficiently, the tests required of the pathology and medical laboratory services.
PA.1.4   There is provision for technologists and other technical personnel, including supervisors, to further their knowledge and skills through hospital-based educational opportunities, such as on-the-job training and in-service education programs, and, as feasible, at least for supervisory personnel, through attendance at outside workshops, institutes, and local, regional, or national society meetings.
PA.1.5   The director, supervisors, and laboratory personnel comply with applicable law and regulations.
PA.1.6   The director of the pathology and medical laboratory services is responsible for the qualifications and performance of the staff.
PA.1.7   A hospital that provides only psychiatric/substance abuse services may provide pathology and medical laboratory services through a contractual agreement with another health care organization that is accredited by the Joint Commission or through a contractual agreement with an independent laboratory that either is approved by the Commission on Laboratory Accreditation of the College of American Pathologists or meets equivalent standards.
PA.2   There are sufficient space, equipment, and supplies within the pathology and medical laboratory services to perform the required volume of work with optimal accuracy, precision, efficiency, timeliness, and safety.
PA.2.1   Provision is made, either on the premises or in a reference laboratory, for the prompt performance of adequate examinations in the fields of anatomic pathology, hematology, chemistry, microbiology, clinical microscopy, parasitology, immunohematology, serology, virology, and, as it relates to the pathology and medical laboratory services, nuclear medicine.
PA.2.2   The laboratory environment is conducive to the optimal performance of personnel and equipment.
PA.2.3   Equipment and instruments are appropriate for the services required.
PA.2.4   The performance of instruments and equipment is evaluated frequently enough to assure that they function properly at all times.
PA.3   Channels of communication within the pathology and medical laboratory services, with other departments/services of the hospital and the medical staff, and with outside services and agencies are appropriate for the size and complexity of the hospital.
PA.3.1   All requests for laboratory tests are made in writing or through electronic means.
PA.3.2   To assure that the specimens are satisfactory for the tests to be performed, written procedures are developed for those who collect specimens.

PA.3.3 Communication systems within the pathology and medical laboratory services and between it and other departments/services efficiently accomplish both the urgent and the regular transfer of information.

PA.3.4 There is assurance of the direct transfer of information between the pathologist performing an operating-room consultation, with or without a "frozen section," and the operating surgeon.

PA.4 Required records and reports are maintained and, as appropriate, are filed in the patient's medical record and in the pathology and medical laboratory services.

PA.4.1 Authenticated, dated reports of all examinations performed by the pathology and medical laboratory services are made part of the patient's medical record.

PA.4.2 The pathologist is responsible for the preparation of a descriptive diagnostic report of gross specimens received and of autopsies performed.

PA.4.3 Reports of all anatomic and clinical laboratory tests and examinations performed are readily available to the individual ordering the tests.

PA.4.4 The pathology and medical laboratory services maintain a record of the daily accession of specimens and an appropriate system for the identification of each.

PA.4.5 Duplicate copies of the reports of all anatomic and clinical laboratory tests and examinations performed are retained in the laboratory in a readily retrievable manner.

PA.5 Quality control systems and measures of the pathology and medical laboratory services are designed to assure the medical reliability of laboratory data.

PA.5.1 The laboratory and, as appropriate, each of its components are licensed as required.

PA.5.2 There is a documented quality control program in effect for each section of the pathology and medical laboratory services.

PA.5.3 General quality controls required of and practiced by the pathology and medical laboratory services include, but need not be limited to, the following

PA.5.4 When histocompatibility testing is performed by the pathology and medical laboratory services, appropriate control systems and validation methods are used.

PA.5.5 Mixed lymphocyte cultures or other recognized methods to detect cellular-defined antigens are performed in accordance with prescribed methods.

PA.5.6 Quality control records are retained for at least two years.

PA.5.7 Equipment maintenance records are retained for the life of each instrument used.

PA.5.8 More specific quality controls are described under the other standards of this chapter of this *Manual.*

PA.6 Specific requirements are observed where anatomic pathology, blood transfusion, and clinical pathology services are offered.

PA.6.1 Anatomic Pathology

PA.6.2 Blood Transfusion Service

PA.6.3 Clinical Pathology

PA.6.4 Decentralized Laboratory Testing

PA.7 As part of the hospital's quality assurance program, the quality and appropriateness of pathology and medical laboratory services are monitored and evaluated in accordance with Standard QA.3 and Required Characteristics QA.3.1 through QA.3.2.8 in the "Quality Assurance" chapter of this *Manual.*

PA.7.1 The physician director of the pathology and medical laboratory department/service is responsible for implementing the monitoring and evaluation process.

PA.7.2 When an outside source(s) provides pathology and medical laboratory services, or when there is no designated pathology and medical laboratory department/service, the medical staff is responsible for implementing the monitoring and evaluation process.

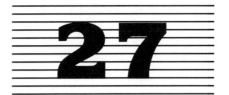

The Microbiology Laboratory

Michael A. Pfaller, M.D.

In general, quality assurance in medicine begins with an assessment of the distribution and determinants of desirable health care in the hospital or clinic setting (1). Clinical laboratories have long been involved in certain aspects of quality assessment (QA), primarily with regards to quality control of laboratory functions. Likewise, laboratory physicians and scientists have been leaders in assessing the diagnostic usefulness of new technologies and in critically evaluating the appropriateness of certain test-ordering procedures. This experience is now being brought to bear with the current emphasis on QA in medicine. Although considerable time and effort in the early 1980s was concentrated on cost-effective utilization of laboratory resources (2), more recently the impact of laboratory testing and diagnostic procedures on the *quality* of care and specifically the *outcome* of diagnostic and therapeutic efforts has come under close scrutiny (3–5). Thus, both laboratory scientists and clinicians must now be concerned with the difficult assessment of the true value of laboratory tests in the diagnostic and therapeutic process and their contribution to quality patient care and outcome.

The general approach of the clinical diagnostic laboratories to the QA process is described in a previous chapter. In addition to this general description, specific examples and observations on the QA process from the perspective of an individual laboratory section is both useful and necessary. The clinical microbiology laboratory is a natural choice for this focused perspective due to its long-standing role in the infection control process, a process considered by some to be the paradigm for QA (1).

QUALITY ASSESSMENT

There are several key issues to consider in assessing the quality of laboratory services and their impact on the process and outcome of medical care. These issues include (*a*) *access* to laboratory services; (*b*) the *process* of delivering laboratory services; (*c*) the *outcome* associated with laboratory test results; and (*d*) the *consequences* attributable to the outcome (Table 27.1). In each case it is essential that endpoints be identified, definitions established, and surveillance carried out with a goal to calculate rates and to identify determinants (risk factors) of quality (1). Taken to their logical conclusions, these efforts should stimulate subsequent clinical investigation and intervention based on the identified risk factors, with a goal of improved health care (outcome). Unfortunately, most laboratories are currently immersed in addressing only one aspect of QA, namely the *process* of delivering labo-

Table 27.1.
Key Issues in Assessing Quality in Clinical Microbiology

Access
  Access to STAT laboratory
    Gram stain
    Antigen detection
  Access to routine diagnostic laboratory
    Culture
    Antibiotic susceptibility testing
  Access to specialty laboratory
    Antibiotic assays
    Susceptibility testing (minimal bactericidal
      concentration, synergy testing)
    Typing studies
    Special stains
Process
  Turnaround time
    STAT results within 45–60 min
    Culture and susceptibility results within 24
      hours
  Accurate results
    Quality control
    Proficiency testing
  Laboratory consultation
    Appropriate specimen
    Specimen collection
    Alternative tests
    Interpretation
  Assistance in detecting nosocomial infection
  Product evaluation
Outcome
  Diagnosis made
  Appropriate therapy administered
  Nosocomial infection detected
    Infection control efforts initiated
  Cure
  Failure
Consequence of outcome
  Discharge without sequelae
  Discharge with sequelae
  Excess stay
    Excess cost
    Additional nosocomial events
  Nosocomial infection prevented
    Decreased cost (LOS)
    Decreased morbidity/mortality
  Death

care. Thus, laboratory physicians and scientists must expand their efforts to evaluate the issues of access and outcome, as well as process, as they relate to the QA of laboratory services. Such efforts will necessitate considerable collaboration, cooperation, and communication among laboratory workers and clinicians and should impact favorably on the quality of medical care.

The remainder of this chapter will focus on each of the four key issues regarding QA in clinical microbiology and infectious diseases (Table 27.1). Examples will be provided of areas where clinical microbiology laboratories have appropriately addressed each of these issues, and measures that laboratories may take in order to improve their function with respect to each issue and the question of QA as a whole will be discussed.

Access

Access to laboratory services has not been a common monitor in laboratory QA. This is surprising since patient access to medical care is generally assumed to be an important component of quality medical care (1). Access to laboratory services is worthy of closer examination as we attempt to improve and optimize delivery of quality diagnostic testing services.

Access to diagnostic microbiology laboratory services is usually somewhat more restricted than access to other services such as clinical chemistry, hematology, or surgical pathology. This has been justified traditionally by the fact that most microbiology tests require the growth of an organism and thus are rarely of immediate value. With the advent of truly rapid methods for detection, identification, and susceptibility testing plus an ever expanding spectrum of pathogens and antimicrobial agents, this pattern of limited hours of service may need to change. A rapid test result may have little clinical impact if it is restricted to the hours of 8 AM to 5 PM. Likewise, access to more specialized laboratory testing (Table 27.1) may be justified increasingly, and in fact may warrant routine availability, as the patient population becomes enriched for the seriously ill pa-

ratory services. This is important and flows naturally from long experience with internal quality control and QA activities. However, as difficult and time consuming as these efforts may be, they fall far short of providing any information regarding the impact (usefulness) of laboratory testing on the quality and outcome of medical tient at high risk for infection. Thus, microbiology laboratories must go to the consumers of their services, the clinicians, and discuss the diagnostic tests available and the clinical needs for microbiology services in order to come to a *consensus agreement* concerning which tests are to be offered where and when in order to maximize clinical usefulness.

At the present time there are very few truly stat tests in clinical microbiology. These include Gram stains of sterile body fluids, certain antigen detection assays, and occasionally special stains and procedures for direct detection of microbial pathogens in specimens obtained from immunocompromised patients. The need for these tests should be ascertained in consultation with the appropriate clinicians and consideration to be given to shifts in staffing and workflow within the laboratory in order to provide optimal service. Similarly, specialized and nonroutine procedures (Table 27.1) should be examined critically for their clinical usefulness and decisions made as to whether they should be offered on-site, referred to an outside laboratory, or not offered at all. Of course the laboratory response to these needs may be limited by available financial and personnel resources; however, the *consensus* recommendations of the laboratory and clinical staff should be presented to hospital administration in an effort to obtain the resources necessary to improve the quality and efficiency of the diagnostic operation.

The establishment of a QA monitor with respect to access to clinical microbiology services may begin by focusing on a single procedure such as the emergent (stat) evaluation of a normally sterile body fluid or bronchoalveolar lavage specimen from an immunocompromised patient. Initially, clinicians may be surveyed by questionnaire concerning their views on current availability, timeliness, and extent of analysis. An assessment by the laboratory of the frequency, time of day (or night), and distribution of test requests within the hospital will provide additional data upon which to base further discussion with the appropriate physician groups. A consensus agreement may require some concessions by each group but should provide a working protocol, which can then be monitored. Subsequent monitoring of frequency and appropriateness of test requests, specimen quality, timeliness of results (turnaround time), and impact on diagnostic and therapeutic decision making and clinical outcome all flow from this initial effort and will be discussed in subsequent sections. Thus, it is apparent that a number of QA monitors can arise by focusing on a single test procedure, and it all begins with the consideration of *access*. The cooperation between clinical and laboratory services in this effort is essential and will result in improved patient care as well as a useful QA monitor.

Process

Most of the effort in establishing QA programs in the clinical laboratory has concentrated on *process*-oriented monitors. This focus on process monitors is not unique to laboratory QA programs. Very few QA programs in general have expanded beyond process to include the evaluation on access and outcome (1). Unfortunately, many laboratory QA programs have settled on *monitoring the mundane* by dutifully collecting and reporting data such as the number of mislabeled specimens, incomplete requisitions, and broken tubes. This is not to say that this information, and the resolution of these problems, is not important in delivering quality laboratory services; however, laboratories must be willing to think more creatively and expand beyond these obvious monitors in order to realize the potential of QA to improve the quality of laboratory services and its impact on medical care.

Turnaround Time

The monitoring of turnaround times for laboratory test results must begin when the test is ordered by a physician and end when the results of that test are received by a physician who can take action based upon the results of the test. Thus, the concept of turnaround time encompasses the time required for test ordering, specimen collection, transport, analysis, and reporting of results. Monitoring of turnaround times for specific laboratory tests is a routine QA function in clinical chemistry and hematology laboratories, but has not received as much attention in the clinical microbiology laboratory, largely due to the relative lack of truly stat microbiology tests.

The clinical rationale for avoiding prolonged turnaround times for certain tests is intuitively obvious. The availability of data is crucial to the process of medical decision making. Thus, it is likely that the test results that most influence patient management are those that are available the earliest (6). For example, in a true medical emergency such as bacterial meningitis, prompt, accurate diagnosis is essential to prevent death or permanent neurologic sequelae. The immediate performance of a Gram-stained smear of cerebrospinal fluid (CSF), properly interpreted, is invaluable and more useful clinically than the results of culture, biochemical identification, and antimicrobial susceptibility profile, which may be available 3 days later. Given this level of importance, it seems reasonable to monitor the turnaround times of stat Gram stain test results as a means of ensuring quality diagnostic services to the clinician. Specific guidelines for the rapidity of urgent test results such as CSF Gram stains should use as a goal the provision of results within 1 hour of the time that the specimen was obtained from the patient. To this end, a recent survey of over 400 clinical laboratories, conducted as part of the College of American Pathologists (CAP) Q-Probe Quality Assurance Program, showed that the median turnaround time for processing, examining, and reporting CSF Gram-stained smears was 45 min (7).

The data accumulated as a result of monitoring turnaround time for rapid smears and related microbiologic tests can be used to make physicians aware of the likely turnaround times for these tests, thus making it more likely that they will use them in clinical decision making. Furthermore, this QA monitor should also be coupled to follow-up studies to ensure that the smear results are properly reported, interpreted, and utilized in serious infections. Thus, the laboratory may routinely correlate Gram stain results with culture results, administration of appropriate antimicrobial therapy, and, in collaboration with clinical colleagues, monitor the outcome of therapy.

The importance of turnaround time for the identification and susceptibility testing of microbial pathogens in the clinical microbiology laboratory is less obvious. Over the past decade there has been increasing emphasis on rapid methods for identification and susceptibility testing of bacterial pathogens, particularly those isolated from blood cultures (8–11). The rationale was that the earlier results would have a greater impact on medical decision making and, in addition, that the more rapid availability of microbiology results could contribute to a reduction in the length of hospital stay for treatment of infectious diseases. Although the application of instrumentation and automation to microbiology has decreased the time required for identification and antimicrobial susceptibility testing from days to hours, the clinical relevance of the information generated has been less well documented (9).

The documentation of decreased turnaround time for microbiologic testing using modern rapid methods and its impact on patient care would appear to be an excellent focus for QA activities. Unfortunately, this has been largely neglected due to the difficulty in organizing and conducting such studies. Bartlett (12) examined the impact of rapid antimicrobial susceptibility testing on clinical behavior at Hartford Hospital and found that 54% of results reported 24 hours earlier than routine testing were considered by clinicians to be useful. Antibiotic therapy was altered appropriately as a result of 38% of the early reports; however, no proof of improved outcome, decreased cost, or length of stay (LOS) in hospital could be documented as a result of these actions. Matsen (6, 13) at the University of Utah, found that earlier (24 hours) antimicrobial susceptibility test results influenced the choice of antibiotic employed in 50% of patients not already on therapy and in 20% of patients who were already receiving antimicrobial therapy.

He was able to document a decreased length of stay in hospital that could be attributable to these actions in 9% of patients. More recently, Trenholme et al. (8) reported a striking impact of rapid identification and susceptibility testing on the care of patients with bacteremia. They found that identification and susceptibility test results were available within 8 hours using rapid testing methods but not for as long as 48 hours using routine testing methods. When compared with that provided by the routine methods, the information provided by the rapid methods was significantly more likely to result in the initiation of antibiotic therapy, a change to more effective therapy, or a change to less expensive therapy. On a more pessimistic note, Edwards et al. (14) found that physicians acknowledged the results of microbiology reports in the medical record less than 4% of the time, suggesting that, despite rapid testing, the results were not available at the time of medical decision making and therefore were not used or documented. Similarly, data from the University of Iowa, where rapid testing and on-line computer reporting was employed routinely, indicated that physicians acknowledged only 24% of Gram stain results, 52% of culture results (78% of positive culture results), and only 10% of antimicrobial susceptibility results. One interpretation of these findings is that the current rapid technologies are still not rapid enough to provide results in a clinically relevant time frame. An alternative interpretation, and an issue for QA, is that microbiologists have not done enough to inform the clinicians of the rapid capabilities of the microbiology laboratory. In order for the results of rapid microbiology tests to actualize their full impact on medical decision making, the microbiologist must condition the clinician to be aware of the likely turnaround times for the various tests and to expect the results of rapid tests to be communicated in a timely fashion that is complementary to their practice habits.

These data are examples of QA studies that extend beyond the concept of process and attempt to establish a measure of the clinical usefulness of current microbiologic testing. In general, the data are positive in suggesting that rapid microbiologic testing (shorter turnaround time) influences medical decision making in a favorable way; however, the extension of these studies to examine the influence on clinical outcome remains a challenge. Nevertheless, performance of these QA studies and feedback of the results to clinicians are necessary steps in evaluating and improving the quality of care.

Accurate Results

The accuracy of laboratory test results is assured in part by a combination of internal quality control monitoring and external proficiency testing and inspection. Quality control (QC) may be defined as a surveillance process in which the performance of laboratory personnel, equipment, and reagents is observed and documented in a consistent manner (15). An effective QC program not only records the consistency of performance but also provides a record of the corrective action taken when defects or errors are detected. QC monitoring has been widely employed in clinical microbiology laboratories since the establishment of the Clinical Laboratory Improvement Act of 1967 (CLIA-67) and includes monitoring of the performance of culture media, reagents, instruments, and equipment. The assumption underlying this monitoring is that all materials, procedures, and equipment are potentially subject to deficiencies and should be monitored each time they are used. The wisdom of such comprehensive monitoring has been questioned as laboratories have begun to evaluate critically the usefulness and cost-effectiveness of QC activities. With experience, clinical microbiologists have observed that some QC monitors do detect deficiencies whereas others never detect deficiencies and are a waste of time and money. Thus, in recent years clinical microbiologists have endeavored to identify and focus attention on the more useful QC activities, those monitors which are more likely to detect problems. The assumption being that detection of a problem will lead to corrective action and will either improve the accuracy of the test or will prevent the reporting of misleading information. The importance of QC activities continues to be emphasized in the recent CLIA-88 rules (5), with an increased emphasis being placed on proficiency testing (discussed below). Interestingly enough, there are little or no data documenting (*a*) the influence of *specific* QC measures on the accuracy of test results or (*b*) actual health care benefits derived from QC activities (15–17). These are issues of great relevance to the quality assurance effort and should be a major goal of laboratory QC and QA activities.

Critical evaluation of QC activities by Bartlett and co-workers (16, 17) has provided guidance in identifying those QC monitors that are most useful and cost-effective in identifying deficiencies in the clinical microbiology laboratory. In order to delineate those QC practices that were expensive and that detected few deficiencies from those that were less expensive and detected a greater number of deficiencies, Bartlett developed a cost-effectiveness index (CEI) defined as the percent deficiencies detected divided by the cost of preventing a deficient operation. The value of the CEI in ranking the QC practices in five functional areas in clinical microbiology is shown in Table 27.2. The data illustrate that, although most kinds of QC surveillance procedures can detect deficiencies, surveillance of equipment and personnel are the most useful and cost-

effective (highest CEI), whereas monitoring of reagents is least productive. By critically evaluating QC practices in this manner, laboratories can eliminate QC practices that are ineffective and focus on those that are most productive and most likely to result in the improvement of laboratory practice.

The data of Bartlett and co-workers (16, 17) emphasize the importance of monitoring personnel performance as a QC activity and suggest that this may be a significant source of real error in laboratory testing (Table 27.2). Detection and control of personnel performance error may be difficult but can be effectively monitored by well-designed programs of internal (Table 27.3) and external (see below) proficiency testing. Bartlett (17) has shown that an internal proficiency testing program involving evaluation of blind unknowns, monitoring of direct smear interpretation, and submission of mock specimens is both efficient in detecting deficiencies and cost-effective (Table 27.3).

Tests of technologist performance evaluate all components of the analytical system and reflect a movement in laboratory QC from the monitoring of individual test components to the consideration of the overall quality of the end product. This is not to say that all component testing should be abandoned. QC surveillance of equipment and certain media appears to be both necessary and effective (Table 27.2). Likewise, whenever a problem is detected in the evaluation of the testing process, the

Table 27.2.
Quality Control in Clinical Microbiology: Functions Monitored[a]

Function Monitored	No. of QC Surveillance Procedures	No. of QC Procedures Detecting Deficiencies	CEI (Mode)
Equipment	4	4	250
Personnel performance	4	4	40
Media	35	27	3.4
Antimicrobial susceptibility	6	6	1
Reagents	13	1	0.2

[a]Data from Bartlett RC. Quality control in microbiology. In: Smith JW, ed. The role of clinical microbiology in cost-effective health care. Skokie, IL: College of American Pathologists, 1984:537–550.

Table 27.3.
Monitoring of Personnel Performance[a]

Monitor	Deficiencies	CEI	Annual Cost
	%		
Blind unknowns	31	1992	257
Direct smear interpretation	16	65	531
Mock specimens	3	17	116
Reference laboratory, comparative analysis	12	0.21	793

[a]Data from Bartlett RC. Quality control in microbiology. In: Smith JW, ed. The role of clinical microbiology in cost-effective health care. Skokie, IL: College of American Pathologists, 1984:537–550.

individual components of the process must be evaluated to determine the cause of the problem and develop an effective solution. Consistent with this logic, CAP has placed less emphasis in their proficiency testing and inspection programs on daily testing of *components* and more on the *overall procedure.* This is exemplified by data obtained from the CAP survey of disk susceptibility QC practices from 1981 to 1989 (18). In 1981, 68% of participants performed daily QC, and only 18% performed weekly QC. In contrast, by 1989 the proportion of laboratories performing weekly QC had increased to 68% compared to only 26% performing daily QC (Table 27.4). This shift in QC frequency was also related to an increase in conformance with standard QC guidelines published by the National Committee for Clinical Laboratory Standards (NCCLS) (59% in 1981 and 99% in 1989).

Evidence that less frequent QC monitoring was not associated with decreased accuracy of disk diffusion testing is provided by the observation that in 1981 15% of laboratories had >2% of QC results judged to be out of control compared to only 2% of laboratories in 1989 (Table 27.4). An additional and very striking example of the importance of evaluating the overall procedure rather than just the individual

technical components of the test is provided by results from the CAP proficiency testing program (18, 19). In 1981 the CAP submitted an isolate of *Streptococcus pneumoniae* relatively resistant to penicillin to its survey participants. Although 95% of the participants correctly determined the zone of inhibition around the oxacillin test disk to be equal to or less than 19mm, only 17% correctly interpreted the result as resistant (Table 27.5). Thus, the individual technical *components* of the test were correctly and accurately performed but the *overall process* failed due to an error in interpretation. This would be classified as a *very major* clinical error because a resistant organism would have been reported as susceptible. By comparison, the testing of a similar organism in 1987, when 67% of laboratories performed *weekly* QC, revealed no decrease in the level of technical performance (95% correctly measured a zone of equal to or less than 19mm), and 98% of participants correctly interpreted the result as resistant. This reflects both the educational effect of the CAP proficiency testing program as well as the emphasis between 1981 and 1987 on evaluation of the entire process rather than just the individual technical components. Similar data have been presented by Bartlett (17) indicating that 10 times the number of deficiencies were detected by monitoring the disk diffusion test for both materials deficiencies and errors in performance and interpretation than were detected by moni-

Table 27.4.
CAP Bacteriology Survey Participant Disk Susceptibility Quality Control Practices for 1981–1989[a]

Parameter	Subscribers by Year				
	1981	1984	1987	1988	1989
Frequency of QC					
Daily	68	53	29	28	26
Weekly	18	37	67	69	68
Laboratories with equal to or less than 2% out-of-control results	85	96	97	97	98
Laboratories using NCCLS QC guidelines	59	83	97	97	99

[a]Data adapted from Jones RN, Edson DC. Antimicrobial susceptibility testing (AST) trends and accuracy in the United States: A review of the College of American Pathologists microbiology surveys 1972–1989. Arch Pathol Lab Med 1991;115:429–436.

Table 27.5.
CAP Surveys *Streptococcus pneumoniae* Testing Results, 1981–1987[a]

Year of Survey	Specimen	Participants with Zone ≤19mm	Participants with Correct Interpretation (Resistant)
		%	%
1981	D-10	95	17
1983	D-16	99	70
1987	D-17	95	98

[a]Data adapted from Jones RN, Edson DC. Antimicrobial susceptibility testing (AST) trends and accuracy in the United States: A review of the College of American Pathologists microbiology surveys 1972–1989. Arch Pathol Lab Med 1991;115:429–436.

toring materials alone. Thus, QC activities in clinical microbiology have shifted from an all-encompassing series of component monitors with little obvious clinical relevance toward more selective component monitoring and increasing emphasis on a more clinically relevant monitoring of the whole analytical system.

External QC efforts, such as proficiency surveys and laboratory inspections, have been shown to be effective in improving laboratory performance. These include teaching specimens such as those distributed by the American Society of Clinical Pathologists (ASCP check sample) as well as the graded CAP proficiency testing surveys and Laboratory Inspection and Accreditation Program. Again, as described above, such external proficiency testing tends to emphasize monitoring of the entire analytical system than individual technical components. Using the CAP's proficiency testing data as an example, it can be demonstrated that laboratory performance in antimicrobial susceptibility testing is measurable and that proficiency surveys have had a beneficial effect (19). CAP survey results have documented (a) shifts in the frequency of QC performance (Table 27.4), (b) performance defects and subsequent improvement following constructive criticisms and critique (Table 27.5), and (c) the overall excellent accuracy of both broth dilution and disk diffusion susceptibility testing (Table 27.6). Furthermore, CAP survey results have served to monitor and educate participants relative to the importance of compliance with essential methodologic and technical aspects of standardized test methods and have documented the favorable impact of these efforts (Table 27.7). Likewise, Duckworth (21) has documented an improvement in inspection scores in laboratories that participate voluntarily in the CAP Laboratory Inspection and Accreditation Program. Finally, the CAP Q-Probe Quality Assurance Program is beginning to generate useful information concerning quality assurance issues in clinical microbiology including blood culture utilization, turnaround time, nosocomial infections, error reports, and comparison of antibiotic susceptibility patterns. The Q-Probe pro-

Table 27.6.
Comparative Performance Accuracy of Broth and Disk Methods of Antimicrobial Susceptibility Testing for CAP Bacteriology Surveys from 1981–1983 and 1989[a]

Susceptibility Test Method	Percent Accuracy	
	1981–1983	1989
Broth dilution	96.2	96.5
Disk diffusion	96.3	98.2

[a]Data adapted from Jones RN. Review of interlaboratory antimicrobial susceptibility testing proficiency from the College of American Pathologists (CAP) microbiology surveys program 1972–1983. In: Smith JW, ed. The role of clinical microbiology in cost-effective health care. Skokie, IL: College of American Pathologists, 1984:237–249; and Jones RN, Edson DC. Antimicrobial susceptibility testing (AST) trends and accuracy in the United States: A review of the College of American Pathologists microbiology surveys 1972–1989. Arch Pathol Lab Med 1991;115:429–436.

gram will provide interlaboratory assessment of QA data and should serve as a useful guide in establishing specific QA monitors as well as a means of educating clinical microbiologists on issues relative to QA. Thus, the impact of proficiency surveys on clinical microbiology has been multifaceted and favorable (19). As evidenced by the new CLIA-88 rules (5), participation in such programs is becoming one of the most important aspects of laboratory QC. Measurement of performance on proficiency testing specimens appears to be one of the better means of assessing the quality of service provided by a given laboratory; however, the impact of these efforts on the overall quality of medical care and patient outcome remains to be determined.

Laboratory Consultation

As stated by Howie (22), the most important part of the microbiologist's work is consultative, designed to help in the diagnosis and therapy of the patient. This type of consultative and collaborative interaction, and its documentation, is essential in expanding laboratory QA to address the broader issues of quality medical care. This means that the clinical microbiologist must function in a much broader role than just making recommendations regarding purchase of equipment and supplies, quality control, new testing methods, or person-

Table 27.7.
CAP Bacteriology Survey Participant Conformance with the NCCLS M2-A4 (1990) Essential Methodologic or Technical Details for the Disk Diffusion Tests for 1972–1989[a]

Method Detail	Laboratories in Conformance		
	1972	1979	1984–1989[b]
	%		
Inoculum			
3–5 colonies picked, Adjusted to 0.5	72	83	88
McFarland standard	74	88	96
Cotton swab inoculated	97	92	92
Agar medium			
Mueller-Hinton medium	96	98	>99
Correct pH measured	44	72	90
Agar depth at 3–5 mm	73	86	96
Disks stored properly	80	81	94

[a]Data adapted from Jones RN, Edson DC. Antimicrobial susceptibility testing (AST) trends and accuracy in the United States: A review of the College of American Pathologists microbiology surveys 1972–1989. Arch Pathol Lab Med 1991; 115:429–436.
[b]No significant variations were identified from 1984 through 1989.

nel problems and must be seen in view of providing clinically useful and relevant information in the areas of diagnosis, identification, and therapeutic recommendations. Microbiologists, whether physicians or medical scientists, must be well versed not only in the methodologies of the laboratory but must have a good understanding of the pathophysiologic consequences of their activities and must apply this knowledge in their communications with clinicians.

What clinicians need most is for the clinical microbiologist to teach and guide them in the appropriate use of the microbiology laboratory, not merely to offer new examinations or to function solely as a restraining force on diagnostic and therapeutic services under the guise of cost-effective laboratory utilization. Microbiologists must interact continuously, tactfully yet assertively, with clinicians in a way that will allow the development of patterns of practice that will be efficient and also to the patient's advantage (2). Person-to-person interaction is a highly effective

means of educating the clinician who has requested an examination of questionable indication or for which the test results are likely to be misinterpreted. Thus, as noted by Reller (23), a personal visit by the microbiologist to the operating room or hospital ward to discuss a patient with the attending physician and nurses does more to increase the proportion of appropriately obtained specimens sent to the laboratory than multiple memoranda. Although this may be labor intensive for the clinical microbiologist, the prospect for improving physician test-ordering habits are excellent when consultation is offered by a colleague (24).

In the interest of improving the quality and clinical usefulness of laboratory services, the laboratory needs to assume a leadership role, in collaboration with clinical colleagues, to develop a *consensus* opinion for the indications for and interpretation of both newly developed and previously accepted microbiology tests, which may be expensive, time consuming, or nonstandardized diagnostic procedures. These consensus guidelines can be applied as criteria for QA monitoring of the use of laboratory services as they relate to patient care. Thus, improved communication and consultation is the cornerstone for enhancing and evaluating the clinical usefulness of the laboratory services.

One area in which laboratory consultation and guidance is clearly indicated concerns specimen quality. It is well recognized that the usefulness of the microbiology report can be no better than the quality of the specimen received. Although the technical aspects of the clinical microbiology laboratory are increasing in reliability, the health care value of the information generated is significantly compromised by unnecessary submissions, excessive frequency of submissions, delays in transportation of specimens to the laboratory, and processing of contaminated or poorly collected specimens. Specimens that are not collected or transported properly, even when handled optimally within the laboratory, are likely to provide misleading results. As stated by Bartlett and co-workers (16, 17, 25), control of these problems is an inherent component of the overall responsibility of the clinical microbiologist to assure that the information being generated by the laboratory is of sufficient quality to support sound diagnostic and therapeutic decision making. Thus, the microbiologist must spend more time teaching proper selection of specimens and intelligible reporting and interpretation of results rather than concentrating on their voluminous generation (23). It should be kept in mind that the clinician has as little interest in acting on incorrect or irrelevant data as the microbiologist has in generating and reporting such information (26). Such data may lead to further unnecessary testing as well as to inappropriate therapy or diagnostic procedures, which may prolong hospitalization and increase morbidity and potential mortality.

Because of the potential for poor specimen quality and inappropriate testing to impact adversely on the quality of medical care, the monitoring of specimen quality, the transportation time, and appropriateness of test submissions are all useful QA activities. The results of these QA monitors can be used to develop specific *consensus* protocols to assess specimen quality. In general such protocols and the supporting data will be welcomed by clinicians as will renewed attempts to define and correct problems that have led to poor specimens. Two examples from the microbiology QA program at the Iowa City Veterans Affairs Medical Center (IC-VAMC) serve to illustrate these points. In the first example, we wanted to assess the degree to which routine stool examination for enteric pathogens (bacterial and parasitic) may be inappropriately ordered on hospitalized patients. This investigation was stimulated by a report by Siegel et al. (27), which indicated that the yield of routine stool

cultures and ova and parasite examination was extremely low when performed on patients hospitalized more than 3 days. We conducted a retrospective study of all stool specimens submitted for culture or ova and parasite examination during 1989 (Table 27.8). Our findings were consistent with those of Siegel et al. (27) and documented that enteric pathogens were extremely rare in stool specimens obtained from hospitalized patients at the IC-VAMC. These results, along with the data of Siegel et al. (27), were discussed with the medical staff and resulted in the establishment of a policy restricting the ordering of routine stool culture and ova and parasite examination without additional justification, on patients hospitalized more than 3 days. The result of this effort has been to decrease stool submissions by approximately 40%. A follow-up investigation will be conducted in order to document the positive (increased efficiency, cost savings) or negative (missed or delayed diagnosis, additional more costly tests) effects of this policy.

The second example concerns the problem of delayed transport of specimens to the laboratory. A review of the time lapse between the collection of specimens and arrival time in the microbiology laboratory revealed that 35% of all specimens arrived in the laboratory more than 1 hour after collection (Fig. 27.1). Because this delay was considered excessive for optimal recovery of potential pathogens, a memorandum was sent to the medical staff describing the problem and informing them that thereafter all specimens of sputum, urine, and feces would be rejected if not received within 1 hour of collection. The laboratory director also met with the members of the medical service in order to clarify the

Table 27.8.
Summary of Results of Stool Analysis for Combined Outpatient and Inpatient Groups for 1989, IC-VAMC

Procedure	Specimens Submitted	Specimens (Patients) Positive for Enteric Pathogens	Specimens (Patients) Positive after ≥3 Days Hospitalization
Culture	600	7 (3)	0
Ova and parasites	300	3 (3)	1 (1)
Total	900	10 (6)	1 (1)

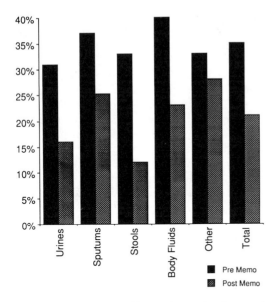

Figure 27.1. The effect of monitoring and feedback on delayed specimen transport at the Iowa City Veterans Affairs Medical Center, January through April, 1990.

policy and to enlist their support. The results of follow-up studies revealed a significant decrease in the number of specimens of all types arriving in the laboratory more than 1 hour after collection and provided documentation of the positive effect of this QA activity. These examples demonstrate that the professional communication of QA data can result in clinical support for rational changes in microbiology test ordering and specimen handling. Follow-up studies are part of the QA process and serve to document the impact of QA-based policies and protocols on laboratory and clinical services.

Assistance in Detecting Nosocomial Infection

There is no question that nosocomial infections represent a leading cause of death in the United States (28), are associated with significant morbidity (29–33), and carry an impressive economic burden (34). The epidemiologic activities involved in nosocomial infection control serve as excellent examples of QA and include assessment of access to medical care, identification of risk factors, and both prevention and control of adverse nosocomial

events. In this regard, it is particularly noteworthy that infection control is the only activity on QA that has been shown to be efficacious (35). Thus, it is not surprising that infection control has been described as the premier program for QA in United States hospitals today (1, 36).

The prevention and control of nosocomial infections is a team effort requiring the cooperation of the hospital epidemiologist, infection control practitioner, and members of the clinical microbiology laboratory. The clinical microbiology laboratory plays a key role in the diagnosis of nosocomial infections and is consulted frequently to assist in the epidemiologic investigation of nosocomial infection problems. In addition to performing routine isolation and identification of nosocomial pathogens from clinical material, the microbiology laboratory must also (*a*) participate fully as a member of the infection control committee; (*b*) organize and report microbiologic data relevant to infection control in a timely manner; (*c*) provide microbiologic support for surveillance and other activities necessary for the investigation of infection control problems; (*d*) provide more detailed (subspecies) characterization of selected nosocomial pathogens as needed to help define an epidemic; (*e*) provide additional microbiologic services such as cultures of patients, hospital personnel, and the environment as indicated in the context of an epidemiologic investigation; and (*f*) serve as a resource for microbiologic training and education of hospital and infection control personnel. This degree of cooperation between clinical and laboratory services is a prime example of the extensive and constructive interactions necessary to build an effective QA program with measurable clinical impact. Such communication and collaboration is essential for quality medical care and should be a goal for laboratories at all levels.

Product Evaluation

Critical evaluation of new technologies and diagnostic testing methods are standard practice for most clinical microbiology laboratories. In many cases these studies are extended beyond technical comparisons of test methods to address the practical clinical application of new and established diagnostic (8–10, 37–39) and therapeutic (39–42) strategies for the care of patients with infectious diseases. Such clinical and laboratory research is an important QA activity and is essential to improve the database on which laboratory consultation in clinical microbiology and infectious diseases is based. Again, collaboration with clinical colleagues can enhance the clinical relevance of these studies and provide an additional means of addressing QA issues in a positive fashion. The results of these studies can and should be used to establish policies and protocols designed to improve laboratory utilization and patient care.

Outcome

Few QA programs in any area of health care explicitly evaluate outcomes, and this is certainly true of laboratory QA programs. Although the science of quantitative medical decision making is beginning to make it possible to estimate the economic cost of making incorrect diagnostic and therapeutic decisions that could result from laboratory errors, it has been more difficult to estimate the morbidity and mortality attributable to laboratory error (17). The few studies mentioned previously that have examined the impact of rapid microbiology test results on patient care have focused largely on medical decision making (6, 8, 9, 12–14). Specifically, they have addressed the impact of rapid antimicrobial susceptibility testing on antibiotic utilization. These studies have extended laboratory QA in the right direction but have yet to address the impact of laboratory services on *outcome* of medical care.

Perhaps the relationship of the clinical microbiology laboratory to infection control provides the best example of the importance of microbiology in a QA activity that has been shown to be efficacious. Nosocomial infection surveillance is currently considered to be an important component of an effective hospital program associated with reduction in the rates of (and thus in the morbidity, mortality, and

cost of) nosocomial infection (1, 33–36). This surveillance effort depends in large part on culture and antimicrobial susceptibility data supplied by the clinical microbiology laboratory. The review of the microbiology laboratory reports is the single most common case-finding method employed routinely for nosocomial infection surveillance (43). Thus, the clinical microbiology laboratory contributes in a major way to the detection of nosocomial infections and initiation of control efforts. Furthermore by extending the laboratory support of infection control at the University of Iowa to include epidemiologic typing of nosocomial pathogens, we have shown that the clinical microbiology laboratory can *enhance* the effectiveness of infection control efforts (44, 45). Thus, the clinical microbiology laboratory is essential for the detection of nosocomial infections and in facilitating infection control efforts, the outcome of which results in improved quality of care in the hospital.

Consequence of Outcome

The consequences attributable to the outcomes of microbiology laboratory services could include (*a*) survival and discharge from the hospital with or without sequelae, (*b*) excess stay in the hospital and the associated costs, (*c*) prevention of nosocomial infections and projected savings in terms of decreased LOS and decreased morbidity and mortality, and (*d*) death (Table 27.1). There are little or no data relating these issues to laboratory testing. Conceivably, QA monitors focusing on clinically important stat tests such as special stains of bronchoscopy specimens in immunocompromised patients with pneumonia could provide this information. For example, studies of timeliness and accuracy of special stain results could be extended to examine diagnostic utility, relationship of test results to therapy, outcome, and sequelae. These studies are necessary and important yet remain neglected.

Although it has been difficult to document the direct impact of laboratory testing on morbidity, mortality, and LOS in the hospital, consideration of data obtained from studies of nosocomial infections provides some insight into the consequences of detecting and controlling nosocomial infections and thus may relate indirectly to microbiology laboratory services. Nosocomial infections add significant mortality, morbidity, and economic burden to the outcomes expected from the underlying diseases alone. It is estimated that nosocomial infections are directly responsible for at least 20,000 deaths and contribute to an additional 60,000 deaths annually (46, 47). Studies employing a matched design to control for confounding variables such as severity of underlying disease have indicated that the mortality directly attributable to nosocomial bloodstream infections ranges from 14% for bloodstream infections due to coagulase-negative staphylococci (32) to 38–50% for bloodstream infections due to *Candida* spp. (31, 48). These data suggest that nosocomial infections, particularly bloodstream infections, carry a significant mortality and constitute a major cause of death nationwide (28).

In addition to an important attributable mortality, nosocomial infections result in excess costs primarily due to a prolonged LOS in the hospital. It is estimated that each nosocomial infection results in an additional 5–10 days of hospitalization, producing a financial burden in the United States of 5–10 billion dollars annually. At the University of Iowa, we have documented excess LOS of 8 and 30 days (median values) for nosocomial bloodstream infections due to coagulase-negative staphylococci and *Candida* spp., respectively (31, 32). Likewise, we have found that nosocomial infections due to *Staphylococcus aureus* resulted in a mean excess LOS of 8.2 days and additional costs of hospitalization in excess of $3000 (1985 dollars) per patient (49).

Given these data, it is not surprising that the prevention and control of nosocomial infections has drawn the attention of hospital epidemiologists, clinicians, clinical microbiologists, and hospital administrators alike. Through such combined efforts it is becoming increasingly clear that a sizeable proportion of nosocomial infections can be eliminated through effective infection control methods. Specifically, data obtained from the Study of the Efficacy of Nosocomial Infection Control (SENIC) indicated that the presence of an active surveillance and infection control system was associated with a 32% decrease in nosocomial infection rates (35). In contrast, the rate of infection *increased* by 18% among hospitals with minimal or poor infection control practices. Thus, effective infection control efforts, of which clinical microbiology is an important component, result in decreased morbidity, mortality, and LOS and contribute in a major way to improved patient care by decreasing the risk of nosocomial infection.

SUMMARY AND CONCLUSIONS

The assessment of quality in medical care is a complex issue that has only just begun to be addressed by workers in laboratory medicine. Issues of internal quality control and quality assessment are familiar to laboratorians; however, laboratory workers must extend their efforts beyond examination of the process of laboratory testing in order to assess the true impact of laboratory testing on medical care and patient outcome. This effort will require considerable collaboration with clinical colleagues and should address issues of access, process, and outcome as they relate to the clinical usefulness of diagnostic testing. Such collaboration will accomplish far more than merely satisfying regulation. It will result in improved patient care.

Acknowledgments

The author acknowledges the excellent secretarial skills of Ruth Kjaer. This work was supported in part by the Department of Veterans Affairs.

References

1. Wenzel RP. Quality assessment: An emerging component of hospital epidemiology. Diagn Microbiol Infect Dis 1990;13:197–204.
2. Smith JW, ed. *The role of clinical microbiology in cost-effective health care.* Skokie, IL: College of American Pathologists, 1984.
3. Schifman RB. Quality assurance in microbiology.

In: Howanitz P, Howantiz J, eds. Laboratory quality assurance. New York: McGraw-Hill, 1987;244–269.

4. Schifman RB. Microbiology quality assurance. In: McClatchey KD, ed. Clinical laboratory medicine. Baltimore: Williams & Wilkins, 1992 in press.

5. Wilensky GR. Medicare, Medicaid and CLIA Programs: Revision of the laboratory regulations for the Medicare, Medicaid and Clinical Laboratories Improvement Act of 1967 Programs. Federal Register 1990;55:9538–9610.

6. Matsen JM. Means to facilitate acceptance and use of rapid test results. Diagn Microbiol Infect Dis 1985;3:735–785.

7. Steindel S. Analytical turn-around time. College of American Pathologists Q-Probes, 1990;90–16A.

8. Trenholme GM, Kaplan RL, Karakusis PH, et al. Clinical impact of rapid identification and susceptibility testing of bacterial blood culture isolates. J Clin Microbiol 1989;27:1342–1345.

9. Doern GV, Scott DR, Rashad AL. Clinical impact of rapid antimicrobial susceptibility testing of blood culture isolates. Antimicrob Agents Chemother 1982;82:1023–1024.

10. Moore DF, Hamada SS, Marso E, Martin WJ. Rapid identification and antimicrobial susceptibility testing of Gram-negative bacilli from blood cultures by the AutoMicrobic System. J Clin Microbiol 1981;13:934–939.

11. Pfaller MA, Automated instrument approaches to clinical microbiology. Diagn Microbiol Infect Dis 1985;3:15S–23S.

12. Bartlett RC. Medical microbiology: How far to go—How fast to go in 1982. In: Lorian V, ed. Significance of medical microbiology in the care of patients. Baltimore: Willams & Wilkins, 1982: 12–44.

13. Matsen J. Rapid reporting of results—impact on patient, physician, and laboratory. In: Tilton RC, ed. Rapid methods and automation in microbiology. Washington, D.C.: American Society for Microbiology, 1982:98–102.

14. Edwards LD, Levin S, Balagtas R, et al. Ordering patterns and utilization of bacteriologic culture reports. Arch Intern Med 1973;132:678–682.

15. Sommers HM. Towards more effective quality control. In: Smith JW, ed. The role of clinical microbiology in cost-effective health care. Skokie, IL: College of American Pathologists, 1984:533–536.

16. Bartlett RC, Rutz CA, Konopacki N. Cost-effectiveness of quality contol in bacteriology. Am J Clin Pathol 1982;77:184–190.

17. Bartlett RC. Quality control in microbiology. In: Smith JW, ed. The role of clinical microbiology in cost-effective health care. Skokie, IL: College of American Pathologists, 1984:537–550.

18. Jones RN, Edson DC. Antimicrobial susceptibility testing (AST) trends and accuracy in the United States: A review of the College of American Pathologists microbiology surveys 1972–1989. Arch Pathol Lab Med 1991;115:429–436.

19. Fuchs PC, Jones RN. The impact of proficiency survey programs on laboratory antimicrobial susceptibility testing. Antimicrob Newsletter 1984; 1:93–98.

20. Jones RN. Review of interlaboratory antimicrobial susceptibility testing proficiency from the College of American Pathologists (CAP) microbiology surveys program 1972–1983. In: Smith JW, ed. The role of clinical microbiology in cost-effective health care. Skokie, IL: College of American Pathologists, 1984:237–249.

21. Duckworth JK. Effect of voluntary accreditation on performance in microbiology. In: Smith JW, ed. The role of clinical microbiology in cost-effective health care. Skokie, IL: College of American Pathologists, 1984:561–565.

22. Howie J. Medical microbiology for the patient and community. J Clin Pathol 1972;25:921–926.

23. Reller LB. Consultative role of the clinical microbiology laboratory: A clinician's viewpoint. In: Smith JW, ed. The role of clinical microbiology in cost-effective health care. Skokie, IL: College of American Pathologists, 1984:581–583.

24. Kleiman MB. What the physician needs from the clinical microbiology laboratory in the next three years. In: Smith JW, ed. The role of clinical microbiology in cost-effective health care. Skokie, IL: College of American Pathologists, 1984:597–601.

25. Bartlett RC. Making optimum use of the microbiology laboratory. I. Use of the laboratory. JAMA 1982;247:857–859.

26. McGowan JE Jr. Rational use of the laboratory: The clinician's perspective. In: Smith JW, ed. The role of clinical microbiology in cost-effective health care. Skokie, IL: College of American Pathologists, 1984:79–84.

27. Siegel DL, Edelstein PH, Nachamkin I. Inappropriate testing for diarrheal diseases in the hospital. JAMA 1990;263:979–982.

28. Wenzel RP. The mortality of hospital-acquired bloodstream infections: Need for a new vital statistic? Int J Epidemiol 1988;17:225–227.

29. Rose R, Hunting KJ, Townsend TR, Wenzel RP. Morbidity/mortality and economics of hospital-acquired bloodstream infections: A controlled study. South Med J 1977;70:1267–1269.

30. Townsend TR, Wenzel RP. Nosocomial bloodstream infections in a newborn intensive care unit. A case matched control study of morbidity, mortality and risk. Am J Epidemiol 1981;114:73–80.

31. Wey SB, Mori M, Pfaller MA, Woolson RF, Wenzel RP. Hospital-acquired candidemia: The attributable mortality and excess length of stay. Arch Intern Med 1988;148:2642–2645.

32. Martin MA, Pfaller MA, Wenzel RP. Coagulase-negative staphylococcal bacteremia. Mortality and hospital stay. Ann Intern Med 1989;110:9–16.

33. Green MS, Rubenstein E, Amit P. Estimating the effects of nosocomial infections on the length of hospitalization. J Infect Dis 1982;145:667–672.

34. Dixon RE. Costs of nosocomial infections and benefits of infection control programs in prevention and control of nosocomial infections. In: Wenzel RP, ed. Prevention and control of nosocomial infections. Baltimore: Williams & Wilkins, 1987:19–25.

35. Haley RW, Culver DH, White JW, et al. The efficacy of infection surveillance and control programs in preventing nosocomial infections on U.S. hospitals. Am J Epidemiol 1985;121:182–205.

36. Wenzel RP, Pfaller MA. Infection control: The premier quality assessment program in United States hospitals. Am J Med 1991, in press.
37. Pfaller M, Ringenberg B, Rames L, Hegeman J, Koontz F. The usefulness of screening tests for pyuria in combination with culture in the diagnosis of urinary tract infecion. Diagn Microbiol Infect Dis 1987;6:207–215.
38. Doebbeling BN, Bale M, Koontz FP, et al. Prospective evaluation of the Gen-Probe DNA probe assay for detection of Legionellae in respiratory specimens. Eur J Clin Microbiol Infect Dis 1988;7:748–752.
39. Cabezudo I, Pfaller M, Gerarden T, et al. The usefulness of the Cand-Tec candida antigen assay in the diagnosis and therapy of systemic candidiasis in high risk patients. Eur J Clin Microbiol Infect Dis 1989;8:770–777.
40. Massanari RM, Pfaller MA, Wakefield DS, et al. Implications of acquired oxacillin resistance for the management and control of *Staphylococcus aureus* infections. J Infect Dis 1988;158:702–709.
41. DeGroote MA, Martin MA, Densen P, Pfaller MA, Wenzel RP. Serum tumor necrosis factor levels in patients with presumed Gram-negative sepsis treated with antilipid-A antibody or placebo. JAMA 1989;262:249–251.
42. Doebbeling BN, Pfaller MA, Kuhns KR, et al. Cardiovascular surgery prophylaxis: A randomized, controlled comparison of cefazolin and cefuroxime. J Thorac Cardiovasc Surg 1990; 99:981–989.
43. Schifman RB. Nosocomial infections data analysis and critique. College of American Pathologists Q-Probes, 1990;89–07A.
44. Pfaller MA, Wakefield DS, Hollis R, et al. The clinical microbiology laboratory as an aid in infection control: The application of molecular techniques in epidemiologic studies of methicillin resistant *Staphylococcus aureus*. Diagn Microbiol Infect Dis 1991;14:209–217.
45. Pfaller MA, Hollis RJ. The use of plasmid profiles and restriction endonuclease analysis of plasmid DNA as epidemiologic and diagnostic tools in the clinical microbiology laboratory. Clin Microbiol Newsletter 1989;11:137–141.
46. Spengler RF, Greenough WE III. Hospital costs and mortality attributed to nosocomial bacteremias. JAMA 1987;240:2455–2458.
47. Gross PA, Neu HC, Aswapokee P, Van Antwerpen C, Aswapokee N. Deaths from nosocomial infections: Experience in a university hospital and a community hospital. Am J Med 1980;68:219–223.
48. Bross J, Talbot GH, Maislin G, Hurwitz D, Strom BL. Risk factors for nosocomial candidemia: A case-control study in adults without leukemia. Am J Med 1989;87:614–620.
49. Wakefield DS, Helms CM, Massanari RM, Mori M, Pfaller M. The cost of nosocomial infection: Relative contributions of laboratory, antibiotic, and per diem costs in serious *S. aureus* infections. Am J Infect Cont 1988;16:185–192.

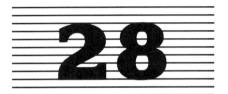

The Pharmacy and Drug Usage

John P. Burke, M.D., and Stanley L. Pestotnik, R.Ph.

"Quis custodiet ipsos custodes?"

The pharmacy is the focal point for the procurement, distribution, and control of drugs used in the hospital. It is also the principal source of information concerning drug usage. However, the pharmacy itself is only part of the pharmaceutical care system, which also includes prescribers, nurses, ward clerks, and transportation couriers (1, 2). The hospitalwide nature of drug-related issues and the involvement of many levels of hospital personnel create diffusion of responsibility, variation in patient care, and complexity in quality assessment (Fig. 28.1). These characteristics also create numerous opportunities for the application of epidemiologic methods aimed at identifying variation, improving systems for drug distribution and use, and improving patient care and outcomes, as well as reducing costs.

The efforts of epidemiologists in meeting these challenges have thus far been limited, some of the most effective programs having been restricted to antibiotic usage (3). Information about nonantibiotic drug usage and drug prescribing practices of physicians is fragmentary, at best, and is largely based on reports published more than two decades ago. In recent years, a few large hospitals with computerized information systems have begun to develop comprehensive drug surveillance programs that promise to become potent tools for epidemiology (4).

The present gaps in our knowledge are illustrated by the problem of adverse drug events (ADEs). The magnitude of the rate of ADEs cannot be stated with the same confidence as the rate of hospital-acquired infections. It is reasonable to conjecture that, among the approximately 40 million admissions to acute care hospitals in the United States each year, there are several hundred million different drug exposures, resulting in ADEs being experienced by 2 to 12 million patients annually (5, 6). One recent report found that complications from drug therapy were the most common adverse events in hospitalized patients (7).

The Joint Commission on Accreditation of Healthcare Organizations (JCAHO) has required hospitals to perform drug usage evaluations that include monitoring ADEs. The ability of hospitals to respond to this requirement is unknown, but it is disturbing that 88% of hospitals accredited by the Joint Commission in 1989 did not fully comply with the existing standards for drug usage evaluation (8). The possible reasons for this high rate of noncompliance include either a lack of understanding of the Joint Commission requirements, inade-

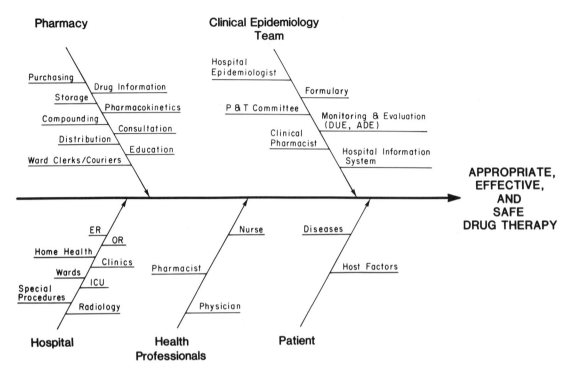

Figure 28.1.   The pharmaceutical care system.

quate resources, or fundamental disagreement with the approach being taken by the Joint Commission.

The purpose of this chapter is to explore the current Joint Commission standards relating to drug usage evaluation, focusing on the responsibilities of the medical staff, and to emphasize the role of the hospital epidemiologist in the quality assessment of drug usage.

INTERPRETING CURRENT JCAHO STANDARDS

The Joint Commission is committed to the principle that continuous quality improvement should be the goal of every hospital (9). The monitoring and evaluation process is viewed as the cornerstone of quality assurance and is described in the "Quality Assurance" chapter of the 1991 *Accreditation Manual for Hospitals (AMH)* as a 10-step process (10). This process is described as an ongoing one and not as time-limited studies of selected topics. The 10 steps represent a common-sense ap-

proach to problem solving that resembles the method advocated by the Centers for Disease Control for the investigation of disease outbreaks. The Joint Commission views these 10 steps as a means to help hospitals focus on high priority quality-of-care issues and to use quality assurance resources more effectively; it is also seen as an essential process for accreditation with the requirement that each of the 10 steps must be documented (11, 12). The overall intent of these 10 steps is to require health care organizations to identify problems in a systematic fashion, to utilize these problems to take appropriate actions, and to demonstrate that the actions were effective in resolving the problems (13).

The pharmaceutical services are addressed by an entire section of the 1991 *AMH*. This section comprises six separate standards, of which five deal with the structure and process of pharmacy services such as staffing, training, and licensing requirements; space, equipment, and supplies; and need for written policies and procedures. These standards require the participation of the pharmacy with the medical staff, through its pharmacy and therapeutics committee, for the development and maintenance of a formulary list and for the monitoring and evaluation of the quality and appropriateness of patient services provided by the pharmacy. The pharmacy is also required to participate with the hospital's quality assurance program in matters relating to drug utilization and effectiveness, determining drug usage patterns, and setting drug use criteria.

The development of drug-monitoring services with the capacity to prevent drug interactions or incompatibilities, e.g., interdicting the use of penicillin in a patient with a history of penicillin allergy, is encouraged by these standards, "within the limits of available resources" (10). Similarly, the reporting of adverse drug reactions and medication errors must be "in accordance with written procedures" (10). It is apparent that the Joint Commission recognizes that existing hospital programs for monitoring ADEs are hampered by incomplete reporting and that comprehensive, effective programs remain in the future for most hospitals.

The sixth and final standard for pharmaceutical services is more problematic and far-reaching, and requires that the pharmacy department, using the 10-step process, monitor and evaluate the quality and appropriateness of patient care services. This quality assurance standard is not entirely satisfied by drug usage evaluations and is the responsibility of the pharmacy director.

In order to satisfy this requirement, hospital pharmacies should itemize the types of care provided, e.g., all aspects of drug procurement, distribution, and information, as well as clinical components of care such as pharmacokinetic services. From this list the pharmacy staff should identify those aspects of care that are high volume, high risk, or problem-prone. From this "short list," objective measurable indicators must be selected that provide information about the quality of care. The indicators may be related either to the structure, process, or outcome of care. These indicators may be either sentinel events that identify substandard care or patterns of care. In the evaluation of pat-

terns of care, thresholds must be selected to define substandard care. It is vital that the pharmacy staff itself design and agree with the choice of indicators, thereby ensuring "ownership" and maximum cooperation in the monitoring and evaluation process. Finally, the effectiveness of this 10-step process must be assessed through continual monitoring of care with resetting of thresholds as necessary.

In addition to these standards, there are two additional standards that apply to pharmaceutical services and that are under the auspices of the medical staff. These medical staff standards concern drug usage evaluation (MS.6.1.3) and the pharmacy and therapeutics function (MS.6.1.6).

MS.6.1.3. "Drug usage evaluation is performed by the medical staff as a criteria-based, ongoing, planned and systematic process for monitoring and evaluating the prophylactic, therapeutic, and empiric use of drugs to help assure that they are provided appropriately, safely, and effectively" (10).

The concept of drug usage evaluation (DUE) was originally described as a drug usage review (DUR) process in 1968 as part of the final report of the task force on prescription drugs submitted by the secretary of Health, Education, and Welfare (14). Brodie and Smith (15) in 1976 further developed these ideas and proposed the first conceptual model of DUR. During the past decade, the philosophy, emphasis, and terminology have changed from a process-oriented focus (DUR) to an outcome-oriented strategy (DUE) (16). Evaluations that were originally designed to be quantitative in focus have been shifted to a qualitative orientation, that is, appropriateness of drug therapy and associated outcomes are now the major emphasis (17). The Joint Commission's previous requirement for antibiotic use review is now considered to be included in overall drug usage evaluation and is no longer addressed in the infection control standards.

The medical and pharmacy staffs of institutions are responsible for ensuring that all drugs in all patient care settings are used appropriately. DUE is an outcome-oriented monitoring and evaluation tool that is used to examine the appropriateness of drug use in institutions. DUE is a quality assurance process that is explicitly designated as a medical staff activity performed in cooperation with pharmacy, nursing, and other allied health care professionals. Since DUE is an activity involving a peer review process, it is, as are all drug use issues in the hospital, under the aegis of the pharmacy and therapeutics committee, a medical staff committee. Nonetheless, for all practical purposes DUEs are performed by the pharmacy, while the pharmacy and therapeutics committee, acting as a representative of the medical staff, assumes overall responsibility for the process and oversees, approves, and reviews the results of such activities.

Drug use evaluation, by design, should involve a monitoring and evaluation process that examines the prophylactic, therapeutic, and empiric uses of the major classes of drugs in the organization, including both antibiotic and nonantibiotic drugs. The goal of the DUE program is to assure the appropriate, effective, and safe use of drugs in the hospital. Drug therapy is considered appropriate when valid clinical indications are present to warrant the prescribing of the drug. The effectiveness is enhanced when the appropriate drugs are prescribed in the correct dose, frequency, and duration for an individual patient. Safety is partly assured when prescribers identify important risk factors in individual patients that predispose them to drug interactions and adverse events. Attendant to the issues of effectiveness and safety is the requirement that the prescriber monitor both clinical and laboratory parameters that will enhance the effectiveness of the drug therapy and avoid toxicity. DUEs should be qualitative in focus and evaluate specific patient outcomes associated with the appropriate, effective, and safe use of drugs in individual patients.

Appropriate design and conduct of drug use evaluations is required if such a program is going to succeed in improving patient care and outcomes. A fundamental understanding of study design and epidemiological surveillance is necessary to perform legitimate and useful DUEs. The 10-step process should also be used to perform drug use evaluations in a logical and systematic fashion. These efforts will enable those responsible for the DUE process to describe the drugs used, the patients treated, the practitioners involved, including the prescribers, dispensers, and administrators of the drugs, as well as the circumstances and locale of specific drug use within the institution. In other words, all aspects of drug use can be identified and delineated when proper surveillance techniques are employed. Once this information is available, investigators can identify and select specific drugs or drug classes as topics for DUE. The Joint Commission guidelines suggest that these DUE topics be selected based on high volume, high risk, and high cost issues.

The process is then expanded to identify and select the proper indicators necessary to monitor and evaluate appropriate and effective drug use. Indicators are measurable variables that provide information about specific patient outcomes as they relate to the use of a particular drug or drug class. These outcome measures address drug therapy issues such as: the indication for the drug, dosage, duration of therapy, drug interactions, adverse drug events, contraindications, amelioration of symptoms, cure of disease, prevention of symptoms or disease, or slowing of the disease process. Indicators should be based on the literature and expert input. The criteria that are then developed through these resources will define the standard of care as applied to that particular drug therapy. Key features of these defined standards are that they are reliable, reproducible, objective, and tied to the specific institution (18). For example, DUE criteria for the empiric use of antibiotics in neutropenic patients with unexplained fever should be based on sound, expert advice (19), but be refined for a particular institution's case mix, formulary, and antimicrobial susceptibility patterns.

Wible (18) has reviewed the steps required in implementing a DUE as well as the data collection techniques that can be employed. Data can be gathered retrospectively (with respect to treatments already completed), prospectively (planned and executed before the initiation of therapy), or concurrently (with respect to treatments as they occur) (20). Each of these methods has its own set of advantages and disadvantages. For instance, retrospective review can be performed at a convenient time interval when both the investigator and the records are available. The disadvantages of this type of an approach are numerous. One obvious disadvantage is that neither the patient nor the prescriber is easily available. The medical record is the only source of information, and there is no opportunity to influence patient outcomes. From a DUE standpoint, prospective review has the greater potential to impact patient outcomes. That is because this method allows for data collection before therapy is initiated, and detected discrepancies can be acted upon in a real-time fashion. However, this method is demanding because the investigator must be available 24 hours a day. Concurrent review shares many of the advantages and disadvantages of a retrospective approach. However, it does offer more flexibility in terms of investigator, prescriber, and patient data availability than the retrospective method. Additionally, concurrent monitoring allows for a positive influence on patient outcomes if therapies are evaluated early in the treatment course.

Traditionally, data are collected and complied through a variety of different means. The information is then analyzed to determine the prescribing trends in the institution and the effects of prescribing on patient outcomes. Summaries of these analyses should be disseminated to appropriate departments, committees, and individuals involved. Since continuous quality improvement (CQI) is the ultimate objective of DUE, problems or deficiencies that are detected should instigate corrective action. The Joint Commission recognizes the concept of DUE as a formal, focused, and legitimate means of monitoring and evaluating the prophylactic, therapeutic, and empiric use of drugs. It is important to note that DUE is an ongoing process. The appropriate, safe, and effective use of drugs is a CQI subject that requires continuous monitoring, evaluation, and action when necessary. It is equally important to underscore the notion that drug therapy is

a critical and integral component and determinant of hospital care and patient outcomes.

The standard for DUE is now a key factor in the accreditation decision process. Nonetheless, the precise requirements appear to be flexible, and there is no requirement for the minimum numbers of drugs or patients to be reviewed or the duration of individual studies.

MS.6.1.6. "The pharmacy and therapeutics function is performed by the medical staff, in cooperation with the pharmaceutical department/service, the nursing department/service, management and administrative services, and, as required, other departments/services and individuals" (10).

The pharmacy and therapeutics committee is a medical staff committee that functions in an advisory capacity on all drug issues to the medical staff and hospital at large and is responsible for the development of the hospital formulary. The pharmacy and therapeutics committee determines policy on the matters of drug selection, procurement, handling, distribution, use, and administration, including investigational drugs in the hospital. It is the responsibility of the committee to monitor and review all adverse drug events as well as to oversee, approve, and review all DUE activities. Formulation of educational programs to meet the drug information needs of the professional staff is also a function of the committee.

The formulary system is a method by which the medical staff of a hospital objectively evaluates and selects the most beneficial drug products based on therapeutic merit, safety, and cost for its particular institution. Petrie and Scott (21) have described the functions and goals of hospital formularies: to provide local guidelines on using the principal drugs, to contain costs, to highlight those drugs with which prescribers should be thoroughly familiar to ensure effective treatment and to avoid unnecessary drug-induced disease, to develop more predictable patterns of prescribing and purchasing, and to ensure immediate availability of drugs that are used as suggested in the formulary. The American Society of Hospital Pharmacists

(ASHP) has published practice standards on formularies and on pharmacy and therapeutics committees (22, 23).

SPECIFIC EXAMPLES

The Joint Commission has developed scoring guidelines for selected standards and required characteristics in the "Pharmaceutical Services" chapter of the *AMH*. In addition, more complete scoring guidelines for drug usage evaluation and the pharmacy and therapeutic functions are provided in the medical staff standards. The Joint Commission also publishes two volumes of examples to illustrate how quality assurance activities can be designed using the 10-step process to address monitoring and evaluation in the pharmacy (nonclinical services) and drug usage evaluation and the pharmacy and therapeutics functions (clinical services) (9, 24). The unsettled and rapidly evolving nature of the Joint Commission's approach is further illustrated by its recent publication, *Primer on Clinical Indicator Development and Application* (25). As the publication of this volume suggests, while the Joint Commission has embraced continuous quality improvement concepts, with a shift away from traditional quality assurance approaches that seek to identify and deal with outliers, it is continuing to develop clinical indicators to measure outcomes.

The Joint Commission's Agenda for Change seems to promise more flexibility for various approaches and has also created a growing market for consultants offering either simple or detailed step-by-step approaches to standards that appear vague and idealistic. As one example, Drug Usage Evaluation$_{TM}$ is "a screening criteria manual for use in concurrent drug usage evaluation" that provides monitoring forms for 55 individual drugs (26). A commercial newsletter (27) suggests a "proactive" approach in drug usage evaluation with recommendations that at least 30 drugs be monitored during each 12-month period and that "simple" standards taken from *Physicians' Desk Reference* or *The Medical Letter On Drugs and Therapeutics* be used, with the admonition that "it's not

necessary to monitor every aspect of each drug. . . . That kind of thoroughness can be counterproductive by providing too much data for analysis and discussion." Further, this newsletter recommends a small sample size of 10–15 records per study to compare the records against the basic criteria. While the scientific standards of such approaches are weak, it also seems that such recommendations have helped individual hospitals satisfy the Joint Commission's surveyors.

Even though DUEs are the responsibility of the medical staff, it is the pharmacist who usually does most of the work. Accordingly, the pharmacy literature is replete with recommended approaches. The ASHP has published *Criteria for Drug Use Evaluation* (28) as well as an ongoing section on DUE criteria in its journal, *Clinical Pharmacy*. The ASHP has also published guidelines on the pharmacists' role in DUE (20). Pharmacists need straightforward examples of monitoring and evaluation activities, in addition to these formal statements. Adachi (8) expressed the view that many professionals have tended to overcomplicate DUEs, and he presented examples of concurrent review centered around daily operations using a "Pharmacist Activities Documentation Form."

EPIDEMIOLOGIC CONSIDERATIONS

Fraser has proposed a broadened definition of epidemiology as the comparison of rates of occurrence of phenomena in various populations so as to increase understanding of the human situation (29). He further proposed that, as a "low technology" science that emphasizes method rather than arcane knowledge, epidemiology is readily accessible to nonspecialists. However, this accessibility also may increase the potential dangers from misapplication of epidemiology. For example, in the current wave of enthusiasm on the part of the hospital administrators and accrediting agencies for the rapid implementation of comprehensive programs for quality assurance, sound epidemiologic principles may be compromised without suitable definitions and means of measuring the occurrence of indicators and without consideration of sampling techniques, denominator data, and methods of analysis (30).

The concept of DUE with its qualitative focus on appropriateness of therapy owes much to the successful efforts of hospital epidemiologists in the evaluation of antibiotic use. Indeed, antibiotic drugs account for 20–50% of hospital pharmacy costs, and many hospitals have realized substantial cost savings in improved antibiotic use by programs to alter prescribing behavior (31–38). However, the lack of a suitable scientific foundation for broad-scope quality assurance activities such as DUE is one of many stumbling blocks (30). The results achieved (and achievable) from DUEs of antibiotic drugs in a readily delineated group of diseases cannot be readily extrapolated to all other drug classes in the present state of medical knowledge. The Joint Commission is targeting appropriate elements for surveillance such as the selection of important adverse events that might be preventable. However, much remains to be done.

Monitoring and intervention to improve processes of care may result in no discernible differences in clinical outcome. For example, surveillance for medication errors is mandated by the Joint Commission even though the clinical impact of such errors is slight. The time and resources spent on this surveillance effort may be poorly invested (30). Similarly, most of the suggested DUE programs include criteria and thresholds for monitoring nephrotoxicity due to aminoglycoside antibiotics, which, in the vast majority of instances, is clinically trivial. Sample size also needs considerable attention that is lacking in most recommended DUE programs. It makes little sense to monitor 10–15 patient records to identify rates of nephrotoxicity that may be on the order of 2–4% (6). On the other hand, an epidemiologic approach may focus on drug-induced renal failure as a more appropriate "target" for surveillance. It may thus seem curious that the Joint Commission gives far more detailed attention to DUEs than to ADEs, a focus that is doubtless due to the greater practicality of identifying patients receiving specific targeted drugs than patients experiencing adverse drug events.

"Primum non nocere" (first of all do no harm) is a strong argument for the scientifically immature field of hospital quality assurance to focus first on the avoidance of complications of drug therapy rather than on optimal outcomes. ADEs have many similarities to nosocomial infections as causes of morbidity, mortality, and prolongation of hospital stays—with staggering economic consequences (39). ADEs are "rateable" events that can be studied by epidemiologic methods (40). The distinction can also be made between endemic and epidemic adverse drug events, and intriguing drug-related epidemics have been described (41–45).

Pharmacoepidemiology is a relatively new discipline that has been defined as the application of epidemiologic knowledge, methods, and reasoning to study the effects (beneficial and adverse) and uses of drugs in human populations (46). To date, this field has focused on the use of large automated databases to identify serious and rare side effects of drugs used in large outpatient populations and on meeting the needs for postmarketing drug surveillance mandated by the Food and Drug Administration (FDA). The increasing availability of computer databases linking the medical records of hospitalized patients and the pharmacy will create new opportunities for surveillance of medication outcomes and for assessing the quality of drug use in hospitals (4, 47).

INTERACTING WITH THE STAFF

The prompt feedback of information, conclusions, and recommendations from surveillance to appropriate individuals or organizational components is both a tenet of the Joint Commission's 10-step process and a guiding principle of hospital epidemiology. "Sentinel health events," such as major medication prescription or administration errors, should be corrected immediately. Nonetheless, whenever adverse events are perceived as "confirmed quality problems," the efforts of the hospital epidemiologist to monitor and record such events will be undermined. A "no-fault" approach to surveillance has been largely responsible for the success of hospital infection surveillance and control programs (30). The Joint Commission also has embraced the concept of continuous quality improvement using the industrial model with its focus on processes rather than individuals as a counter balance to this weakness of traditional quality assurance activities.

The pharmacy and therapeutics committee is the formal mechanism for involving the medical and nursing staff in drug-related quality assurance activities. Some issues relating to inappropriate prescribing need to be approached by direct communication through the clinical department chairperson with the involved practitioners, e.g., a physician who prescribes inappropriate antibiotic prophylaxis for surgical procedures. However, a tactful approach by a clinical pharmacist may be perceived as far less threatening by physicians. At the LDS Hospital in Salt Lake City, a computerized medication monitoring system has been used to generate alerts that warn of potential drug interactions, allergies, and adverse drug reactions. A pharmacist notifies the physician immediately ˇwhen an alert results from a new drug prescription. The response to these alerts with direct communication from the pharmacy has been clearly favorable, with more than 90% of the alerts being judged clinically relevant and resulting in a change of therapy (48, 49). Using decision support functions of this integrated hospital information system, pharmacists have effectively intervened to correct inappropriate therapeutic and prophylactic uses of antibiotics (50–52).

In large hospitals, an interested, well-trained clinical pharmacist should be recruited to take responsibility for drug-related quality assurance issues. This individual can function in a manner analogous to the infection control practitioner, and the successful model of the infection control program can be replicated by a pharmacoepidemiology team comprising the clinical pharmacist, the hospital epidemiol-

ogist, and the pharmacy and therapeutics committee.

SPECIFIC INSTRUCTIONS FOR IMPLEMENTING A QUALITY ASSURANCE PROGRAM

The development of internal quality control in the pharmacy should be accomplished using the 10-step process and accompanied by a written plan. Monitoring should be incorporated into the daily tasks in the pharmacy so that ongoing records are available for incident reports, dispensing errors, accounting for controlled substances, etc.

The quality assurance literature and the various publications of the Joint Commission contain an enormous number of recommendations that deal with evaluating the quality and appropriateness of patient care services provided by the pharmacy. Eickhoff's statement regarding the status of infection control recommendations has broad relevance in this regard: "Taken individually, each of the recommendations may have some intrinsic merit or rationale. Viewed collectively, it is frankly appalling and wholly devoid of any indication of relative importance or priority" (53). The present atmosphere of frustration and confusion is compounded by the delay and rethinking surrounding the Joint Commission's Agenda for Change as it seeks to incorporate the trendy principles of continuous quality improvement and total quality management in the framework of traditional quality assurance using clinical indicators.

Accordingly, specific instructions for quality assurance must be without scientific justification in many instances. In general, it seems wise to attempt to apply the successful model of infection control, which has already been responsible for more work in hospitals on antibiotic prescription practices than has been done with any other class of drugs (54, 55).

Simple approaches with a conscientious effort to determine "what works" seem preferable to large-scale well-intentioned and too-often misguided programs for drug use evaluation. It remains disturbing that the leading "thinkers" in quality assessment are unable to support their recommendations with sound clinical evidence and seem preoccupied by the semantics of quality. Cynics are probably correct that, despite the rhetoric about concerns over quality, the underlying motive has been cost control, often without emphasis on the cost-effectiveness of the review process (56).

In order to have an effective program for drug monitoring, a database is needed that defines prescribing practices. Pharmacies, with or without computer support, can provide useful quantitative information about drug utilization. The evaluation of these data is "vintage epidemiology" (54). Tracking drug use over time can provide evidence for prescribing changes that can lead to well-focused investigation. The development of improved programs for reporting adverse drug events can also lead to concurrent or prospective DUEs. Examples of this process can be found in recent experiences with seizures reported in patients receiving imipenem-cilastatin and with respiratory arrests in patients receiving midazolam (57, 58).

The revolution in computer technology is certain to benefit quality assurance programs as the field overcomes the lack of adequate data systems (59–61). Advanced computerized hospital information systems will provide access to patient information and, in addition, will help with decisions about patient data. For example, physicians often overlook or fail to notice adverse drug effects, even when the evidence is present in the paper chart (62). Computer-generated alerts have been used as signals for ADEs at the LDS Hospital, resulting in the verification of 731 ADEs in contrast to 9 ADEs reported by traditional means during an 18-month period (63). In addition, computers are perhaps the only means to help prevent random prescribing errors that are due to human limitations, and protocol-based computer reminders can be expected to play an important role both in quality assessment and quality improvement (64).

The integrated patient database at the LDS Hospital permits the automated linkage of antibiotic susceptibility reports with antibiotic prescriptions so that alerts can be generated to identify patients whose antibiotic therapy is inappropriate in relation to microbiology culture and susceptibility data. In a prospective study, these "therapeutic antibiotic alerts" were evaluated by a clinical pharmacist and were used to inform physicians of recent susceptibility test results (50). In nearly one-half of the clinically relevant alerts, the physicians were not previously aware of the results. Physicians often altered therapy because of these alerts, and the monitoring provided an important new clinical role for pharmacists. Similar computer-generated reminders have been used to identify and correct errors in prophylactic antibiotic use in surgery (51, 52).

Clearly, the potential is great for the development of computer reminders for all aspects of drug therapy. At present, however, most hospitals do not have fully integrated computerized information systems, and the tasks that can be done efficiently with computer support are often simply not cost-effective when attempted by manual methods. The task of the hospital epidemiologist is to bring his/her special perspective to help set priorities for the quality assurance of drug therapy. For this, there is no substitute for "shoe leather" epidemiology in the hospital. Shoe leather epidemiology refers to that type of data collection that depends upon the presence and judgment of the epidemiologist as an active observer in the patient care setting. The infection control experience in hospitals has repeatedly confirmed the critical importance of the physical presence of the hospital epidemiologist and the infection control team on the hospital wards. If infection control had depended only on reviews of the paper medical records of infected patients and on committee meetings with department chairpersons, no progress would have been possible. The "thinkers" in quality assurance and the "doers" in hospital epidemiology must join forces in order to develop effective programs to improve drug therapy.

CONCLUSIONS

The pharmaceutical care system and drug usage are complex hospitalwide concerns. In the past, efforts to assure quality have focused on the pharmacy itself and on medical staff responsibility for optimal prescribing. However, many other individuals and hospital services have shared responsibilities for the effectiveness of drug therapy—such as nursing, the emergency room, home care services, and ambulatory care services. These services, and the interfaces between them, should also be the subject of quality assurance activities. The pharmacy and therapeutics committee is the key organizational unit through which quality assurance initiatives must be coordinated, and the development of a formulary is the single most important tool to improve prescribing and to reduce variation in drug usage.

The Joint Commission has formulated a 10-step process for drug usage evaluation that in practice has often become the responsibility of the pharmacy without the collaboration of epidemiologists or physicians, even though the pharmacy and therapeutics committee oversees and reviews this activity. The Joint Commission has required that medical staffs perform DUEs and monitor ADEs, but a scientific foundation for these activities is lacking. One of the most established models for DUE has heretofore been the antibiotic monitoring and control activities initiated by infection control units. This model is based on the collaboration of the hospital epidemiologist, the infection control practitioner, and the infection control committee. A similar team for drug usage evaluation should be created, comprising the hospital epidemiologist, a clinical pharmacist, and the pharmacy and therapeutics committee. A major focus of this team's activities should be ADEs, which are the most frequent complications in hospitalized patients and which resemble hospital-acquired infections as causes of morbidity, mortality, increased lengths of stay, and excess costs of hospitalization. Shoe leather epidemiology is needed to better define ADEs, to determine the benefits that may accrue from efforts to prevent ADEs, and to use this knowledge to guide well-focused DUEs.

References

1. Hepler CD, Strand LM. Opportunities and responsibilities in pharmaceutical care. Am J Hosp Pharm 1990;47:533–543.
2. Laffel G, Blumenthal D. The case for using industrial quality management science in health care organizations. JAMA 1989;262:2869–2873.
3. Marr JJ, Moffet HL, Kunin CM. Guidelines for improving the use of antimicrobial agents in hospitals: A statement by the Infectious Diseases Society of America. J Infect Dis 1988;157:869–876.
4. Burke JP, Tilson HH, Platt R. Expanding roles of hospital epidemiology: Pharmacoepidemiology. Infect Control Hosp Epidemiol 1989;10(6):253–254.
5. Cluff LE, Caranasos GJ, Stewart RB. Clinical problems and drugs (Major problems in internal medicine. Vol. 5). Philadelphia: WB Saunders, 1975.
6. Platt R, Stryker WS, Komaroff AL. Pharmacoepidemiology in hospitals using automated data systems. Am J Prev Med 1988;4(Suppl 1):39–47.
7. Leape LL, Brennan TA, Laird N, et al. The nature of adverse events in hospitalized patients. Results of the Harvard medical practice study II. N Engl J Med 1991;324:377–384.
8. Adachi W. A simplistic approach to establishing drug-usage/quality assurance programs. Hosp Pharm 1990;25:541–559.
9. Joint Commission on Accreditation of Healthcare Organizations. Examples of monitoring and evaluation in pharmaceutical services. 2nd ed. Chicago: Joint Commission on Accreditation of Healthcare Organizations, 1990.
10. Joint Commission on Accreditation of Healthcare Organizations. Accreditation manual for hospitals. Chicago: Joint Commission on Accreditation of Healthcare Organizations, 1991.
11. Enright SM. Assessing patient outcomes. Am J Hosp Pharm 1988;45:1376–1378.
12. Penna RP. Pharmaceutical care: Pharmacy's mission for the 1990s. Am J Hosp Pharm 1990;47:543–549.
13. O'Leary DS. The Joint Commission looks to the future [Editorial]. JAMA 1987;258:951–952.
14. Department of Health, Education, and Welfare. Final report—Task Force on Prescription Drugs. Washington, D.C.: United States Government Printing Office, 1968.
15. Brodie DC, Smith WE. Constructing a conceptual model of drug utilization review. Hospitals, 1976;50:143–149.
16. Myers CE. Keeping up-to-date with Joint Commission requirements: The case of drug-use evaluation. Am J Hosp Pharm 1988;45:64, 69.
17. Wible DA. Drug usage evaluation blueprints. Hosp Ther 1988;13:25–35.
18. Wible DA. Steps in implementing a DUE. Hosp Ther 1989;14:48–62.
19. Hughes WT. Guidelines for the use of antimicro-

bial agents in neutropenic patients with unexplained fever. J Infect Dis 1990;161:381–396.

20. American Society of Hospital Pharmacists. ASHP guidelines on the pharmacist's role in drug use evaluation. Am J Hosp Pharm 1988;45:385–386.

21. Petrie JC, Scott AK. Drug formularies in hospitals [Editorial]. Br Med J 1987;294:919.

22. American Society of Hospital Pharmacists. ASHP statement on the pharmacy and therapeutics committee. Am J Hosp Pharm 1984;41:1621.

23. American Society of Hospital Pharmacists. ASHP statement on the formulary system. Am J Hosp Pharm 1983;40:1384–1385.

24. Joint Commission on Accreditation of Healthcare Organizations. Examples of drug usage evaluation. Chicago: Joint Commission on Accreditation of Healthcare Organizations, 1989.

25. Joint Commission on Accreditation of Healthcare Organizations. Primer on clinical indicator development and application. Chicago: Joint Commission on Accreditation of Healthcare Organizations, 1990.

26. Gutshall EL, Davidson HE, Davis SK. Drug usage evaluation. A screening criteria manual for use in concurrent drug usage evaluation. HPI Publishing, 1988.

27. Anonymous. Take a proactive approach to drug usage evaluation. Briefings on JCAHO. Alternative perspectives on accreditation. January 1991:8–9 (Opus IV Communications, Marblehead, MA).

28. American Society of Hospital Pharmacists. Criteria for drug use evaluation. Vol. 1. Bethesda, MD: American Society of Hospital Pharmacists, 1989.

29. Fraser DW. Epidemiology as a liberal art. N Engl J Med 1987;316:309–314.

30. McGeer A, Crede W, Hierholzer WJ Jr. Surveillance for quality assessment. II. Surveillance for non-infectious processes: Back to basics. Infect Control Hosp Epidemiol 1990;11:36–41.

31. Avorn J, Soumerai SB, Taylor W, Wessels MR, Janousek J, Weiner M. Reduction of incorrect antibiotic dosing through a structured educational order form. Arch Intern Med 1988;148:1720–1724.

32. Woodward RS, Medoff G, Smith MD, Gray JL III. Antibiotic cost savings from formulary restrictions and physician monitoring in a medical school affiliated hospital. Am J Med 1987;83:817–823.

33. Hirschman SZ, Meyers DR, Bradbury K, Mehl B, Gendelman S, Kimelblatt B. Use of antimicrobial agents in a university teaching hospital. Evolution of a comprehensive control program. Arch Intern Med 1988;148:2001–2007.

34. Briceland LL, Nightingale CH, Quintiliani R, Cooper BW, Smith KS. Antibiotic streamlining from combination therapy to monotherapy utilizing an interdisciplinary approach. Arch Inter Med 1988;148:2019–2022.

35. Recco RA, Gladstone JL, Friedman SA, Gerken EH. Antibiotic control in a municipal hospital. JAMA 1979;241:2283–2286.

36. Durbin WA Jr, Lapidas B, Goldmann DA. Improved antibiotic usage following introduction of a novel prescription system. JAMA 1981;246:1796–1800.

37. Pelletier LL. Hospital usage of parenteral antimicrobial agents: A graduated utilization review and cost-containment program. Infect Control 1985;6:226–230.

38. Moleski RJ, Andriole VT. Role of the infectious disease specialist in containing cost of antibiotics in the hospital. Rev Infect Dis 1986;8:488–493.

39. Melmon KL. Preventable drug reactions—causes and cures. N Engl J Med 1971;284:1361–1368.

40. Lynch P, Jackson MM. Monitoring for nosocomial noninfectious complications: A classification system that parallels the NNIS definitions for infectious complications. Am J Infect Control 1990;18:391–398.

41. Buehler JW, Smith LF, Wallace EM, Heath CW Jr, Kusiak R, Herndon JL. Unexplained deaths in a children's hospital. An epidemiologic assessment. N Engl J Med 1985;313:211–216.

42. Sacks JJ, Stroup DF, Will ML, Harris EL, Israel E. A nurse-associated epidemic of cardiac arrests in an intensive care unit. JAMA 1988;259:689–695.

43. Istre GR, Gustafson TL, Baron RC, Martin DL, Orlowski JP. A mysterious cluster of deaths and cardiopulmonary arrests in a pediatric intensive care unit. N Engl J Med 1985;313:205–211.

44. Solomon SL, Wallace EM, Ford-Jones EL, et al. Medication errors with inhalant epinephrine mimicking an epidemic of neonatal sepsis. N Engl J Med 1984;310:166–170.

45. Rothman KJ. Sleuthing in hospitals [Editorial]. N Engl J Med 1985;313:258–259.

46. Porta MS, Hartzema AG. The contribution of epidemiology to the study of drugs. Drug Intell Clin Pharm 1987;21:741–747.

47. Strom BL. Pharmacoepidemiology: Current status, prospects and problems [Editorial]. Ann Intern Med 1990;113:179–181.

48. Gardner RM, Evans RS, Andrews RD. Impact of a clinical information system on hospital costs. In: Kuhn RL, ed. Frontiers of medical information science. New York: Praeger, 1987:81–89.

49. Hulse RK, Clark SJ, Jackson JC, Warner HR, Gardner RM. Computerized medication monitoring system. Am J Hosp Pharm 1976;33:1061–1064.

50. Pestotnik SL, Evans RS, Burke JP, Gardner RM, Classen DC. Therapeutic antibiotic monitoring: Surveillance using a computerized expert system. Am J Med 1990;88:43–48.

51. Larsen RA, Evans RS, Burke JP, Pestotnik SL, Gardner RM, Classen DC. Improved perioperative antibiotic use and reduced surgical wound infections through use of computer decision analysis. Infect Control Hosp Epidemiol 1989;10:316–320.

52. Evans RS, Pestotnik SL, Burke JP, Gardner RM, Larsen RA, Classen DC. Reducing the duration of prophylactic antibiotic use through computer monitoring of surgical patients. DICP, Annals of Pharmacotherapy 1990;24:351–354.

53. Eickhoff TC. Nosocomial infections—A 1980 view: Progress, priorities, and prognosis. Am J Med 1981;70:381–388.

54. Wenzel RP. Quality assessment. An emerging component of hospital epidemiology. Diag Microbiol Infect Dis 1990;13:197–204.

55. Garibaldi RA, Burke JP. Surveillance and control of antibiotic use in the hospital. Am J Infect Control 1991;19:164–170.

56. Morehead MA. Assessing quality of care: Another step forward [Editorial]. Am J Public Health 1989;79:415–416.

57. Classen DC, Pestotnik SL, Stevens LE, Evans RS, Burke JP. Midazolam use and associated respiratory arrests in the hospital population. Presented at the Fourth International Conference on Pharmacoepidemiology. Minneapolis, MN, September, 6–9, 1988.

58. Pestotnik SL, Classen DC, Stevens LE, Evans RS, Burke JP. Prospective monitoring for seizures associated with imipenem-cilastatin therapy. Abstracts of the 28th Interscience Conference on Antimicrobial Agents and Chemotherapy, Los Angeles, CA, October, 23–26 1988, Abstract 553.

59. Shortliffe EH. Computer programs to support clinical decision making. JAMA 1987;258:61–66.

60. McDonald CJ, Tierney WM. Computer-stored medical records. Their future role in medical practice. JAMA 1988;259:3433–3440.

61. Haynes RB, Walker CJ. Computer-aided quality assurance. A critical appraisal. Arch Intern Med 1987;147:1297–1301.

62. Shapiro S, Slone D, Lewis GP, Jick H. Fatal drug reactions among medical inpatients. JAMA 1971;216:467–472.

63. Classen DC, Pestotnik SL, Evans RS, Burke JP. Computerized surveillance of adverse drug events in hospital patients, Clin Res 1991; 39:373A.

64. McDonald CJ. Protocol-based computer reminders, the quality of care and the non-perfectibility of man. N Engl J Med 1976;295:1351–1355.

Index

Page numbers in *italics* denote figures; those followed by "t" denote tables.